PHILLIPS' SCIENCE OF DENTAL MATERIALS

PHILLIPS' SCIENCE OF DENTAL MATERIALS

TENTH EDITION

Kenneth J. Anusavice, D.M.D., Ph.D.

Professor and Chairman
Department of Dental Biomaterials
College of Dentistry
University of Florida
Gainesville, Florida

W.B. SAUNDERS COMPANY
A Division of Harcourt Brace & Company
Philadelphia London Toronto Montreal Sydney Tokyo

W.B. SAUNDERS COMPANY
A Division of Harcourt Brace & Company

The Curtis Center
Independence Square West
Philadelphia, Pennsylvania 19106

Library of Congress Cataloging-in-Publication Data

Phillips' science of dental materials / [edited by] Kenneth J. Anusavice.—10th ed.

p.   cm.

Rev. ed. of: Skinner's science of dental materials / Ralph W. Phillips. 9th ed. 1991.

Includes bibliographical references and index.

ISBN 0–7216–5741–9

1. Dental materials.   I. Anusavice, Kenneth J.   II. Phillips, Ralph W.
    Skinner's science of dental materials.   [DNLM: 1. Dental Materials.
    WU 190 P5625 1996]

RK652.5.P495   1996   617.6'95—dc20

DNLM/DLC   96–4885

PHILLIPS' SCIENCE OF DENTAL MATERIALS   ISBN 0–7216–5741–9

Last digit is the print number: 9   8   7   6   5   4   3   2

Contributors

Kenneth J. Anusavice, D.M.D., Ph.D.
Professor and Chairman, Department of Dental Biomaterials, College of Dentistry, University of Florida, Gainesville, Florida.
Performance Standards for Dental Materials; Physical Properties of Dental Materials; Mechanical Properties of Dental Materials; Solidification and Microstructure of Metals; Constitution of Alloys; Dental Amalgam: Technical Considerations; Direct Filling Gold and Its Manipulation; Dental Casting Alloys; Casting Procedures for Dental Alloys; Dental Ceramics; Soldering; Wrought Base Metal and Gold Alloys

Charles F. DeFreest, D.D.S.
Assistant Chairman, Fixed Prosthodontics, Wilford Hall USAF Medical Center, Lackland Air Force Base, Texas.
Finishing and Polishing Materials

Jack Ferracane, M.S., Ph.D.
Professor and Chair, Department of Biomaterials and Biomechanics, Oregon Health Sciences University, Portland, Oregon.
Dental Implants

J. Rodway Mackert, Jr., D.M.D., Ph.D.
Professor, Dental Materials, Department of Oral Rehabilitation, School of Dentistry, Medical College of Georgia, Augusta, Georgia.
Dental Ceramics

Miroslav Marek, Ph.D.
Professor, School of Materials Science and Engineering, Georgia Institute of Technology, Atlanta, Georgia.
Corrosion

Victoria A. Marker, M.S., Ph.D.
Associate Professor, Department of Biological Materials Science, Baylor College of Dentistry, Dallas, Texas.
Hydrocolloid Impression Materials; Nonaqueous Elastomeric Impression Materials

Grayson W. Marshall, Jr., D.D.S., M.P.H., Ph.D.
Professor, Restorative Dentistry, and Chair, Biomaterials Division, University of California, San Francisco, San Francisco, California.
Dental Amalgam: Structures and Properties

Sally J. Marshall, Ph.D.
Professor and Vice Chair—Research, Department of Restorative Dentistry, University of California, San Francisco, San Francisco, California.
Dental Amalgam: Structures and Properties

Robert Neiman, B.S., M.S.
Vice President, Research, Whip Mix Corporation, Louisville, Kentucky.
Gypsum Products: Chemistry of Setting, Basic Principles, and Technical Considerations; Inlay Casting Wax; Investments for Small Castings

Rodney D. Phoenix, D.D.S., M.S.
Assistant Professor, Department of Prosthodontics, University of Texas Health Science Center at San Antonio, San Antonio, Texas.
Denture Base Resins: Technical Considerations and Processing Techniques

Chiayi Shen, M.S., Ph.D.
Associate Professor, Department of Dental Biomaterials, College of Dentistry, University of Florida, Gainesville, Florida.
Hydrocolloid Impression Materials; Inelastic Impression Materials; Dental Cements for Restorations and Pulp Protection; Dental Cements for Bonding Applications

Karl-Johan Söderholm, D.D.S., M.Phil., Odont.Dr.
Professor, Department of Dental Biomaterials, College of Dentistry, University of Florida, Gainesville, Florida.
Structure of Matter and Principles of Adhesion; Chemistry of Synthetic Resins; Restorative Resins; Bonding

Harold R. Stanley, B.S., M.S., D.D.S., D.Sc(Hon)
Professor Emeritus, Department of Oral Diagnostic Sciences, College of Dentistry, University of Florida, Gainesville, Florida.
Biocompatibility of Dental Materials

Preface

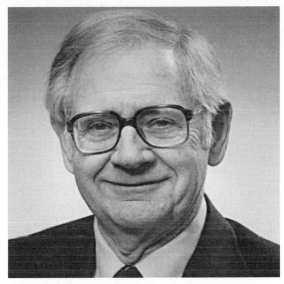

Dr. Ralph W. Phillips

On May 17, 1991, the dental community lost one of its premier leaders in research and education. Dr. Ralph W. Phillips died after a bout with cancer and, with his loss, dental materials scientists and educators have shared with the Phillips family and close friends enduring memories of the wonderful interactions that we had experienced with Dr. Phillips. Our best wishes for the future are extended to family members and his many friends, who will carry on some of his hopes for the future.

Dr. Ralph Phillips had long been recognized as the eminent scholar of dental materials science. He was one of the first dental researchers to investigate the relationship between laboratory research and clinical performance of restorative materials. He also emphasized safety of the patient and the dentist, not the physical properties of the material, as the principal criterion for its success. Because of his foresight in human safety issues and the recent heightened awareness of this topic, the chapter on biocompatibility (Chapter 5) has been expanded significantly. His pioneering studies of the influence of fluoride solutions on the acid solubility and hardness of enamel later led to his demonstration that fluoride could be added to restorative materials to increase their anticariogenic potential In the 1960s, he coordinated the first workshop on adhesive dental materials. During his illustrious career he published more than 300 scientific papers and books, including *Skinner's Science of Dental Materials*, which is one of the most widely used and translated dental textbooks in history. He published the Ninth Edition in March 1991, less than 3 months before his death.

I am honored to have been recommended by Dr. Phillips and selected by the publisher to continue his work as the editor of this text. Dr. Phillips left a great legacy as a researcher and as a scholar. He will long be remembered for his leadership role in research studies of restorative dental materials and for the international recognition of his achievements and contributions to the dental profession. He was greatly respected by his peers because he had uncompromising standards and a willingness to share his expertise and his humor with others. It is an extreme honor to follow in his footsteps and to try to uphold his high standards of dental materials science.

The new *Phillips' Science of Dental Materials* has been modified significantly to expand the chapters that represent the material characteristics and principles of critical importance to general dentistry as we approach the twenty-first century—biocompatibility, adhesion, bonding, composites, ceramics, impression materials, denture base materials, alternatives to dental amalgam, cementation agents, restorative cements, and finishing materials. An outline of major topics at the beginning of each chapter provides a logical overview of its contents, and in many chapters terminology and definitions are presented to enhance their usefulness to readers, who range from first-year predoctoral students to practicing clinicians, graduate students, clinical faculty, materials scientists, dermatologists, and other health care professionals. Most chapters can be easily understood by a college graduate who has completed basic chemistry, mathematics, and physics courses. The basic science presented in some chapters is quite advanced and must be supplemented by lectures, continuing education courses, and consultations with research faculty. Because the authors of chapters over the years have focused on the most fundamental basic science principles of dental materials as well as the clinical relevance of these principles, this text has been the most widely used reference and teaching source of its kind in dental colleges throughout the world for many years.

Practicing general dentists during the past two decades have experienced a barrage of new materials for restorative dentistry. Many of these materials have been developed over relatively short periods to meet the increasing demands by the dental community for products that will ensure excellent aesthetics and durability. If these dentists examine their supply closets, they will realize that many of these materials generally have a short product life of 3 years or less. Furthermore, several of these materials such as dentin bonding agents, composites, resin-based glass ionomers, and ceramics are highly technique sensitive; that is, they exhibit marked changes in performance or quality when relatively small changes are made in their manipulation. The changes in the Tenth Edition are designed to enhance the general understanding by students, clinicians, and researchers of the principles that control the success or failure of restorative materials. Through a fundamental mastery of these principles, the reader will become better equipped to analyze technical reports and scientific publications on new products such that major errors in judgment of their potential clinical performance will be minimized.

The Tenth Edition comprises 30 chapters, starting with "Performance Standards for Dental Materials," which describes the roles of the American Dental Association, the U.S. Food and Drug Administration, the International Organization for Standardization, and the Fédération Dentaire Internationale in ensuring the safety and efficacy of materials used for dental and medical materials and devices. Chapter 2 addresses the "Structure of Matter and Principles of Adhesion." This introductory chapter and the following three chapters, "Physical Properties of Dental Materials" (Chapter 3), "Mechanical Properties of Dental Materials" (Chapter 4), and "Biocompatibility of Dental Materials" (Chapter 5), prepare the reader with a foundation in materials principles that will facilitate an understanding of subsequent chapters on the composition, structure, and properties of dental materials. Chapters 3 and 4 were formed by dividing the previous Chapter 3 into two separate chapters because of the challenging nature of these topics. Chapter 5 has been greatly expanded to reflect the increased emphasis around the world on biological safety issues and the environment. Chapter 6 ("Hydrocolloid Impression Materials"), Chapter 7 ("Nonaqueous Elastomeric Impression Materials"), Chapter 8 ("Inelastic Impression Materials"), and Chapter 9 ("Gypsum Products: Chemistry of Setting, Basic Principles, and Technical Considerations") are presented in a sequence that reflects the general order in which these materials are taught in a dental school. Likewise, Chapter 10

("Chemistry of Synthetic Resins"), Chapter 11 ("Denture Base Resins: Technical Considerations and Processing Techniques"), Chapter 12 ("Restorative Resins") and Chapter 13 ("Bonding") represent the principles of polymer chemistry and the chief polymeric materials that are used in resin-based restorations and dentures. Chapters 14 through 20 present the principles of metals and alloys that are used in restorative dentistry. Chapters 21 through 23 cover casting technology and supplement Chapters 9, 14, and 15. Chapters 24 and 25 describe current and traditional restorative cements and resin-based cementation agents, respectively. Chapter 26 ("Dental Ceramics") has been updated and expanded. Chapter 28 ("Wrought Base Metals and Gold Alloys") was formed by combining the previous Chapters 14 and 28. Chapter 29 ("Dental Implants") has been revised to more completely describe bioactive materials. Finally, Chapter 30 ("Finishing and Polishing Materials") has been expanded significantly because of the importance of finishing procedures on the clinical performance of restorative materials. Many of these chapters have been improved by introducing a greater number of diagrams, schematic illustrations, charts, and tables. In addition, a much greater clinical emphasis has been introduced in many of the chapters.

I believe that the Tenth Edition represents the most current and comprehensive text of its kind. Previous editions have withstood the test of time. This trend should continue since the principles proposed will ensure that the practicing clinicians will be better prepared to select materials that also pass their most critical test—the test of time.

KENNETH J. ANUSAVICE, D.M.D., PH.D.

Acknowledgments

The newest edition of *Skinner's Science of Dental Materials* has been renamed *Phillips' Science of Dental Materials* for the Tenth Edition in honor of Dr. Ralph Phillips, who served as editor of the book until he passed away in 1991. His contributions to this book will long be remembered. As the new editor of this book I deeply appreciate the efforts of Dr. Phillips and his colleagues, who established a level of excellence and credibility for the book that has withstood the test of time. It is my intention to ensure that the worldwide recognition of this highly regarded textbook will be maintained. The contributors to the Tenth Edition have made many significant changes that will advance the knowledge base in this field. Thus, I am thankful to all those individuals who assisted Dr. Phillips and those who have provided input to the Tenth Edition for having facilitated my efforts in updating the 30 chapters of the book.

Previous contributors include M. L. Swartz, B. K. Moore, R. J. Schnell, J. C. Setcos, M. W. Beatty, B. F. Rhodes, H. E. Clark, A. H. Kafrawy, C. J. Goodacre, C. Munoz, J. L. McDonald, Jr., D. R. Avery, H. Z. Henderson, M. A. Cochran, R. Neiman, C. E. Ingersoll, G. W. Marshall, Jr., S. J. Marshall, W. P. Naylor, A. J. Goldberg, J. R. Mackert, Jr., J. L. Ferracane, J. W. Stanford, H. R. Stanley, L. L. Miller, P. D. Hammesfahr, G. J. Mount, J. W. McLean, M. Durda, H. F. Morris, R. L. Erickson, D. G. Singleton, and W. Dasch. Some of the previous contributors have also participated in the revision of the Tenth Edition. These individuals include R. Neiman, G. W. Marshall, Jr., S. J. Marshall, J. Ferracane, and H. R. Stanley. I would also like to express my appreciation to Carolyn Kramer, Clyde Ingersoll, and Ed Reetz for their input and suggestions regarding the content of several chapters.

The graphs, schematic illustrations, and other figures were prepared by the authors as well as by R. B. Lee, J. S. Anusavice, and the artist staff of the Learning Resource Center of the Health Science Center of the University of Florida.

I especially appreciate the assistance of my wife Sandi in proofreading the galley proofs of the 30 chapters. Through her assistance the readability and continuity of text in the individual chapters of the book have been greatly improved.

Thanks are given to P. L. Fan of the American Dental Association for his constructive suggestions on standards programs for the testing of dental biomaterials.

Finally, the excellent assistance of L. McGrew, R. Kersey, S. Reilly, R. Gagliardi, D. LeMelledo, and other staff members of the W.B. Saunders Company has been instrumental in the processing of all activities related to the preparation of the Tenth Edition.

KENNETH J. ANUSAVICE

Contents

Color Plates

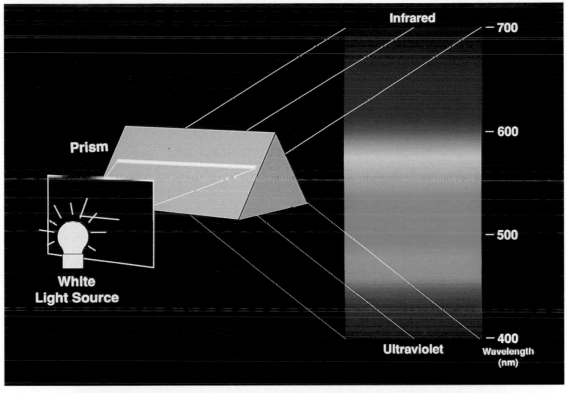

Figure 3–3. Spectrum of visible light ranging in wavelength from 400 nm (violet) to 700 nm (red). The most visually perceptible region of the equal energy spectrum under daylight conditions is between wavelengths of 540 and 570 nm, with a maximum value of visual perceptibility at 555 nm (see Fig. 3–4).

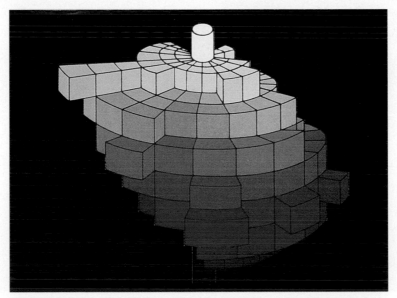

Figure 3–5. Color solid that is used to describe the three dimensions of color. Value increases from black at the bottom center to white at the top center. Chroma increases from the center outward, and hue changes occur in a circumferential direction. (Courtesy of Minolta Corporation, Instrument Systems Division, Ramsey, NJ.)

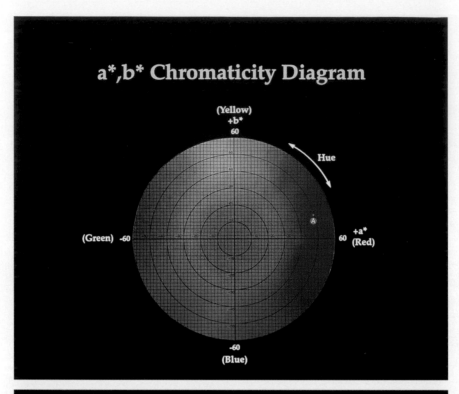

a*,b* Chromaticity Diagram

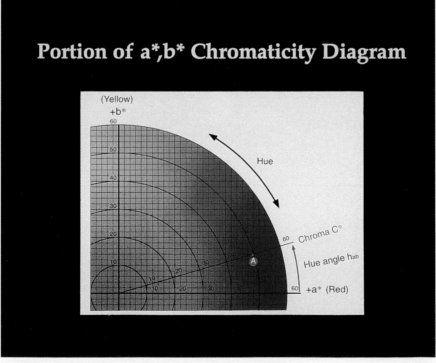

Portion of a*,b* Chromaticity Diagram

Figure 3–6. L*a*b* color chart showing the color of a red apple at point A (top and bottom). For this chart, the appearance is expressed by L* (value) = 42.83; a* (red-green axis) = 45.04; and b* (yellow-blue axis) = 9.52. In contrast, the color of shade A2 porcelain can be described by L* = 72.99; a* = 1.00; and b* = 14.41. (Courtesy of Minolta Corporation, Instrument Systems Division, Ramsey, NJ.)

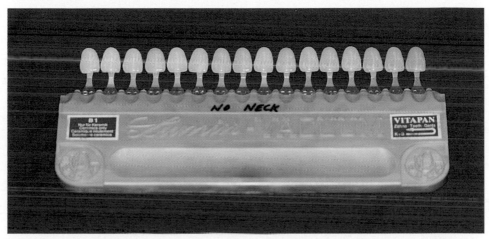

Figure 3–7. Dental shade guide tabs of the Vita Lumin type arranged in decreasing order of value (lighter to darker). The necks of the tooth-shaped tabs have been ground away to facilitate the selection of tooth shades.

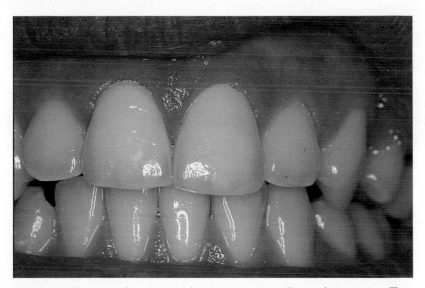

Figure 3–8. Two central incisor metal-ceramic crowns with porcelain margins. The value (L^*) of these crowns is higher than that of the adjacent lateral incisor teeth.

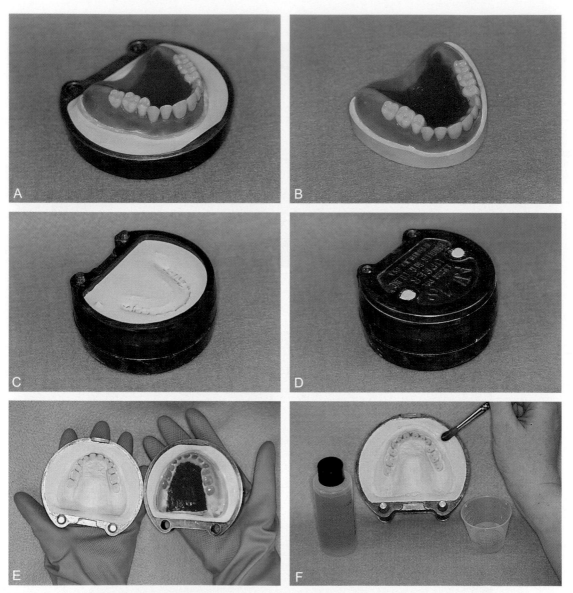

Figure 11–3. Steps in mold preparation (compression-molding technique). *A,* Completed tooth arrangement prepared for the flasking process. *B,* Master cast embedded in properly contoured dental stone. *C,* Occlusal and incisal surfaces of the prosthetic teeth are exposed to facilitate subsequent denture recovery. *D,* Fully flasked maxillary complete denture. *E,* Separation of flask segments during wax elimination process. *F,* Placement of alginate-based separating medium.

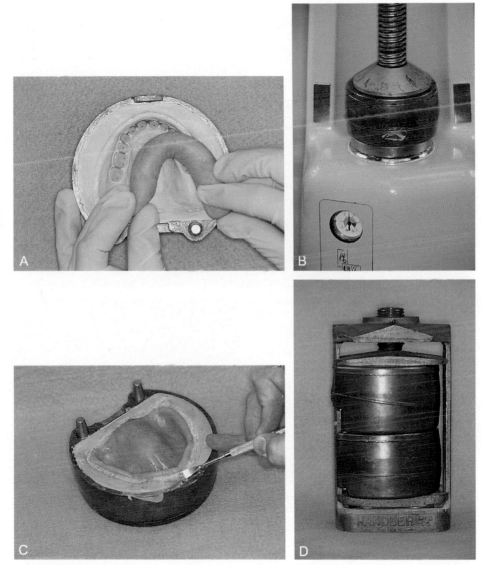

Figure 11–4. Steps in resin packing (compression-molding technique). *A*, Properly mixed resin is bent in a horseshoe shape and placed into the mold cavity. *B*, The flask assembly is placed into a flask press, and pressure is applied. *C*, Excess material is carefully removed from the flask. *D*, The flask is transferred to a flask carrier that maintains pressure on the assembly during processing.

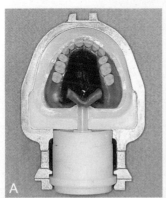
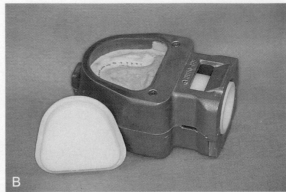
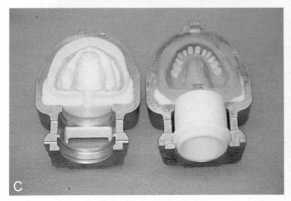
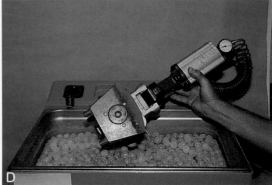

Figure 11–6. Steps in mold preparation (injection-molding technique). *A,* Placement of sprues for introduction of resin. *B,* Occlusal and incisal surfaces of the prosthetic teeth are exposed to facilitate denture recovery. *C,* Separation of flask segments during wax elimination process. *D,* Injection of resin and placement of assembly into water bath.

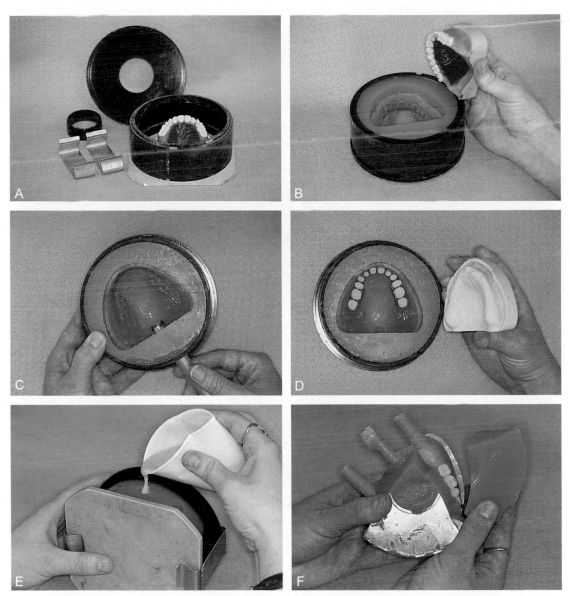

Figure 11–10. Steps in mold preparation (fluid resin technique). *A,* Completed tooth arrangement positioned in a fluid resin flask. *B,* Removal of tooth arrangement from reversible hydrocolloid investment. *C,* Preparation of sprues and vents for the introduction of resin. *D,* Repositioning of the prosthetic teeth and master cast. *E,* Introduction of pour-type resin. *F,* Recovery of the completed prosthesis.

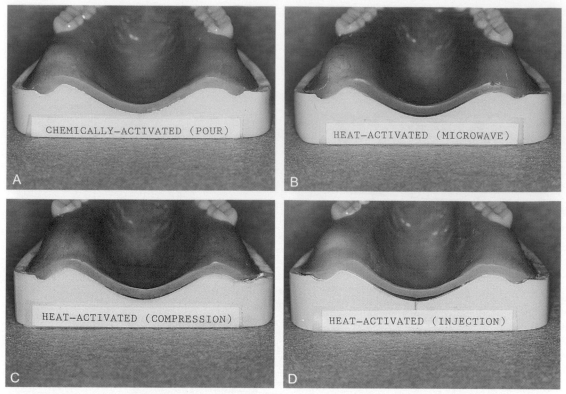

Figure 11–12. Dimensional changes resulting from polymerization. *A,* Chemically activated resin (pour technique). *B,* Microwave resin (compression-molding technique). *C,* Conventional heat-activated resin (compression-molding technique). *D,* Heat-activated resin (injection-molding technique).

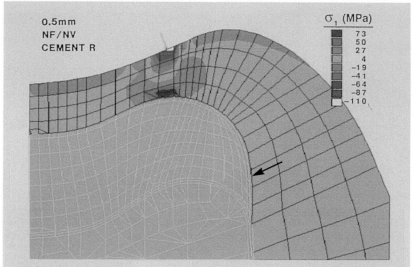

Figure 26–11. Stress distribution computed by finite element analysis in a 0.5-mm-thick molar Dicor glass-ceramic crown loaded on the occlusal surface, just within the marginal ridge area. The maximum tensile stress of 73 MPa is located directly below the point of applied force along the internal surface of the crown adjacent to the 50-μm-thick layer of resin luting agent *(arrow).*

1 *Performance Standards for Dental Materials*

- Historical Use of Restorative Materials
- ADA Acceptance Program
- Federal Regulations and Standards
- International Standards
- Other Standards Organizations
- How Safe Are Dental Restorative Materials?
- Scope of the Book
- Aim of the Book
- Need for the Book

HISTORICAL USE OF RESTORATIVE MATERIALS

The principal goal of dentistry is to maintain or improve the quality of life of the dental patient. This goal can be accomplished by preventing disease, relieving pain, improving mastication efficiency, enhancing speech, and improving appearance. Because many of these objectives require the replacement or alteration of existing tooth structure, the main challenges for centuries have been the development and selection of biocompatible prosthetic materials that can withstand the adverse conditions of the oral environment. Historically, a wide variety of materials have been used as tooth replacements, including animal teeth, human teeth, seashells, ivory, bone, hydroxyapatite, cobalt-chromium alloy, and titanium, although the latter three materials have not been used for tooth implants until the past several decades. Materials for the replacement of missing portions of tooth structure have evolved more slowly over the past several centuries. The four possible materials groups used include metals, ceramics, polymers, and composites. In spite of recent improvements in the physical properties of these materials, none of these are *permanent*. Dentists and materials scientists will continue the search into the twenty-first century for the "Holy Grail" of restorative dentistry, that is, the restorative material that bonds permanently to all tooth structures, aesthetically matches tooth structure, exhibits properties similar to those of tooth enamel and dentin, and initiates tissue repair. To predict future trends, it is useful to look to the past.

Dentistry as a specialty is believed to have begun about 3000 B.C. Although inscriptions on Egyptian tombstones indicate that tooth doctors were considered to be medical specialists, they are not known to have performed restorative dentistry. Gold bands and wires were used by the Phoenicians (after 2500 B.C.) and the Etruscans (after 800 B.C.) for the construction of partial dentures. The gold bands were used to position extracted teeth in place of missing teeth. Gold foil has also been employed for dental restorative purposes, and its initial use is attributed to Johannes Arcelanus of the University of Bologna (Italy) in 1498. The earliest documented evidence of tooth implant materials is attributed to the Etruscans as early as 700 B.C. In about 600 A.D. the Mayans used implants consisting of seashell segments that were placed in anterior tooth sockets. However, tooth coloring for decorative purposes occurred much earlier (Ring, 1985). Hammered gold inlays and stone or mineral inlays also were placed for aesthetic purposes or traditional ornamentation by the Mayans and later by the Aztecs. The Incans also performed tooth mutilations using hammered gold, but the material was not placed for decorative purposes.

Even though the practice of dentistry antedates the Christian era, comparatively little historical data exist on the science of dental materials. Modern dentistry began in 1728, when Fauchard (1678–1761), the "father of dentistry," published a treatise describing many types of dental restorations, including a method for the construction of artificial dentures made from ivory. In 1756 Pfaff described a method for making impressions of the mouth in wax, from which he constructed a model with plaster of Paris. In 1792 de Chamant patented a process for the construction of porcelain teeth. The porcelain inlay was introduced soon thereafter in the early 1800s. The use of fluoride to prevent tooth demineralization originated from observations in 1915 of low decay rates of people in areas of Colorado whose water supplies contained significant fluoride concentrations. In 1935 polymerized acrylic resin was introduced as a denture base material to support artificial teeth. Controlled water fluoridation (1 ppm) to reduce tooth decay (demineralization) began in 1944, and the incidence of tooth decay in children who had access to fluoridated water has decreased by 50% since then. The recent use of pit and fissure sealants and fluoride-releasing restorative materials has reduced the caries incidence even further.

Little scientific information about dental restorative materials has been available until recently. Their use was entirely an art, and the only testing laboratory was the mouth of the patient. Some of this testing still occurs today in the mouths of our patients in spite of the availability of sophisticated technical equipment and the development of standardized testing methods. The reasons for this situation are diverse. In some instances, products are approved for human use without being tested in animal or human subjects. In other instances, dentists use materials for purposes that were not indicated by the manufacturer, for example, a ceramic product for posterior fixed partial dentures (FPDs) when the product has been recommended only for inlays, onlays, crowns, and anterior three-unit FPDs.

The first important awakening of scientific interest occurred during the middle of the nineteenth century, when research studies on amalgam began. At about the same time there were some reports in the literature of studies on porcelain and gold foil. These sporadic advances in knowledge finally culminated in the investigations of G. V. Black, which began in 1895. There is hardly a phase of dentistry that was not explored and advanced by this pioneer in restorative dentistry.

The next great advance in the knowledge of dental materials and their manipulation began in 1919. During that year, the U.S. Army requested the National

Bureau of Standards (now known as the *National Institute of Standards and Technology* [NIST]) to set up specifications for the evaluation and selection of dental amalgams for use in federal service. This research was done under the leadership of Wilmer Souder, and an excellent report on this study was published in 1920. The information contained in the report was received enthusiastically by the dental profession, and similar testing data were then requested for other dental materials.

At the time, the U.S. government could not allocate sufficient funds to continue the work, so a fellowship was created and supported by the Weinstein Research Laboratories. Under such an arrangement, the sponsor provided money for the salaries of research associates and a certain amount of equipment and supplies. The associates then worked in the National Bureau of Standards under the direction of the staff members. They were for all practical purposes members of the staff, supported by private interests. All findings were published and became common property under this particular arrangement.

Working under Dr. Souder's direction, several research associates investigated the properties of dental wrought gold materials, casting gold alloys, and accessory casting materials. This phase of the work resulted in the publication of an extensive and valuable research report.

In 1928, the Dental Research Fellowship at the National Bureau of Standards was assumed by the American Dental Association (ADA). The research carried out by the ADA research associates in conjunction with the staff members of NIST has been of inestimable value to the dental profession, and it has earned for this group an international reputation. People such as Wilmer Souder, George C. Paffenbarger, and William T. Sweeney will undoubtedly be remembered historically as the pioneer researchers whose work began a new era of intense research in the field of dental materials. It was the enthusiasm of these men that prompted the organization of the first courses in dental materials that were taught in the dental schools of the United States and abroad.

ADA ACCEPTANCE PROGRAM

The work at the ADA is divided into a number of categories, including the measurement of the physical and chemical properties of dental materials that are of clinical significance and the development of new materials, instruments, and test methods. Until 1965, one of the primary objectives of the facility at NIST was to formulate standards or specifications for dental materials. However, when the ADA Council on Dental Materials and Devices (now known as the *Council on Scientific Affairs*) was established in 1966, it assumed responsibility for standards development and initiated the certification of products that meet the requirements of these specifications.

Such specifications are standards by which the quality and properties of particular dental materials can be gauged. They identify the requirements for the physical and chemical properties of a material that ensure satisfactory performance if it is properly used by the dental laboratory technician and the dentist. The Acceptance Program of the Council on Scientific Affairs incorporates these specifications in the evaluation of dental products, and the products are tested for compliance with specification requirements. When a product is classified as *acceptable*, the manufacturer is permitted to signify on the label of the product the notation "ADA Accepted."

The ADA Council on Scientific Affairs also is the administrative sponsor of a standards-formulating committee operating under the direction of the American

National Standards Institute. The Accredited Standards Committee (ASC) MD156 develops specifications for all dental materials and devices, with the exception of drugs and x-ray films. Thus, the Council on Scientific Affairs is also responsible for the evaluation of drugs and therapeutic agents used in dentistry and dental x-ray film.

On the basis of advice from the subcommittees of ASC MD156, specifications are formulated. When a specification has been approved by the ASC MD156, it is submitted to the American National Standards Institute. On acceptance by that body, it becomes an American National Standard. Thus, the Council on Scientific Affairs also has the opportunity of accepting it as an ADA specification.

New specifications are continually being developed to apply to new program areas. Likewise, existing specifications are periodically revised to reflect changes in product formulations and new knowledge about the behavior of materials in the oral cavity, as for example, the ADA Specification No. 1 for dental amalgam, which has been revised periodically.

FEDERAL REGULATIONS AND STANDARDS

On May 28, 1976, legislation was signed into law that gave the U.S. Food and Drug Administration (FDA) the regulatory authority to protect the public from hazardous or ineffective medical (and dental) devices. This legislation was the culmination of a series of attempts to provide safe and effective products, beginning with the passage of the Food and Drug Act of 1906, which did not include any provision to regulate medical device safety or the claims made for devices.

This newer legislation, named the *Medical Device Amendments of 1976,* requires the classification and regulation of all noncustomized medical devices that are intended for human use. According to the Federal Register, the term *device* includes

[A]ny instrument, apparatus, implement, machine, contrivance, implant, or *in vitro* re-agent used in the diagnosis, cure, mitigation, treatment, or prevention of disease in man and which does not achieve any of its principal intended purposes through chemical action within or on the body of man or other animals and which is not dependent upon being metabolized for the achievement of any of its principal intended purposes.

Some dental products, such as those with fluoride, are considered drugs, but most products used in the operatory are considered to be devices and are thus subject to control by the FDA Center for Devices and Radiological Health. Also encompassed are over-the-counter products sold to the public, such as toothbrushes, dental floss, and denture adhesives.

The classification of all medical and dental items is developed by panels composed of nongovernmental dental experts as well as representatives from industry and consumer groups. The Dental Products Panel identifies any known hazards or problems and places the item into one of three classification groups based on relative risk factors. Class I devices are considered to be of low risk, and they are subject to general controls, including matters such as the registration of the manufacturer's products, adherence to *good manufacturing practices,* and certain record-keeping requirements. If it is believed that such general controls are not in themselves adequate to ensure safety and effectiveness as claimed by the manufacturer, then the device is placed into the Class II category. Products that fall into this class are required to meet performance standards established by the FDA or appropriate ones from other authoritative bodies, such as those of the ADA. These performance standards may relate to components, construction, and properties of a device, and they may also indicate specific testing requirements to ensure that lots or individual products conform to the regulatory requirement.

Class III, the most stringent category, requires that the device be approved for safety and effectiveness before it is marketed. All implanted or life-supporting devices are placed in this premarket clearance category. Specific data must be provided to demonstrate safety and efficacy before marketing. In certain instances, the product or device may be substantially equivalent to other approved products, and under this situation, only the demonstration of equivalence is necessary. Any item that does not have adequate clinical or scientific information available to permit the formulation of a performance standard is placed in the premarket approval category. For example, one of these devices, the endosseous implant for prosthetic attachment, is considered a high priority relative to the necessity for adequate data to demonstrate safety and effectiveness. Manufacturers of this device now need to submit premarket approval applications for their implants. These are then evaluated by the Dental Products Panel to determine whether the preamendment implants can stay on the market or whether new implants can be marketed. Guidelines that have been developed by the FDA are available to all interested parties to provide the preclinical and clinical requirements for the preparation of a premarket approval application.

More than 160 dental items have been classified into one of these three classes. The FDA program, in conjunction with the ADA Acceptance Program for dental products, provides a crucial framework for standards developments and provides initial evidence that the product will be safe and effective as claimed. Other countries have national government agencies comparable to the FDA that also include dental materials and devices within the jurisdiction of their regulatory authority.

INTERNATIONAL STANDARDS

For many years there has been great interest in the establishment of specifications for dental materials on an international level. Two organizations, the Fédération Dentaire Internationale (FDI) and the International Organization for Standardization (ISO), are working toward that goal. Originally, the FDI initiated and actively supported a program for the formulation of international specifications for dental materials. As a result of that activity, several specifications for dental materials and devices have been adopted.

The ISO is an international, nongovernmental organization whose objective is the development of international standards. This body is composed of national standards organizations from more than 80 countries. The American National Standards Institute is the U.S. member. The request by the FDI to the ISO that they consider FDI specifications for dental materials as ISO standards led to the formation of an ISO committee, TC106-Dentistry. The responsibility of this committee is to standardize terminology and test methods, and to determine specifications for dental materials, instruments, appliances, and equipment.

Several FDI specifications have now been adopted as ISO standards. Since 1963, more than 40 new standards have been developed or are currently under development in ISO TC106 through cooperative programs with the FDI. Thus, considerable progress has already been realized in achieving the ultimate goal of a broad range of international specifications for dental materials and devices.

The benefit of such specifications to the dental profession has been invaluable, since the supply and demand for dental materials, instruments, and devices are worldwide. The dentist is provided with criteria for selection that are impartial and reliable. In other words, if dentists use only those materials that meet the appropriate specifications, they can be confident that the material will be satisfactory. Probably no other single factor has contributed as much to the high level of dental practice as has this specification program. An awareness by dental laboratory technicians and dentists of the requirements of these specifications is important to emphasize the limitations of the dental material with which they are working. As is discussed frequently in the chapters to follow, no dental material is perfect in its restorative role, any more than an artificial arm or leg can serve as well as the original body member that it replaces.

The Acceptance Program of the ADA Council on Scientific Affairs applies to products for which safety and effectiveness have been established by biologic, laboratory, and clinical evaluations, if appropriate, or where physical standards or specifications do not currently exist. Specific guidelines for acceptance of each generic product, for example, pit and fissure sealants or powered toothbrushes, are formulated by the Council.

Research on dental materials supervised by the ADA Council on Scientific Affairs is of vital concern in this textbook on dental materials. The ADA specifications for dental materials are referred to throughout the following chapters, although specific details regarding the test methods employed are omitted. For those products sold in other countries, the counterpart ISO standards, if applicable, should be used as a reference source. It is assumed for the discussions in this textbook that the student has access to a collection of specifications and Acceptance Program guidelines of the ADA or other national or international standards.

OTHER STANDARDS ORGANIZATIONS

The work at the National Institute of Standards and Technology has stimulated comparable programs in other countries. The Australian Dental Standards Laboratory was established in 1936. H. K. Worner and A. R. Docking, the first two directors, are recognized for their leadership in the development of the Australian specifications for dental materials. Until 1973 this facility was known as the *Commonwealth Bureau of Dental Standards*. Other countries that have comparable organizations for developing standards and certifying products are Canada, Japan, France, Czech Republic, Germany, Hungary, Israel, India, Poland, and South Africa. Also, by agreement among the governments of Denmark, Finland, Iceland, Norway, and Sweden, the Scandinavian Institute of Dental Materials, better known as NIOM (Nordisk Institutt for Odontologisk Materialprøvning), was established in 1969 for testing, certification, and research regarding dental materials and equipment to be used in the five countries. NIOM became operational in 1973. In Europe the Comité Européen de Normalisation (CEN) established Task Group 55 to develop European standards. After the establishment of the European Economic Community, the CEN was given the charge to outline recommendations of standards for medical devices, including dental materials. In fact, the proper term for *dental materials, dental implants, dental instruments, and dental equipment* in Europe is *medical devices used in dentistry*. The CE marking on product labels denotes the European mark of conformity with the Essential Requirements in the Medical Device Directive that became effective on January 1, 1995. All medical devices marketed in the European Union countries* must

*The European countries include Austria, Belgium, Denmark, Finland, France, Germany, Greece, Ireland, Italy, The Netherlands, Portugal, Luxembourg, Spain, Sweden, and the United Kingdom.

have the CE mark of conformity. For certain products, some countries may enforce their own standards when other countries or the international community have not developed mutually acceptable requirements for certain products. For example, Sweden restricts the use of nickel in cast dental alloys because of biocompatibility concerns, whereas no such restriction applies to those alloys in the United States. Iceland, Liechtenstein, and Norway are also signatories of the European Economic Area Agreement and require the CE marking and NIOM's Notified Body registration number on medical device packaging.

An increasing number of universities in the United States and abroad have established laboratories for research in dental materials. In the past few years, this source of basic information on the subject has exceeded that of all other sources combined. Until recently, dental research activities in universities were centered solely in those that had a dental school, with most of the investigation being done in the dental school itself and by the dental faculty. Now, however, research in dental materials is also being conducted in some universities that do not have dental schools. This dental-oriented research in areas such as metallurgy, polymer science, materials science, engineering, and ceramics is being conducted in basic science departments. These expanding fields of research in dental materials illustrate the interdisciplinary aspects of the science. Since the final criterion for the success of any material or technique is its service in the mouth of the patient, there have been countless contributions to this field by dental clinicians. The observant clinician contributes invaluable information by his or her keen observations and analyses of failures and successes. Accurate record-keeping and well-controlled practice procedures form an excellent basis for good clinical research.

The importance of clinical documentation for claims made relative to the *in vivo* performance of dental materials is now readily apparent. For example, the Acceptance Program of the Council on Scientific Affairs requires clinical data, whenever appropriate, to support the laboratory tests for physical properties. Thus, the past decade has seen an escalation in the number of clinical investigations designed to correlate specific properties to performance and to establish the precise behavior of a given material or system. In the chapters that follow, frequent reference is made to such investigations.

Another source of information is derived from manufacturers' research laboratories. The far-sighted manufacturer recognizes the value of a research laboratory relative to the development and production control of products, and unbiased information from such groups is particularly valuable. As in the previous edition of this book, the counsel of scientists from dental and nondental industries was called on during this revision. In this way the product formulations described in the succeeding chapters reflect with greater accuracy the commercial materials used by the dentist.

This diversity of research activity is resulting in an accelerating growth in the body of knowledge related to dental materials. For example, in 1978 approximately 10% of all U.S. support for dental research was focused on restorative dental materials. The percentage would no doubt be considerably higher if the money spent by industry for the development of new materials, instruments, and appliances were included. This growing investigative effort is resulting in a marked increase in the number of new materials, instruments, and techniques being introduced to the profession. For these and other reasons, an intimate knowledge of the properties and behavior of dental materials is imperative if the modern dental practice is to remain abreast of changing developments.

HOW SAFE ARE DENTAL RESTORATIVE MATERIALS?

Specifications and standards have been developed to aid producers, users, and consumers in the evaluation of the safety and effectiveness of dental products. However, the decision of producers to test their materials according to national and international tests is purely voluntary. The existence of materials evaluation standards does not preclude anyone from manufacturing, marketing, buying, or using dental or medical devices that do not meet these standards. However, producers or marketers of products and devices are expected to meet the safety standards established for those products in the countries in which they are sold. Thus, it is possible for a producer to be given premarket approval by the U.S. FDA to sell a dental device such as a dental restorative material without the device being approved by the ADA in accordance with the specification or Acceptance Program requirements. Nevertheless, these agencies are becoming increasingly dependent on one another to ensure that all products marketed in the United States are safe and effective.

No dental device (including restorative materials) is absolutely safe. Safety is relative, and the selection and use of dental devices or materials are based on the assumption that the benefits of such use far outweigh the known biologic risks. However, there is always uncertainty over the probability that a patient will experience adverse effects from dental treatment. The two main biologic effects are allergic and toxic reactions. Paracelsus (1493–1541), a Swiss physician and alchemist, formulated revolutionary principles that have remained an integral part of the current field of toxicology. He stated that "all substances are poisons; there is none which is not a poison. The right dose differentiates a poison from a remedy" (Gallo and Doull, 1991).

The major routes by which toxic agents enter the body are through the gastrointestinal tract (ingestion), lungs (inhalation), skin (topical, percutaneous, or dermal) and parenteral routes (Klaassen and Eaton, 1991). Exposure to toxic agents can be subdivided into acute (less than 24 hours), subacute (repeated, 1 month or less), subchronic (1 to 3 months), and chronic (longer than 3 months). For many toxic agents, the effects of a single exposure are different from those associated with repeated exposures.

Like toxicity, chemical allergy may also be dose dependent, but it often results from low doses of chemical agents once sensitization has occurred. For a dental restorative material to produce an allergic reaction, most chemical agents or their metabolic products function immunologically as haptens and combine with endogenous proteins to form an antigen. The synthesis of sufficient numbers of antibodies takes 1 to 2 weeks. A later exposure to the chemical agent can induce an antigen-antibody reaction and clinical signs and symptoms of an allergy. Munksgaard (1992) concluded that occupational risks in dentistry are low and that patient risk to the side effects of dental treatment are extremely low. Adverse reactions to dental materials have been reported to occur in only 1 in 700 general patients (Kallus and Mjör, 1991) and in 1 in 300 prosthetic patients (Hensten-Pettersen and Jacobsen, 1991).

SCOPE OF THE BOOK

Not all the materials used in dentistry are included in this book. For example, anesthetics, medicaments, and therapeutic agents such as chlorhexidine are not within the scope of this book. The science of dental materials generally comprises natural oral tissues (enamel, dentin, cementum, pulp tissue, periodontal ligament, cartilage, and bone) and the synthetic materials that are used for prevention of dental caries, for periodontal therapy, and for reconstruction of missing, damaged, or unaesthetic oral structures. These categories include materials employed in dental specialties such as operative dentistry, oral and maxillofacial surgery, orthodontics, periodontology, pediatric dentistry, and prosthodontics. One of the aims of this book is to introduce dental materials to people with little or no dental background and to facilitate the study of their physical and chemical properties as such properties are related to proper selection and use by the dentist. However, certain biologic considerations are also included. It is assumed that the reader possesses a basic knowledge of physics as well as inorganic and organic chemistry.

The engineering curriculum of most major universities includes the discipline of *materials science*. This is concerned with the internal structure of materials and with the dependence of properties on these internal structures. The sequence of instruction generally progresses from atomic to macroscopic structures, from the simple to the more complex. Knowledge in this field is derived from various disciplines, such as physical chemistry, solid state physics, polymer science, ceramics, engineering mechanics, and metallurgy. Because it is the fundamentals that govern the properties of all materials, it is logical to study the microstructural characteristics before proceeding to the macrostructural features.

This importance of relating properties of a material to its atomic or crystalline structure is emphasized in Chapter 2, which deals with the structure of matter and certain principles of materials science that are not always included in a college physics course. These principles are in turn related to the properties of dental materials, as discussed in Chapters 3 and 4.

The requirements placed on dental structures and materials are demanding and unique. It is unfortunate that the dentist and the patient are too often unaware of the limitations involved and the demanding conditions imposed in the oral cavity. These factors are also discussed in Chapters 3 and 4. One should be increasingly aware of the difficulties involved in producing a satisfactory dental material or in designing a technique that is usable and practical, as is continually emphasized in the discussions that follow on specific materials. It is obvious from the earlier discussion of the regulatory agencies in dentistry, such as the ADA Council on Scientific Affairs and the FDA, that the precursor to the marketing or selection of a dental material is its biocompatibility with oral tissues. These biologic considerations are also covered in Chapter 5 and are noted thereafter throughout the text.

Following these chapters on the structure of matter and the physical and biologic properties of dental materials are chapters dealing with the chemistry and manipulation of gypsum products and impression materials. The chemistry of synthetic resins is presented as an introduction to the study of the various types of polymeric materials used for the construction of dental restorations and appliances.

Before the metallic dental materials are described, a short discussion of the principles of metallography, physical metallurgy, and tarnish and corrosion is presented as applied to dental materials and procedures. The basic science of physical metallurgy is concerned with the properties of metals and alloys, whereas the study of metallography involves the constitution and structure of metallic substances. One will find that the subject matter in Chapter 2 is used as source information in many of these discussions.

Dental amalgam and gold foil as well as their manipulation are then described. This discussion is followed by a consideration of the noble and base metal alloys used in dentistry and the materials and techniques employed in dental casting procedures. The cements used as restorations and associated materials such as liners, bases, and varnishes are the subject of Chapter 24. The cements that are used for placement of restorations, in particular those based on polyacrylic acid, are covered in Chapter 25.

A chapter on dental ceramics is followed by a description of soldering (brazing) materials and procedures. The remainder of the book addresses miscellaneous materials, including dental implants, materials used in orthodontics, and the principles of abrasion and polishing.

Many branches of science are incorporated in the presentation of the information and various specialized branches of chemistry are applied. Practically all the engineering applied sciences have contributed to the subject. There is also an increasing awareness by the dentist that the biologic properties of dental materials cannot be divorced from their mechanical and physical properties. Thus, interwoven throughout the book are discussions of the pertinent biologic characteristics to be considered in the selection and use of dental materials. However, the subject of dental materials is a basic science unto itself.

AIM OF THE BOOK

The aim of this textbook and reference source is to present the basic properties of dental materials as they are related to clinical manipulation by the dentist. It is intended to bridge the gap between the knowledge obtained in the basic courses in materials science, chemistry, and physics and the dental operatory. As previously noted, a dental technique does not need to be an empirical process, but rather it can be based on sound scientific principles as more information is available from further research. In any basic science, principles should be emphasized over practice. The discussions that follow deal more with why the materials react as they do and why the manipulation variables should receive attention.

NEED FOR THE BOOK

One of the differences between a professional and a tradesman is that the former possesses basic knowledge with which he or she can establish conditions for a situation such that a prediction of eventual success of a project is reasonably ensured. A riveter must be responsible for the joined beams in a bridge, but the engineer is responsible for the design of the bridge, especially where the rivets and every truss and beam are to be placed and joined, and for the selection of the materials with which the structure is constructed. If the engineer knew nothing about the physical and chemical properties of the steels and other metals with which the bridge is made, the structure would be more likely to fail.

The dentist and the engineer have much in common. Dentists must analyze the stresses present in a dental bridge that they will build and be guided by such analyses in the design of the bridge. They should possess a sufficient knowledge of the physical properties of the different types of materials that they use so that they can exercise the best judgment possible in their selection. For example, they must know whether the dental operation requires the use of a gold alloy, a cement, or a synthetic resin. Only if they know the physical and chemical properties of each of these materials are they in a position to make such a judgment. In addition to the mechanical requirements of the materials, there are also certain aesthetic and physiologic requirements that often complicate the situation beyond the difficulties usually experienced by the engineer.

Once the dentist has selected the type of material to be used, a commercial product must be chosen. It is the intention of the best dental manufacturers to cooperate with dentists in supplying them with materials of high quality in an ethical manner. The competition is keen, however, and the dentist should be able to evaluate the claims of the respective manufacturers in an intelligent manner. It is unfortunate that there are a few unprincipled dental manufacturers who make preposterous claims and who exploit the dentist for their own profit. For their own protection and for the protection of their patients, dentists must be able to recognize spurious practices of this sort. Along with other aims, courses in dental materials attempt to provide dentists with certain criteria of selection so as to enable them to discriminate between fact and propaganda.

Furthermore, it is hoped that students of dental materials are given an appreciation of the broad scientific scope of their chosen profession. Because a great deal of the daily practice of dentistry involves the selection and use of dental materials, either for the treatment procedure or in the instrumentation required, it is obvious that the science of dental materials is critically important.

The advances being made in dental materials science suggest that intriguing changes will continue to occur in the practice of dentistry. Based on your knowledge of materials science principles, you should be prepared to analyze the benefits and limitations of these materials products and to make rational decisions on their selection and use in a clinical practice.

Acknowledgment

I extend my appreciation to Dr. P. L. Fan of the American Dental Association for his helpful suggestions on standardization programs.

SELECTED READING

Coleman RL: Physical Properties of Dental Materials. National Bureau of Standards Research Paper No. 32. Washington, DC, US Government Printing Office, 1928.
This publication is the first major effort to relate physical properties of dental materials to the clinical situation. The American Dental Association specification program was established based on this historical review of the philosophy and the content of the facility created at the National Bureau of Standards.
Federal Register: Medical Devices; Dental Device Classification; Final Rule and Withdrawal of Proposed Rules. August 12, 1987, p 30,082.
A listing of the dental materials and devices classified in Category III by the Food and Drug Administration as of that date.
Gallo MA, and Doull J: History and scope of toxicology. In: Casarett and Doull's Toxicology. New York, Pergamon Press, 1991, pp 3–11.
Hensten-Pettersen A, and Jacobsen N: Perceived side effects of biomaterials in prosthetic dentistry. J Prosthet Dent 65:138, 1991.
Kallus T, and Mjör IA: Incidence of adverse effects of dental materials. Scand J Dent Res 99:236, 1991.
Klaassen CD, and Eaton DL: Principles of toxicology. In: Casarett and Doull's Toxicology. New York, Pergamon Press, 1991, pp 12–49.
Munksgaard EC: Toxicology versus allergy in restorative dentistry. In: Advances in Dental Research. Bethesda, International Association for Dental Research, September 1992, pp 17–21.
Phillips RW: Changing trends of dental restorative materials. Dent Clin North Am 33(2):285, 1989.
A review of the trends in biomaterials that are influencing dental restorative procedures, particularly in aesthetic dentistry. Emphasis is on bonding technology and its application.
Ring ME: Dentistry: An Illustrated History. New York, Harry N Abrams, 1985.

2

Structure of Matter and Principles of Adhesion

- Change of State
- Interatomic Primary Bonds
- Interatomic Secondary Bonds
- Interatomic Bond Distance and Bonding Energy
- Thermal Energy
- Crystalline Structure
- Noncrystalline Structure
- Diffusion
- Adhesion and Bonding
- Adhesion to Tooth Structure

CHANGE OF STATE

Several material properties must be considered when dental materials are selected for clinical use. These considerations include (1) biocompatibility, (2) physicochemical properties, (3) handling characteristics, (4) aesthetics, and (5) economy. Of these properties, biocompatibility determines whether the material can be used intraorally. Within the group of biocompatible materials, the other four considerations will then determine the acceptability of the physicochemical properties, the ease of processing, the aesthetic potential, and the cost effectiveness.

To gain an understanding of dental materials, we need a basic knowledge of matter, particularly solids, and its behavior during handling and use in the oral environment. Unfortunately, our understanding of the behavior of materials in the oral environment is still incomplete. Because environmental factors are critically important for clinical success, extrapolation of *in vitro* information, often presented in textbooks and research articles, to *in vivo* conditions should be approached with extreme caution.

Despite a need for better understanding of the clinical behavior of dental materials, we can conclude that the performance of all dental materials, whether they are ceramic, plastic, or metal, is based on their atomic structure. The collective reactions of the atoms, whether physical or chemical, determine the properties of the material. Therefore, a short review of matter is justified to lay a foundation for a basic understanding of dental materials.

Atoms and molecules are held together by atomic interactions. When water boils, energy is needed to transform the liquid to vapor, and this quantity of energy is known as the *heat of vaporization.* During condensation of water vapor, the same amount of heat is released to the environment and thus satisfies the conservation of energy. The heat of vaporization is defined as the amount of heat needed to evaporate 1 g of liquid to the vapor state at a given temperature and pressure. For example, 540 cal of heat is required to vaporize 1 g of water at 100° C and a pressure of 1 atm. Thus, one can conclude that the gaseous state possesses more kinetic energy than does the liquid state.

Although molecules in the gaseous state exert a certain amount of mutual attraction, they can move readily because of their high kinetic energy. This is also the reason why gaseous molecules need to be confined to avoid dispersion. Atoms present in a liquid can also diffuse, but because their mutual attractions are greater in the liquid state than in the gaseous state, kinetic energy must be increased to achieve separation in the liquid state. If the kinetic energy of a liquid decreases sufficiently when its temperature is decreased, a second transformation in state may occur and the liquid can change to a solid. Kinetic energy is released in the form of heat when the liquid freezes. In this instance, the energy released is known as the *latent heat of fusion.* For example, when 1 g of water freezes, 80 cal of heat are released. If 1 g of a solid is changed to a liquid, the reverse is true and an input of energy is required. For certain solids, such as pure metals, the temperature at which this change occurs is known as the *melting temperature.*

Because energy is required for a change from the solid to the liquid state, one can conclude that the attraction between atoms (or molecules) in the solid state is greater than that in either the liquid or the gaseous state. If this were not true, atoms would separate easily. In addition, metals would deform readily, and they would exist in the vapor phase at low temperatures.

The temperature at which a liquid boils or solidifies depends partly on the environmental pressure. A liquid can vaporize (or evaporate) at any temperature between its freezing and boiling temperatures provided that the space above the liquid is not already saturated or supersaturated with the vapor. As the vapor density above the liquid increases, the vapor pressure produced by the molecules in the gaseous state develops within a closed container. This vapor density, as well as the resulting vapor pressure, attains a constant value in equilibrium, because the molecules are entering and leaving the liquid phase at an equal rate. Although it is possible for some solids to transform directly to a gas phase through the process of sublimation, this phenomenon is of little practical importance with respect to dental materials currently in use.

With this brief discussion of the variables that affect change of state, considerations involving atomic or molecular attractions are discussed in the following sections.

INTERATOMIC PRIMARY BONDS

The forces that hold atoms together are called cohesive forces. These interatomic bonds may be classified as primary or secondary. The strength of these bonds, as well as their ability to reform after breakage, determines the physical properties of the material. Primary atomic bonds (Fig. 2–1) may be of three different types: (1) ionic, (2) covalent, and (3) metallic.

Ionic Bonds. These primary bonds (Fig. 2–1*A*) are of the simple chemical type, resulting from the mutual attraction of positive and negative charges. The classic example is sodium chloride (Na^+Cl^-). Because the sodium atom contains one

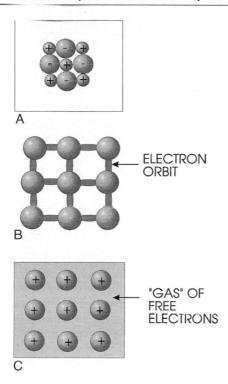

A

ELECTRON ORBIT

B

"GAS" OF FREE ELECTRONS

C

Figure 2–1. *A,* Ionic bond formation—characterized by electron transfer from one element (positive) to another (negative). *B,* Covalent bond formation—characterized by electron sharing and very precise bond orientations. *C,* Metallic bond formation—characterized by electron sharing and formation of a "gas" of electrons that bonds the atoms (which become positively charged because of the electron gas formation) together in a lattice.

valence electron in its outer shell and the chlorine atom has seven electrons in its outer shell, the transfer of the sodium valence electron to the chlorine atom results in the stable compound Na^+Cl^-. Ionic bonds result in crystals whose atomic configuration is based on a charge and size balance. In dentistry, ionic bonding exists in certain crystalline phases of some dental materials, such as gypsum and phosphate cements.

Covalent Bonds. In many chemical compounds, two valence electrons are shared by adjacent atoms (Fig. 2–1*B*). The hydrogen molecule, H_2, is an example of covalent bonding. The single valence electron in each hydrogen atom is shared with that of the other combining atom, and the valence shells become stable. Covalent bonding occurs in many organic compounds, such as dental resins, where they link to form the backbone structure of hydrocarbon chains. The carbon atom has four valence electrons forming an sp^3 hybrid configuration (Fig. 2–2) and can be stabilized by combining with hydrogen. A typical characteristic of covalent bonds is their directional orientation.

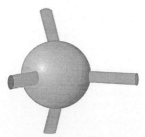

Figure 2–2. Carbon atom with an sp^3 orbit formation. This type of hybrid configuration is also common for silicon.

Metallic Bonds. The third type of primary atomic interaction is the *metallic bond* (Fig. 2–1C). The metallic bond can be understood best by studying a metallic crystal such as pure gold. Typically, such a crystal consists only of gold atoms. Like all other metals, gold atoms can easily donate electrons from their outer shell and form a "gas" of free electrons. The contribution of free electrons to this cloud results in the formation of positive ions that can be neutralized by acquiring new valence electrons from adjacent atoms.

Because of their ability to donate and recover electrons, atoms in a metal crystal exist as clusters of positive metal ions surrounded by a gas of electrons. This structure is responsible for the excellent electrical and thermal conductivity of metals and also for their ability to deform plastically. The electrical and thermal conductivities of metals are controlled by the ease with which the free electrons can move through the crystal, whereas their deformability is associated with slip along crystal planes, and thus the ability of the electrons to easily regroup and still retain the cohesive nature of the metal as deformation occurs.

INTERATOMIC SECONDARY BONDS

In contrast with primary bonds, secondary bonds (Fig. 2–3) do not share electrons. Instead, charge variations among molecules or atomic groups induce polar forces that attract the molecules. Since there are no primary bonds between water and glass, it would be difficult to understand how water drops, when they freeze to ice crystals, can bond to an automobile windshield. However, the concepts of hydrogen and secondary bonding—two types of bonds that exist between water and glass—allow us to explain this adhesion.

Hydrogen Bonding. This bond can be understood by studying a water molecule (Fig 2–4). Attached to the oxygen atom are two hydrogen atoms. These bonds are covalent because the oxygen and hydrogen atoms share electrons. As a consequence, the protons of the hydrogen atoms pointing away from the oxygen atom are not shielded efficiently by the electrons. Thus, the proton side of the water molecule becomes positively charged. On the opposite side of the water molecule, the electrons that fill the outer orbit of the oxygen provide a negative charge. Thus, a permanent dipole exists that represents an asymmetric molecule. The hydrogen bond, which is associated with the positive charge of hydrogen caused by polarization, is an important example of this type of secondary bonding.

When a water molecule intermingles with other water molecules, the hydro-

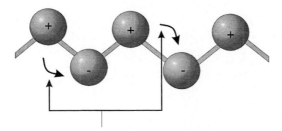

DIFFERENCES IN ELECTRON DENSITIES
RESULT IN CHARGE VARIATIONS
ALONG THE MOLECULE

Figure 2–3. Secondary bond formation. Charge variations along molecules induce polar forces that attract other molecules.

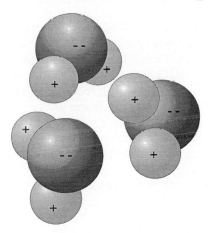

Figure 2-4. Hydrogen bond formation between water molecules. The polar water molecule ties up adjacent water molecules via an H···O interaction between molecules.

gen (positive) portion of one molecule is attracted to the oxygen (negative) portion of its neighboring molecule, and hydrogen bridges are formed. Polarity of this nature is important in accounting for the intermolecular reactions in many organic compounds, for example, the sorption of water by synthetic dental resins.

van der Waals Forces. These forces form the basis of a dipole attraction (Fig. 2-5). For example, in a symmetric molecule, such as occurs in an inert gas, the electron field is constantly fluctuating. Normally, the electrons of the atoms are distributed equally around the nucleus and produce an electrostatic field around the atom. However, this field may fluctuate so that its charge becomes momentarily positive and negative, as shown in Figure 2-5. A fluctuating dipole is thus created that will attract other similar dipoles. Such interatomic forces are quite weak.

INTERATOMIC BOND DISTANCE AND BONDING ENERGY

Bond Distance. Regardless of the type of matter, there is a limiting factor that prevents the atoms or molecules from approaching each other too closely, that is, the distance between the center of an atom and that of its neighbor is limited to the diameter of the atoms involved. Although the atom, for convenience, is treated as a discrete particle with boundaries and volume, its boundaries are

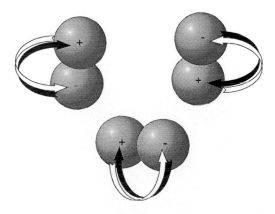

Figure 2-5. Fluctuating dipole binding inert gas molecules together. The *arrows* show how the fields may fluctuate so that the charges become momentarily positive and negative.

rather vaguely established by the electrostatic fields of the electrons. If the atoms approach too closely, they are repelled from each other by their electron charges. On the other hand, forces of attraction tend to draw the atoms together. The position at which these forces of repulsion and attraction become equal in magnitude (but opposite in direction) is the equilibrium position of the atoms shown in Figure 2–6. In this position, the repelling forces are equal in magnitude to the attracting forces. Atom B can be displaced to position B′ by a disturbing mechanical, thermal, or electrical force. A disturbing force may also cause the atoms to move more closely together (B″ in Fig. 2–6). As the forces of attraction increase, the interatomic space decreases. On the other hand, the forces of repulsion remain relatively inactive until the atoms are sufficiently close to each other. The sum or resultant of the two forces is indicated by the broken line in Figures 2–6 and 2–7. As noted, the resultant force becomes zero, that is, the magnitudes of the two forces are equal at the intersection of the broken line with the horizontal axis, labeled by the distance a. This is the interatomic distance at equilibrium, and it represents the distance between the centers of the atoms involved.

Bonding Energy. Because conditions of equilibrium are usually described in terms of energy rather than interatomic forces, the relationships in Figure 2–7 can be more logically explained in terms of interatomic energy. According to the laws of physics, *energy* can be defined as a force integrated over a distance. If the resultant force (F), represented by the dashed line in Figure 2–7, is integrated over the interatomic distances (a), the graph shown in Figure 2–8 will result. As shown in Figure 2–7, the horizontal axis is the interatomic spacing, but interatomic or bonding energy is plotted on the vertical axis in Figure 2–8, where a represents the normal interatomic distance. In contrast with the resultant force plotted in Figure 2–6, the energy does not change a great deal initially as two atoms come closer together. As the resultant force approaches zero (see Fig. 2–7),

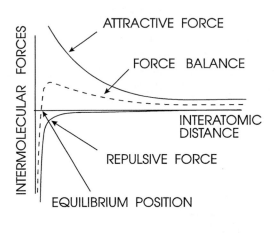

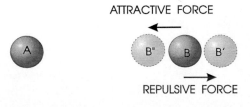

Figure 2–6. Attractive and repulsive forces balance each other, and atom B attains its equilibrium position.

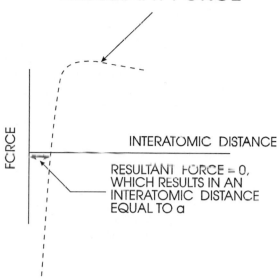

Figure 2-7. When the equilibrium position is reached, the interatomic distance is a. By moving the atom from that position, either a negative (repulsive) or a positive (attractive) force is required to move the atom back to its equilibrium position as shown in Figure 2–6.

the energy decreases (see Fig. 2–8). The energy finally reaches a minimum when the resultant force becomes zero. Thereafter, the energy increases rapidly (see Fig. 2–8), because the resultant repulsive force (see Fig. 2–7) increases rapidly with little change in interatomic distance. The minimal energy corresponds to the condition of equilibrium and defines the equilibrium interatomic distance.

THERMAL ENERGY

Thermal energy is accounted for by the kinetic energy of the atoms or molecules at a given temperature. The atoms in a crystal at temperatures above absolute zero temperature are in a constant state of vibration, and the average amplitude will be dependent on the temperature; the higher the temperature, the greater the amplitude and, consequently, the greater the kinetic or internal energy. Further consideration of Figure 2–7 and Figure 2–8 in particular can provide some interesting interpretations of these phenomena.

Thus, for a certain temperature, the minimal energy is the energy at equilibrium and is denoted by the bottom of the trough in Figure 2–8. As the temperature increases, the amplitude of the atomic (or molecular) vibration increases. It follows also that the mean interatomic spacing increases (see Figs. 2–8 and 2–9)

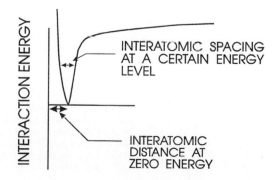

Figure 2–8. By multiplying the force shown in Figure 2–7 by the atomic displacement from its equilibrium position, the energy change can be plotted as a function of displacement in either direction.

as well as the internal energy. The overall effect represents the phenomenon known as *thermal expansion* (Fig. 2–9).

If the temperature continues to increase, the interatomic spacing will increase, and eventually a change of state will occur. The solid changes to a liquid, and the liquid subsequently changes to a gas. It follows from Figures 2–9A and B that the deeper the trough in the curve, the greater the amount of energy required to achieve melting and boiling, and consequently the higher the melting and boiling temperatures. By the same reasoning, it can be argued that the deeper the energy trough, the lower the thermal expansion per degree increase in temperature, because the interatomic spacing does not necessarily increase as the depth of the trough increases. In other words, the linear coefficient of thermal expansion (α) of materials with similar atomic or molecular structures tends to be inversely proportional to the melting temperature.

Shown in Figures 2–7 and 2–8 is another interesting relationship between the melting temperature and the force required to move atoms away from their equilibrium spacing. As shown in Figure 2–7, the net force on the atoms at the equilibrium spacing is zero, but small displacements result in rapidly increasing forces that maintain the equilibrium spacing. The stiffness of the material is proportional to the rate of change of the force with a change in displacement that is measured by the slope of the net force curve near a. A greater slope of the force curve implies a narrower, deeper trough in the energy curve (see Fig. 2–8). Hence, a high melting point is usually accompanied by a greater stiffness.

Thermal conductivity is related to interatomic spacing only to the extent that the heat is conducted from one atom or molecule to the next as adjacent basic structural units are affected by the kinetic energy of their neighbors. However, the number of "free" electrons in the material influences its thermal conductivity. As discussed earlier, the metallic structure contains many free electrons, and most metals are good conductors of heat as well as electricity. On the other hand, nonmetallic materials do not include many free electrons, and, consequently, they are generally poor thermal and electrical conductors.

The preceding principles represent generalities, and exceptions do occur. Nev-

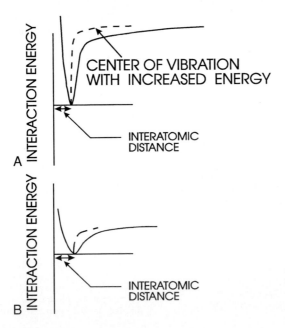

Figure 2–9. The depth of the energy curve is determined by the magnitude of the attractive-repulsive forces. Thus, for a shallow curve *(B)*, less energy is needed compared with the deeper curve *(A)* to separate the atoms.

ertheless, they allow one to estimate the influence of temperature on the properties of most of the dental materials to be discussed in subsequent chapters.

CRYSTALLINE STRUCTURE

Thus far we have generally assumed the presence of only two atoms or molecules. Obviously, dental materials consist of many millions of such units. But one questions how the structural units are arranged in a solid and how they are held together.

In 1665, Robert Hooke (1635–1703) simulated the characteristic shapes of crystals by stacking musket balls in piles. It was 250 years later before anyone knew that he had created an exact model of the crystal structure of many familiar metals, with each ball representing an atom.

The atoms are, of course, bonded by either primary or secondary forces. In the solid state, they combine in a manner that ensures minimal internal energy. For example, sodium and chlorine share one electron as previously described. In the solid state, however, they do not simply form only pairs, but, in fact, all of the positively charged sodium ions attract all of the negatively charged chlorine ions. The result is that they form a regularly spaced configuration known as a *space lattice* or *crystal*. A space lattice can be defined as any arrangement of atoms in space such that every atom is situated similarly to every other atom. Space lattices may be the result of primary or secondary bonds.

There are 14 possible lattice types or forms, but many of the metals used in dentistry belong to the cubic system; that is, the atoms crystallize in cubic arrangements. The simplest cubic space lattice is shown in Figure 2–10, with the spheres representing the positions of the atoms. Their positions are located at the points of intersection of three sets of parallel planes, each set being perpendicular to the other two sets of planes. These planes are often referred to as *crystal planes.*

Shown in Figure 2–11A is one unit cell of the simple cubic space lattice. The cells are repeated in three-dimensional space as indicated in Figure 2–10. The simple cubic arrangements in Figures 2–10 and 2–11A are only hypothetical. No real material has this structure. The arrangements shown in Figures 2–11B and C represent the cubic space lattices of practical importance. Also, Figures 2–10 and 2–11 are diagrammatic only. The atoms are actually closely packed so that

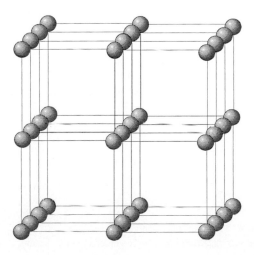

Figure 2–10. Simple cubic space lattice.

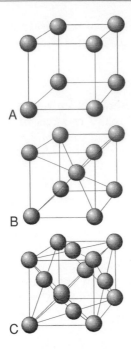

Figure 2–11. Single cells of cubic space lattices: *A*, simple cubic; *B*, body-centered cubic; and *C*, face-centered cubic.

the interatomic spacing is equal to the sum of their radii. The closer packing arrangement for a model of the less closely packed structure of a body-centered cubic structure is shown in Figure 2–12, and a similar model for a face-centered cubic lattice is pictured in Figure 2–13.

The type of space lattice is defined by the length of three of the unit cell edges (called the *axes*) and the angles between the edges. For example, the cubic space lattice (see Fig. 2–11*A*) is characterized by axes that are all of equal length and meet at a 90-degree angle. Other types of space lattices are diagrammed in Figure 2–14.

NONCRYSTALLINE STRUCTURE

There are structures other than the crystalline form that can occur in the solid state. For example, some of the waxes used by a dentist or laboratory technician may solidify as amorphous materials such that the molecules are distributed at random. Even in this instance, there is a tendency for the arrangement to be regular.

Glass is also considered to be a noncrystalline solid, since its atoms tend to develop a short-range order instead of the long-range order characteristic of crystalline solids. In other words, the ordered arrangement of the glass is more

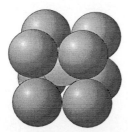

Figure 2–12. Model of a body-centered cubic crystal.

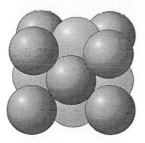

Figure 2–13. Model of a face-centered cubic crystal.

or less locally interspersed with a considerable number of disordered units. Because this arrangement is also typical of liquids, such solids are sometimes called *supercooled liquids.*

The structural arrangements of the noncrystalline solids do not represent such low internal energies as do crystalline arrangements of the same atoms and molecules. They do not have a definite melting temperature, but rather they gradually soften as the temperature is raised. The temperature at which there is an abrupt increase in the thermal expansion coefficient, indicating increased molecular mobility, is called the *glass transition temperature* (T_g) and it is characteristic of the particular glassy structure. Occasionally, the term is shortened to

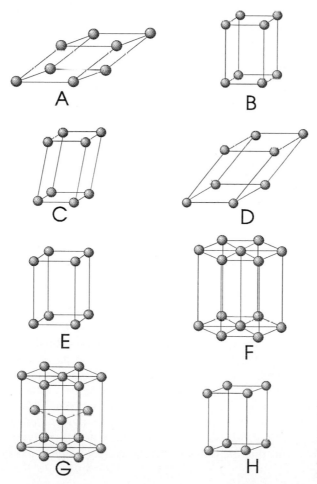

Figure 2–14. Other simple lattice types of dental interest: *A,* rhombohedral; *B,* orthorhombic; *C,* monoclinic; *D,* triclinic; *E,* tetragonal; *F,* simple hexagonal; *G,* close-packed hexagonal; and *H,* rhombic.

glass temperature. Below T_g, the glassy structure loses its fluid characteristics and has significant resistance to shear deformation. Synthetic dental resins are examples of materials that often have glassy structures.

DIFFUSION

The diffusion of molecules in gases and liquids is well known. However, molecules or atoms diffuse in the solid state as well. As previously described, the atoms in a space lattice are constantly in vibration about their centers. The average kinetic energy of vibration over the entire crystal is related to the temperature. At absolute zero the vibration ceases, the energy becomes zero, and the atom occupies the center of vibration (see Fig. 2–9).

An understanding of diffusion in a solid requires two new concepts. At any temperature above absolute zero, the atoms (or molecules) of a solid possess some amount of kinetic energy, as previously discussed. In this regard, one new concept is that all the atoms do not possess the same amount of energy. Rather, there is a distribution of a number of atoms with a particular energy that varies from very small to quite large, with the average energy related to the absolute zero temperature. Even at very low temperatures, some atoms have large energies. If the energy of a particular atom exceeds the bonding energy, it can move to another position in the lattice. In a noncrystalline solid with only short-range order, there is a strong probability that a high-energy atom will be located adjacent to a vacant position. This is the second concept that is required to describe solid-state diffusion. In crystalline solids at any temperature above the absolute zero temperature, there are a finite number of missing atoms (called *vacancies*) that represent *holes* through which diffusion can occur.

Atoms change position in pure solids even under equilibrium conditions; this process is known as *self-diffusion*. However, such diffusion is generally not of practical importance, because no visible or measurable dimensional changes occur.

As with any diffusion process, the atoms or molecules diffuse in the solid state in an attempt to reach an equilibrium state. For example, a concentration of sugar molecules in solution tends to diffuse to achieve a uniform concentration. As discussed later, a concentration of atoms in a metal can also be redistributed through the diffusion process.

Diffusion may also occur in the other direction to produce a concentration of atoms in a solution. For example, if the sugar in the water becomes supersaturated, the molecules of sugar diffuse toward each other, and the sugar crystallizes out of solution. In the same manner, too many copper atoms in a solid alloy of copper and silver may cause supersaturation and diffusion of the copper atoms to increase the concentration of copper locally, causing them to precipitate out of solution.

Diffusion rates for a given substance depend mainly on temperature. The higher the temperature, the greater the rate of diffusion. The diffusion rate varies with the atom size, interatomic or intermolecular bonding, lattice imperfections, and similar phenomena. In other words, various media exhibit different characteristic diffusion rates. The diffusion constant, uniquely characteristic of the given element, compound, crystal, and so forth in a particular substrate (medium), is known as the *diffusion coefficient*, usually designated as D. It can be defined as the amount of diffusion that takes place across a given unit area (e.g., 1 cm^2), through a unit thickness of the substance (e.g., 1 cm), in one unit of time (e.g., 1 s).

The diffusion coefficients of most crystalline solids at room temperature are very low. Diffusion in dental alloys is so slow at room temperature that it cannot be detected in a practical sense. Yet, at a temperature a few hundred degrees higher, the properties of the metal may be changed radically by atomic diffusion. Diffusion in a noncrystalline material may occur at a more rapid rate and often may be evident at room or body temperature. The disordered structure enables the molecules to diffuse more easily with less activation energy.

ADHESION AND BONDING

The phenomenon of adhesion is involved in many situations in dentistry. For example, leakage adjacent to dental restorative materials is affected by the adhesion process. The retention of artificial dentures is probably dependent, to some extent, on adhesion between the denture and saliva and between the saliva and soft tissue. Certainly, the attachment of plaque or calculus to tooth structure can be partially explained by an adhesion mechanism. Therefore, an understanding of the fundamental principles associated with the phenomenon is important to the dentist.

When two substances are brought into intimate contact with each other, the molecules of one substance adhere or are attracted to molecules of another. This force is called *adhesion* when unlike molecules are attracted and *cohesion* when molecules of the same kind are attracted. The material or film added to produce the adhesion is known as the *adhesive*, and the material to which it is applied is called the *adherend*.

In the broadest sense adhesion is simply a surface attachment process, but the term is usually qualified by specifying the type of intermolecular attraction that may exist between the adhesive and the adherend.

Mechanical Bonding. Strong attachment of one substance to another can also be accomplished by mechanical bonding or retention rather than by molecular attraction. Such structural retention may be gross in nature, as evidenced by applications involving the use of screws, bolts, or undercuts. Mechanical bonding may also involve more subtle mechanisms such as the penetration of the adhesive into microscopic or submicroscopic irregularities (e.g., crevices and pores) in the surface of the substrate. A fluid or semiviscous liquid adhesive is best suited for such a procedure, because it readily penetrates into these surface defects. On hardening, the multitude of adhesive projections embedded in the adherend surface provides the anchorage for mechanical attachment (retention).

This mechanism has been commonly used in dentistry, in the absence of truly adhesive cements or restorative materials. For example, retention of cast restorations, such as a cast gold alloy crown or a base metal endodontic post and core, is enhanced by mechanical attachment of the cementing agent into irregularities that exist on the internal surface of the casting and those that are present in the adjoining tooth structure.

A more recent example of mechanical bonding is that of resin (plastic) restorative materials. Because these resins do not have the capability of truly adhering to tooth structure, leakage adjacent to the restoration may pose a major problem. Such leakage patterns contribute to marginal stain, secondary caries, and irritation of the pulp.

To minimize the risks of deleterious agents that may migrate toward the pulp, the following technique for placement of such materials is used. Before insertion of the resin, the enamel of the adjoining tooth structure is treated with phosphoric acid for a short period. This is referred to as the *acid-etching* technique. The acid produces minute pores in the enamel surface into which the resin subsequently flows when it is placed into the preparation. On hardening, these resin projections provide improved mechanical retention of the restoration, thereby reducing the possibility of interfacial marginal leakage.

Thus, the acid-etching technique is an example of how bonding between a dental material and tooth structure can be attained through mechanical mechanisms, not through molecular adhesion. The principles of adhesion and the factors associated with this phenomenon are discussed further in the following sections.

Surface Energy. For adhesion to exist, the surfaces must be attracted to one another at their interface. Such a condition may exist regardless of the phases (solid, liquid, or gas) comprising the two surfaces, with the exception that adhesion between two gases is not expected because of the lack of an interface.

The energy at the surface of a solid is greater than that of its interior. For example, consider the space lattice shown in Figure 2–15. Inside the lattice, all the atoms are equally attracted to each other. The interatomic distances are equal, and the energy is minimal. At the surface of the lattice, the energy is greater because the outermost atoms are not equally attracted in all directions, as diagrammed in Figure 2–15. The interior atom A has a balanced array of nearest neighbors surrounding it, whereas surface atom B has an unbalanced number of adjacent atoms.

The increase in energy per unit area of surface is referred to as the *surface energy* or *surface tension*. A soap film contracts and drops of a liquid form spherical shapes by minimizing surface area because this surface tension condition represents the state of lowest energy.

The surface atoms of a solid tend to form bonds to other atoms that are in close proximity to the surface and reduce the surface energy of the solid. This attraction across the interface between unlike molecules is called *adhesion*. For example, molecules in the air may be attracted to the surface and become *adsorbed* on the material surface. Silver, platinum, and gold adsorb oxygen readily. With gold, the bonding forces are of the secondary type, but in the case of silver the attraction may be controlled by chemical or primary bonding, and silver oxide may form.

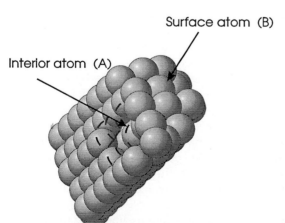

Surface atom (B)

Interior atom (A)

Figure 2–15. Comparing an atom under the surface (A) with one on the surface (B) reveals that a bond balance exists around A, while B can develop bonds to atoms or molecules approaching the surface at B.

When primary bonding is involved, the adhesion is termed *chemisorption*, as compared with physical bonding by van der Waals forces. In chemisorption, a chemical bond is formed between the adhesive and the adherend. As previously noted, an example of this type of adhesion is an oxide film formed on the surface of a metal. Thus, van der Waals forces are weaker than primary bonding because they are intermolecular rather than intramolecular.

The development of van der Waals forces invariably precedes chemisorption. As the distance between the adhesive and the adherend diminishes, primary bonding may become effective. However, chemisorption is limited to the monolayer of adhesive present on the adherend. The surface energy and the adhesive qualities of a given solid can be reduced by any surface impurity, such as adsorbed gas or an oxide as previously described. The functional chemical groups available or the type of crystal plane of a space lattice present at the surface may affect the surface energy. In summary, the greater the surface energy, the greater the capacity for adhesion.

Wetting. It is difficult to force two solid surfaces to adhere. Regardless of how smooth these surfaces may appear, they are likely to be extremely rough when they are viewed on the atomic or molecular scale. Consequently, when they are placed in apposition, only the "hills" or high spots are in contact. Because these areas usually constitute only a small percentage of the total surface, no perceptible adhesion takes place. The attraction is generally negligible when the surface molecules of the attracting substances are separated by distances greater than 0.7 nm (0.0007 μm).

One method of overcoming this difficulty is to use a fluid that flows into these irregularities and thus provides contact over a greater part of the surface of the solid. For example, when two polished glass plates are placed one on top of the other and are pressed together, they exhibit little tendency to adhere for reasons previously described. However, if a film of water is introduced between them, considerable difficulty is encountered in separating the two plates. The surface energy of the glass is sufficiently great to attract the molecules of water.

To produce adhesion in this manner, the liquid must flow easily over the entire surface and adhere to the solid. This characteristic is referred to as *wetting*. If the liquid does not wet the surface of the adherend, adhesion between the liquid and the adherend will be negligible or nonexistent. If there is a true wetting of the surface, adhesion failures cannot occur. Failure in such instances actually occurs cohesively in the solid or in the adhesive itself, not along the interface where the solid and adhesive are in contact.

The ability of an adhesive to wet the surface of the adherend is influenced by a number of factors. As previously noted, the cleanliness of the surface is of particular importance. A film of water only one molecule thick on the surface of the solid may lower the surface energy of the adherend and prevent any wetting by the adhesive. Likewise, an oxide film on a metallic surface may also inhibit the contact of an adhesive.

The surface energy of some substances is so low that few, if any, liquids wet their surfaces. For example, some organic substances are of this type. Close packing of the structural organic groups and the presence of halogens may prevent wetting. Teflon (polytetrafluoroethylene), a commercial synthetic resin, is often used when it is desirable to prevent the adhesion of films to a surface.

Metals, on the other hand, interact vigorously with liquid adhesives because of their high surface energy.

In general, the comparatively low surface energies of organic and most inorganic liquids permit them to spread freely on solids of high surface energy. Thus, formation of a strong adhesive joint requires good wetting.

Contact Angle of Wetting. The extent to which an adhesive wets the surface of an adherend may be determined by measuring the contact angle between the adhesive and the adherend. The contact angle is the angle formed by the adhesive with the adherend at their interface. If the molecules of the adhesive are attracted to the molecules of the adherend as much as or more than they are to themselves, the liquid adhesive will spread completely over the surface of the solid, and no angle (θ = 0 degrees) will be formed (Fig. 2–16A). Thus, the forces of adhesion are stronger than the cohesive forces holding the molecules of the adhesive together.

However, if the energy of the surface of the adherend is reduced slightly by

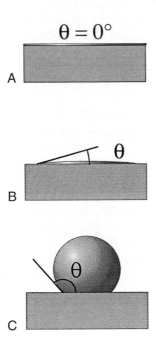

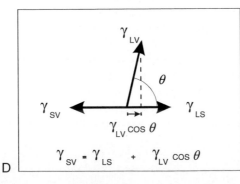

Figure 2–16. Adhesion depends on wetting the surface. *A,* When the contact angle (θ) is 0 degrees, the liquid contacts the surface completely and spreads freely. *B,* Small contact angle on slightly contaminated surface. *C,* Large angle formed by poor wetting. *D,* The relationships among the surface tension of the solid (γ_{SV}), the liquid (γ_{LV}), and the contact angle (θ) can be used to determine the surface tension between the liquid and the solid (γ_{LS}) according to the equation shown.

contamination or other means (the surface tension of the solid [γ_{SV}] decreases) and a slight increase in the contact angle (Θ) can be measured (Fig. 2–16*B*). This increase in Θ retains the force balance shown in Figure 2–16*D*. Note that as Θ increases from 0 to 90 degrees, the value of cos Θ decreases from 1 to 0. If a monolayer film of a contaminant is present over the entire surface, a medium angle might be obtained, whereas a very high angle would result on a solid of low surface energy (γ_{SV}), such as polytetrafluoroethylene (Fig. 2–16*C*). Because the tendency for the liquid to spread increases as the contact angle decreases, the contact angle is a useful indicator of spreadability or wettability (Fig. 2–16*D*).

Thus, the smaller the contact angle between an adhesive and an adherend, the better the ability of the adhesive to fill in irregularities on the surface of the adherend. Also, the fluidity of the adhesive influences the extent to which these voids or irregularities are filled.

Solid "flat" surfaces are not actually planar. Surface imperfections represent a potential impediment to the achievement of an adhesive bond. Air pockets may be created during the spreading of the adhesive that prevent complete wetting of the entire surface (Fig. 2–17). When the adhesive joint is subjected to thermal changes and mechanical stresses, *stress concentrations* develop around these voids. The stress may become so great that it initiates a separation in the adhesive bond adjacent to the void. This crack may propagate from one void to the next, and the joint may separate under stress as if it had a built-in "zipper."

ADHESION TO TOOTH STRUCTURE

The fundamental principles of adhesion can be readily related to dental situations. For example, when contact angle measurements are used to study the wettability of enamel and dentin, it is found that the wettability of these surfaces is markedly reduced after the topical application of an aqueous fluoride solution. Transferring this information to the clinical setting, it is found that the fluoride-treated enamel surface retains less plaque over a given period, presumably because of a decrease in surface energy. Thus, it is not inconceivable that fluoride products may be effective in reducing dental caries by providing a tooth surface that stays cleaner over a longer period, in addition to the recognized mechanism of reduced enamel solubility in an acidic environment.

Similarly, because of the higher surface energy of many restorative materials compared with that of the tooth, there is a greater tendency for the surface and margins of the restoration to accumulate debris. This may in part account for the relatively high incidence of marginal caries seen around dental restorations.

In the following chapters, leakage that occurs between tooth structure and dental restorations is discussed. It is shown that, under certain instances, recurrent caries, pulpal sensitivity after placement of the restoration, and deterioration at the margins of the restoration can be associated with a lack of adhesion between the restorative material and the tooth. Extensive research is in progress to develop adhesives that adhere to tooth structure. In subsequent chapters, we

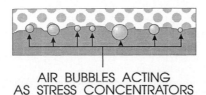

AIR BUBBLES ACTING
AS STRESS CONCENTRATORS

Figure 2–17. Air pockets created in surface irregularities. Such regions contribute to propagation of adhesive failure by concentration of stress at these points.

shall see how traditional dental restorative procedures are affected by such adhesive systems.

However, if one applies the principles that influence adhesion to dental structures, it is obvious that the problems are indeed complex. Tooth composition is not homogeneous. Both organic and inorganic components are present in different amounts in dentin than they are in enamel. A material that can adhere to the organic components may not adhere to the inorganic components, and an adhesive that bonds to enamel may not adhere to dentin to the same extent.

After the dentist has completed a cavity preparation, tenacious microscopic debris covers the enamel and dentin surfaces. This surface contamination, called the *smear layer*, reduces wetting. In addition, the instruments used to cut the cavity leave a rough surface that also may increase air entrapment at the interface.

The greatest problem associated with bonding to tooth surfaces is water or saliva contamination. The inorganic components of tooth structure have a strong affinity for water. To remove the water, the enamel and dentin would have to be heated to an unacceptable temperature. This means that a tooth cannot be safely dried at mouth temperature with the devices and agents currently available to the dentist. The presence of at least a monolayer of water on the surface of the prepared cavity must be accepted. This water layer reduces the surface energy and thus may reduce the wetting of the adhesive restorative material.

In addition, there is fluid exchange through certain components of the tooth. The dental adhesive must displace the water, react with it, or wet the surface better than the water that is already present on and within the tooth structure. Furthermore, the adhesive must sustain long-term adhesion to tooth structure in an aqueous environment.

Although the obstacles are formidable, the progress of research in the field of adhesive materials is promising. To enhance adhesive bonding, attempts are being made to use more hydrophilic resins that are not as sensitive to the presence of moisture as materials currently in use. Certainly, these goals are worthy of the challenges presented. A truly adhesive filling material can replace many of those used in restorative dentistry. Likewise, the technique for placement of the material can be simplified, because the mechanical retention of the material in the cavity preparation would be unnecessary.

More intriguing is the possibility of developing a material capable of forming a thin, durable film on the tooth surface that could be topically applied to the intact enamel surface. Such a film with low surface energy could serve as a barrier to the formation of plaque, the development of caries, and even the deposition of calculus.

SELECTED READING

Buonocore MG: The Use of Adhesives in Dentistry. Springfield, IL, Charles C Thomas, 1975.
  The problems associated with dental adhesives are nicely illustrated. It is of interest that many of the procedures using bonding technology discussed in this text have become commonplace.
Glantz P: On wettability and adhesiveness. Odont Rev 20:1(Suppl 17):1, 1969.
  The first in a series of publications by this author suggesting that another mechanism is involved in reduction of dental caries because of topical fluorides, that is, lowering of the surface energy of tooth structure and thereby reducing plaque accumulation over a given interval.
Gordon JE: The New Science of Strong Materials, or Why You Don't Fall Through the Floor? 2nd ed. Princeton, NJ, Princeton University Press, 1984.
  A general discussion of the strength of materials from a fundamental base. Sections on biologic structural materials, timber, cellulose, teeth, and bone are particularly interesting.
Phillips RW, and Ryge G (eds): Proceedings on Adhesive Restorative Dental Materials. Spencer, IN, Owen Litho Service, 1961.

These transactions resulted from the first workshop on the problems and potential solutions to the development of adhesive dental materials. The recommendations for critically important areas of research have provided an impetus for investigations in this area.

Van Vlack LH: Elements of Materials Science and Engineering, 5th ed. Reading, MA, Addison-Wesley, 1985.

An excellent text on materials science. Recommended for a more in-depth coverage of materials structure and properties.

Zisman WA: Influence of constitution on adhesion. Ind Eng Chem 55:19, 1963.

One of the pioneers in surface phenomena discusses parameters that influence wetting. Zisman was a leader in the use of contact angle measurements to screen the potential wetting of adhesives to selected adherends.

3 *Physical Properties of Dental Materials*

- • What Are Physical Properties?
- • Abrasion and Abrasion Resistance
- • Viscosity
- • Structural and Stress Relaxation
- • Creep and Flow
- • Color and Color Perception
- • Thermophysical Properties

WHAT ARE PHYSICAL PROPERTIES?

Physical properties are based on the laws of mechanics, acoustics, optics, thermodynamics, electricity, magnetism, radiation, atomic structure, or nuclear phenomena. *Hue, value, chroma,* and *translucency* are physical properties that are based on the laws of optics, which is the science that deals with phenomena of light, vision, and sight. *Thermal conductivity* and *coefficient of thermal expansion* are physical properties that are based on the laws of thermodynamics. This chapter offers a brief description of physical properties, although some of these topics are presented in more detail in the chapters on specific materials. For example, color and coefficient of thermal expansion are also discussed in the chapter on dental ceramics.

This chapter addresses properties that are defined in several other scientific fields. For example, *viscosity* is related to the fields of materials science and mechanics. *Color* is a sensation of light reaching the eye that is based on the laws of optics. Mechanical properties are a subset of physical properties that are based on the laws of mechanics and are discussed in Chapter 4.

CRITICAL QUESTION *Hardness is a property that is often used to predict the wear resistance of a material and its ability to abrade opposing dental structures. What factors other than hardness may be responsible for excessive wear of natural tooth enamel or prosthetic surfaces by a harder material?*

ABRASION AND ABRASION RESISTANCE

Hardness has often been used as an index of the ability of a material to resist abrasion or wear. However, abrasion is a complex mechanism in the oral environment that involves an interaction between numerous factors. For this reason, the reliability of hardness as a predictor of abrasion resistance is limited. Often it is valid for comparing materials within a given classification, such as one brand of cast metal with another brand of the same type of casting alloy. However, it may be invalid for evaluating different classes of materials, such as a metallic material with a synthetic resin, as discussed in the chapter on synthetic resins.

A reliable *in vitro* test for abrasion resistance is one that is designed to simulate as closely as possible the particular type of abrasion to which the material will eventually be subjected *in vivo*. However, a simple *in vitro* wear test does not usually predict *in vivo* wear performance accurately because of the greater complexity of the clinical environment. The wear of enamel by ceramic and other restorative materials is well known. However, the hardness of a material is only one of many factors that affects the wear of the contacting enamel surfaces. Other major factors include biting force, frequency of chewing, abrasiveness of the diet, composition of liquids, temperature changes, roughness of each surface, physical properties of the materials, and surface irregularities such as fine anatomic grooves, pits, or ridges. The excessive wear of tooth enamel by an opposing ceramic crown is more likely to occur in the presence of high biting forces and a rough ceramic surface. Although clinicians cannot control the bite force of a patient, they can polish the abrading ceramic surface to reduce the rate of destructive enamel wear.

VISCOSITY

Up to this point, discussion of the physical properties of dental materials has been devoted to the room-temperature or oral-temperature behavior of solid materials that were subjected to various types of stress. However, many, if not most, of these metals are liquid at some stage in their dental application. Moreover, the success or failure of a given material may be as dependent on its properties in the liquid state as it is on its properties as a solid. For example, later we will study materials like cements and impression materials that undergo a liquid-to-solid transformation in the mouth. Gypsum products used in the fabrication of models and dies, and casting alloys are materials that are formed as liquids into structures that solidify outside the mouth. Amorphous materials such as waxes and resins appear solid but actually are supercooled liquids that flow plastically (irreversibly) or elastically (reversibly) under small stresses. The ways in which these materials deform or flow when subjected to stress are important to their use in dentistry. The study of matter flow characteristics is the basis for the science of *rheology*.

Although a liquid at rest cannot support a shear stress (shearing force per unit of shearing area), most liquids, when placed in motion, resist imposed forces that cause them to move. This resistance to motion is called *viscosity*, and it is controlled by internal frictional forces within the liquid. Viscosity is a measure of the consistency of a fluid and its inability to flow. A highly viscous fluid flows slowly because of its high viscosity. Dental materials have different viscosities when prepared for their intended clinical application. This viscosity difference is familiar to dental assistants, dentists, and dental students who have compared the flow properties of glass ionomer cement, which is more viscous than zinc phosphate cement, when both have been properly mixed as luting agents.

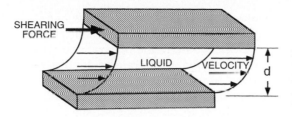

Figure 3–1. Shear of a viscous liquid between two rigid plates separated by distance d. The top plate is moving under the influence of a shearing force to the right at a velocity V relative to the lower plate.

To put this concept on a quantitative basis, consider Figure 3–1. A liquid occupies the space between two metal plates; the lower plate is fixed and the upper plate is being moved to the right with a certain velocity (V). A force (F) is required to overcome the drag produced by the friction (viscosity) of the liquid. As will be discussed more completely in Chapter 4, stress is the force per unit area that develops within a structure when an external force is applied. The stress produced causes a deformation or strain to develop that is calculated as a change in length divided by the initial reference length. If the plates have area A, a shear stress (τ) can be defined as $\tau = F/A$. The shear strain rate, or rate of change of deformation, is $\dot{\epsilon} = V/d$, where d is the distance between the two plates and V is the velocity of the liquid. For each different F value, we get a new value for V, and a curve can be obtained for force versus velocity analogous to the load versus displacement curves that are derived from static measurements on solids.

Similarly, a shear stress versus strain rate curve can be plotted. Typical examples are shown in Figure 3–2. An "ideal" fluid demonstrates a shear stress that is proportional to the strain rate, and thus the plot is a straight line. Such behavior is called *newtonian*. Because the viscosity (η) is defined as the shear stress divided by the strain rate, $\sigma_s/\dot{\epsilon}$, a newtonian fluid has a constant viscosity and exhibits a constant slope of shear stress plotted against strain rate (a straight line in Fig. 3–2). The plot is a straight line and resembles the elastic portion of a stress-strain curve (see Chapter 4), with viscosity the analog of the elastic modulus. Viscosity is measured in units of MPa per second (centipoise [cP]) and, obviously, the higher the value, the more viscous is the material. For example, pure water at 20° C has a viscosity of 1.0 cP, whereas the viscosity of molasses is approximately 300,000 cP and is approximately the same as that of tempered agar hydrocolloid impression material (281,000 cP at 45° C). Of the elastomeric impression materials, light-body polysulfide has a viscosity of 109,000 cP compared with a value of 1,360,000 cP for heavy-body polysulfide at

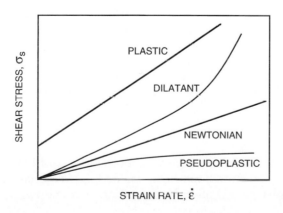

Figure 3–2. Shear stress versus shear strain rate for fluids exhibiting different types of rheologic behavior.

36° C. Many dental materials exhibit *pseudoplastic* behavior, as illustrated in Figure 3–2. Their viscosity decreases with increasing shear rate until it reaches a nearly constant value. Liquids that show the opposite tendency are called *dilatant*. These liquids become more rigid as the rate of deformation increases.

Finally, some classes of materials behave like a rigid body until some minimum value of shear stress is reached. These are referred to as *plastic*. Catsup is a familiar example—a sharp blow to the bottle is usually required to produce an initial flow.

The viscosity of most liquids decreases rapidly with increasing temperature. Viscosity may also depend on previous deformation of the liquid. A liquid of this type that becomes less viscous and more fluid under pressure is referred to as *thixotropic*. Dental prophylaxis pastes, plaster, resin cements, and some impression materials are thixotropic. The thixotropic nature of these materials is beneficial because the impression material does not flow out of a tray until placed over dental tissues, and a prophylaxis paste does not flow out of a rubber cup until it is rotated against the teeth to be cleaned. If these materials are stirred rapidly and the viscosity is measured, a lower value is obtained than that for a sample that has been left undisturbed.

The viscosity of a dental material may determine its suitability for a given application. Likewise, the nature of the shear stress–strain rate curve can be important in determining the best way to manipulate a material. As explained later, the viscosity as a function of time can also be used to measure the working time of a material that undergoes a liquid-to-solid transformation.

STRUCTURAL AND STRESS RELAXATION

After a substance has been permanently deformed (plastic deformation), there are trapped internal stresses. For example, in a crystalline substance the atoms in the space lattice are displaced, and the system is not in equilibrium. Similarly, in amorphous structures, some molecules are too close together and others too far apart after the substance has been permanently deformed.

It is understandable that such a situation is unstable. The displaced atoms are not in equilibrium positions. Through a solid-state diffusion process driven by thermal energy, they slowly move back to their equilibrium positions. The result is a change in the shape or contour of the solid as a gross manifestation of the rearrangement in atomic or molecular positions. The material *warps* or *distorts*. Such a relief of stress is known as *relaxation*.

The rate of relaxation increases with an increase in temperature. For example, if a wire is bent, it may tend to straighten out if it is heated to a high temperature. At room temperature, any such relaxation or diffusion may be negligible. On the other hand, there are many noncrystalline dental materials, such as waxes, resins, and gels, that, when manipulated and cooled, can then undergo relaxation (distortion) at an elevated temperature. Considerable attention is given to this phenomenon in succeeding chapters, because such dimensional changes by relaxation may result in an inaccurate fit of the dental appliance.

CREEP AND FLOW

Engineers who design structures to withstand both stress and high temperature are faced with the rheologic (or flow) behavior of solid materials. If a metal is held at a temperature near its melting point and is subjected to a constant applied stress, the resulting strain will increase as a function of time. *Creep* is defined as the time dependent plastic strain of a material under a static load or constant stress. The related phenomenon of *sag* is the deformation potential of long-span metal bridge structures at porcelain-firing temperatures under the influence of the mass of the prosthesis. For a given thickness, a higher bridge mass is related to greater flexural stress and, thus, greater *flexural creep*. Metal creep usually occurs as the temperature approaches within a few hundred degrees of the melting range. Metals used in dentistry for cast restorations or substrates for porcelain veneers have melting points that are much higher than mouth temperature and thus are not susceptible to creep deformation except when they are heated to very high temperatures. The most important exception is dental amalgam, which has components with melting points only slightly above room temperature. Because of its low melting range, dental amalgam can slowly creep from a restored tooth site under periodic sustained stress such as would be imposed by patients who clench their teeth. Because *creep* produces continuing plastic deformation, the process can be destructive to a dental restoration. The relationship of this property to the behavior of the amalgam restoration is discussed in Chapters 17 and 18. A creep test is required in American National Standards Institute/American Dental Association Specification No. 1 and Addendum 1a for dental amalgam products.

A somewhat synonymous term is *flow*. It will be recalled that flow was used in the discussion of rheologic behavior of liquids and is now applied to amorphous materials, which is not surprising in consideration of their structure. Silly Putty is a good example of such a substance. It fractures at a rapid stretching rate; however, if it is placed as a sphere on the table, it will flatten out under its own weight over time.

The term flow, rather than creep, has generally been used in dentistry to describe the rheology of amorphous materials such as waxes. The flow of wax is a measure of its potential to deform under a small static load, even that associated with its own mass. Although creep or flow may be measured under any type of stress, compression is usually employed in the testing of dental materials. A cylinder of prescribed dimensions is subjected to a given compressive stress for a specified time and temperature. The creep or flow is measured as the percentage of shortening in length that occurs under these testing conditions. Creep is an important consideration for any dental material that must be held at a temperature near its melting point for an extended period.

COLOR AND COLOR PERCEPTION

The preceding sections have been concerned with those properties that are necessary to permit a material to restore the function of damaged or missing natural tissues. Another important goal of dentistry is to restore the *color* and appearance of natural dentition. Aesthetic considerations in restorative and prosthetic dentistry have assumed a high priority within the past several decades. For example, the search for an ideal general purpose, direct-filling, tooth-colored restorative material is one of the challenges of current dental materials research.

Since aesthetic dentistry imposes severe demands on the artistic abilities of the dentist and technician, a knowledge of the underlying scientific principles of dental materials is essential. This is especially true for the increasingly popular restorations that involve ceramic materials (see Chapter 26). A more comprehensive treatment of this subject can be found in other texts (see the Selected Reading list at the end of this chapter).

Light is electromagnetic radiation that can be detected by the human eye. The eye is sensitive to wavelengths from approximately 400 (violet) to 700 nm (dark red), as shown in Figure 3–3 (see also the color section in the front of the book). The reflected light intensity and the combined intensities of the wavelengths present in a beam of light determine the appearance properties (hue, value, and chroma). For an object to be visible, it must reflect or transmit light incident on it from an external source. The latter is the case for objects that are of dental interest. The incident light is usually polychromatic, that is, some mixture of the various wavelengths. Incident light is selectively absorbed or scattered or both at certain wavelengths. The spectral distribution of the transmitted or reflected light resembles that of the incident light, although certain wavelengths are reduced in magnitude.

The phenomenon of vision, and certain terminology, can be illustrated by considering the response of the human eye to light coming from an object. Light from an object that is incident on an eye is focused on the retina and is converted into nerve impulses that are transmitted to the brain. Cone-shaped cells in the retina are responsible for color vision. These cells have a threshold intensity required for color vision and also exhibit a response curve related to the wavelength of the incident light. Such curves are shown in Figure 3–4 for a normal person and a color-deficient person. The normal observer curve shown in Figure 3–4 indicates the human visual responsiveness to light coming from a particular

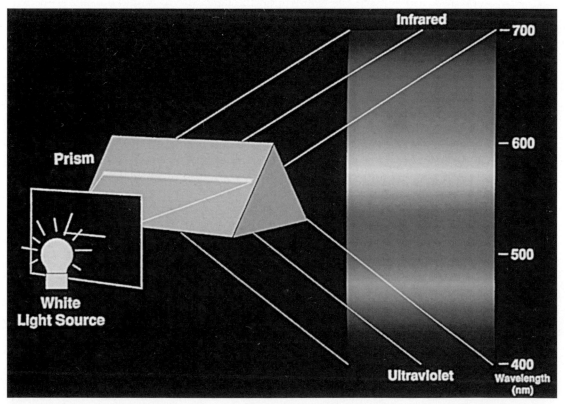

Figure 3–3. Spectrum of visible light ranging in wavelength from 400 nm (violet) to 700 nm (red). The most visually perceptible region of the equal energy spectrum under daylight conditions is between wavelengths of 540 and 570 nm, with a maximum value of visual perceptibility at 555 nm (see Fig. 3–4). (See also color section.)

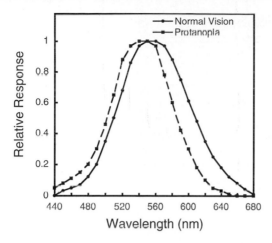

Figure 3–4. Relative visual response of humans to wavelength of light for a normal observer and one with protanopia (red-green) color blindness. Protanopia is experienced by 1% of the male population and 0.02% of the female population.

source or object. This figure indicates that the eye is most sensitive to light in the green-yellow region (wavelength of 550 nm) and least sensitive at either extreme, that is, red or blue.

Because a neural response is involved in color vision, constant stimulation by a single color may result in color fatigue and a decrease in the eye's response. The signals from the retina are processed by the brain to produce the psychophysiologic perception of color. Defects in certain portions of the color-sensing receptors result in the different types of color blindness and, thus, people vary greatly in their ability to distinguish colors. In a scientific sense, one might liken the normal human eye to an exceptionally sensitive differential colorimeter, a scientific instrument that measures the intensity and wavelength of light. Although the colorimeter is more precise than the human eye in measuring slight differences in colored objects, it can be extremely inaccurate when used on rough or curved surfaces. The eye is able to differentiate between two colors seen side by side on smooth or irregular surfaces, whether curved or flat.

Three Dimensions of Color. Verbal descriptions of color are not precise enough to describe the appearance of teeth. To describe a brownish-purple color called "puce," Webster's Third New International Dictionary defines the word as "a dark red that is yellower and less strong than cranberry, paler and slightly yellower than average garnet, bluer, less strong, and slightly lighter than pomegranate, and bluer and paler than average wine." This definition is far too complex to describe the desired color of a dental crown to a laboratory technician. The *New Webster's Dictionary and Thesaurus* describes puce as brownish purple. Thus, a written description does not clearly and unambiguously allow one to perceive the color. To accurately describe our perception of a beam of light reflected from a tooth or restoration surface, three variables must be measured. Quantitatively, the color and appearance must be described in three-dimensional color space by measurement of hue, value, and chroma. *Hue* describes the dominant color of an object, for example, red, green, or blue. This refers to the dominant wavelengths present in the spectral distribution. The continuum of these hues creates the color solid shown in Figure 3–5 (see also the color section in the front of the book). Value increases toward the top (whiter) and decreases toward the bottom (darker or more black).

Teeth and other objects can be separated into lighter shades (higher value) and darker shades (lower value). For example, the yellow of a lemon is lighter

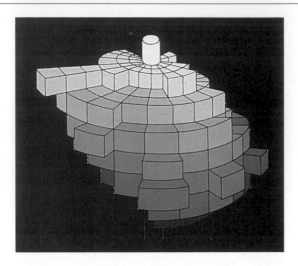

Figure 3–5. Color solid that is used to describe the three dimensions of color. Value increases from black at the bottom center to white at the top center. Chroma increases from the center outward, and hue changes occur in a circumferential direction. (Courtesy of Minolta Corporation, Instrument Systems Division, Ramsey, NJ.) (See also color section.)

than is the red of a cherry. For a light-diffusing and light-reflecting object such as a tooth or dental crown, or luminous reflectance, *value* is the lightness or darkness of a color, which can be measured independently of the hue. Examine Figure 3–6 (see also the color section in the front of the book), which represents a horizontal plane though Figure 3–5. This color chart is based on the CIE L*a*b* color space in which L* represents the value of an object, a* is the measurement along the red-green axis, and b* is the measurement along the yellow-blue axis. The color of a red apple is shown by the letter A in the upper and lower charts. Its color appearance can be expressed by L* = 42.83, a* = 45.04, and b* = 9.52. In comparison, a dental body (gingival) porcelain of shade A2 can be described by a higher (lighter) L* of 72.99, a lower a* of 1.00, and a higher b* of 14.41.

The yellow color of a lemon is more "vivid" than that of a banana which is "dull" yellow. This is a difference in the color intensity or its strength. *Chroma* represents this degree of saturation of a particular hue. Just as value varies vertically, chroma varies radially (see Fig. 3–6, *bottom*). Colors in the center are dull (gray). In other words, the higher the chroma, the more intense is the color. Chroma cannot exist by itself but is always associated with hue and value. The adjustments on a color television set make use of these principles.

In the dental operatory or laboratory, color matching is usually done by the use of a *shade guide* like that shown in Figure 3–7 (see also the color section in the front of the book) to select the color of ceramic veneers, inlays, or crowns to be made by a laboratory technician. The neck region of these shade tabs has been removed because its shade is darker and its presence would complicate the matching of the correct shade. Unfortunately, although a reasonable match can be achieved between the tooth or restoration of interest and one of the shade guide tabs from a set of tabs, it is difficult to relate this information to a laboratory technician who may not have a chance to see the patient. Furthermore, the thickness of the shade tab may be quite different from that of the prosthesis to be made, and the shade of one porcelain crown may look different from that of another crown made from the same jar of porcelain powder. Also, the porcelain of a given shade made by the same manufacturer may vary from batch to batch. Thus, the challenges are formidable for the dentist and technician who work as a team to restore the proper appearance to teeth that are damaged, decayed, or defective.

As stated previously, the shade guide shown in Figure 3–7 has been specially

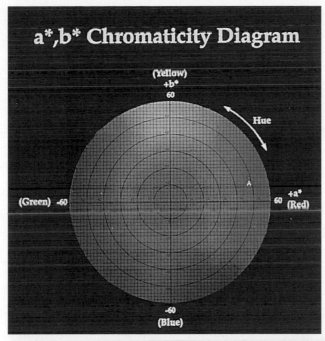

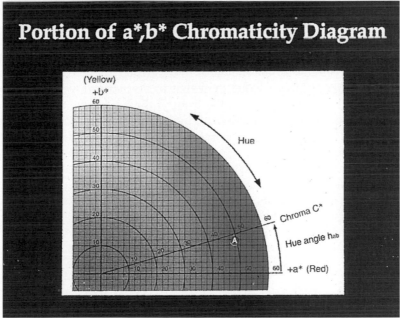

Figure 3–6. L*a*b* color chart showing the color of a red apple at point A (top and bottom). For this chart, the appearance is expressed by L* (value) = 42.83; a* (red-green axis) = 45.04; and b* (yellow-blue axis) = 9.52. In contrast, the color of shade A2 porcelain can be described by L* = 72.99; a* = 1.00; and b* = 14.41. (Courtesy of Minolta Corporation, Instrument Systems Division, Ramsey, NJ.) (See also color section.)

prepared by grinding away the necks of the porcelain tabs because the correct shade is determined from the gingival half of the tab and not from the neck. These are used in much the same way as paint chips are used to select the color for house paint. Using these shade tabs, one can specify the color to the techni-

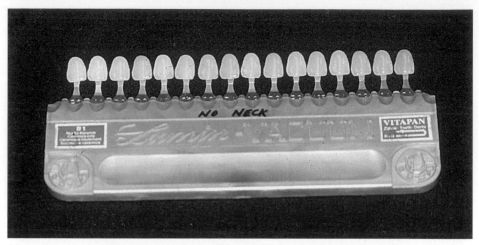

Figure 3–7. Dental shade guide tabs of the Vita Lumin type arranged in decreasing order of value (lighter to darker). The necks of the tooth-shaped tabs have been ground away to facilitate the selection of tooth shades. (See also color section.)

cian who will produce the proper shade in the laboratory. The tooth-shaped tabs in Figure 3–7 have been arranged in decreasing order of value (lightest to darkest) from left to right rather than the standard grouping by hue (A1 to D4). This technique is based on the perception that the matching of tooth shades is simplified by the arrangement of tabs by value.

Obviously, if the technician can see the actual teeth, the probability of achieving an acceptable color match is even greater. However, patients often desire restorations of higher value than that of the natural teeth. As shown in Figure 3–8 (see the color section in the front of the book), the shade of the two central incisor metal-ceramic crowns with porcelain butt-joint margins is higher in value than that of the lateral incisor teeth. However, the patient was pleased with this result.

As stated earlier, signals of color are sent to the human brain from three sets of receptors in the retina called *cones*. The cones are especially sensitive to red, blue, and green. Factors that interfere with the true perception of color generally include low or high light levels, fatigue of the color receptors, sex, age, memory, and cultural background. However, there appears to be no effect of observer age, sex, or clinical experience relative to the accuracy of dental shade matching, according to a recent study (Anusavice and Barrett, 1995).

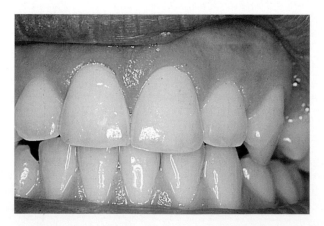

Figure 3–8. Two central incisor metal-ceramic crowns with porcelain margins. The value (L*) of these crowns is higher than that of the adjacent lateral incisor teeth. (See also color section.)

At low light levels, the rods of the human eye are more dominant than the cones and color perception is lost. As the brightness becomes too intense, color appears to change (Bezold-Brucke effect). Also, if one looks at a red object for a reasonably long time, receptor fatigue causes a green hue to be seen when one looks at a white background. For this reason, if a patient is visualized against an intense-colored background, a tooth shade may be selected with a hue that is shifted somewhat toward the complementary color of the background color, for example, a blue background shifts color selection toward yellow, and an orange background shifts the color selection toward blue-green. Unfortunately, 8% of men and 0.5% of women exhibit color blindness. Most commonly, these people cannot distinguish red from green because of the lack of either green-sensitive or red-sensitive cones. However, this deficiency may not affect the shade selection of natural teeth.

Although the range of hue, chroma, and value ordinarily found in human teeth represents only a small portion of the standard color space (such as that shown in Fig. 3–5), the selectivity of the human eye is sufficient to make accurate color matching difficult when using a shade guide (see Fig. 3–7) that contains only a small number of shades. Spectrophotometric analysis of commercial shade guides has also demonstrated the absence of large regions of hue, value, and chroma when compared with the color space determined from measurements of human teeth.

Because the spectral distribution of the light reflected from or transmitted through an object is dependent on the spectral content of the incident light, the appearance of an object is quite dependent on the nature of the light by which the object is viewed. Daylight, incandescent, and fluorescent lamps are common sources of light in the dental operatory or laboratory, and they have different spectral distributions. Objects that appear to be color matched under one type of light may appear different under another light source. This phenomenon is called *metamerism*. Thus, if possible, color matching should be done under two or more different light sources, one of which should be daylight, and the laboratory procedures should be performed under the same lighting conditions.

In addition to the processes already discussed, natural tooth structure absorbs light at wavelengths too short to be visible to the human eye. These wavelengths between 300 and 400 nm are referred to as *near-ultraviolet radiation*. Natural sunlight, photoflash lamps, certain types of vapor lamps, and ultraviolet lights used in decorative lighting are sources containing substantial amounts of near-ultraviolet radiation. The energy that the tooth absorbs is converted into light with longer wavelengths, in which case the tooth actually becomes a light source. This phenomenon is called *fluorescence*. The emitted light, a blue-white color, is primarily in the 400- to 450-nm range. Fluorescence makes a definite contribution to the brightness and vital appearance of a human tooth. A person with ceramic crowns or composite restorations that lack a fluorescing agent appears to be missing teeth when viewed under a black light in a nightclub. Thus, the researcher developing a tooth-colored restorative material and the dentist and technician who fabricates them must be concerned with color matching under light sources that contain a sufficient near-ultraviolet component. Incandescent lighting contains little ultraviolet radiation. The dentist and laboratory technician must be aware of the importance of color matching under more than one source of light. Additional information on color and color perception is presented in Chapter 26 and in several reference books on color applications in dentistry.

THERMOPHYSICAL PROPERTIES

Thermal Conductivity. Heat transfer through solid substances most commonly occurs by means of conduction. The conduction of heat occurs through the interactions of lattice vibrations and by the motion of electrons and their interaction with atoms. *Thermal conductivity* (κ) is a thermophysical measure of how well heat is transferred through a material by the conductive flow. The rate of heat flow through a structure is proportional both to the area (perpendicular to the heat flow direction) through which the heat is conducted and to the temperature gradient across the structure. Thus, if significant porosity exists in the structure, the area available for conduction is reduced and the rate of heat flow is reduced. The thermal conductivity, or *coefficient of thermal conductivity*, is the quantity of heat in calories per second that passes through a specimen 1-cm thick having a cross-sectional area of 1 cm^2 when the temperature differential between the surfaces perpendicular to the heat flow of the specimen is 1° C. According to the second law of thermodynamics, heat flows from points of higher temperature to points of lower temperature.

Materials that have a high thermal conductivity are called *conductors*, whereas materials of low thermal conductivity are called *insulators*. The typical International System (SI) unit for thermal conductivity is watts per meter per degree Kelvin (W · m^{-1} · K^{-1}). The higher the value, the greater is the ability of the substance to transmit thermal energy, and vice versa. Compared with a resin-based composite that has a low thermal conductivity, heat is transferred more rapidly away from the tooth when cold water contacts a metallic restoration because of its higher thermal conductivity. This increased conductivity of the metal compared with that of the resin, induces greater pulpal sensitivity, which is experienced as a negligible, mild, moderate, or extreme discomfort, depending on previous tooth trauma and the pain response of the patient.

Thermal Diffusivity. The value of thermal diffusivity of a material controls the time rate of temperature change as heat passes through a material. It is a measure of the rate at which a body with a nonuniform temperature reaches a state of thermal equilibrium. Although the thermal conductivity of zinc oxide–eugenol is slightly less than that of dentin, its diffusivity is more than twice that of dentin. The square root of thermal diffusivity is indirectly proportional to the thermal insulation ability, whereas the thickness of the cement base is directly related to its benefit as an insulator. Thus, the thickness of the liner is a more important thermal insulation factor than the thermal diffusivity. The relevance of thermal diffusivity is explained below.

However, the temperatures are not held constant. Generally, there is an unsteady state, because the thermal transfer through the material decreases the thermal gradient. Under such conditions, *thermal diffusivity* is important. The mathematic formula that relates thermal diffusivity (h) to thermal conductivity is

$$h = \frac{\kappa}{c_p \rho}$$

where κ is the thermal conductivity, c_p is the temperature-dependent specific heat capacity, and ρ is the temperature-dependent density. Heat capacity is numerically equal to the more commonly used term *specific heat*. The SI unit of thermal diffusivity units is one that is typical of diffusion processes, that is, square meters per second. However, the unit of square centimeters per second is often used. Typical values of diffusivity in units of 10^{-6} m²/s are pure gold, 119; amalgam, 9.6; composite, 0.68; enamel, 0.47; zinc phosphate cement, 0.29; and dentin, 0.18. Thus, for a patient drinking ice water, the low specific heat of amalgam and its high thermal conductivity suggest that the higher thermal diffusivity favors a thermal shock situation more than is likely to occur when only natural tooth structure is exposed to the cold liquid.

For a given volume of material, the heat required to raise the temperature a given amount depends on its *heat capacity* (calories per gram per degrees centigrade) and the density (grams per cubic centimeter). When the product of heat capacity and density ($c_p\rho$) is high, the thermal diffusivity may be low, even though the thermal conductivity is relatively high. Therefore, both thermal conductivity and thermal diffusivity are important parameters in predicting the transfer of thermal energy through a material. Because an unsteady state of heat transfer exists during the ingestion of hot or cold foods and liquids, the thermal diffusivity of a dental restorative material may be more important than its thermal conductivity. As noted in Table 3–1, enamel and dentin are effective thermal insulators. Their thermal conductivity and thermal diffusivity compare favorably with silica brick and water in contrast with the markedly higher values for metals.

However, as for any thermal insulator, tooth structure must be present in sufficient thickness for insulating dental cements to be effective. When the layer of dentin between the bottom of the cavity floor and the pulp is too thin, the dentist should place an additional layer of an insulating base, as discussed in the chapter on dental cements. The effectiveness of a material in preventing heat transfer is directly proportional to the thickness of the liner and inversely proportional to the square root of the thermal diffusivity. Thus, the thickness of the remaining dentin and the base is as important as, if not more than, the thermal properties of the materials.

The low thermal conductivity of enamel and dentin aids in preventing thermal shock and pulpal pain when hot or cold foods are taken into the mouth. However, the presence of oral restorations of any type tends to change the situation. As discussed later, many restorative materials are metallic. Because of the free electrons present in solid metal (see Chapter 2), these materials are such good thermal conductors that the tooth pulp may be adversely affected by thermal changes. In many instances it is necessary to insert a thermal insulator between the restoration and the tooth structure. In this respect, a restorative material that exhibits a low thermal conductivity is more desirable.

On the other hand, artificial teeth are held in a denture base that ordinarily is constructed of a synthetic resin, a poor thermal conductor. In the upper denture,

TABLE 3–1. Thermal Properties of Enamel and Dentin as Compared with Other Commonly Recognized Conductors and Insulators

	Density $(g \cdot cm^{-3})$	Specific Heat $(cal/g \cdot C)$	Thermal Conductivity $(W \cdot m^{-1} \cdot K^{-1})$	Thermal Diffusivity $(cm^2 \cdot s^{-1})$
Enamel*	2.9	0.18	0.87	0.0042
Dentin*	2.1	0.28	0.59	0.0026
Silver	10.5	0.056	385	1.67
Copper	8.96	0.092	370	1.14
Water (20° C)	1.0	1.0	0.55	0.0014

*Data from Braden M: Heat conduction in normal human teeth. Arch Oral Biol 9:479, 1964.

this base usually covers most of the roof of the mouth (hard palate). Its low thermal conductivity tends to prevent heat exchange between the supporting soft tissues and the oral cavity itself. Thus, the patient partially loses the sensation of hot and cold while eating and drinking. The use of a metal denture base may be more comfortable and pleasant from this standpoint.

Coefficient of Thermal Expansion. A thermal property that is sometimes important to the dentist is the *linear coefficient of thermal expansion*, which is defined as the change in length per unit of the original length of a material when its temperature is raised 1° C (see the section on thermal energy in Chapter 2). Linear expansion coefficients of some materials of interest in dentistry are presented in Table 3–2. The unit of α can be expressed also as $\mu m/cm° C$.

A tooth restoration may expand or contract more than the tooth during a change in temperature; thus, the restoration may leak, or it may debond from the tooth. According to the values in Table 3–2, restorative materials may change in dimension up to 4.4 times more than the tooth enamel for every degree of temperature change. However, while the dimensions of a wax pattern may change markedly when the temperature changes by 20° C, the relative contraction of an amalgam restoration that is 10 mm wide is only 5 μm when the oral temperature decreases by 20° C since the tooth enamel contracts by about 2.2 μm. Thus, the net difference is only 2.7 μm, which is much smaller than the dimensional change of 220 μm between cusps that are subjected to mechanical stresses during the polymerization of resin-based composites.

The high expansion coefficient of inlay wax is also important because it is highly susceptible to temperature changes. For example, an accurate wax pattern that fits a prepared tooth contracts significantly when it is removed from the tooth or from a die in a hot area and then stored in a cooler area. This dimensional change is transferred to a cast restoration that is made from the lost-wax process. Similarly, denture teeth that may have been set in denture base wax in a relatively warm laboratory may shift appreciably in their simulated intraoral positions after the denture base is moved to a cooler room before the processing of a denture.

Thermal stresses produced from a thermal expansion or contraction difference are also important in the production of metal-ceramic restorations. Consider a porcelain veneer that is fired to a metal substrate (coping). It may contract to a

TABLE 3–2. Linear Coefficients of Thermal Expansion (α) of Dental Materials Relative to the Tooth Enamel

Material	α ($10^{-6}/°$ C)	$\alpha_{material}/\alpha_{tooth}$
Aluminous porcelain	6.6	0.58
Dentin	8.3	0.75
Commercially pure titanium	8.5	0.77
Type II glass ionomer	11.0	0.96
Tooth (crown enamel)	**11.4**	**1.00**
Gold-palladium alloy for PFM crown	13.5	1.18
Pure gold	14.0	1.23
Palladium-silver alloy for PFM crown	14.8	1.30
Dental amalgam	25.0	2.19
Resin-based composite	14–50	1.2–4.4
Denture resin	81.0	7.11
Pit and fissure resin	85.0	7.46
Inlay wax	400.0	35.1

greater extent than the metal during cooling and induce tangential tensile stresses or tensile hoop (circumferential) tensile stresses in the porcelain that may cause immediate or delayed crack formation. Although these thermal stresses cannot be eliminated completely, they can be reduced appreciably by selection of materials whose expansion or contraction coefficients are matched fairly closely (within 4%).

SELECTED READING

American Dental Association: Esthetic dentistry: A new direction. J Am Dent Assoc Dec (Special issue), 1987.
A series of papers covering the many facets of selecting materials and clinical procedures used in aesthetic dentistry. Depicted are the improved services available through bonding technology, with particular emphasis on the organization of color in the design and fabrication of restorative materials.
Anusavice KJ, and Barrett AA: Color/shade matching performance of dental students and faculty dentists. J Dent Res 74:Abstr No. 1788, 235.
Barna GJ, Taylor JW, King GE, and Pelleu GB Jr: The influence of selected light intensities on color perception within the color range of natural teeth. J Prosthet Dent 46:450, 1981.
The influence of light intensity on the ability to discriminate color differences within the color range of natural teeth was studied. A significant number of the dentists were found to be color defective. In such instances, the dentist should obtain assistance when matching tooth shades.
Goldstein RE: Change Your Smile, 2nd ed. Chicago, Quintessence, 1988.
Although this book is written for the patient, it is a useful reference for dentists to illustrate aesthetic and reconstructive changes that are possible. The color illustrations before and after restorative treatment are evidence of the satisfactory end result when based on an appreciation of parameters involved in color phenomena, as discussed in this chapter.
Judd DB, and Wyszecki G: Color in Business, Science, and Industry. New York, John Wiley & Sons, 1975.
This book, developed for a variety of businesses, reviews the principles of color vision, color matching, color deficiencies, colorimetry, and the physics of colorant layers.
McLean JW: The Science and Art of Dental Ceramics. Vol. 1: The Nature of Dental Ceramics and Their Clinical Use. Amador City, CA, Quintessence, 1979.
Essential reading for those interested in an in-depth discussion of principles of color as related to dental ceramics. Basic fundamentals are clearly interwoven with clinical procedures.
Miller LL: A Scientific Approach to Shade Matching. In: Proceedings of the Fourth International Symposium on Ceramics. Chicago, Quintessence, 1988, p 193.
It is unfortunate that commercial shade guides do not cover all the areas of value, hue, and chroma present in tooth structure. A definitive analysis of the problem is presented.

4 *Mechanical Properties of Dental Materials*

WHAT ARE MECHANICAL PROPERTIES?

This chapter focuses on the mechanical properties of materials. Mechanical properties are defined by the laws of mechanics, that is, the physical science that deals with energy and forces and their effects on bodies. The discussion centers primarily on static bodies—those at rest—rather than dynamic bodies that are in motion.

An important factor in the design of a dental prosthesis is *strength*, a mechanical property of a material that ensures that the prosthesis serves its intended functions effectively, safely, and for a reasonable period. In a general sense, *strength* refers to the ability of the prosthesis to resist applied forces (loads) without fracture or excessive deformation. Excessive deformation can result when a limiting stress (force per unit area) within the prosthesis is exceeded or because of inadequate stiffness (modulus of elasticity) of the prosthetic material.

By the end of the section on stress concentration factors, you should have developed some concept of the causes of fracture of restorative materials and an understanding of design modifications that will improve the fracture resistance of restorations and prostheses in the oral environment. This knowledge will also assist you in the diagnosis of the potential causes of clinical failures, whether they are caused by material deficiencies, human errors, or patient factors.

An analysis of the failure potential of a prosthesis under applied forces must be related to the mechanical properties of the prosthetic material. Mechanical properties are the measured responses, both elastic (reversible on force removal) and plastic (irreversible or nonelastic), of materials under an applied force or distribution of forces. A category of physical properties is the group of mechanical properties that are expressed most often in units of stress and strain. They can represent measurements of (1) elastic or reversible deformation, that is, *proportional limit*, *resilience*, and *modulus of elasticity*; (2) plastic or irreversible deformation, for example, *percentage of (percent) elongation*; or (3) a combination of elastic and plastic deformation, such as *toughness* and *yield strength*. To discuss these properties, one must first understand the concepts of stress and strain.

STRESSES AND STRAINS

Stress is the force per unit area acting on millions of atoms or molecules in a given plane of a material. Except for certain flexural situations, such as four-point bending specimens, and certain nonuniform object shapes, stress typically decreases as a function of distance from the area of the applied force or applied pressure. The *strength* of a material is defined as the average level of stress at which a material exhibits a certain amount of plastic deformation or at which fracture occurs in several test specimens of the same shape and size. However, the clinical strength of brittle materials (such as ceramics, amalgams, composites, and cements) may appear to be low when large flaws are present or if stress concentration areas exist because of improper design of a prosthetic component (such as a notch across a section of a clasp arm on a partial denture). Under these conditions a clinical prosthesis may fracture at a much lower applied force because the localized stress exceeds the strength of the material at the critical location of the flaw or stress concentration.

When a patient chews with a gold crown in place, the atomic structure of the crown is slightly deformed by the forces of mastication. If only elastic deformation occurs, the surface of the crown will recover completely when the forces are removed. Elastic stresses in ductile materials such as the gold alloy do not cause permanent damage. Plastic stresses, on the other hand, cause permanent deformation and may be high enough to produce a fracture. However, for brittle materials that exhibit only elastic deformation and no plastic deformation, stresses at or slightly above the maximum elastic stress result in fracture. These mechanical properties of dental materials are important for the dentist to understand when designing a restoration or making adjustments to a prosthesis. The differences between mechanical properties are easier to visualize through the use of a stress-strain diagram, as described later.

When an external force acts on a solid body, a reaction occurs to oppose this force that is equal in magnitude but opposite in direction to the external force. The applied force divided by the area over which it acts within the body is the value of stress produced within the structure. A tensile force produces *tensile stress*; a compressive force produces *compressive stress*; and a shear force produces *shear stress*. A flexural force can produce all three types of stress in a structure, but in most cases fracture occurs because of the tensile component. In this situation, the tensile and compressive stresses are principal stresses, whereas the shear stress is a combination of tensile and compressive components.

Whenever a stress is present, deformation or strain is induced. As an illustration, assume that a stretching or tensile force of 200 N is applied to a wire 0.000002 m² in cross-sectional area. The *tensile stress* (σ), by definition, is the tensile force per unit area perpendicular to the force direction,

$$\sigma = \frac{200\,\text{N}}{0.000002\,\text{m}^2} = 100 \times 10^6\,\frac{\text{N}}{\text{m}^2} = 100\,\frac{\text{MN}}{\text{m}^2} = 100\,\text{MPa}$$

Because the wire has fractured at this stress level, the tensile strength of this wire is 100 MPa. In the English system of measurement, the stress is expressed in pounds per square inch. However, the megapascal unit is preferred because it is consistent with the SI system of units. (SI stands for Système International d' Unités [International System of Units] for length, time, electric current, temperature, luminous intensity, mass, and amount of substance.)

If the wire above is 0.1 m long, and if it stretches 0.001 m under the load, the strain (ϵ), by definition, is the change in length, Δl, per unit original length, l_o, or

$$\epsilon = \frac{\Delta l}{l_O} = \frac{0.001 \text{ m}}{0.1 \text{ m}} = 0.0001 \, \frac{\text{m}}{\text{m}} = 0.0001 = 0.01\%$$

Now we can conclude that the wire fractures at a tensile stress of 100 MPa and at a *tensile strain* of 0.01%. Note that although strain is a dimensionless quantity, units such as meter per meter or centimeter per centimeter are often used to remind one of the system of units employed in the actual measurement. The accepted equivalent in the English system is inch per inch, foot per foot, and so forth.

CRITICAL QUESTION *Why is the maximum elastic strain of a cast alloy for an inlay or crown an important factor when burnishing a margin? Use a sketch of a gap between a crown and the tooth margin or a stress–strain diagram to explain your answer.*

Strain may be either elastic or plastic or a combination of the two. *Elastic strain* is reversible: it disappears when the force is removed. *Plastic strain* represents a permanent deformation of the material that never recovers when the force is removed. When a prosthetic component such as a clasp arm on a partial denture is deformed past the elastic limit into the plastic deformation region, only the elastic strain is recovered when the force is removed. Thus, when an adjustment is made by bending an orthodontic wire and the force is released, a margin of a metal crown, or a denture clasp, the plastic strain is permanent, but the wire, margin, or clasp springs back a certain amount as elastic strain recovery occurs.

As previously described, a stress must be defined according to its type and magnitude. By means of their directions of force application, three types of "simple" stresses can be classified: *tensile*, *compressive*, and *shear*. Complex stress conditions that are produced by flexural or torsional forces are discussed in the section on flexural stress.

Tensile Stress. A *tensile stress* is caused by a load that tends to stretch or elongate a body. A tensile stress is always accompanied by *tensile strain*. There are few pure tensile stress situations in dentistry and tensile stress components can be generated when structures are flexed and even when compressive loads are applied. The deformation of a bridge and the diametral compression of a cylinder that are described later represent examples of these complex stress situations. In fixed prosthodontics clinics, a candy called *Jujubes* is used because of its adhesive nature to remove crowns by means of a tensile force when patients attempt to open their mouths. However, tensile, compressive, and shear stresses can also be produced by a bending force as shown in Figure 4–1 and as discussed in the following sections.

Compressive Stress. If a body is placed under a load that tends to compress or shorten it, the internal resistance to such a load is called a *compressive stress*. A compressive stress is associated with *compressive strain*. To calculate either tensile stress or compressive stress, the applied force is divided by the cross-sectional area perpendicular to the force direction.

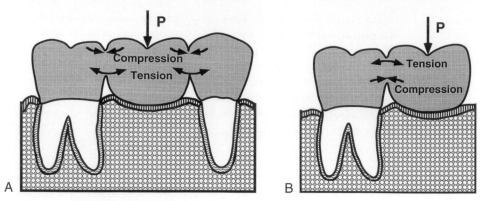

Figure 4–1. Stresses induced in a three-unit bridge *(A)* by a flexural force (P). Stresses induced in a two-unit cantilever bridge are shown in *B*. Note that the tensile stress develops on the gingival side of the three-unit bridge and on the occlusal side of the cantilever bridge.

CRITICAL QUESTION

Although the shear bond strength of dental adhesive systems is often advertised, most dental prostheses and restorations are not likely to fail because of pure shear stresses. Which two factors tend to prevent the occurrence of pure shear failure?

Shear Stress. A *shear stress* tends to resist the sliding of one portion of a body over another. Shear stress can also be produced by a twisting or torsional action on a material. For example, if a force is applied along the surface of tooth enamel by a sharp-edged instrument parallel to the interface between the enamel and an orthodontic bracket, the bracket may debond by shear stress failure of the resin luting agent. Shear stress is calculated by dividing the force by the area parallel to the force direction.

In the oral environment shear failure is unlikely to occur for many of the brittle materials because restored tooth surfaces are generally rough in surface morphology and they are not planar. The presence of chamfers, bevels, or changes in curvature of a bonded tooth surface would make shear failure of a bonded material highly unlikely. Furthermore, to produce shear failure the applied force must be located immediately adjacent to the interface, as shown in Figure 4–2B. This is quite difficult to accomplish, even under experimental conditions when flat interfaces are used. The farther away from the interface the load is applied, the more likely that tensile failure rather than shear failure would occur because the potential for bending stresses would increase. Because the convex surface indicates a stretching action, tensile stress is produced. Because the tensile strength of brittle materials is usually well below their shear strength values, shear failure is less likely to occur.

CRITICAL QUESTION

Why do structures that are flexed usually fail on the surface that is increasing in convexity?

Flexural (bending) Stress. Examples of *flexural stress* that is produced in a three-unit bridge and a two-unit cantilever bridge are illustrated in Figures 4–1A and 4–1B, respectively. It is produced by bending forces in dental appliances in one of two ways: (1) by subjecting a structure such as a fixed partial denture to three-point loading, whereby the endpoints are fixed and a force is applied between these endpoints, as in Figure 4–1A; and (2) by subjecting a cantilevered structure that is supported at only one end to a load along any part of the unsupported section Figure 4-1B. Also, when a patient bites into an apple, the anterior teeth receive forces that are at an angle to their long axes, thereby creating flexural stresses within the teeth.

As shown in Figure 4–1A, tensile stress develops on the tissue side of the bridge, and compressive stress develops on the occlusal side. Between these two areas is the neutral axis that represents a state of no tensile stress and no compressive stress. For a cantilevered bridge such as shown in Figure 4–1B, the maximum tensile stress develops on the occlusal surface or the surface that is becoming more convex (indicating a stretching action). If you can visualize this unit bending downward toward the tissue, the upper surface becomes more convex or stretched (tensile region), and the opposite surface becomes compressed. As explained in the section on stress concentration, these areas of tension represent potential fracture initiation sites in most materials, but especially in brittle materials that have little or no plastic deformation potential.

Shown in Figure 4–2 is a bonded two-material system with the white atoms of material A shown above the interface and the shaded atoms of material B shown below the interface. The atoms are represented over six atom planes, although dental structures have millions of atom planes. However, the principles of stress and strain apply in both cases. In the upper section of Figure 4–2A a shear force is applied at a distance d/2 from interface A-B. As this force increases in magnitude, it first produces an elastic shear strain that would return to zero if the shear force was removed (lower section). As shown in Figure 4–2B, if the shear force on the external surface is increased sufficiently, a permanent or plastic deformation will be produced. In this case the force is applied closer to or along interface A-B and not at a distance away, as shown in Figure 4–2A. Because of this application of force along the interface, shear stress and shear strain develop only within the interfacial region, and only localized plastic deformation has occurred. In the lower section of Figure 4–2B, the force has been removed, and a permanent strain of one atom space has occurred.

MECHANICAL PROPERTIES BASED ON ELASTIC DEFORMATION

There are several important mechanical properties and parameters that are measures of the *elastic* or *reversible deformation* behavior of dental materials. These

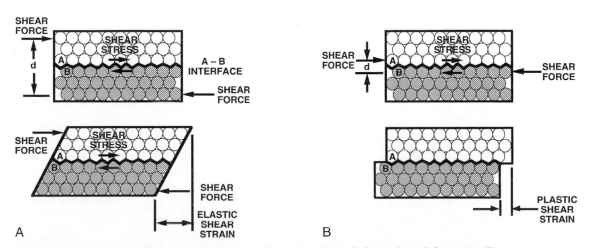

Figure 4–2. Atomic model illustrating elastic shear deformation *(A)* and plastic shear deformation *(B)*.

are *elastic modulus (Young's modulus* or *modulus of elasticity), dynamic Young's modulus* (determined by measurement of ultrasonic wave velocity), *shear modulus, flexibility, resilience,* and *Poisson's ratio.* Other properties that are determined from stresses at the end of the elastic region of the stress-strain plot and at the beginning of plastic deformation region *(proportional limit, elastic limit,* and *yield strength)* are described in the following section on strength properties.

Elastic Modulus (Young's modulus or modulus of elasticity). The term *elastic modulus* describes the relative stiffness or rigidity of a material, which is measured by the slope of the elastic region of the stress-strain diagram. Shown in Figure 4–3 is a stress-strain diagram for a stainless steel orthodontic wire that has been subjected to a tensile test. The ultimate tensile strength, yield strength (0.2% offset), proportional limit, and elastic modulus are shown in the figure. This figure represents a plot of *true stress* versus strain because the force has been divided by the changing cross-sectional area as the wire was being stretched. The straight-line region represents reversible elastic deformation, because the stress remains below the proportional limit of 1020 MPa, and the curved region represents irreversible plastic deformation that is not recovered when the wire fractures at a stress of 1625 MPa. However, the elastic deformation is fully recovered when the force is removed or when the wire fractures. We can see this easily by bending a wire in our hands a slight amount and then reducing the force. It straightens back to its original shape as the force is decreased to zero and assuming that the induced stress has not exceeded the proportional limit.

This principle of elastic recovery is illustrated in Figure 4–4 for a burnishing procedure of an open metal margin (top, left) where a dental abrasive stone is shown rotating against the metal margin (top, right) to close the marginal gap as a result of elastic plus plastic strain. However, after the force is removed, the margin springs back an amount equal to the total elastic strain. Only by removing the crown from a tooth or die can total closure be accomplished. Because we must provide at least 25 μm of clearance for the cement, total burnishing on the tooth or die is usually adequate since the amount of elastic strain recovery is relatively small.

A stress-strain diagram is shown in Figure 4–5 for enamel and dentin that

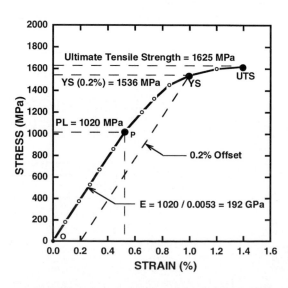

Figure 4–3. Stress-strain plot for a stainless steel orthodontic wire that has been subjected to tension. The proportional limit (PL) is 1020 MPa. Although not shown, the elastic limit is approximately equal to this value. The yield strength (YS) at a 0.2% strain offset from the origin (O) is 1536 MPa and the ultimate tensile strength (UTS) is 1625 MPa. An elastic modulus value (E) of 192,000 MPa (192 GPa) was calculated from the slope of the elastic region.

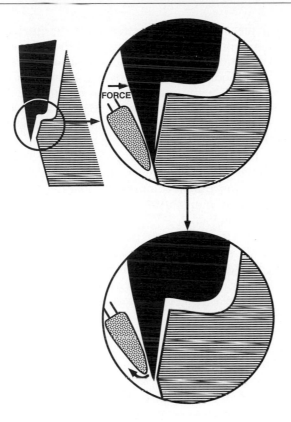

Figure 4–4. Schematic illustration of a procedure to close an open margin of a metal crown *(top, left)* by burnishing with a rotary instrument *(top, right).* Note that after the rotating stone is removed *(bottom),* the elastic strain has been recovered and a slight marginal discrepancy remains.

have been subjected to a simulated compressive test. These curves were constructed from typical values of elastic moduli, proportional limit, and ultimate compressive strength reported in the scientific literature. If the tensile stress below the proportional limit in Figure 4–3 or the compressive stress (below the proportional limit) in Figure 4–5 is divided by its corresponding strain value, that is, tensile stress/tensile strain or compressive stress/compressive strain, a constant of proportionality will be obtained that is known as the *elastic modulus,*

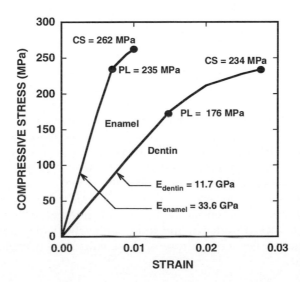

Figure 4–5. Stress-strain plot for enamel and dentin that have been subjected to compression. The ultimate compressive strength (CS), proportional limit (PL), and elastic modulus (E) values are shown. (Data from Stanford JW, Weigel KV, Pattenbarger GD, and Sweeney WT: Compressive properties of hard tooth tissue. J Am Dent Assoc 60:746, 1960.)

modulus of elasticity, or *Young's modulus.* These terms are designated by the letter E. The slope of the straight-line region (elastic range) of the stress-strain diagram is a measure of the relative *rigidity* or *stiffness* of a material. Differing values of proportional limit, elastic modulus, and ultimate compressive strength have been reported for enamel and dentin, depending on the area of the tooth from which they were obtained. Note that the proportional limit, ultimate compressive strength, and elastic modulus of enamel are greater than the corresponding values for dentin (see Fig. 4–5). In fact, the elastic modulus of enamel is about three times greater than that of dentin and, depending on the study cited, it can be as much as seven times higher. However, dentin is capable of sustaining significant plastic deformation under compressive loading before it fractures. Thus, enamel is a stiffer and more brittle material than dentin. Conversely, dentin is more flexible and tougher.

The elastic modulus of a material is a constant and is unaffected by the amount of elastic or plastic stress that can be induced in a material. Thus, it is independent of the ductility of a material, and it is not a measure of its strength. Although a compressive test was selected to measure the properties of tooth structures in Figure 4–5, the elastic modulus can also be measured by means of a tensile test.

Because the elastic modulus represents the ratio of the elastic stress to the elastic strain, it follows that the lower the strain for a given stress, the greater the value of the modulus. For example, if one wire is much more difficult to bend than another of the same shape and size, considerably higher stress must be induced before a desired strain or deformation can be produced in the stiffer wire. Such a material would possess a comparatively high modulus of elasticity. Modulus of elasticity is given in units of force per unit area, typically, giganewtons per square meter (GN/m^2), or gigapascals (GPa). This property is indirectly related to other mechanical properties. For example, two materials may have the same proportional limit but may have elastic moduli that differ considerably.

The elastic modulus of a tensile test specimen can be calculated as follows:

Let E = elastic modulus
            P = applied force or load
            A = cross-sectional area of the material under stress
            Δl = increase in length
            l_o = original length

By definition   Stress = P/A = σ
                 Strain = $\Delta l/l_o$ = ϵ

Thus, $$E = \frac{\text{Stress}}{\text{Strain}} = \frac{\sigma}{\epsilon} = \frac{P/A}{\Delta l/l_o}$$

Dynamic Young's Modulus. Elastic modulus can be measured by a dynamic method as well as the static techniques that were described in the previous section since the velocity at which sound travels through a solid can be readily measured by ultrasonic longitudinal and transverse wave transducers and appropriate receivers. Based on this velocity and the density of the material, the *elastic modulus* and *Poisson's ratio* can be determined. This method of determining dynamic elastic moduli is less complicated than conventional tensile or compressive tests, but the values are often found to be higher than the values obtained by static measurements. For most purposes, these values are acceptable.

If, instead of uniaxial tensile or compressive stress, a shear stress was induced, the resulting shear strain could be used to define a shear modulus for the material. The shear modulus (G) can be calculated from the elastic modulus (E) and Poisson's ratio (v). It is determined by the equation,

$$G = \frac{E}{2(1 + v)} = \frac{E}{2(1 + 0.3)} = 0.38E$$

A value of 0.3 for Poisson's ratio is typical. Thus, the shear modulus is usually about 38% of the elastic modulus.

Flexibility. In the case of dental appliances and restorations, a high value for the elastic limit (the stress above which a material will not recover to its original state when the force is removed) is a necessary requirement for the materials from which they are fabricated, because the structure is expected to return to its original shape after it has been stressed. Usually a moderately high modulus of elasticity is also desirable, because only a small deformation will develop under a considerable stress, such as in the case of an inlay.

There are instances, however, in which a larger strain or deformation may be needed with a moderate or slight stress. For example, in an orthodontic appliance, a spring is often bent a considerable distance under the influence of a small stress. In such a case, the structure is said to be *flexible* and it possesses the property of *flexibility*. The *maximum flexibility* is defined as the strain that occurs when the material is stressed to its proportional limit.

Resilience. As previously pointed out, as the interatomic spacing increases, the internal energy increases. As long as the stress is not greater than the proportional limit, this energy is known as *resilience*. Popularly, the term *resilience* is associated with "springiness," but it connotes something more than this. On the basis of the previous discussion, resilience can be defined as the amount of energy absorbed by a structure when it is stressed to its proportional limit. The resilience of two or more materials can be compared by observing the areas under the elastic region of their stress-strain plots, assuming that they are plotted on the same scale. The material with the larger elastic area has the higher resilience.

Shown in Figure 4–6 is a stress-strain diagram that illustrates the concepts of resilience and toughness. The area bounded by the elastic region is a measure of resilience, and the total area under the stress-strain curve is a measure of toughness. This figure is explained further in the following section.

As noted in the previous chapter, work is the product of the force and the distance through which the force acts. When work is performed on a body, energy is imparted to it. Consequently, when a dental restoration is deformed, it absorbs energy. If the induced stress is not greater than the proportional limit, and the oral structure is not permanently deformed, only the absorbed energy associated with elastic deformation is developed.

When a dental restoration is deformed during mastication, the chewing force acts on the tooth structure, the restoration, or both, and the magnitude of the structure's deformation is determined by the induced stress. In most dental restorations, large strains are precluded because of the proprioceptive response of neural receptors in the periodontal ligament. The pain stimulus causes the force to be decreased and the induced stress to be reduced, thereby preventing damage to the teeth or restorations. For example, a proximal inlay might cause

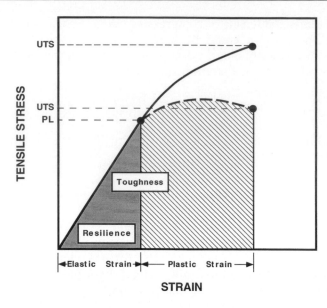

Figure 4–6. Conventional tensile stress-strain curve *(bold dashed line)* in the plastic deformation region calculated on the basis of the initial cross-sectional area of a rod. The *solid line* (above the *dashed line*) represents the calculated stress values based on the actual reduced area of the rod as deformation increases. The resilience can be calculated by measuring the area within the elastic region. The toughness is related to the total area within the elastic and plastic regions.

excessive movement of the adjacent tooth if large proximal strains developed during compressive loading on the occlusal surface. Hence, the restorative material should exhibit a moderately high elastic modulus and low resilience, thereby limiting the elastic strain that is produced.

Poisson's Ratio. When a tensile force is applied to an object, the object becomes longer and thinner. Conversely, a compressive force acts to make an object shorter but thicker. If an axial tensile stress, σ_z, in the z (a long vertical axis) direction of a mutually perpendicular *xyz* coordinate system produces an elastic tensile strain, and accompanying elastic contractions in the x and y directions (ϵ_x and ϵ_y, respectively), the ratio of ϵ_x/ϵ_z or ϵ_y/ϵ_z is an engineering property of the material called *Poisson's ratio* (ν).

$$\nu = -\frac{\epsilon_x}{\epsilon_z} = -\frac{\epsilon_y}{\epsilon_z}$$

Poisson's ratio can be similarly determined in an experiment involving an axial compressive stress. Poisson's ratio is related to the nature and symmetry of the interatomic bonding forces described in Chapter 2. For an ideal isotropic material of constant volume, the ratio is 0.5. Most engineering materials have values of approximately 0.3.

CRITICAL QUESTION *Is it possible for a stiff material with its high modulus of elasticity to fail with no plastic deformation and at stresses much lower than a more flexible material? Explain your answer.*

STRENGTH PROPERTIES

Strength is the stress that is necessary to cause fracture or a specified amount of plastic deformation. When we describe the strength of an object or a material, we are most often referring to the ultimate stress that is required to cause fracture. Both types of deformational behavior can be described by strength properties, but we must use proper strength terms to differentiate between the maximum stress to produce permanent deformation and that required to produce fracture.

For specific dental materials, particularly metals, we are equally interested in the maximum stress that a structure can sustain before it becomes permanently or plastically deformed. This stress can be described either by the *proportional* or *elastic limit*. At stresses above these limits, plastic deformation occurs.

The strength of a material can be described by one or more of the following properties: (1) *proportional limit*, the stress above which stress is no longer proportional to strain; (2) *elastic limit*, the maximum stress a material can withstand before it becomes plastically deformed; (3) *yield strength* or *proof stress*, the stress required to produce a given amount of plastic strain; and (4) *ultimate tensile strength, shear strength, compressive strength*, and *flexural strength*, each of which is a measure of stress required to fracture a material. Strength is not a measure of individual atom-to-atom attraction or repulsion, but rather it is a measure of the interatomic forces collectively over the entire wire, cylinder, implant, crown, pin, or whatever structure is stressed. Furthermore, the ultimate strength may not necessarily be equal to the actual instantaneous average stress at fracture if the original cross-sectional area has changed in size.

Shown in Figure 4–6 is a stress-strain plot of a typical metal rod that has been subjected to a tensile test. The stress is often calculated by dividing the applied force at any instant by the original cross-sectional area and is represented as the bold dashed line above the lightly shaded area. However, the diameter actually decreases as the metal is stretched. The actual stress is calculated as the force divided by the actual cross-sectional area at each measured strain value and is represented in Figure 4–6 by the bold line in the plastic deformation region above the dashed line. At stresses above the proportional limit (point PL), the actual stress curve (dashed line) terminates at the higher UTS (ultimate tensile strength) value, or the stress at the point of fracture. The corresponding point for the stresses calculated from the initial cross-sectional area (solid line) is the lower UTS value.

It is evident that the cross section of the wire decreases as it lengthens under tensile stress. Consequently, the stress calculated for testing purposes (force per unit initial area) decreases, and the ultimate tensile strength based on the initial area (lower UTS value) as indicated in Figure 4–6 is less than the maximum tensile stress that occurs at the peak of the curve.

Had the decrease in cross-sectional area of the wire been taken into consideration when the stress beyond tensile stress was calculated, the actual or true stress-strain curve would be indicated by the upper solid line, and the ultimate tensile strength (UTS) would be higher than that for the stress calculated using the initial area of the rod specimen. For a compressive stress test, however, the cross-sectional area increases, and the ultimate tensile strength based on the actual cross-sectional area is lower compared with the compressive strength if it was calculated using the initial cross-sectional area.

Although the actual or true stress-strain curve represents the situation more accurately, the stress-strain curve as indicated by the solid line in Figure 4–6 is commonly used. When we calculate the tensile strength of a certain wire, we wish to know the maximum stress it supports in tension without regard to the small changes that may occur in cross-sectional area. The ultimate tensile strength is, therefore, defined as the tensile stress within a structure at the point of rupture.

Brittle materials have a tensile strength that is markedly lower than the corresponding compressive strength, because of their inability to plastically deform and reduce the tensile stress at flaw tips. This is true of all brittle dental materials, such as amalgams, composites, cements, and ceramics. The failure of these materials in clinical usage is most often associated with their low tensile strengths and the presence of flaws within the tensile stress region.

Proportional Limit. As the wire in the previous section is stretched steadily in tension, the wire eventually fractures. However, in dentistry we are interested in the stress at which plastic deformation begins to develop. One method to determine this point is to plot a stress-strain diagram similar to that in Figures 4–3, 4–5, or 4–6. If the material obeys Hooke's law, the elastic stress will be proportional to elastic strain. For such a material, the stress-strain diagram shown in Figure 4–3 starts from the origin (O) as a straight line. Along this linear path the material behaves elastically, and it springs back to its initial shape and size at the instant the force is removed. After a certain stress value at point P is exceeded, the line becomes nonlinear, and stress is no longer proportional to strain. If a ruler is laid along the straight-line portion of the curve from O to P, the stress value at P, the point above which the curve digresses from a straight line, is known as the *proportional limit*.

For a material to satisfy Hooke's law, the elastic stress must be directly proportional to the elastic strain; that is, the initial region of the stress-strain plot must be a straight line. Because direct proportionality between two quantities is graphically represented by a straight line, the linear portion of the graph in Figures 4–3, 4–5, and 4–6 satisfies this law. Because the proportional limit (stress corresponding to point P) is the greatest elastic stress possible in accordance with this law, it represents the maximum stress above which stress is no longer proportional to the strain. For the stress-strain curve of dentin that is shown in Figure 4–5, the strain corresponding to the proportional limit is important because it represents the percent deformation that can be sustained in dentin before it becomes damaged permanently.

Elastic Limit. If a small tensile stress is induced in a wire, the wire will return to its original length when the load is removed. If the load is increased progressively in small increments and then released after each increase in stress, a stress value will be reached at which the wire does not return to its original length after it is unloaded. At this point the wire has been stressed beyond its *elastic limit*. The elastic limit of a material is defined as the greatest stress to which a material can be subjected such that it returns to its original dimensions when the force is released. Although tensile stress was used in the example, similar elastic limit measurements can be made for any type of stress, although different values of elastic limit are obtained in tension, compression, and shear.

CRITICAL QUESTION *Yield strength is a commonly reported property for metals and alloys but not for ceramics. Why is it not possible to measure the yield strength of ceramics or other purely brittle materials? Use a stress-strain plot to explain your answer.*

Yield Strength (proof stress). The conditions assumed for the definitions of elastic limit and proportional limit are not always realized under practical conditions. If the measuring instruments are sufficiently sensitive, irregularities on the straight-line region of the stress versus strain plot represent minor deviations from Hooke's law and cause some uncertainty in determining the precise point at which the selected line deviates from linearity (proportional limit point). Thus, a different property, *yield strength*, is used in such cases when the proportional limit cannot be determined with sufficient accuracy.

Yield strength often is a property that represents the stress value at which a small amount (0.1% or 0.2%) of plastic strain has occurred. A value of either 0.1% or 0.2% of the plastic strain is often selected and is referred to as the *percent offset*. The yield strength is the stress required to produce the particular offset strain (0.1% or 0.2%) that has been chosen. As seen in Figure 4–3, the yield strength for 0.2% offset is generally greater than that associated with an offset of 0.1%. If yield strength values for two materials tested under the same conditions are to be compared, identical offset values should be used. To determine the yield strength for a material at 0.2% offset, a line is drawn parallel to the straight-line region (see Fig. 4–3), starting at a value of 0.002, or 0.2% of the plastic strain, along the strain axis, and is extended until it intersects the stress-strain curve. The stress corresponding to this point is the yield strength. Although the term *strength* implies that the material has fractured, it actually is intact but has sustained a small amount of plastic deformation. For brittle materials such as composites and ceramics, the stress-strain plot is a straight line with little or no plastic region. Thus, a determination of yield strength is not possible for brittle materials at either a 0.1% or 0.2% strain offset because there can be no intercept of a parallel straight line.

Elastic limit, proportional limit, and *yield strength* are defined differently, but their values (of stress) are fairly close to each other in many cases. Elastic and proportional limits are usually assumed to be identical, although their experimental values may differ slightly. As shown in Figure 4–3, the yield strength (proof stress) is usually greater than the proportional limit. These values are important in the evaluation of dental materials, because they represent the stress at which permanent deformation of the structure begins. If they are exceeded by mastication stresses, the restoration or appliance may no longer function as originally designed.

Permanent (plastic) Deformation. As shown in Figure 4–3, the stress-strain curve is no longer a straight line above the proportional limit (PL) but rather curves until the structure fractures. The stress-strain curve shown in Figure 4–3 is more typical of actual stress-strain curves for ductile materials. Unlike the linear portion of the graph at stresses below the proportional limit, the shape of the curve above P is not possible to predict. In addition, the stress is no longer proportional to the strain.

If the material is deformed by a stress to a point above the proportional limit before fracture, the removal of the applied force will reduce the stress to zero, but the strain does not decrease to zero because plastic deformation has occurred. Thus, the object does not return to its original dimension when the force is removed. It remains bent, stretched, compressed, or otherwise plastically deformed.

Diametral Tensile Strength. Tensile strength is generally determined by subjecting a rod, wire, or dumbbell-shaped specimen to tensile loading (a uniaxial tension test). Since such a test is quite difficult to perform for brittle materials because of alignment and gripping problems, another test has become popular for determining this property for many dental materials. It is referred to as the *diametral compression test*, which is represented schematically in Figure 4–7. This test should be used only for materials that exhibit predominantly elastic deformation and little or no plastic deformation.

In this method, the compressive load is placed by a flat plate against the side of a short cylindrical specimen (disk), as illustrated in Figure 4–7. The vertical

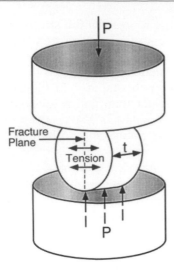

Figure 4–7. Diametral compression test. Although a compressive force is applied along the side of the disk, a tensile fracture is produced. The tensile strength is calculated from the fracture load P, the disk diameter D, and the thickness t.

compressive force along the side of the disk produces a tensile stress that is perpendicular to the vertical plane that passes through the center of the disk. Fracture occurs along this vertical plane (the dashed vertical line on the disk). In such a situation, the tensile stress is directly proportional to the compressive load applied. It is computed by the following formula:

$$\text{Tensile stress} = \frac{2P}{\pi \times D \times t}$$

where P = load
D = diameter
t = thickness

This test is simple to conduct and provides excellent reproducibility of results. However, use of this test on materials that exhibit appreciable plastic deformation before fracture results in erroneously high tensile strength determinations. The fracture of the specimen into several pieces rather than the ideal fragmentation into two segments suggests an unreliable test result.

Flexure Strength. *Flexure strength, transverse strength,* or *modulus of rupture,* as this property is variously called, is essentially a strength test of a bar supported at each end, or a thin disk supported along a lower support circle, under a static load. For the disk specimen the failure stress value is referred to as the *biaxial flexure strength* and the theory involved is beyond the scope of this textbook. However, for a bar subjected to three-point flexure, the mathematical formula for computing the flexure strength is as follows:

$$\sigma = \frac{3Pl}{2bd^2}$$

where σ = flexural strength
l = distance between the supports
b = width of the specimen
d = depth or thickness of the specimen
P = maximum load at the point of fracture

The units of stress are force per unit area, most often given in SI units of megapascals. This test is, in a sense, a collective measurement of tensile, compressive, and shear stresses simultaneously; however, for sufficiently thin specimens, it is usually dominated by the tensile stress that develops along the lower surface. When the load is applied, the specimen bends. The resulting strain is represented by a decrease in length of the top surface (compressive strain) of a bar specimen (or a decrease in diameter of a disk specimen) and an increase in the length or diameter of the lower surface (tensile strain). Consequently, the principal stresses on the upper surface are compressive, whereas those on the lower surface are tensile. Obviously, the stresses change direction within the specimen between the top and the bottom surfaces, with both stress and strain being zero at the region of change. This neutral surface does not change in dimension and is known as the *neutral axis*. Shear stress is also produced near the supported ends of the specimen, but it does not play a significant role in the fracture process. For brittle materials such as ceramics, flexure tests are preferred to the diametral compressive test because they more closely simulate the stress distributions in dental prostheses such as cantilevered bridges and multiple-unit bridges.

Fatigue Strength. Strength values obtained from a measurement of the failure load based on a steady increase in force described earlier may be quite misleading if they are used to design a structure that is subjected to repeated or cyclic loading. Few clinical fractures occur during try-in procedures that represent a single-load application. If try-in fractures were common, these products would be withdrawn from the market soon after their introduction. This is a good reason why one should not be the first to buy a new restorative material, but rather allow others to experience the initial clinical failures. Most prosthetic and restoration fractures develop progressively over many stress cycles after initiation of a crack from a critical flaw and subsequently by propagation of the crack until a sudden, unexpected fracture occurs. Stress values well below the ultimate tensile strength can produce premature fracture of a dental prosthesis because microscopic flaws grow slowly over many cycles of stress. This phenomenon is called *fatigue failure*. Normal mastication can induce thousands of stress cycles per day within a dental restoration. For glasses and certain glass-containing ceramics, the induced tensile stress and the presence of an aqueous environment cause an extension of the microscopic flaws by chemical attack and further reduce the number of cycles to cause dynamic fatigue failure.

Fatigue behavior is determined by subjecting a material to a cyclic stress of a maximum known value and determining the number of cycles that are required to produce failure. As shown in Figure 4–8, a plot of the failure stress versus the number of cycles to failure enables calculation of a *maximum service* stress level or an *endurance limit*—the maximum stress that can be maintained without failure over an infinite number of cycles. For brittle materials with rough surfaces, the endurance limit is lower than it would be if the surfaces were more highly polished (see Fig. 4–8). For a given applied stress, the rougher material would fail in fewer cycles of stress.

Some materials or prosthetic appliances exhibit *static fatigue*, a phenomenon attributed to the interaction of a constant tensile stress with structural flaws over time. The influence of flaw size on the stress to cause failure is shown in Figure 4–9. Note that for a given flaw size, less stress is required to produce failure if the stress is dynamically cycled between high and low values. Furthermore, aqueous solutions are known to corrosively degrade dental ceramics by length-

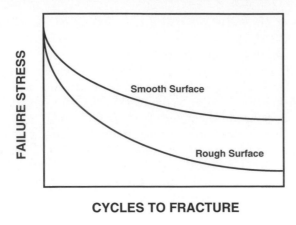

Figure 4–8. Dynamic fatigue failure stress for a brittle material as a function of surface roughness and number of stress cycles.

ening surface flaws over time in the presence of tensile stress. This environmental factor further reduces the magnitude of tensile stress that can be sustained by ceramics over time. Ceramic orthodontic brackets and activated wires within the brackets represent a clinical system that can exhibit *static fatigue failure*. The delayed fracture of molar ceramic crowns that are subjected to periodic cyclic forces may be caused by *dynamic fatigue failure*. Thus, dental restorative materials can exhibit either static or dynamic fatigue failure, depending on the nature of the loading situation. In either case, the failure begins as a flaw that slowly propagates until catastrophic fracture occurs.

Impact Strength. Impact strength may be defined as the energy required to fracture a material under an impact force. The term *impact* is used to describe the reaction of a stationary object to a collision with a moving object. A Charpy-type impact tester is usually used to measure impact strength. A pendulum is released that swings down to fracture the center of a specimen that is supported at both ends. The energy lost by the pendulum during the fracture of the specimen can be determined by a comparison of the length of its swing after the impact with that of its free swing when no impact occurs. The energy units are joules, foot-pounds, inch-pounds, and so forth. Unlike most mechanical tests, the dimensions, shape, and design of the specimen to be tested should be identical for uniform results.

For another impact device, called the *Izod impact tester,* the specimen is clamped vertically at one end. The blow is delivered at a certain distance above

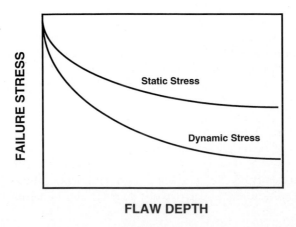

Figure 4–9. Dynamic and static fatigue failure stress for a brittle material as a function of flaw depth.

the clamped end instead of at the center of the specimen supported at both ends as described for the Charpy impact test.

With appropriate values for the velocities and masses involved, a blow by a fist to the lower jaw can be considered an impact situation. A blow from an external object such as a baseball bat to the teeth is another example. In the impact process, the external forces and resulting stresses change rapidly, and a static property such as the proportional limit is not useful in predicting the resulting deformations. However, a moving object possesses a known amount of kinetic energy. If the struck object is not permanently deformed, it stores the energy of the collision in an elastic manner. This ability is reflected by the *resilience* of a material, which is measured by the area under the elastic region of the stress-strain diagram. Thus, a material with a low elastic modulus and a high tensile strength is more resistant to impact forces. However, a low elastic modulus and a low tensile strength suggest low-impact resistance. For dental materials of low-impact resistance, the elastic moduli and tensile strengths, respectively, are as follows:

- Dental porcelain—40 GPa and 50 to 100 MPa
- Amalgam—21 GPa and 60 MPa
- Resin-based composite—17 GPa and 30 to 90 MPa
- Polymethylmethacrylate—3.5 GPa and 60 MPa

Although the tensile strength of alumina ceramic is moderately high (120 MPa), its elastic modulus is also high (350 GPa). Thus, its impact resistance is only fair.

MECHANICAL PROPERTIES OF TOOTH STRUCTURE

Many of the mechanical properties of human tooth structure have been measured, but the reported values vary markedly from one study to another. Undoubtedly, the differences are attributed to the technical problems associated with preparing and testing such minute specimens, which in some instances are less than 1 mm in length. The results reported in one study are shown in Table 4–1. Because the teeth are subject more to dynamic than static stress, the modulus of resilience is also included in the table.

Although the data in Table 4–1 indicate a variation in the properties of enamel and dentin from one type of tooth to another, the difference probably is more the result of variations within individual teeth than between molar and cuspid teeth, for example. The properties of enamel vary somewhat with its position on the tooth, cuspal enamel being stronger than enamel on the side of the tooth.

TABLE 4–1. Compressive Properties of Tooth Structure

Tooth	Structure	Modulus of Elasticity		Proportional Limit		Modulus of Resilience		Strength	
		$MPa \times 10^4$	$psi \times 10^5$	MPa	psi	MJ/m^3	$in\text{-}lb/in^3$	MPa	psi
Molar	Dentin	1.2	17	148	21,500	0.94	136	305	44,200
	Enamel (cusp)	4.6	67	224	32,500	0.55	79	261	37,800
Bicuspid	Dentin	1.4	20	146	21,200	0.77	112	248	36,000
	Enamel	—	—	—	—	—	—	—	—
Cuspid	Dentin	1.4	20	140	20,300	0.71	103	276	40,100
	Enamel (cusp)	4.8	69	194	28,200	0.41	58	288	41,800
Incisor	Dentin	1.3	19	125	18,000	0.60	85	232	33,700

From Stanford JW, Weigel KV, Paffenbarger GC, and Sweeney WT: Compressive properties of hard tooth tissue. J Am Dent Assoc 60:746–756, 1960.

Also, the properties vary according to the histologic (microscopic) structure. For example, enamel is stronger under longitudinal compression than when subjected to lateral compression. On the other hand, the properties of dentin appear to be independent of structure, regardless of the direction of compressive stress.

The tensile properties of tooth structure have also been measured. Dentin is considerably stronger in tension (50 MPa) than is enamel (10 MPa). Although the compressive strengths of enamel and dentin are comparable, the proportional limit and modulus of elasticity of enamel are higher than the corresponding values for dentin. The higher modulus of elasticity results in less resilience of enamel in comparison with dentin.

MASTICATION FORCES AND STRESSES

Because of their dynamic nature, the actual biting stresses during mastication are difficult to measure. A number of studies have been made to determine the biting force. The *Guinness Book of Records* (1994) lists the highest biting force as 4337 N (975 pounds) sustained for 2 seconds. The average maximum sustainable biting force is approximately 756 N (170 pounds). However, it varies markedly from one area of the mouth to another and from one individual to another. In the molar region, it may range from 400 to 890 N (90 to 200 pounds); in the premolar area, from 222 to 445 N (50 to 100 pounds); on the cuspids, from 133 to 334 N (30 to 75 pounds); and on the incisors, from 89 to 111 N (20 to 55 pounds). Although there is considerable overlapping, biting force generally is higher for males than for females and is greater in young adults than in children.

It is assumed that if a force of 756 N (170 pounds) is applied to a cusp tip over an area equivalent to 0.039 cm^2 (0.006 square inch), the compressive stress would be 193 MPa (28,000 psi). If the area is smaller, then the stress within the cusp would be proportionately greater.

Normally, the energy of the bite is absorbed by the food bolus during mastication, as well as by the teeth, periodontal ligament, and bone. Nevertheless, the design of the tooth is an engineering marvel in that the tooth is generally able to absorb such static as well as dynamic (impact) energies. As can be seen in Figure 4–5 and Table 4–1, the modulus of resilience of dentin is greater than that of enamel and thus is better able to absorb impact energy. Enamel is a brittle substance with a comparatively high modulus of elasticity, a low proportional limit in tension, and a low modulus of resilience. However, although it is supported by dentin with significant ability to deform elastically, teeth seldom fracture under normal occlusion.

OTHER MECHANICAL PROPERTIES

Toughness. *Toughness* is defined as the amount of elastic and plastic deformation energy required to fracture a material and it is a measure of the resistance to fracture. As previously noted, the modulus of resilience is the energy required to stress a structure to its proportional limit, and it can be measured as the area under the elastic, straight-line portion of the stress-strain curve. By the same token, toughness can be measured as the total area under the stress-strain curve (such as shown in Fig. 4–3) from zero stress to the fracture stress. Toughness depends on strength and ductility. The higher the strength and the higher the ductility (total plastic strain), the greater the toughness. Thus, it can be concluded that a tough material is generally strong, although a strong material is not necessarily tough.

Fracture Toughness. The strength of ductile materials such as gold alloys and some composites is useful for determining the maximum stress that restorations made of these materials can withstand before plastic deformation or fracture occurs. For brittle materials such as dental ceramic, strength values are of only limited value in the design of ceramic prostheses. Small defects (porosity and microcracks) are randomly distributed in location and in size throughout a ceramic, causing large strength variations in otherwise identical ceramic specimens. Furthermore, surface flaws caused by grinding, such as from coarse-grit, medium-grit, or fine-grit diamond particles, can greatly weaken an otherwise strong ceramic, especially in the presence of tensile stress in the area of these flaws. The strength is inversely proportional to the square root of the flaw depth into the surface. Fracture toughness is a mechanical property that describes the resistance of brittle materials to the catastrophic propagation of flaws under an applied stress. *Fracture toughness* is given in units of stress times the square root of crack length, that is, $MPa \cdot m^{1/2}$ or the equivalent form, $MN \cdot m^{-3/2}$.

CRITICAL QUESTION *Is it possible for a stiff material (high elastic modulus) to fail at a lower stress than a more flexible material? Explain your answer by sketching a stress-strain plot.*

Brittleness. Shown in Figure 4–10 are three stress-strain curves of materials with variable strength, elastic modulus, and percent elongation. Material A is stronger, stiffer, and more ductile than materials B or C. Material B has less ductility than material A and is thus more brittle. Material C has no ductility and is the most brittle of the three materials; it is also the weakest material. *Brittleness* is the relative inability of a material to sustain plastic deformation before fracture of a material occurs. For example, amalgams, ceramics, and composites are brittle at oral temperatures (5° to 55° C). They sustain little or no plastic strain before they fracture. In other words, a brittle material fractures at or near its proportional limit. This behavior is shown by material C in Figure 4–10.

However, a brittle material is not necessarily weak. For example, cobalt-

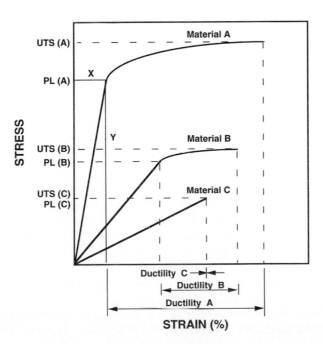

Figure 4–10. Stress-strain plots of materials that exhibit different mechanical properties. UTS, ultimate tensile stress; PL, proportional limit.

chromium partial denture alloy has 1.5% elongation but an ultimate tensile strength of 870 MPa. The tensile strength of a glass-infiltrated alumina core ceramic (In-Ceram) is moderately high (450 MPa), but it has 0% elongation. If the glass is drawn into a fiber with very smooth surfaces and insignificant internal flaws, its tensile strength may be as high as 2800 MPa (400,000 psi), but it will have no ductility (0% elongation). Thus, dental materials with low or zero percent elongation, including amalgams, composites, ceramics, and nonresin luting agents, will have little or no burnishability, because they have no plastic deformation potential.

CRITICAL QUESTION

What is the difference in appearance between a stress-strain plot for a material that has high strength, high stiffness, and high ductility and a plot for a material that is weak, flexible, and more brittle?

Ductility and Malleability. When a structure is stressed beyond its proportional limit, it becomes permanently deformed. If a material sustains tensile stress and considerable permanent deformation without rupture, it is ductile. *Ductility* represents the ability of a material to sustain a large permanent deformation under a tensile load without rupture. A metal that may be drawn readily into a wire is said to be *ductile.*

Examples of three materials with different amounts of ductility (percent elongation) are shown in Figure 4–10. Material A is the most ductile as shown by the longest plastic strain range (curved region). Material C is typical of brittle materials because no plastic deformation is possible and fracture occurs at the proportional limit.

The ability of a material to sustain considerable permanent deformation without rupture under compression, as in hammering or rolling into a sheet, is termed *malleability.* It is not as dependent on strength as is ductility.

Gold is the most ductile and malleable pure metal, and silver is second. Of the metals of interest to the dentist, platinum ranks third in ductility, and copper ranks third in malleability.

Ductility is the maximum plastic deformation a material can withstand when it is stretched at room temperature. It is quite important from a dental standpoint. Its magnitude can be assessed by the amount of permanent deformation indicated by the stress-strain curve. For example, the plastic strain indicated in Figure 4–10 is an estimation of the ductility of the substance. After fracture, the mechanical stress is reduced to zero, and the residual strain represents the amount of permanent deformation that has been produced in the object.

Measurement of Ductility. There are three common methods for measurement of ductility: (1) the percent elongation after fracture; (2) a reduction in area in the fractured region ends; and (3) the cold bend test.

Probably the simplest and most commonly used method is to compare the increase in length of a wire or rod after fracture in tension to its length before fracture. Two marks are placed on the wire or rod a specified distance apart and this distance is designated the *gauge length*. For dental materials, the standard gauge length is usually 51 mm. The wire or rod is then pulled apart under a tensile load. The fractured ends are fitted together, and the gauge length is again measured. The ratio of the increase in length after fracture to the original gauge length, expressed in percent, is called the *percent elongation* and represents the quantitative value of ductility.

Another manifestation of ductility is the necking or cone-shaped constriction that occurs at the fractured end of a ductile wire after rupture under a tensile load. The percentage of decrease in cross-sectional area of the fractured end in comparison to the original area of the wire or rod is called the *reduction in area*.

A third method for the measurement of ductility is known as the *cold bend test*. The material is clamped in a vise and bent around a mandrel of a specified radius. The number of bends to fracture is counted, and the greater the number, the greater the ductility. The first bend is made from the vertical to the horizontal, but all subsequent bends are made through angles of 180 degrees.

CRITICAL QUESTION *Hardness is a property that is used to predict the wear resistance of a material and its ability to abrade opposing dental structures. What other factors may be responsible for excessive wear of natural tooth enamel or prosthetic surfaces by a hard material?*

Hardness. The term *hardness* is difficult to define. In mineralogy the relative hardness of a substance is based on its ability to resist scratching. In metallurgy, and in most other disciplines, the concept of hardness that is most generally accepted is the "resistance to indentation." It is on this precept that most modern *hardness* tests are designed.

The indentation produced on the surface of a material from an applied force of a sharp point or an abrasive particle results from the interaction of numerous properties. Among the properties that are related to the hardness of a material are strength, proportional limit, and ductility.

Knowledge of the hardness of materials is useful to the engineer and furnishes valuable information to the dentist. Hardness tests are included in numerous American Dental Association (ADA) specifications for dental materials. There are several types of surface hardness tests. Most are based on the ability of the surface of a material to resist penetration by a point under a specified load. The tests most frequently used in determining the hardness of dental materials are known by the names *Barcol, Brinell, Rockwell, Shore, Vickers,* and *Knoop.* The selection of the test should be determined by the material being measured.

The Brinell hardness test is one of the oldest tests employed for determining the hardness of metals. In the Brinell test, a hardened steel ball is pressed under a specified load into the polished surface of a material, as diagrammed in Figure 4–11. The load is divided by the area of the projected surface of the indentation, and the quotient is referred to as the *Brinell hardness number,* usually abbreviated as BHN. Thus, for a given load, the smaller the indentation, the larger is the number, and the harder is the material.

The Brinell hardness test has been used extensively for determining the hardness of metals and metallic materials used in dentistry. In addition, the BHN is related to the proportional limit and the ultimate tensile strength of dental gold alloys. Because the test is a relatively simple one, it may often be conveniently used as an index of properties that involve more complicated test methods.

The Rockwell hardness test is somewhat similar to the Brinell test in that a steel ball or a conical diamond point is used, as diagrammed in Figure 4–11. Instead of measuring the diameter of the impression, the depth of penetration is measured directly by a dial gauge on the instrument. A number of indenting points with different sizes are available for testing a variety of different materials. The *Rockwell hardness number* (usually abbreviated as RHN) is designated according to the particular indenter and load employed.

The convenience of the Rockwell test, with direct reading of the depth of the indentation, has led to its wide usage in industry. Neither the Brinell test nor the Rockwell test is suitable for brittle materials.

The Vickers hardness test employs the same principle of hardness testing that

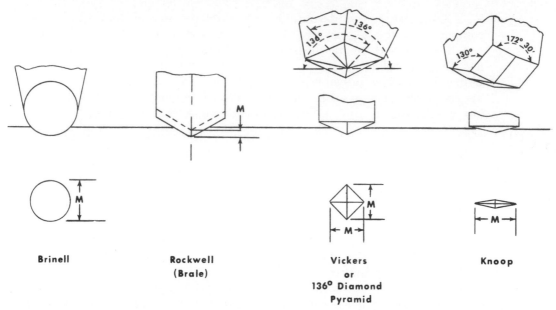

Brinell   **Rockwell**   **Vickers**   **Knoop**
                (Brale)   **or**
                                 136° Diamond
                                 Pyramid

Figure 4–11. Shapes of hardness indenter points *(upper row)* and the indentation depressions left in material surfaces *(lower row)*. The measured dimension M that is shown for each test is used to calculate hardness. The following tests are shown: *Brinell test*—a steel ball is used, and the diameter of the indentation is measured after removal of the indenter. *Rockwell test*—a conical indenter is impressed into the surface under a minor load *(dashed line)* and a major load *(solid line)*, and M is the difference between the two penetration depths. *Vickers* or *136-degree diamond pyramid test*—a pyramidal point is used, and the diagonal length of the indentation is measured. *Knoop test*—a rhombohedral pyramid diamond tip is used, and the long axis of the indentation is measured.

is used in the Brinell test. However, instead of a steel ball, a diamond in the shape of a square-based pyramid is used (see Fig. 4–11). Although the impression is square instead of round, the method for computation of the *Vickers hardness number* (usually abbreviated as VHN) is the same as that for the BHN in that the load is divided by the projected area of indentation. The lengths of the diagonals of the indentation are measured and averaged. The Vickers test is employed in the ADA specification for dental casting gold alloys. The test is suitable for determining the hardness of brittle materials; therefore, it has been used for measuring the hardness of tooth structure.

The Knoop hardness test employs a diamond indenting tool that is cut in the geometric configuration shown in Figure 4–11. The impression is rhombic in outline, and the length of the largest diagonal is measured. The projected area is divided into the load to give the *Knoop hardness number* (usually abbreviated as KHN). When the indentation is made, and the indenter is subsequently removed, the shape of the Knoop indenter causes elastic recovery of the projected impression to occur primarily along the shorter diagonal. The stresses are therefore distributed in such a manner that only the dimensions of the minor axis are subject to change by relaxation. Thus, the hardness value is virtually independent of the ductility of the material tested. The hardness of tooth enamel can be compared with that of gold, porcelain, resin, and other tooth restorative materials. Also, the load may be varied over a wide range, from 1 g to more than 1 kg, so that values for both exceedingly hard and soft materials can be obtained by this test.

The Knoop and Vickers tests are classified as microhardness tests in comparison with the Brinell and Rockwell macrohardness tests. Both Knoop and Vickers tests employ loads less than 9.8 N. The resulting indentations are small and are limited to a depth of less than 19 μm. Hence, they are capable of measuring the hardness in small regions of very thin objects. The Rockwell and Brinell tests give average hardness values over much larger areas. Other less sophisticated measurement methods, such as the Shore and the Barcol tests, are sometimes employed for measuring the hardness of dental materials, particularly rubbers and plastics. These tests use compact portable indenters of the type generally used in industry for quality control. The principle of these tests is also based on resistance to indentation. The equipment generally consists of a spring-loaded metal indenter point and a gauge from which the hardness is read directly. The hardness number is based on the depth of penetration of the indenter point into the material.

STRESS CONCENTRATION FACTORS

CRITICAL
QUESTION

Why do prostheses sometimes fail under a very small force, even though the strength of the prosthetic material is as high as advertised by the manufacturer?

Although dental prostheses are designed to resist plastic deformation and fracture, unexpected fractures occur occasionally even when high-quality materials have been used. As stated previously, these failures result from localized high stresses in specific areas even though the average stress in the structure is low. The cause of this strength reduction is the presence of small microscopic flaws or microstructural defects on the surface or within the internal structure. These flaws are especially critical in brittle materials in areas of tensile stress because the stress at the tips of these flaws is greatly increased and may lead to crack initiation and broken bonds. Shown in Figure 4–12 is the tensile stress distribution in a brittle and a ductile material. Although the tensile stress has increased at the flaw tip in each case, it has increased by a smaller amount in the ductile material (center illustration of Fig. 4–12) in which plastic deformation has occurred with subsequent widening of the flaw tip, thereby reducing the localized tensile stress. As shown on the left side of Figure 4–12, the tensile stress in a brittle material cannot be relieved by plastic deformation at the flaw tip and cracks develop as the stress increases to a critical level. Note the increased level of tensile stress at the tip of the flaw. However, the stress at areas far away from these flaws will be much lower if flaws are absent in these areas. The flaw

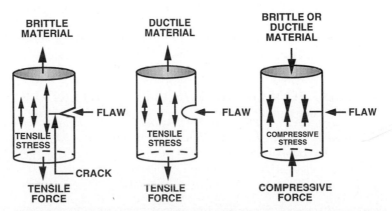

Figure 4–12. Influence of tensile and compressive stresses on flaws in brittle and ductile materials.

does not play a significant role when the material is subjected to an external compressive force, as shown on the right side of Figure 4–12. In this case the compressive stress that develops in the material tends to close the crack, and this stress distribution is more uniform.

There are two important aspects of these flaws: (1) the stress intensity increases with the length of the flaw, especially when it is oriented perpendicular to direction of tensile stress, and (2) flaws on the surface are associated with higher stresses than are flaws of the same size in interior regions. Thus surface finishing of brittle materials such as ceramics, amalgams, and composites is extremely important in areas subjected to tensile stress.

Localized areas of stress enhancement can also result from factors other than the inherent microscopic flaws on the surface or interior of a material. Areas of high stress concentration are caused by one or more of the following factors:

1. Large surface or interior flaws, such as porosity, grinding roughness, and machining damage
2. Sharp changes in shape, such as the point of attachment of a clasp arm to the partial denture framework or the sharp internal angle at the pulpal-axial line angle of a tooth preparation for an amalgam restoration
3. The interface region of a bonded structure in which the elastic moduli of the two components are quite different
4. The interface region of a bonded structure in which the thermal expansion or thermal contraction coefficients of the two components are quite different
5. A load applied at a point to the surface of a brittle material (called the *Hertzian point load*)

There are several ways to minimize stress concentrations and thus reduce the risk of clinical fracture. Relative to factor 1, the surface can be finely polished to reduce the depth of the flaws. Little can be done for interior flaws other than to improve the quality of the structure or increase the size of the object. For factor 2, the design of any prosthesis should vary gradually rather than abruptly. Notches should be avoided. Internal line angles of tooth preparations should be well rounded to minimize the risk of cusp fracture. For factor 3, the most brittle material should have the lower elastic modulus so that more stress is transferred to the material with the higher elastic modulus. If this is not possible, the elastic moduli of the two materials should be more closely matched. For factor 4, the materials must be closely matched in their coefficients of expansion or contraction. If a thermal mismatch cannot be avoided, the weaker, more brittle material should have a slightly lower expansion or contraction coefficient so that a protective compressive stress is sustained in its structure next to the interface. Relative to factor 5, the cusp tip of an opposing crown or tooth should be well rounded such that occlusal contact areas in the brittle material are large.

CRITERIA FOR SELECTION OF RESTORATIVE MATERIALS

CRITICAL QUESTION *Fracture toughness is a more precise measure of the fracture resistance of a brittle material than is tensile strength. Why is tensile strength of brittle materials such as dental amalgam, composite, ceramic, and inorganic cements so variable, and which one of a series of reported tensile strength values should be used when considering the selection of a new product of one of these materials?*

We have discussed the variability of tensile strength in earlier sections. Because brittle materials are so susceptible to surface flaws and internal defects when tensile stresses are present and because they cannot plastically deform to reduce stress concentrations, their tensile strengths are far lower than their compressive strengths. For convenience compressive strengths are reported even though most brittle materials rarely fail under compressive stresses. However, compressive strength values are of importance when comparisons are made among relative strength values of a similar family of brittle materials, such as amalgams or cements.

The compressive properties of some popular restorative materials used in operative dentistry are presented in Table 4–2. The modulus of resilience of the gold alloy is the lowest of the materials considered. It has a relatively high proportional limit and high ductility, both of which contribute to its toughness. When the gold alloy is subjected to high stress it tends to deform rather than fracture. Amalgam has a higher modulus of resilience than does gold, but it is a brittle material, and, in instances of extreme stress, it fractures rather than deforms because of its low toughness and ductility.

Because the physical properties described earlier have been obtained using specimen shapes and sizes quite different than those of tooth restorations, we should question how dental materials can be selected by the dentist on the basis of these properties. Engineers employ similar criteria for the selection of materials to be used for the construction of a bridge. Engineers have an advantage over dentists in this respect, because they know beforehand the maximum "average" stresses that structures are expected to sustain before fracture occurs. Furthermore, these expected stress values are multiplied by a "safety factor" to ensure that the structure may be able to withstand a certain amount of excess stress. However, the tensile strength values reported for restorative materials represent the average stress values below which 50% of the test specimens have fractured and above which only 50% have survived. Because this is an unacceptable failure rate for restorative dentistry, the range of measured values should be known. From an ultraconservative viewpoint the lowest strength values should be used to compare materials and also to design a prosthesis to resist fracture at a high level of confidence.

It is unfortunate that the magnitudes of mastication forces are not known for any given patient to the extent that the dentist can predict the stresses that will be induced in restorative appliances. However, knowledge of the relationships between the properties of restorative materials that are known to exhibit excellent long-term survival performance is reinforced by clinical experience. As is true for the field of engineering, the dental profession is also aware that the best test of a successful restorative material is the test of time.

TABLE 4–2. Compressive Properties of Some Dental Restorative Materials

Material	Modulus of Elasticity		Proportional Limit		Modulus of Resilience		Strength	
	GPa*	psi × 10⁶	MPa	psi	MJ/m³	in-lb/in³	MPa	psi
Unfilled acrylic resin	1.9	0.27	44	6,400	0.52	76	76	11,000
Resin-based composite	14.0	2.0	161	23,400	0.93	137	235	34,000
Zinc phosphate	13.7	2.0	153	22,000	0.87	126	161	23,300
Amalgam	34.0	5.0	340	49,000	1.7	247	423	61,300
Inlay gold	77.0	11.3	166	24,100	0.18	26	—	—

*1 GPa = 10^3 MPa.

Certain data from Stanford JW, Weigel KV, Paffenbarger GC, and Sweeney WT: Compressive properties of hard tooth tissue. J Am Dent Assoc 60:746–756, 1960.

When clinical survival data over a 3-year period or longer are not known on a recently introduced product, we should first investigate whether reliable short-term (<3-year) clinical data are available. In the absence of clinical data on a material for at least a 3-year period, a new material should be evaluated on the basis of whether it meets minimal property requirements identified in dental materials specifications and standards such as those that have been developed by the ADA and the International Organization for Standardization. If a new material meets these requirements, dentists can be reasonably confident that the material will perform satisfactorily if it is used properly.

SELECTED READING

Guinness Book of Records, 1994 edition, New York, Facts on File, p. 168.

O'Brien WJ: Dental Materials: Properties and Selection. Chicago, IL, Quintessence, 1989.
The appendix contains a complete listing of tabulated values of the physical and mechanical properties of dental materials and tooth structures.

Stanford JW, Weigel KV, Paffenbarger GD, and Sweeney WT: Compressive properties of hard tooth tissue. J Am Dent Assoc 60:746, 1960.
Although this study dates from 1960, it remains the most authoritative on mechanical properties of tooth structure.

Van Vlack LH: Elements of Materials Science and Engineering, 5th ed. Reading, MA, Addison-Wesley, 1985.
This text was also cited in Chapter 2 as the best source on the structure of matter, the properties of materials, and engineering.

5 Biocompatibility of Dental Materials

- Tests for Evaluation of Biocompatibility
- Allergic Responses to Dental Materials
- Minimizing Dental Iatrogenesis
- Pulp Responses to Specific Agents and Techniques
- Pulp Responses to Experimental and Clinical Procedures
- Microleakage
- The Occurrence of Dentin Hypersensitivity
- Pulp Capping
- Endodontic Procedures

Because of the increasing concern of the American Dental Association (ADA) in the early 1960s for the safety and biocompatibility of dental materials and devices, a committee was established in 1963 to develop testing procedures for generalized use. The document for these tests, "Recommended Standard Practices for Biological Evaluation of Dental Materials," was published in 1972. This original document was quite primitive; it was revised and republished in 1979 as Document No. 41. A similar document was produced and published by the Fédération Dentaire Internationale (FDI) in 1984. Currently, a new document is being developed that will meet international needs, particularly those of the nations of the European Union. The draft document is entitled, "Preclinical Evaluation of Biocompatibility of Medical Devices Used in Dentistry-Test Methods" (Table 5–1) (International Standard).[1,*]

In the 1960s the word *biocompatibility* was not commonly used. The word *toxicity* was more frequently applied in discussions of the safety of dental materials. The term *biocompatible* is defined in *Dorland's Illustrated Medical Dictionary* as being harmonious with life and not having toxic or injurious effects on biologic function. In general, biocompatibility is measured on the basis of localized cytotoxicity (such as pulp and mucosal response), systemic responses, allergenicity, and carcinogenicity.

---

*For an explanation of the reference numbers in this chapter, refer to the section entitled "Primary Review Articles" at the end of the chapter.

TABLE 5–1. Dentistry-Preclinical Evaluation of Medical Devices Used in Dentistry-Test Methods*

Nature of Contact	Duration of Contact	Group I Primary (initial) Tests				Group II Secondary Tests							Group III Preclinical Usage Tests		
		Cytotoxicity Test ISO XXXX Clauses 6, 7	Cytotoxicity Test ISO 10993-5	Cytotoxicity Test ISO XXXX Annex A	Genotoxicity Test ISO 10993-3 Clause 4	Acute Systemic Toxicity—Oral Application ISO 10993-11 Clause 6.5.1	Acute Systemic Toxicity—Application by Inhalation ISO 10993-11 Clause 6.5.3	Subchronic Systemic Toxicity—Oral Application ISO 10993-11 Clause 6.7.1	Skin Irritation and Intracutaneous Reactivity ISO 10993-10 Clauses 5.2, 5.4	Sensitization ISO 10993-10 Clauses 6.2, 6.3	Subchronic Systemic Toxicity—Application by Inhalation ISO 10993-11 Clause 6.7.3	Local Effects After Implantation ISO 10993-6 Clauses 4, 5, 6	Pulp and Dentine Usage Test ISO XXXX Clause 8	Pulp Capping and Pulpotomy Test ISO XXXX Clause 9	Endodontic Usage Test ISO XXXX Clause 10
Surface-Contacting Devices	≤24 h	X	X				X		X	X					
	24 h to 30 days	X	X				X	X	X	X	X				
	>30 days	X	X		X		X	X	X	X	X				
External Communicating Devices	≤24 h	X	X	X		X	X		X	X			X	X	X
	24 h to 30 days	X	X	X	X		X	X	X	X	X	X	X	X	X
	>30 days	X	X	X	X		X	X	X	X	X	X			
Implant Devices	≤24 h	X	X						X	X				X	X
	24 h to 30 days	X	X		X			X	X	X		X		X	X
	>30 days	X	X		X			X	X	X		X		X	X

*X in the columns indicates test that shall be considered for use. ISO XXXX in the column heading indicates that the official number will be designated when the ISO grants approval.

This Draft International Standard was developed by a Technical Committee of the International Organization for Standardization (ISO). The American National Standards Institute (ANSI), the U.S. member of ISO, participates in its technical program and administers secretariats of various technical committees and subgroups. ANSI is also ISO's exclusive sale agent in the United States for all ISO standards, Draft International Standards, and Committee Drafts. The excerpt from this Draft International Standard is being distributed by W.B. Saunders Company through an arrangement with ANSI.

This is *not* an approved ISO International Standard. It is distributed for review and comment and may be modified during this process. It is subject to change without notice and may not be referred to as an International or ISO Standard until published as such.

Copyright by the International Organization for Standardization. No part of this publication may be copied or reproduced in any form, electronic retrieval system or otherwise, without the prior written permission of the American National Standards Institute, 11 West 42nd Street, New York, NY 10036, which holds reproduction rights in the United States.

Based on these criteria, the requirements for dental material biocompatibility include the following:

- It should not be harmful to the pulp and soft tissues.
- It should not contain toxic diffusable substances that can be released and absorbed into the circulatory system to cause a systemic toxic response.
- It should be free of potentially sensitizing agents that are likely to cause an allergic response.
- It should have no carcinogenic potential.

In a broad sense, a *biomaterial* can be defined as any substance, other than a drug, that can be used for any period as a part of a system that treats, augments, or replaces any tissue, organ, or function of the body. The science of dental biomaterials must be based on a broad information base of certain biologic considerations that are associated with the use of materials designed for the oral cavity. Strength or resistance to deformation is unimportant if the material is injurious to the pulp or soft tissues.

Dental materials are used in humans for short or long periods. Most dental materials are similar to other specialized materials used in orthopedics, cardiovascular prostheses, plastic surgery, and ophthalmology; that is, they function in close contact with various human tissues. Collectively, these materials must meet the requirements given in the definitions of the terms *biomaterials, biocompatibility, and bioacceptance,* which are relative to all oral tissues. The ability of these materials to satisfy these conditions represents a paramount consideration in the formulation and use of biomaterials. In this regard, the host environment for dental biomaterials is especially complicated because of the presence of bacteria and debris in the oral cavity and the corrosive properties of saliva and other fluids.

When dentists purchase a material, they should know if it is safe, and if it is safe, how safe it is relative to other materials. Dental students should know the most likely side effects of materials, whether they affect dental patients or dental auxiliary personnel and laboratory technicians. They should also recognize mechanisms through which these effects are produced.

TESTS FOR EVALUATION OF BIOCOMPATIBILITY[1]

The purpose of biocompatibility tests is to eliminate any potential product or component of a product that can cause harm or damage to oral or maxillofacial tissues. Biocompatibility tests are classified on three levels (tiers), with the most rapid and economical occurring at the primary level. A product with promising attributes is subjected to the more expensive secondary tests and, finally, to the expensive preclinical (usage) tests in animals or humans. The number of tests and the use of animals have been greatly reduced since 1972.

Group I: Primary Tests. The primary tests consist of cytotoxic evaluations in which dental materials in a fresh or a cured state are placed directly on tissue culture cells or on membranes (barriers such as dentin disks) overlying tissue culture cells that react to the effects of products or components that leach through the barriers. Many products that are judged initially to be quite cytotoxic can be modified or their use can be controlled by the manufacturer to prevent cytotoxicity.

Genotoxicity Test. Mammalian or nonmammalian cells, bacteria, yeasts, or fungi are used to determine whether gene mutations, changes in chromosomal structure, or other deoxyribonucleic acid or genetic changes are caused by the test materials, devices, and extracts from materials (AAMI Standards, 1994).

Group II: Secondary Tests. At this level the product is evaluated for its potential to create systemic toxicity, inhalation toxicity, skin irritation and sensitization, and implantation responses. In the systemic toxicity tests such as the oral median lethal dose (LD_{50}) test, the test sample is administered daily to rats for 14 days either by oral gavage or by dietary inclusion. If 50% of the animals survive, the product has passed the test. Efforts are being made to develop other systemic toxicity tests that require far fewer animals.

The dermal toxicity test is important because of the great number of chemical substances, not only dental products, that we contact daily. A primary irritant is capable of producing an inflammatory response in most susceptible people after the first exposure. Once a toxic material, product, or component is identified, it can be replaced, diluted, neutralized, and chelated to reduce the risk for toxicity. In addition, irritation and sensitization must be differentiated. *Irritation* is defined as an inflammation brought about without the intervention of an antibody or immune system, whereas *sensitization* is an inflammatory response requiring the participation of an antibody system specific for the material allergen in question.

To simulate dermal toxicity, the test material is held in contact with the shaved skin of albino rats for periods ranging from 24 (one exposure) to 90 days (with repeated exposures). The animal must receive an occlusive covering to prevent mechanical loss of the contacting agent, even by evaporation.

The guinea pig is the laboratory animal used to establish allergic contact sensitization. An *allergen* is defined as a substance that is not primarily irritating on the first exposure but produces reactions more rapidly in animals of appropriate genetic constitution on subsequent exposure to similar concentrations.

The test material is introduced intradermally on the shaved intrascapular region. After 24 hours, the resulting dermal reaction is assessed. For the main test, the highest concentration of the test material that causes no more than slight erythema and edema is selected. After an interval of 7 days, the test material of the same concentration is placed on gauze patches and applied to cover the previously injected sites. Fourteen days later, the test material is applied to the shaved flank of the animals. After removal of the dressings at 24, 48, and 72 hours, the skin reactions at the challenged skin sites are evaluated and graded.

The inhalation toxicity tests are performed on rats, rabbits, or guinea pigs in an exposure chamber with aerosol preparations by releasing the spray material around the head and upper trunk of the animals. The animals are subjected to 30 seconds of continuous spray released at 30-minute intervals. After 10 consecutive exposures, the animals are observed over a 4-day period. If any animal dies within 2 to 3 minutes, the agent is considered very toxic. If none of the animals die, the agent is not likely to be hazardous to humans (Stanley, 1985).

Implantation Tests. The use of *in vivo* implantation techniques also takes into consideration the physical characteristics of the product, such as form, density, hardness, and surface finish, that can influence the character of the tissue response.

The animal species is selected according to the size of the implant test specimen and the intended duration of the test in relation to the life span of the animal. For short-term tests ($\leq$12 weeks) in subcutaneous tissue or muscle, animals such as mice, rats, hamsters, guinea pigs, and rabbits are commonly used. For long-term tests ($\geq$12 weeks) in muscle or bone, animals such as rabbits, dogs, sheep, goats, and subhuman primates with a relatively long life expectancy are used. The use of smaller animals of lower-order species is the most conservative approach, considering today's responsible animal-use climate.

For subcutaneous and muscle implantation, the test implant material is packed into various types of plastic tubes (variations of polyethylene or Teflon). For bone implantation, the lateral cortex of a femur or a tibia or both are exposed, and holes are drilled using low-speed, intermittent cutting under profuse irrigation with physiologic saline solution to prevent overheating of the bone. Cylinders of the test implant material are inserted into the drilled holes by finger pressure to allow a tight press fit. The diameter of the implant and the implant bed in the bone must match well enough to avoid the ingrowth of fibrous connective tissue and mobility of the implant. Histopathologically, one evaluates the formation of new bone onto the surface of the test implant material without intervening connective tissue.

Group III: Preclinical Usage Tests. A product can be approved by the US Food and Drug Administration (FDA) after it successfully passes the primary and secondary tests on the basis that the product would not be harmful to humans. With regard to drugs, the FDA is most concerned that efficacy and usage tests are thoroughly conducted and scrutinized. However, in regard to dental materials, the manufacturer has as long as 7 years to prove efficacy after the product has reached the open market with FDA approval.

A dental practitioner should not assume that a dental product that can be purchased or is promoted in prominent dental publications necessarily fulfills all the advertised claims. It is better at this time to determine if the product has the ADA Seal of Acceptance that is granted when sufficient data are available to provide evidence of safety and efficacy through biologic, laboratory, and clinical evaluations. Because the FDA has recently experienced problems with this philosophy in dealing with implant materials, it is now requiring more long-term data on the efficacy of such products.

Pulp and Dentin Usage Test. This test is designed to assess the biocompatibility of dental materials placed in dentin adjacent to the dental pulp. Nonrodent mammals (subhuman primates, dogs, ferrets, and miniature pigs) are selected to ensure that their dentition contains recently erupted, intact permanent teeth. Class V cavity preparations are cut on the buccal or labial surfaces or both using sharp burs with an adequate air-water spray to leave 1 mm or less of tubular dentin between the floor of the cavity preparation and the pulp. The appropriate number of cavities are restored, and some are retained for control specimens. As a negative control, some form of zinc oxide–eugenol (ZOE) is used. For a positive control, a restorative material is selected that consistently induces a moderate to severe pulp response. If a product is to be used as a luting agent, a Class V cavity preparation is cut to receive suitable inlays. These are then luted under pressure for the length of time necessary for the initial set of the luting agent to simulate the hydraulic forces produced during cementation of full crowns, inlays, or onlays.

The animals are sacrificed after 7 days, 28 ± 3 days, and 70 ± 5 days. After routine histopathologic processing, the specimens are graded for degree of inflammatory response, the prevalence of reparative dentin formation in the pulp, and the number of micro-organisms (microleakage) entrapped in the surrounding cavity walls and cut dentinal tubules.

Promising test materials induce the least inflammatory response in the pulp, and if a response is produced, the time required to disappear is also measured.

As a rule, the less reparative dentin that is subsequently formed the better, because more bulk vital pulp tissue is available to deal with future episodes of caries and dental treatment.

Pulp Capping and Pulpotomy Usage Tests. The testing procedures here are similar to those just described except that the pulp is merely exposed for the pulp capping evaluation and is partially removed for the pulpotomy assessment. A calcium hydroxide (CH) product is used as a negative control. The animals are sacrificed after 7 ± 2 days and 70 ± 5 days.

Observations are made of dentinal bridge formation adjacent to or subjacent to the applied capping material. The quality or structure of the covering dentinal bridge is determined. It is preferred to find a bridge directly against the capping material, implying minimal destruction of pulp tissue at the time the pulp capping agent was applied.

Endodontic Usage Test. For this test the same types of animals are used, but the pulp is completely or almost completely removed from the pulp chamber and root canals and replaced by the obturating test material and control material. ZOE alone or ZOE combined with a sealer (usually Grossman's sealer) is used as a control material. The animals are sacrificed after 28 ± 3 days and 13 ± 1 weeks. The teeth are removed together with their surrounding apical periodontal (soft and hard) tissues in a single block. The degree of inflammation is evaluated in the periapical tissues. For a biocompatible material, one should observe minimal or no response and the shortest resolution time if a response is detected. This time is affected by the resistance of the test material to degradation and dissolution. When the latter occurs, tissue fluid accumulates in the porous areas of the obturation material, and it may contribute to the growth of microorganisms, recurrent infection, and clinical failure.

ALLERGIC RESPONSES TO DENTAL MATERIALS[2]

Allergic Contact Dermatitis. Allergic contact dermatitis is commonly seen first by primary physicians. Such effects are often experienced in the workplace. In fact, allergic contact dermatitis now ranks as the most common occupational disease.

The interval between exposure to the causative agent and the occurrence of clinical manifestations usually varies between 12 and 48 hours, although it may be as short as 4 hours or as long as 72 hours. The incubation period may be as short as 2 days (poison ivy) or as long as several years (for a weak sensitizer such as a chromate). Dermatitis usually occurs where the body surface makes direct contact with the allergen. In some instances, however, the relationship is not quite as straightforward. For example, contact dermatitis of the eyelids is frequently caused by nail polish or hand cream.

A skin condition that is frequently confused with allergic contact dermatitis is primary irritant dermatitis, which is caused by a simple chemical insult to the skin, such as that observed in "dishpan hands." A prior sensitizing exposure is unnecessary. Primary irritant dermatitis is dose dependent, whereas allergic reactions are virtually dose independent.

Personnel and patients involved in orthodontics and pediatric dentistry have the highest incidence of side effects, amounting to 50% of the personnel and 1% of the patients. An allergic contact dermatitis associated with the monomers of bonding agents frequently involves the distal parts of the fingers and the palmar aspects of the fingertips. Similar cases of allergic contact dermatitis have been reported in industry where workers were involved in electronic assembly operations that used polyethylene glycol dimethacrylate as an anaerobic sealant. Similar conditions can develop from artificial acrylic fingernails and acrylic components of dental cements that are well-known as allergic contact sensitizers.

Allergy to Latex Products. On March 29, 1991, the FDA issued a bulletin (US FDA, 1991) in response to the increasing number of latex-related allergic reactions. Although rubber has been identified as a cause of contact sensitivity since the mid-1940s, Malten and associates reported an increasing incidence of hypersensitivity in 1976.

In our modern environment there are many sources of daily latex exposure, including toy balloons, condoms, swim goggles, dishwashing gloves, hairnet elastics, clothing elastics, footwear, cervical diaphragms, hot water bottles, rubber-bulb eyedroppers, rubber sheeting, swimming caps, surgical support stockings, cosmetic sponges, and eyelash curlers.

Hypersensitivity to latex-containing products may represent a true latex allergy or a reaction to accelerators and antioxidants used in latex processing (Rankin et al, 1993). Thiuram is a chemical used in the fabrication of latex articles that has also been reported to cause allergic reactions. March (1988) suggested that the polyether component in latex rubber gloves worn by dentists was the causative agent.

The processing of latex has made identification of specific protein allergens difficult. Natural rubber products are made from latex, a white milky sap harvested from a tree that grows in tropical regions. Ammonia is added to the sap to preserve it, but at the same time it hydrolyzes and degrades the sap proteins to produce allergens. Vulcanization is the process by which liquid latex is hardened into rubber through the use of sulfur chemicals and heat. The final manufacturing process leaches the allergens from the rubber products by soaking them in hot water. The leaching water is changed repeatedly to decrease the concentration of the latex antigens. However, leaching brings the allergens to the surface and places the highest concentration of allergens next to the skin of the wearer (Snyder and Settle, 1994).

In the early 1980s, dental professionals began wearing gloves to reduce the risk of disease transmission. The subsequent increase in the incidence of allergic reactions to natural rubber products has been perplexing and menacing. The FDA (1991) estimated that about 6% to 7% of surgical personnel may be allergic to latex. A survey of periodontists, hygienists, and dental assistants revealed that 42% of these professionals reported adverse reactions to occupational materials, most of which were related to dermatoses of the hands and fingers. Adverse reactions in 3.7% of 323 patients were associated with latex gloves. However, only 8.8% of these patients reported work-related latex glove use.

Reactions vary from simple types such as localized rashes and swelling to more serious types such as wheezing and anaphylaxis (Council on Dental Materials Instruments, and Equipment, 1993). Dermatitis of the hands (eczema) is the most common adverse reaction (Rankin et al, 1993). A history of eczema and a familial history of allergies are predisposing factors. Repeated exposure and duration of exposure play a role in the degree of response, which explains the high incidence of latex allergy among surgical personnel.

The most serious systemic allergic reactions occur when latex-containing products, such as gloves and rubber dams, contact the mucous membranes. In 1984, Blinkhorn and Leggate described generalized angioneurotic edema, chest pains, and a rash on the neck and chest of a 15-year-old boy as a reaction to a dental rubber dam. Axelsson and colleagues (1987) reported an adverse reaction to rubber dam involving respiratory distress. The reported incidence of hypersensitivity reactions to latex products such as rubber dam material and condoms was equal to that associated with gloves. Hypersensitivity responses to rectal and vaginal examinations with latex gloves were exhibited by 5.5% of the population. To avoid these adverse responses to latex products, vinyl gloves or gloves made from other synthetic polymers may be used.

Allergic Contact Stomatitis.[2] Allergic contact stomatitis is by far the most common adverse reaction to dental materials. The adverse reactions may be observed as local or contact-type lesions, but reactions distant from the material site (such as itching on the palms of the hand or soles of the feet) are also reported. The long-term reactions are dependent on the composition of the materials, the toxic components, the degradation products, the concentration of absorbed and accumulated components, and other factors associated with substances leached from these materials.

The most definitive diagnostic test for allergic contact dermatitis or stomatitis is the patch test. The suspected allergen is applied to the skin with the intent to produce a small area of allergic contact dermatitis. The test generally takes from 48 to 96 hours, although a reaction may appear after 24 hours. This reaction may cause hyperemia, edema, vesicle formation, and itching (Slavin and Ducomb, 1989).

Dental materials contain many components known to be common allergens, such as chromium, cobalt, mercury, eugenol, components of resin-based materials, colophonium, and formaldehyde. Minute amounts of formaldehyde may be released as a degradation product of unreacted monomers in dentures made from resin-based composite materials. People who are sensitive to formaldehyde may develop enhanced tissue responses under this condition. Baker and coworkers (1988) demonstrated that the free residual methyl methacrylate monomer in autopolymerized acrylic dentures or appliances can cause allergic reactions, particularly in children, that seldom occur when correctly heat-cured dentures and appliances are used. To avoid this problem, the authors recommended that autopolymerized appliances and dentures should be immersed in water for 24 hours before being worn.

The allergic reactions associated with resin-based materials affect not only patients but also dental personnel working with such materials. Resin-based composite materials consist of inorganic fillers, usually quartz or glass, and an organic matrix composed primarily of polymeric dimethacrylates. The organic matrix contains, in addition to a variety of different dimethacrylates, a number of reactive chemicals to improve their clinical performance or handling properties. These components consist of initiators such as benzoyl peroxide or camphorquinone, accelerators, toluidines, anilines, aminobenzoic acid, inhibitors (hydroquinone monomethylether or 2,6 di-tertiary butyl-*p*-cresol plasticizers) such as dibutylphthalate, and other components, depending on whether the polymerization reaction is chemically or light activated.

The polymerization of composite materials is never complete, that is, a percentage of reactive groups do not participate in polymerization. The incomplete polymerization of a resin restorative material may predispose to material degradation. In addition, any surface layer exposed to air (oxygen) is incompletely polymerized. The same inhibition results in unreacted molecules that form the walls of pores within the bulk material. Degradation and wear of the materials release components of the resin-based materials, and these may cause reactions both locally and systemically.

Although few gingival reactions have been reported following contact with composite materials, the permeability of the gingival epithelium enhances the penetration of leachable components and thus the potential for toxic and allergenic reactions. When the degree of gingival inflammation (crevicular exudate) resulting from contact with resin composite surfaces was compared with that from intact enamel surfaces after 7 days of oral neglect, there were no differences in the performance of 12-month-old resin composite restorations made from different products but much less gingival inflammation against enamel surfaces (Mackert et al, 1988). Podshadley (1969) described greater inflammatory reactions adjacent to unfilled cold-cured acrylic resin than those adjacent to heat-cured resins.

Under extremely rare conditions (1:1 million), patients who have been sensitized to gold may react to gold restorations with burning sensations and lichenoid lesions of the oral mucosa in contact with gold alloy as well as generalized systemic reactions. When patch testing was performed with different gold salts (gold trichloride), 8.5% of the female patients developed papular reactions to the patch substance. Some of these patients had presented lesions of oral lichen planus, and one exhibited the "burning mouth syndrome." Clinical improvement occurred when gold in the dentures was replaced (Laeijendecker and von Joost, 1994).

Lichenoid reactions representing a long-term effect in the oral mucous membrane adjacent to amalgam and resin-based composite materials occur quite often. However, in patients for whom the contact area of the lesion opposed the amalgam, there was a significantly greater proportion of patients allergic to the mercury in the amalgam. In a recent study of patients with oral lichenoid lesions in the buccal mucosa and/or lateral borders of the tongue in contact with amalgam restorations, the lesions disappeared or became less apparent after their replacement (Bratel and Jontell, 1994). If removal of a dental material results in spontaneous healing of a local lesion, it is often considered to be verification of an allergic response. Chemicals that may produce allergic contact stomatitis on a short-term basis can be found also in mouthwashes, dentifrices, and topical medications such as lozenges and cough drops. They can cause burning, swelling, and ulcerations of the oral tissues.

The Mercury Controversy. For many years a controversy has raged over the biocompatibility of amalgam restorations because of the presence of elemental mercury. Another form that has received attention is methyl mercury that is contained in ocean fish. Methyl mercury is generally formed by biologic action on elemental mercury.

The Minamata disaster of the early 1970s in Japan was the result of inorganic mercury methylation from factory effluent by bottom-dwelling organisms in the Minamata Bay of Japan. This methylated mercury accumulated in the food chain and humans were poisoned by eating contaminated fish and shellfish. This incident created quite a stir worldwide, and measurement of mercury in all forms of fish became a focal point for environmental scientists. Later, however, scientists found that fish from uncontaminated ocean waters, particularly tuna and swordfish, had high concentrations of methyl mercury in their tissues. This mercury is derived from areas of undersea volcanic activity and hydrothermal waters. Mercury accumulates in the food chain, and large cold-water fish have concentrations that often exceed FDA limits, even though the mercury is from natural sources. Virtually 100% of methyl mercury is absorbed in the gut. Thus, conversion of elemental mercury to methyl mercury would greatly increase absorption via the gastrointestinal route. This point is moot, however, because all the mercury in seafood is methyl mercury, and all is absorbed. The average contribution of one seafood meal per week to blood mercury levels of methyl mercury is many times that of the average contribution of elemental mercury from the presence of 8 to 10 amalgam restorations in the mouth.

Less than 0.01% of ingested elemental mercury is absorbed. However, it does have a high vapor pressure. Between 65% and 85% of the mercury vapor that is inhaled is retained in the body; therefore, this route is of concern in considering the contribution of mercury absorption from dental amalgam.

Much of the confusion associated with the biocompatibility of amalgam stems from ignorance of the signs and symptoms of mercury poisoning. Headache, one of the symptoms most frequently claimed to disappear on removal of amalgams, is not a symptom of mercury poisoning. The recognized symptoms of chronic mercury poisoning include weakness, fatigue, anorexia, weight loss, insomnia, irritability, shyness, dizziness, and tremors in the extremities. The signs and symptoms of methyl mercury poisoning are distinctly different from those of elemental mercury poisoning: paresthesia of the extremities, lips, and tongue; ataxia (gait disturbances); and concentric constriction of visual fields ("tunnel vision").

When the most recent wave of antiamalgam sentiment began, the claim was made that a few patients can react to extremely small amounts of mercury with the signs and symptoms of mercury poisoning, multiple sclerosis, epilepsy, and other diseases of unknown causes. It was alleged that these patients had a condition that prompted some dentists to diagnose this "micromercurialism hypersensity" through the use of the cutaneous patch test.

In spite of attempts to demonstrate a direct relationship between the presence of dental amalgams and elevated blood levels of mercury, none has been found. The average mercury level in the blood of subjects with amalgams was 0.7 ng/mL (coefficient of variation = 78%), whereas the level in subjects without amalgams was 0.3 ng/mL (coefficient of variation = 77%). In comparison, other investigators reported that ingestion of one saltwater seafood meal per week raised the average blood mercury level from 2.3 to 5.1 ng/mL. Thus, one saltwater seafood meal per week can be expected to contribute seven times more mercury to blood levels than the presence of multiple dental amalgam restorations. The lowest level of total blood mercury at which the earliest nonspecific symptoms occur is 35 ng/mL (after long-term exposures). Thus, the widespread removal of amalgams is unwarranted.

Allergy to Nickel. About 10% of the female population is allergic to nickel, compared with only about 1% of the male population. This disparity is attributed to greater exposure of females to nickel. Nearly all gold-plated jewelry is made with a nickel undercoat beneath the gold plating. Metal parts on clothing and undergarments are nickel plated for corrosion resistance. Only about 30% of those patients with a known nickel allergy develop a reaction to an intraoral nickel-chromium dental alloy. There appears to be little danger of producing an allergic reaction to nickel by placing a nickel-containing alloy intraorally. Fears of producing cancer from nickel alloys in the mouth are unfounded. A higher incidence of nasal and sinus cancer has been found among nickel refinery workers, but this higher incidence has been linked to a nickel carbonyl that is used in the refining process.

Toxicity and Allergenicity of Beryllium. Berylliosis is an inflammatory lung disease resulting from the inhalation of beryllium dust or fumes. Beryllium-containing alloy should be ground only with adequate ventilation (Mackert et al., 1988).

MINIMIZING DENTAL IATROGENESIS[3]

The word *iatrogenesis* is derived from the Greek words *iatros*, meaning physician, and *genesis*, meaning to produce. It is defined as the creation of side effects, problems, or complications resulting from treatment by a physician or dentist.

Although dental products and techniques are approved and certified, the practitioner should follow explicitly the instructions and directions of the manufacturer; any variance in technique and substitution of components with the components of another manufacturer, no matter how subtle the change, may prove detrimental to the long-term success of the treatment. If products have narrow limits for safety, special precautions should be adopted to reduce unnecessary risks or to prevent adverse effects.

The graphs in this chapter represent pulp responses (Fig. 5–1) that have been observed by the author in testing programs and from reviewing the relevant literature. The curves (Fig. 5–2) do not represent experimental data but the general interpretation of existing information.

The curves in Figure 5–2 are based primarily on the presence and density of infiltrating neutrophilic leukocytes (A-acute) (see Fig. 5–1A), mononucleated cells (C-chronic) (see Fig. 5–1B), and reparative dentin formation curve) (see Fig. 5–1C). The slope of the curve represents the percentage of specimens within a category that produce reparative dentin.

Parameters for Assessment. It is desirable to have a remaining dentin thickness (RDT) of 1 mm or less in all categories. Categories and time intervals are compared to determine from the grading of the histopathologic characteristics whether a pulp lesion is resolving, persisting, or intensifying. A favorable situation requires that the intensity of a pulp response, if any, should be higher initially and decrease with increasing postoperative time intervals (PTIs). If the response values in the long-term PTIs are equal to or higher than that for the initial short-term interval, it is indicative of a prolonged side effect and response, a situation that is unacceptable. The number of specimens with no response should increase and the number of specimens with moderate to severe responses should decrease with long PTIs. However, for an increase in PTI, the percentage of specimens exhibiting reparative dentin formation (RDF) may increase, as may the volume of tissue that is formed.

Any system, technique, procedure, or restorative material that creates an abscess or a lesion extending beyond the cut tubules is unacceptable. In addition, if the average response for intensity of inflammatory cells exceeds a minimal to moderate level (1.5-degree),* the material or procedure should be looked on with suspicion, especially in the long-term PTIs, even in the absence of extended lesions or abscess formation.

Cavity Preparation: Effects of Air-water Spray. In most instances, 2 mm of dentin thickness provides an adequate insulating barrier against the more traumatic thermal operative techniques and the irritating components of most

---

*Minimal to moderate level is 1 to 2 degrees; moderate to severe level is 3 to 4 degrees.

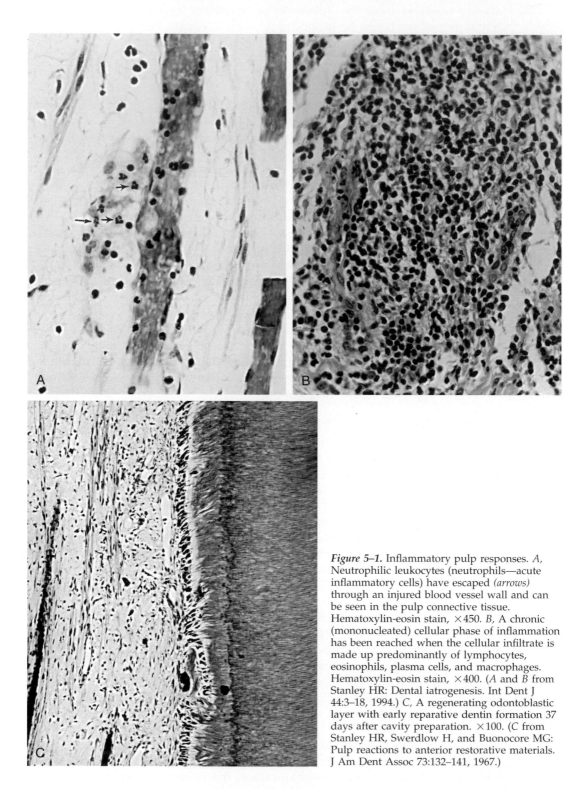

Figure 5–1. Inflammatory pulp responses. *A*, Neutrophilic leukocytes (neutrophils—acute inflammatory cells) have escaped *(arrows)* through an injured blood vessel wall and can be seen in the pulp connective tissue. Hematoxylin-eosin stain, ×450. *B*, A chronic (mononucleated) cellular phase of inflammation has been reached when the cellular infiltrate is made up predominantly of lymphocytes, eosinophils, plasma cells, and macrophages. Hematoxylin-eosin stain, ×400. (*A* and *B* from Stanley HR: Dental iatrogenesis. Int Dent J 44:3–18, 1994.) *C*, A regenerating odontoblastic layer with early reparative dentin formation 37 days after cavity preparation. ×100. (*C* from Stanley HR, Swerdlow H, and Buonocore MG: Pulp reactions to anterior restorative materials. J Am Dent Assoc 73:132–141, 1967.)

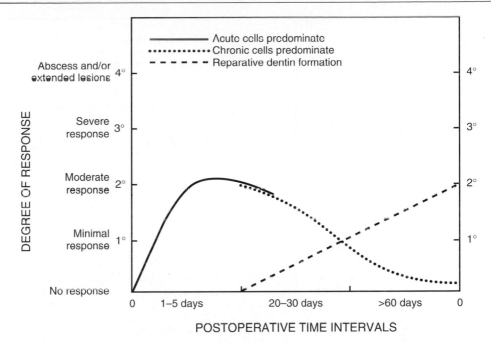

Figure 5–2. Effect of low-speed cutting (6000 to 20,000 rpm) with air-water spray and zinc oxide–eugenol (ZOE) restoration. The acute cells predominate for 10 days, creating a moderate response. After 15 days chronic cells predominate but decrease over time as odontoblasts begin to produce reparative dentin after 20 days. (Redrawn from Stanley HR: Dental iatrogenesis. Int Dent J 44:3–18, 1994.)

restorative materials. At lesser dentin thicknesses, however, inflammatory responses develop and increase in severity as the dentin thickness decreases.

At low handpiece speed (6000 to 20,000 rpm) with an air-water spray, a cavity preparation 2 mm from the pulp elicits a minimal pulp lesion despite restoration with ZOE. As the cavity preparation approaches within 1 mm of the pulp, the intensity of the response increases. The inflammatory response is significant (moderate, 2-degree) in the first 24 hours. Many neutrophils migrate into the superficial and deeper tissues of the pulp, odontoblasts are displaced into the dentinal tubules, and focal hemorrhages occur throughout the affected region.

Despite the apparent severity of this initial lesion, the inflammatory response begins to resolve in a few days as acute inflammatory cells are replaced by mononucleated cells. Because the effect of the cavity preparation is a once-only traumatic episode, little inflammation will be present by 15 days, and by 30 days, reparative dentin will begin to form and reach its maximum thickness after 60 days (see Fig. 5–2).

When a tooth preparation is cut at high speed (≥50,000 rpm) with adequate low-pressure air-water spray and restored with ZOE, the pulp response is greatly reduced as compared with low-speed techniques for preparations of comparable depth (Fig. 5–3).

PULP RESPONSES TO SPECIFIC AGENTS AND TECHNIQUES

Considerable confusion exists regarding the response of pulp to restorative materials because earlier investigations were performed with low-speed cutting

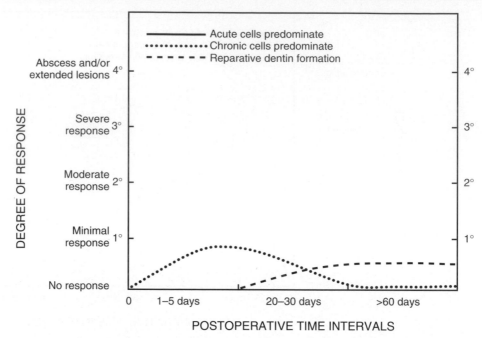

Figure 5–3. Effect of high-speed cutting (50,000 to 300,000 rpm) with air-water spray and zinc oxide–eugenol (ZOE) restoration. There is no significant pulp response, the curves are much flatter, and there are no acute cells present. (Redrawn from Stanley HR: Dental iatrogenesis. Int Dent J 44:3–18, 1994.)

instruments that induced a significant pulp response. High-speed instruments, operating with adequate safeguards, however, permit cavity preparations with minimal pulp responses. Accordingly, the superimposed effects of restorative materials are easier to recognize and interpret.

Amalgam. Conventional amalgam restorations have generally been considered to be either inert or mildly irritating to the pulp. Mercury itself does not seem to contribute to any pulp response.

Swerdlow and Stanley (1962) reported the results of a human study with amalgam condensed by hand or by low-speed mechanical condensers. A common histopathologic feature of amalgam-restored teeth is a dense accumulation of neutrophilic leukocytes between the predentin and the odontoblast layer. The quantity of neutrophils was, in several instances, sufficient to lift the odontoblast layer away from the predentin and press it into the deeper pulpal tissues. Such lesions represent extreme degrees of neutrophilic accumulation and not the conversion of necrotic tissue to abscess formation. Because the pulp responses of the short-term amalgam specimens were greater than those of the ZOE control specimens, it was suggested that the physical insertion of the amalgam is a major contributing factor responsible for the greater responses rather than the toxic, chemical, or thermal properties of amalgam. Despite the increased pulpal responses from amalgam restorations initially, compared with ZOE, definite resolution was found as early as 15 days. It has been shown that the applied load for grinding procedures can contribute to an intensification of the pulp response, even though frictional heat appeared to be neutralized by the use of adequate coolant.

Pulp response to amalgam placement as described earlier is related mainly to

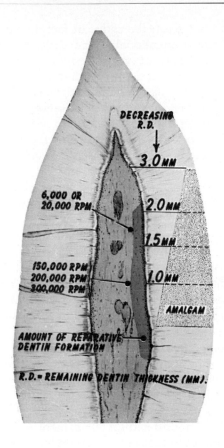

Figure 5–4. The insertion and condensation of amalgam in unlined cavities prepared at high speed increases the pulp response in such a way that the combination of high speed, cutting under air-water spray, and amalgam condensation resembles the pulp response of low-speed cutting under air-water spray. Much of the biological advantage of a high-speed cutting technique is lost. In addition, the production of reparative dentin resembles that of low-speed cutting rather than that of high speed cutting. (From Stanley HR, and Swerdlow H: An approach to biologic variation in human pulp studies. J Prosthet Dent 14:365–371, 1964.)

condensation pressure. Little inflammatory response is elicited when a cavity preparation is cut using a high-speed air-water spray technique. However, if the practitioner places a conventional amalgam restoration after cutting a cavity preparation at high speed, the pressure of condensation will intensify the initial minimal inflammatory response and it will subsequently increase the formation of reparative dentin to a level comparable with that formed after the use of a low-speed air-water spray technique (Fig. 5–4). Practitioners whose work is principally related to indirect restorations that are luted into place are at a disadvantage because their technique precludes the stimulation of RDF and its benefits to protect the health of the pulp. The pulp responses from the insertion of the cohesive and compacted gold are also associated with condensation, whether with hand instruments or with mechanical pneumatic instruments. The responses develop when the condensation occurs over freshly cut dentinal tubules, but not when dentinal tubules are lined with preoperatively formed reparative dentin induced from previous episodes of disease or restorative procedures.

Soremark and associates (1968) showed that radioactive mercury reached the pulp in humans after 6 days if no cavity liner was used. They found that areas in dentin near the amalgam had a high mercury content and that the rate of diffusion into enamel and dentin was inversely related to the degree of mineralization. Generally, this implies that enamel and dentin that were more mineralized in older patients permitted less penetration of mercury ions. The penetration rate was even lower if the water component in enamel and dentin was reduced, as occurs in a nonvital tooth.

Kurosaki and Fusayama (1973) showed that mercury from amalgam restorations in humans and dogs did not reach the pulp. In fact, it did not penetrate dentin that had been demineralized intentionally before placement of the amalgam. They also claimed that the discoloration of the tooth was caused by ions other than mercury in the amalgam. They postulated that, as the γ_2 phase corrodes, mercury does not leach out, as does tin, but instead repenetrates the amalgam and reacts further with previously unreacted alloy particles. Stephen and Ingram (1969) reported similar findings. van der Linden and van Aken (1973), studying human teeth, also found no mercury in the more radiopaque dentin beneath amalgam restorations. Previously, it had been thought that this layer was prominent because of mercury diffusion. Instead, only zinc and tin were found in high concentrations in the dentin beneath the amalgam restoration. These findings were confirmed by Halse (1975), using human teeth.

Chemically Cured Resin Composites. The addition of mineral fillers to the direct-filling, chemically cured resin composites (CCRCs) in the 1960s and 1970s did not reduce their potential for creating severe pulp responses. The filled resin composites, if not properly lined, still cause chronic pulpitis that persists for an indefinite time even in cavities of ordinary depth (dentin thickness of approximately 1 mm). These CCRCs maintained their potential for irritating the pulp because they still required the use of matrix pressure to enhance adaptation to the cavity walls during polymerization.

Unlike the early response of the pulp to low-speed cavity preparation techniques, the response to composite restorations may take several days to 3 weeks to develop a massive pulp lesion. Some moderate to severe degrees of pulp response could be expected no matter which proprietary CCRC is used (Fig. 5–5). In the past, a thin coating of a hard-setting CH cement was recommended for deep cavity preparations and over areas of all freshly cut dentin before any composite materials were placed.

Visible Light-Cured Resin Composites. It is important to obtain as complete a polymerization as possible through the entire composite restoration to minimize pulp responses. The level of the pulp response to resin composite restorations is especially intensified in deep cavity preparations when an incomplete curing of the resin permits an even higher concentration of residual unpolymerized monomer to reach the pulp. As experience revealed the deficiencies and dangers of ultraviolet light-cured (UVLC) systems, visible light-cured (VLC) systems were developed that provided a greater depth of cure, shorter curing times, less porosity, and more wear-resistant composite restorations. The incandescent lamps maintain a more constant energy output and reduce curing problems. The modulus of elasticity of most CCRCs reaches only a fraction of their final value about 10 minutes after mixing, whereas the VLC resin composite restorations approach 24-hour values after only 10 minutes.

Although the visible light source is better controlled than the older UVLC systems, variations in intensity still occur and the effective wavelength is not always constant. It is prudent to use twice the recommended time exposure to light recommended by the manufacturer. These materials cannot be overcured by light, but certainly they can be left undercured.

No matter what types of lamps (ultraviolet or visible light) are developed for the dental profession, insufficient energy is available to cure a large volume or thickness in one application; it must be cured in incremental layers. Generally, an increase in the size of a tooth preparation and the mass of the restoration are associated with greater shrinkage of the restoration. Volumetric shrinkage

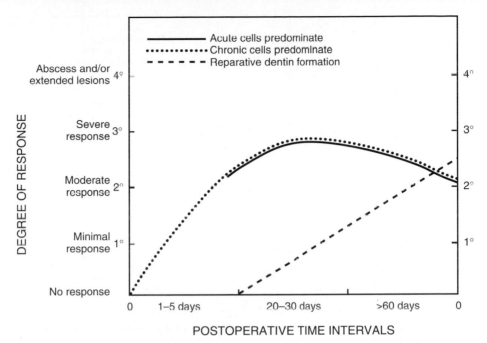

Figure 5–5. Effect of placing a self-cured (chemical-cured) resin composite with the use of pressure on insertion after high-speed cutting with air-water spray; no cavity lining. The material is not particularly toxic initially, so the response begins with a few chronic cells. Acute cells appear after day 5, and a severe response develops subsequently. The reparative dentin formation is excessive. (Redrawn from Stanley HR: Dental iatrogenesis. Int Dent J 44:3–18, 1994.)

accompanying the polymerization reaction, that is, the conversion of the plastic, moldable matrix resin into a solid matrix, is still the overwhelming obstacle in maintaining adhesion and minimizing microleakage. Accordingly, a more conservative cavity preparation with incremental placement of the resin composite is highly recommended for posterior restorations.

Since light-cured techniques with incremental layering were introduced, composites that were previously quite toxic to the pulp have become less so with the elimination of the need for matrices and pressure to gain acceptable adaptation (Fig. 5–6).

Zinc Phosphate Cement. When used as a base, that is, as a thick, puttylike mass, zinc phosphate cement is not a highly toxic substance compared with CCRCs. However, with cementation procedures, a different situation occurs. Few signs of pulp inflammation result when a temporary crown is cemented with a ZOE-type cement after crown preparation using a high-speed air-water technique. However, if a thin mix of zinc phosphate cement is used instead of ZOE to cement a crown or inlay, a strikingly different response occurs. When the patient bites down on a tongue blade to seat the restoration, the phosphoric acid within the mix of zinc phosphate cement is forced into the dentinal tubules in such quantity that it creates, after 3 or 4 days, a widespread three-dimensional lesion involving all the coronal pulp tissue (Fig. 5–7).

A young tooth with wide-open dentinal tubules is more susceptible to such an intense inflammatory response than is an older tooth, which has produced a considerable amount of sclerotic and reparative dentin that blocks the tubules and prevents acids from reaching the pulp. Because the presence of reparative

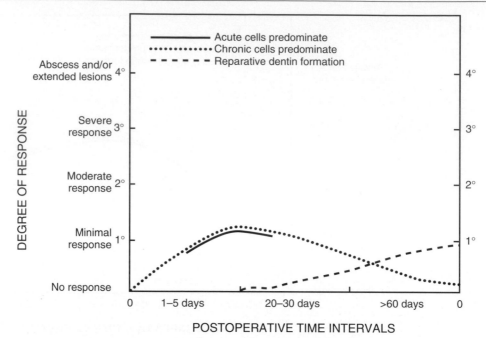

Figure 5–6. Effect of placing a visible light-cured resin composite, with no insertion pressure (incremental layering), high-speed cutting, air-water spray, and no cavity lining. Much flatter curves are shown compared with Figure 5–5. Minimal responses lead to a reduction in magnitudes of all three variables. (Redrawn from Stanley HR: Dental iatrogenesis. Int Dent J 44:3–18, 1994.)

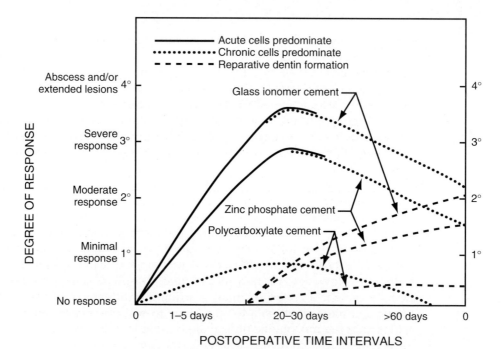

Figure 5–7. Effect of placing luting agents applied with ≤0.5 mm of remaining dentin thickness (RDT). Glass ionomer cement, when used without protective agents as shown here, produces a greater response than zinc phosphate cement. Polycarboxylate cement does not produce such a strong response. (Redrawn from Stanley HR: Dental iatrogenesis. Int Dent J 44:3–18, 1994.)

dentin cannot be predicted, the best protection against phosphoric acid penetration is provided by coating the dentin with two coats of an appropriate varnish, dentin bonding agent, liner, or a thin wash of CH. These procedures eliminate 90% of the severity of the adverse pulp responses. Thus, the pulp response appears similar to those induced by polycarboxylate cements. CH cement mechanically plugs dentinal tubules and neutralizes acids. As mentioned earlier, hydrophilic resin primers may be used to seal tubules and infiltrate the collagen mesh produced by acid-etching the dentin.

Glass Ionomer Cement. When glass ionomer cement (GIC) was first introduced as a restorative material, the pulp responses were classified as bland, moderate, and less irritating than silicate cement, zinc phosphate cement, and CCRC. Nevertheless, several investigators recommended the use of CH in sites close to the pulp.

The blandness of the GIC was attributed to the absence of strong acids and toxic monomers. Polyacrylic acid and related polyacids are much weaker than phosphoric acid and, as polymers, they possess higher molecular weights that may limit their diffusion through the dentinal tubules to the pulp. Later, other acids were added, including itaconic acid, which lowers the viscosity of the solution and increases the reactivity of the polyacrylic acid with the glass particles, and tartaric acid, which extends the working time of the cement and accelerates the setting time. Maleic, mesaconic, and similar unsaturated acids have also been added.

In some water-hardening (water-setting) formulations, the glass powder was blended with polyacrylic acid powder, and the cement was formed by mixing this powder blend with water or diluted tartaric acid solution. The elimination of the viscous polyacid solution from the system yielded a more satisfactory mix that was fluid and easily workable. Ketac-Fil (ESPE-GmbH) is a water-hardening cement product that consists of dried polymaleic acid powder instead of polyacrylic acid, with an aqueous solution of tartaric acid that supposedly leaves little or no unreacted anhydrous polymaleic acid.

Smith and Ruse (1986) compared the initial acidity of GIC with zinc polycarboxylate and zinc phosphate cements and found a general rise in pH for all cements during the first 15 minutes. The liquids in the zinc phosphate and zinc polycarboxylate cements reacted rapidly with the zinc oxide powder, causing the pH to rise to above 2.0 after 1 minute of mixing. However, the initial reactions of the GICs were slower, exhibiting a pH of 2.0 at 5 minutes and a pH of 3.0 after 10 minutes.

When Pameijer and Stanley (1984) permitted an anhydrous GIC to set under continuous pressure (simulating crown cementation), pulp abscesses (4-degree) and intense (severe) hemorrhage (3-degree) occurred when the RDT was 0.5 mm or less. When Duralay Class V resin templates coated with GIC were held under pressure, simulating the hydraulic pressures occurring during crown cementation with GIC, neither abscesses nor severe hemorrhages occurred in those specimens with RDTs less that 1 mm. However, a mean inflammatory cellular pulp response of 1.67 degrees developed and persisted through the 60-day PTI. This value exceeded the acceptable response level of 1.5° and showed the importance of RDT in determining the pulp response to GIC luting agents. GICs, regardless of the technique of mixing, or trituration, appear to be pulp irritants only when used as luting agents. Therefore, it was recommended at that time that a small dab of CH be applied only to areas of extensive crown preparations whenever any site of the preparation was believed to be within 1 mm of the pulp before the cementation procedure was carried out. This provided the required pulp protection to the critical areas without decreasing the overall adhesion benefits of the GIC. Lately, dentin adhesives that seal dentinal tubules and infiltrate etched dentin are being used in addition to CH.

Resin-based Composite Cements (Dual-Cure). Resin-based cements are indicated for all-ceramic crowns, metal-ceramic crowns, ceramic veneers, and porcelain inlays. Because of the relatively low viscosity of resin cements, proper restorative seating with less pressure reduces the possibility for luting voids beneath stress-bearing areas where fractures are most likely to occur. Because of their adhesive and bonding potential, resin-based composite cementation agents appear to increase the fracture resistance of all ceramic crowns by as much as 100% compared with traditional cements.

In 1992, Pameijer and Stanley compared the pulp responses to dual-cured (light-cured and chemically self-cured) resin-based cementation agents. The resin composites were inserted and held under pressure by means of preformed, clear plastic cervical matrices until polymerization was completed. Only when the dual-cure resin cement received no visible light energy did the average pulp response levels exceed the accepted level of biocompatibility and resemble pulp responses associated with the CCRCs developed earlier. When dealing with dual-cure types of resin composites, it is important to use an adequate light-curing time. If the time is inadequate, the self-cure mechanism may not be effective to complete polymerization of the remaining uncured resin that was light cured. Excessive pulp responses may then occur. Adequate light exposure must be ensured buccolingually and interproximally. The increase in exposure time to visible light is not harmful to pulp tissue (Fig. 5–8).

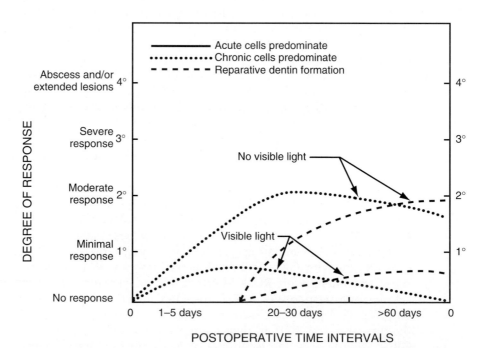

Figure 5–8. Effect of placing dual-cure resin cements (with and without visible light). When these materials are sufficiently cured, the pulpal response curves remain virtually flat. Without the adjunctive use of visible light, the response is greater. (Redrawn from Stanley HR: Dental iatrogenesis. Int Dent J 44:3–18, 1994.)

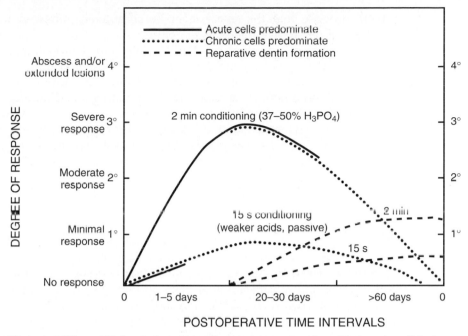

Figure 5–9. Effect of high-speed cutting with air water spray and application of conditioning agents on dentin. The shorter the conditioning time and the weaker the acid, the less marked the pulp response. (Redrawn from Stanley HR: Dental iatrogenesis. Int Dent J 44:3–18, 1994.)

The same physiologic laws that explain the toxicity of zinc phosphate cement also apply to GICs. More acid solution and less powder in the mixture increase the probability of acid diffusion within dentin. In addition, an increase in conditioning time and hydraulic pressure increases the severity of pulp responses (Fig. 5-9). Pulp responses to inlays and crowns of cast metals, porcelain, and ceramics are determined not only by the ingredients of the restorations but also by the type of cementation agent and technique that are used.

Conditioning (etching) Agents.[4] Conditioning procedures are used with both resin composite systems and GICs. Before a resin composite or a GIC restorative material is placed, surface contaminants must be removed to permit the micromechanical attachment or the ionic exchange of the dental material with the tooth structure. When these products were first introduced with etching agents, the same concentrations of enamel-etching acids (37% and 50% phosphoric acid) and the time of application (1 to 2 minutes) used for pit and fissure sealants were used on dentin after tooth preparation. However, these high acid concentrations, when applied for extended intervals, remove the smear unit (the smear layer and dentinal tubule plugs), funnel the orifices of the tubules, deplete the surface ions available for chemical bonding, denature the exposed collagen fibers, and increase the potential for severe pulp responses to restorative materials placed subsequently.

Brännstrom (1981) showed that conditioning of dentin and removal of the smear unit allows the ingress of bacteria and the outward flow of dentinal fluid within the tooth-material interfacial region and possibly contributes to formation of a biofilm that interferes with adhesion. Consequently, some scientists recommend that the smear layer should remain, but in a modified form, whereas others propose that the smear layer be completely removed to optimize the bonding of restorative materials to dentin.

In 1977, Brännstrom and Nordenvall noted no demonstrable differences between dentinal surfaces conditioned for 15 seconds and those conditioned for 2 minutes and thus recommended shorter conditioning times. This change represented the beginning of a new phase in dentin conditioning. Mount (1990) reported that the agent that removes the smear layer in 5 seconds can cause considerable demineralization if left in place for 30 seconds, and it can produce pulp damage if left for 60 seconds. Removal of the smear layer and induction of the desired changes by an etching agent were accomplished in 5 to 10 seconds of exposure for a weak acid and in 5 seconds for a strong acid such as 37% phosphoric acid.

By 1982, numerous *in vitro* and *in vivo* studies had demonstrated that the use of less concentrated acids with higher molecular weights and shorter time intervals for conditioning induced minimal pulp responses. Bowen and colleagues (1982) introduced a mordanting solution (acidified ferric oxalate, subsequently replaced by aluminum oxalate) that appeared to dissolve the original smear layer and replace it with a more uniform "artificial" (altered) smear layer. Stanley and coworkers (1988) and Bowen and associates (1983; 1984; 1989) detected little pulp response because of dentinal tubule closure produced by the creation of the new artificial (altered) smear layer. Blosser and Bowen (1988) and Blosser et al. (1989) reported that solutions of aluminum nitrate (2.5%) and oxalic acid (1.5%) or 2.4% nitric acid and 5.7% *N*-phenyl glycine applied for 60 seconds were equally effective as conditioning agents without the use of ferric or aluminum oxalate. Subsequently, in 1990, Hamlin and colleagues demonstrated that the application of a solution of aluminum nitrate and oxalic acid to dentin of extracted teeth for only 5 seconds was sufficient to remove most of the smear layer and a treatment time of 10 seconds was adequate to remove all of the smear layer without opening and widening the tubules.

Thus, these studies suggest that only the surface of the dentin (10-μm depth) needs to be modified and not its deeper layers. Conditioning techniques that are associated with weaker acids, shorter periods of application, and the elimination of rubbing and scrubbing procedures produce a minimal pulp response and satisfactory bonding (see Fig. 5–9).[4]

Bonding Agents. Bonding agents do not appear to be toxic. Between 1975 and 1992, some studies demonstrated that bonding agents helped reduce the expected pulp responses induced by the subsequent placement of the more toxic resin-based composite materials. Lee Pharmaceutical Corporation in 1975 had produced an "adhesion booster" (used either alone with Enamelite, a resin composite, or in conjunction with 50% phosphoric acid) that reduced the pulp responses, even though the acid evidently removed the smear layer and opened the tubules. Since then, other investigators have found no significant pulp responses to bonding agents (Fig. 5–10).

To enhance bonding to a resin-based composite, a fast-setting VLC, low-viscosity (unfilled) resin primer is applied that infiltrates the demineralized dentin surface (smear layer and tubules) and the exposed collagen mesh to form a hybrid layer. On this layer a bonding resin is placed and cured. The plugging of the dentinal tubules prevents the penetration of toxic components to the pulp from subsequently placed resin-based composite restorations (see Fig. 5–10).

In 1991, Pameijer and Stanley evaluated Prisma Universal Bond-2 (PUB-2), a

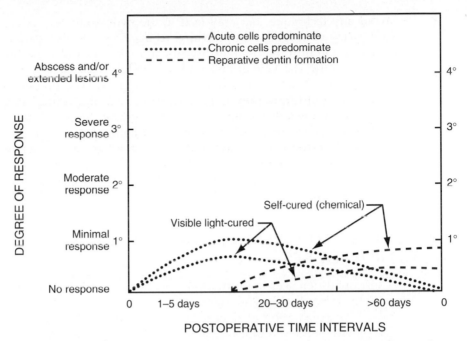

Figure 5–10. Effect of placing a visible light-cured and self-cured (chemical) primers and bonding agents. All the curves are relatively flat and in the minimal or no-response range. (Redrawn from Stanley HR: Dental iatrogenesis. Int Dent J 44:3–18, 1994.)

two-component, no-mix system composed of a dentin primer and an adhesive. The primer contained 30% by weight (30 wt%) hydroxyethyl methacrylate (HEMA), 64 wt% ethanol, and PENTA (Dipent-aerythritol penta-acrylate phosphoric 6 wt% [a patented adhesive promoter]), acid ester 6 wt%. The hydrophilic dentin primer promotes the wettability of the surface; it did not remove the smear layer but modified it by increasing its permeability, thus providing both micromechanical bonding and possibly a chemical interaction with dentin. The adhesive consisted of PENTA and glutaraldehyde (<1%) dispersed in a VLC elastomeric urethane dimethacrylate resin. The adhesive copolymerized chemically with the primer and supposedly to the collagen and hydroxyapatite components of the dentin.

The procedure for using this bonding system consisted of etching the enamel borders of Class V cavity preparations for 60 seconds with a 37% phosphoric acid gel, rinsing for 30 seconds, and drying with oil-free compressed air. The PUB primer was placed into the cavity preparation on all nonenamel surfaces for 30 seconds and allowed to air dry. The adhesive was then placed in the preparations and after slight air thinning was light cured for 10 seconds. Prisma-fil composite was then placed in the cavity and light cured for 40 seconds. Specimens from subhuman primates revealed low-to-average inflammatory cellular response values for all time intervals, despite small-to-average RDT values.

Influence of Patient Age on Pulp Response. Older patients have much less pulp tissue bulk than do younger patients. As permanent teeth endure the effects of abrasion, erosion, caries, and restorative procedures throughout the life span of the host, the pulp becomes reduced in size because of the deposition of primary, secondary, and reparative dentin, the formation of scar tissue, and the ever-increasing size of pulp stones and dystrophic calcifications. It is desirable to avoid any technique that may lead to the overproduction of reparative dentin and excessive reduction in pulp size. At age 55 years, the volume of pulp tissue is about one fifth that at age 25 years and contains only one fifth of its former blood supply. The factors that lead to a reduced vascular component decrease the capacity of the pulp to recover if it is injured. The prognosis for resolution and healing of future pulp lesions increases with the volume of pulp tissue and blood supply whether from disease or iatrogenic causes. Thus, if an inflammatory response develops in the pulp of an aging patient, that pulp has far less defense in resolving a lesion and resisting infection. Clinicians should make every effort to minimize the development of pulp responses and also to treat a tooth in such a way as to help resolve established foci of chronic pulpitis (Stanley, 1990).

PULP RESPONSES TO EXPERIMENTAL AND CLINICAL PROCEDURES

There are differences in pulp responses after experimental procedures compared with those produced by similar procedures in clinical practice. In the experimental cavity preparation of noncarious teeth, reparative dentin does not underlie the patent dentinal tubules, as is usually the case when cavities are prepared in areas of caries or in teeth with older restorations. After cavity preparation, pulps that are covered only with a very thin layer of remaining dentin often receive a liner or base before they are subjected to the direct effects of potentially toxic filling materials. CH products and resin agents, if compatible with a particularly toxic resin-based composite, have been recommended to prevent or modify pulp responses in the past. Dentin bonding procedures are now recommended to seal the dentinal tubules.

Some clinicians have observed that postoperative pulpitis and pulp death result less frequently if indirect restorations are luted with a temporary cement for several months before final cementation. The rationale for this precaution is the belief that permanent cementation should be delayed until reparative dentin forms beneath the patent dentinal tubules that were cut at the time of preparation. This problem has become increasingly significant because mildly traumatic, high-speed, water-cooled cutting techniques have greatly decreased the prevalence of RDF, as shown in Figures 5–2 and 5–3. The average prevalence of RDF for any high-speed, water-cooled technique is 18.7%, and this value decreases as the RDT increases. This is a very low value compared with a prevalence of 40% to 60% with low-speed, water-cooled cutting techniques. Furthermore, if the injured human pulp is not stimulated to form reparative dentin within the first 50 days after a cutting and restorative procedure, reparative dentin will not form from that particular procedure no matter how long one waits.[3] Because the prevalence of RDF is so low with the high-speed, water-cooled techniques, it is unrealistic to wait for reparative dentin to form. More practical approaches include (1) the application of an adequate and effective cavity liner, coating, or base, or (2) sealing the dentin by infiltrating the conditioned dentin with a primer.

MICROLEAKAGE[3]

Brännstrom and colleagues (1971; 1974) have proposed that infection caused by penetration of micro-organisms from marginal leakage around the restoration, and especially beneath it, is a greater threat to the pulp than is the toxicity of the restorative material. Since the classic work of Kakehashi and coworkers (1965) with germ-free animals, an obvious relationship has been established between the presence of micro-organisms and the degree of pulp response.

No doubt pulp lesions that increase in intensity after a PTI longer than 1 week can be caused by the ingress of micro-organisms, but to attribute severe pulpal lesions in short-term experiments to micro-organisms and their by-products without relating such lesions to the potential toxicity of restorative materials themselves is questionable. Unfortunately, the present strong support for the Brännstrom theory has reached a point that many now believe that no restorative material has a toxic potential.

In 1974, Brännstrom and Johnson observed that they could remove most of the smear layer but not the smear plugs in the tubules when they initially scrubbed the surface for 5 seconds with a microbicidal fluoride solution (Tubulicid) and then exposed the dentin to this agent for an additional remaining 60 seconds. This appears to be the first documented evidence that demonstrates one can separate the smear layer from the tubular plugs.

In previous studies, Vojinovic and associates (1973) had observed that the tubular plugs prevented the ingrowth of micro-organisms into the tubules that occurred following the use of demineralizing acids that opened and widened tubular apertures and increased the outward flow of pulp fluid from 10% to 25%. Bergman (1963) had previously demonstrated an outward flow of liquid *in vivo* through the dentinal tubules after drying. The hydrostatic pressure of pulp *in vivo* is higher than that of the mouth, and dentinal fluid moves peripherally through the tubules. Despite this fact, it is presumed that microleakage permits bacteria and their by-products to travel in the opposite direction toward the pulp. This increased amount of moisture can create a biofilm and impair the adhesion potential of subsequently placed restorative materials.

Originally, Brännstrom placed great emphasis on the presence or absence of micro-organisms in the smear layer. Nordenvall and colleagues (1979) predicted that if one micro-organism was left in the smear layer, more than 100 billion organisms could develop within 24 hours if the conditions were favorable. However, Bergenholtz (1982) questioned this view because solitary micro-organisms, particularly anaerobes, with high demands for proper growth conditions, would probably not survive and multiply on the dentin floor where the nutritional supply is poor and where the micro-organisms would be exposed to host-defense factors within the fluid of the dentinal tubules. He also pointed out that although micro-organisms may contribute to the pulp responses beneath restorations, they appear to be unable to sustain a long-standing irritation to the pulp. Unless recurrent caries develops under a clinically defective restoration, the dentin permeability to noxious bacterial agents decreases over time, even under continual bacterial provocation, allowing the pulp to heal. This may partially explain why pulps remain vital in most restored teeth. Consequently, when pulp devitalization occurs after a restorative procedure, it probably results from the combined effect of the mechanical injury induced during cutting of the tooth substance, the toxicity of the restorative materials, and the action of bacteria.

Mejare and coworkers (1987) contaminated cavity preparations by rubbing them with a cotton pellet soaked in saliva, washed the cavities with either a water spray or Tubulicid, and restored them with composite restorations. (One must appreciate that 1 mL [30 drops] of saliva contains approximately 1 billion anaerobes and 100 million aerobes.) The outer half of the composite restoration was then replaced with zinc sulfate cement. Regardless of the cleansing procedure, no bacterial growth occurred. The nutritional supply to the area under a composite restoration sealed with zinc sulfate cement was too poor to allow survival of the bacteria within the smear layer. If growth does occur in the smear layer, it probably is fed from subsequent marginal leakage sources.

Pashley (1990) showed that when cultures of *Streptococcus mutans* colonized the surface of dentin disks *in vitro*, they did not invade the tubules until they generated enough metabolic acids after several days to dissolve away the smear layer and tubular plugs. However, if the dentin disk was first etched with acid to remove the smear unit and some of the peritubular dentin, thereby increasing the dentin permeability more than 50%, the bacteria rapidly invaded the tubules. Similarly, Meryon (1988) demonstrated *in vitro* that *Streptococcus faecalis* was unable to penetrate the smear layer during the first 48 hours and *Escherichia coli* did not penetrate for 96 hours. Generally, most newly placed materials are somewhat toxic and bactericidal but lose their antibacterial effects as they cure and age. In the first few days, amalgam and silicate cement are as antimicrobial as ZOE, but the antibacterial effects of ZOE last much longer.

For the past several years investigators have performed Brown and Brenn staining of specimens in numerous toxicologic pulp studies and have been unable to establish any acceptable correlation between the presence, absence, and quantity of micro-organisms and the presence and intensity of the pulp lesions. For every lesion possibly associated with micro-organisms, one can find lesions with no organisms present. Also, one can find normal pulps with micro-organisms present.

Although it is doubtful that marginal leakage will ever be completely eliminated, it certainly can be controlled. When extensive leakage is associated with a clinically defective restoration, recurrent caries can occur. No one would question the importance of invading micro-organisms under such circumstances, but how important clinically is marginal leakage of a lesser degree? Further research is needed to identify the specific effects of microbial activity associated with microleakage. Greater emphasis on germ-free studies will help resolve this dilemma.

If the pulp is not inflamed, there is absolutely no reason for dental procedures to cause pulp death. All the parameters have been established to guide dentists in their efforts to provide the best treatment.

THE OCCURRENCE OF DENTIN HYPERSENSITIVITY[4]

When one considers the problems and confusion resulting from dentin hypersensitivity studies, several factors must be taken into account that can have a major influence on the results, including (1) the age and sex of the patient; (2) the age of the tooth; (3) the amount of sclerosis present; (4) the proximity to the pulp (RDT); (5) the presence or absence of CH liners; and (6) the depth of carious lesions versus the thickness of reparative dentin formed.

If no postoperative symptoms occur initially, one might assume that the bonding agent and the micromechanical bond are intact and that there is no active leakage. However, the absence of symptoms may be attributed to sclerosis, reparative dentin, and sufficient RDT present to prevent symptoms, although the micromechanical bond may be degrading and microleakage may be occurring.

If symptoms develop soon after the restoration process, they may be associated with insufficient sclerosis, reparative dentin, or RDT for the peripheral dentinal tubules to protect the pulp. Also, when the nerve endings in the superficial pulp tissues, especially in the odontoblastic layer and predentin, are injured by a restorative procedure, the healing process induces an enormous outgrowth of dendrites that temporarily contributes to increased dentin hypersensitivity. Approximately 21 days are required for complete regeneration of the nerve endings, the removal of the excess degenerating dendrites, and a return to a normal level of dentin sensitivity. Such symptoms occur too soon to consider a breakdown of the micromechanical bond and significant microleakage to be the cause. If symptoms disappear over time, for example, after 7 to 12 weeks, this may mean sufficient reparative dentin has subsequently formed in the critical areas (beneath the more recently cut peripheral tubules) to block the tubules and eliminate postoperative sensitivity.

However, if the symptoms develop over a longer period and persist, then it is reasonable to consider factors such as (1) degradation of the micromechanical bond; (2) shrinkage of resin during polymerization and cohesive failure of the liner or base; (3) exposure of patent dentinal tubules; (4) cusp deformation; (5) excessive occlusal loading of Class II posterior resin composites (especially if the cervical margins are on cementum-dentin); (6) flexing during chewing (because of a low elastic modulus); and (7) thermal stimuli (particularly low-temperature effects) that can increase gap width because of the large thermal contraction of the resin and subsequent microleakage.

If the patient experiences prolonged sensitivity and the composite is replaced with a more conventional restorative material, the symptoms may soon disappear. This result suggests that the involved tubules have now been sealed. The circumstances surrounding this tooth and patient were such that reparative dentin would probably never have formed.

Powell and colleagues (1990, 1991), using teeth from adolescents and a few adults, found that the most severe postoperative pain occurred in females. Stanley and coworkers (1983) had previously reported that females produce less dentinal sclerosis and reparative dentin and that some females produce no reparative dentin even in the presence of deep cervical erosive lesions.

Because all material-tooth interfaces tend to sustain leakage over time, can postoperative sensitivity be reduced or avoided? As explained earlier, an understanding of the factors that contribute to sensitivity must be taken into consideration to answer this question. Certainly as bonding systems seal dentinal tubules, the potential for early postoperative sensitivity is reduced or avoided. At this point, it is not known how soon this hybrid zone of collagen and polymer undergoes degradation. If it does not, the protection will be prolonged indefinitely.

With the improved high resistance to solubility of current luting agents (cements), the potential for postoperative sensitivity should be reduced. Until the ideal restorative material is developed that does not contract on polymerization and pull away from the tooth surface, excessive leakage and the risk for secondary caries will continue.

PULP CAPPING[5]

During the 1940s and 1950s it became apparent that the pulp, like any other organ of the body, could heal itself, provided overwhelming adverse conditions were removed.

The possibility of stimulating reparative dentin over pulp exposures challenged investigators and clinicians alike. Many extracted teeth had shown pulp bridging with reparative dentin, but it was not known how to intentionally initiate regeneration and bridging after the primary odontoblasts were lost. The most promising new materials tested contained spicules of dentin and pastes using CH based on Hermann's introduction of CH in 1920. This approach started a new era in the treatment of dental pulp by demonstrating that a calcium mixture induced bridging of the exposed pulp surface with reparative dentin.

Calcium Hydroxide. Despite the growing success of CH in vital-pulp therapy (pulp capping, pulpotomies, root amputation, apexification, and apexogenesis), considerable confusion and condemnation of this material have long persisted because CH in the pure state and in the original formulations actually killed a certain amount of tissue when placed in direct contact with the pulp rather than merely functioning as a biologic dressing. Numerous studies have also shown that CH is extremely toxic to cells in tissue culture. How can something be destructive and beneficial at the same time in terms of healing?

This destructive characteristic has spurred on a great effort to find a formula that stimulates reparative dentin bridging without sacrificing any of the remaining pulp tissue by chemical cauterization, as occurs with many CH products.

The exact mechanism by which CH generates a dentinal bridge is not clear, but the caustic action associated with its high pH, when solubilized, and its induction of superficial necrosis were assumed to be factors involved in the stimulation of secondary dentin formation.

Histology of Healing After Pulp Capping. Because of the recent adjustments made in the pH of CH, two different modes of healing are now proposed. Because dentin bridge formation resulting from the original CH products of high pH (11 to 13) has been described for many years, and some present-day products still maintain a high pH, it is appropriate to describe the healing leading to bridge formation under high pH conditons. It is also useful to describe the CH materials and the variations induced with the newer, less alkaline CH products.

With a cement like Pulpdent (CH and water), healing leading to bridge formation occurs at the junction of the firm, necrotic nonvital layer created by the caustic (high-alkaline pH) CH agent that destroys 1 mm or more of pulp tissue. The bridge is readily visualized with the radiolucent Pulpdent paste because the degenerated, necrotic zone separates the CH layer from the bridge (Fig. 5–11). However, with the original Dycal material (L. D. Caulk, Dentsply International, Inc., Milford, DE), the calcified dentinal bridge forms directly against the CH (the pulp capping agent) and is more difficult to observe radiographically.

Stanley and Lundy (1972) found that Dycal produced the zone of coagulated necrosis (firm necrosis) similar to that produced by CH and water or Pulpdent but that it was rapidly removed by phagocytes and replaced with granulation tissue that quickly organized, matured, and differentiated odontoblasts to produce the dentinal bridge adjacent to the Dycal. When Dycal is used, the tooth has the same quantity of pulp tissue that had existed before the placement of Dycal. This effect is the same as that associated with the more recent CH products.

With some of the new hard-setting formulations, bridging at the CH-pulp interface occurs without the induction of a visible coagulated necrotic layer, an indication of a less extensive initial chemical (caustic) injury than that produced by capping agents of high pH (Fig. 5–12). Because one or two cell layers closest to the CH dressing are affected, there is not enough tissue destruction to require macrophages to phagocytize the dead and wounded cells and to form

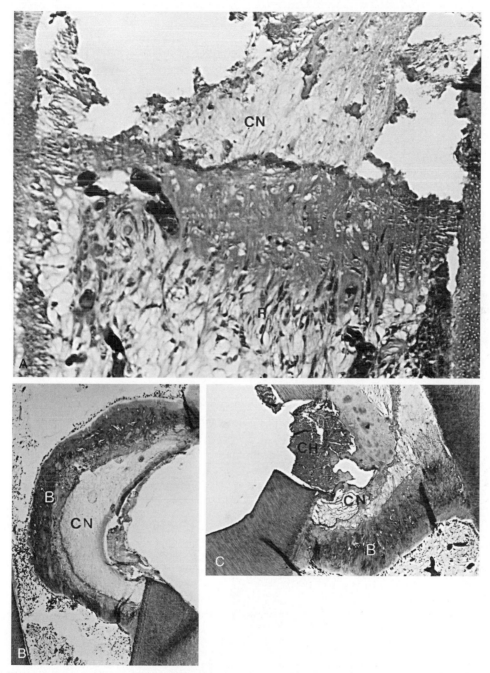

Figure 5–11. A, A line of demarcation can be seen between the chemically cauterized necrotic (CN) tissue created by the application of calcium hydroxide of high pH and the regenerating (R) pulp tissue. Post-treatment period = 7 days. Hematoxylin-eosin stain, ×200. *B,* A mineralized bridge (B) surrounding the remains of coagulated necrotic tissue (CN) pulp tissue. Post-treatment period = 63 days. Hematoxylin-eosin stain, ×80. *C,* Another example of a thick mineralized bridge (B) separated from the calcium hydroxide (CH) by the coagulated necrotic (CN) tissue. Post-treatment period = 60 days. Hematoxylin-eosin stain, ×200. (*B* and *C* from Turner C, Courts FJ, and Stanley HR: A histological comparison of direct pulp capping agents in primary canines. J Dent Child 54:423–428, 1987.)

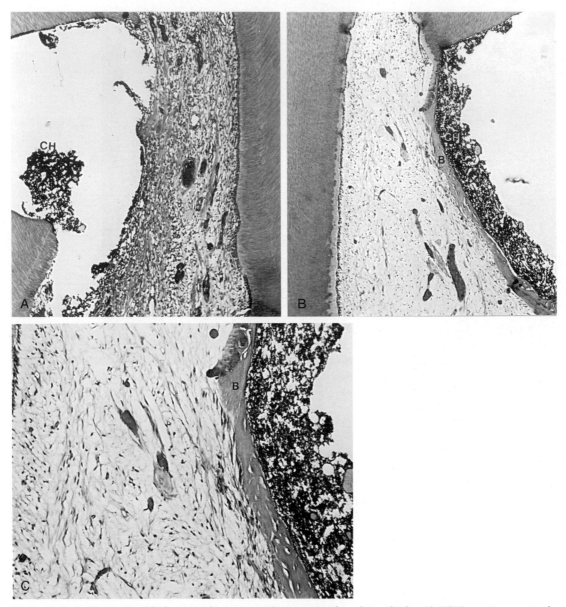

Figure 5–12. A, The porous black material represents the remains of a calcium hydroxide (CH) capping agent of a lower pH where no layer of caustic necrosis exists. Surviving pulp tissue is, however, heavily infiltrated with inflammatory cells. Post-treatment period = 7 days. Hematoxylin-eosin stain, ×80. *B,* A lower magnification view of a mineralized bridge (B) up against the calcium hydroxide (CH) capping agent. The cellular inflammatory infiltrate has disappeared. Post-treatment period = 63 days. Hematoxylin-eosin stain, ×80. *C,* A higher magnification of *B* revealing details of bridge (B) formation butting against the calcium hydroxide capping agent. The subjacent vital pulp tissue has returned to a normal state. Post-treatment period = 63 days. Hematoxylin-eosin stain, ×200. (*B* and *C* from Turner C, Courts FJ, and Stanley HR: A histological comparison of direct pulp capping agents in primary canines. J Dent Child 54:423–428, 1987.)

granulation tissue. Healing and regeneration occur directly against the CH dressing. A sufficient hydroxyl concentration capable of stimulating the differentiation and regeneration of odontoblasts still exists to produce a high-quality dentinal bridge. The capacity to produce a more uniform dentinal bridge adjacent to the capping material is a great advantage.

A capping agent should never be placed on a bleeding pulp. It is also important to control any excessive oozing of serum or plasma that occupies, fills, or creates a space by lifting the pulp capping agent from the pulp tissue. If enough bleeding or oozing occurs under the dressing, it can lift off the dressing and permit the formation of an excessive blood clot or a thick fibropurulent membrane between the dressing and the tissue. This membrane then attracts the elements for granulation tissue replacement and favors organization and differentiation of fibroblasts and odontoblasts to create ectopic RDF in nonideal sites such as in the cavity preparation rather than at the exposure site. While this process is taking place, the clot or stagnated serum is subject to secondary infection, which can lead to complete loss of pulp vitality.

As emphasized previously, hemorrhage must be controlled before application of CH. As one looks at active hemorrhage, one must appreciate that if there are open vessels from the injury to release erythrocytes, there are probably transsectioned venules or venous capillaries capable of transporting particles through the vascular system toward the heart. Sometimes particles of the capping material may enter these channels and travel as emboli until they are lodged somewhere deeper in the pulp tissue. At these sites the caustic effect of the fresh particles of CH (still active chemically) produce perivascular foci of coagulation necrosis and inflammation. If too many embolic phenomena occur in the pulp, these foci may coalesce and cause so much destruction of the pulp that its reparative capacity is lost and the pulp becomes nonvital.

Microbial contamination, dentinal debris, and a lack of a proper peripheral seal can contribute to pulp cap failure. However, another contributing factor may be the operator's inability to perform the proper surgical procedure rather than the inadequacy of the medicament employed. This factor applies also to pulpotomy techniques.

ENDODONTIC PROCEDURES

As a consequence of pathologic changes in the dental pulp, the root canal system can harbor numerous irritants. Depending on the nature and quantity of these irritants, as well as the duration of exposure to the periradicular tissues, destruction of periradicular tissue can occur. As irritants are released from the root canal system into the periradicular tissue, granulation tissue proliferates and replaces normal periradicular tissues. Removal of irritants from the root canal system and its total obturation result in repair of the periradicular tissue to its normal architecture (Fig. 5–13). Grossman grouped obturating materials into plastics, solids, cements, and pastes. He indicated that an ideal root canal filling material should meet the following requirements:

1. It should seal the canal laterally as well as apically.
2. It should not shrink after being inserted.
3. It should be impervious to moisture.
4. It should be bacteriostatic, or at least not encourage bacterial growth.
5. It should not irritate periradicular tissue.
6. It should not provoke an immune response in periradicular tissue.
7. It should be neither mutagenic or carcinogenic.

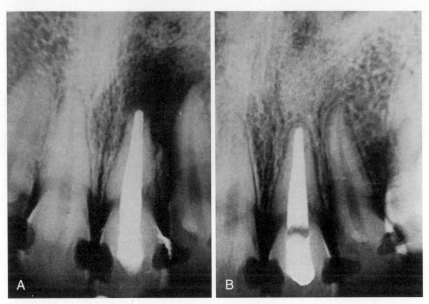

Figure 5–13. A large periradicular lesion in *A* has healed completely within 6 months in a 20-year-old patient, shown in *B*. (From Ingle JJ, and Bakland LK: Endodontics, 4th ed. Baltimore, Williams & Wilkins, 1994, p 32.)

The method most frequently used in filling root canals involves the use of solid-core points that are inserted in conjunction with cementing materials (sealers). The sealers form a fluid-tight seal at the apex by filling (1) the minor interstices between the solid material and the wall of the canal and (2) the patent accessory canals with multiple foramina. Gutta-percha is by far the most universally used solid-core root canal filling material and may be classified as a plastic. Modern plastics have been disappointing as solid-core endodontic filling materials.

Many endondontists believe that filling just short of the radiograph apex is preferred to overfilling. The space between the root filling and the apical tissue surface fills in with new connective tissue within a few months to complete the repair process. A minimal reaction was found when the canal was not overfilled. In contrast, the teeth with overfilled root canals exhibited persistent chronic inflammatory responses. When evaluating the apical responses with experimental products, the clinician should note whether the experimental material was confined within the canal or extended into the apical tissues.

Sealer Efficacy. Although all root canal sealers leak to some extent, there is probably a critical level of leakage that is unacceptable for healing and that may result in endodontic failure. This leakage may occur at the interface of the dentin and sealer, at the interface of the solid core and sealer, through the sealer itself, or by dissolution of the sealer.

All currently available sealers leak, and they are not impermeable. Some leak more than others, mostly through dissolution. The broader the sealer–periradicular tissue interface, the faster the dissolution will take place. Moreover, all sealers shrink slightly on setting. Fortunately, most of the root canal sealers currently used, as well as the solid-core filling materials, are eventually tolerated by the periradicular tissue once the cements have set.

If the apical orifice can be blocked principally by a solid-core material, success is immeasurably improved over time. On the other hand, in most studies in which obturation without sealers was attempted, the leakage results were enormously greater. Thus, sealers are essential for endodontic therapy to be successful.

Percolation of periradicular exudate into incompletely filled canals is the greatest cause of endodontic failure. Nearly 60% of failures are apparently caused by incomplete obliteration of the radicular space (root canals). Many studies indicate that most fillings do not completely fill the root canal system.

It appears safe to assume that the noxious products leaking from the apical foramen act as an inflammatory irritant. It is presently speculated that the transudate constantly leaking into the partially filled canal arises indirectly from the blood serum and consists of a number of water-soluble proteins, enzymes, and salts. It is further speculated that the serum is trapped in the cul-de-sac of the poorly filled canal, away from the influences of the blood stream in which it undergoes degradation. Later, when the degraded serum slowly diffuses to the periradicular tissue, it acts as an irritant to produce the periapical inflammation of chronic apical periodontitis.

Such a sequence of events might well explain the paradox of the periradicular lesion associated with a noninfected pulpless tooth. Periradicular inflammation is presumed to persist under the influence of any noxious substance. Bacteria certainly play a major role in the production of these products in the root canal. However, in the absence of bacteria, degraded serum, per se, may well assume the role of the primary tissue irritant. If the canal is not filled perfectly, serum will seep into it from the apical tissues. With sufficient bacteria present, the situation worsens. The serum may furnish nutrient material for any micro-organisms remaining in the tubules.

Without question, all the materials used to seal root canals irritate periradicular tissue if allowed to escape from the canal or if placed against a pulp stump, as in a partial pulpectomy. The argument seems to be not whether the tissue is irritated but rather the degree of inflammation and for how long the condition has persisted.

Although arborization of the pulp at the periapical area is more likely to happen in dogs and monkeys than in humans, the final filling is no better than its preparation, and if necrotic dentin and debris are left in place, the case stands a greater chance of eventual failure. Even with the best and most experienced clinicians, debris is usually found within the canal when the tooth is examined histopathologically.

Apical Filling with Dentin Chips. Inadvertently, dentin chips may produce an apical plug against which other materials are then compacted. Each apical foramen may actually be occluded by dentin chips produced by the endodontic procedure. To condense dentin chips deliberately constitutes a "new technique" or a "biologic seal" rather than a mechanical-chemical seal.

Such a "plug" can prevent overfilling and can restrict the irrigating solutions and obturating materials to the canal spaces. After the canal is totally débrided and shaped, a drill or file is used to produce dentin powder in the central position of the canal. These dentin chips may then be pushed apically and packed into place. However, when biocompatibility studies are performed with experimental products, care must be taken that a dentin chip plug is not induced so as to not bias the results, because the chemical components of the experimental material will not reach the periapical site in a concentration sufficient to produce a potential lesion.

From the earlier description concerning the problems and deficiencies with endodontic therapy, one can appreciate why there is a continual research endeavor to find the ideal obturating material.

PRIMARY REVIEW ARTICLES

The bulk of the material in this chapter is based on the five review papers listed here. For more detailed information and a greater emphasis on the contribution of the authors, refer to these articles, which are listed by superscripted number in the chapter.

1. Stanley HR: Biological evaluation of dental materials. Int Dent J 42:37, 1992.
2. Stanley HR: Local and systemic responses to dental composites and glass ionomers. Adv Dent Res 6:55, 1992.
3. Stanley HR: Dental iatrogenesis. Int Dent J 44:3, 1994.
4. Stanley HR: Pulpal consideration of adhesive materials. Operat Dent Suppl 5:151, 1992.
5. Stanley HR: Pulp capping: Conserving the dental pulp—Can it be done? Is it worth it? Oral Surg Oral Med Oral Pathol 68:628, 1989.

SELECTED READING

AAMI Standards and Recommended Practices, Vol 4: Biological Evaluation of Medical Devices. Arlington, VA, Association for the Advancement of Medical Instrumentation, 1994, p 40.

Axelsson J, Johansson S, and Wrangsjo K: IgE-mediated anaphylactoid reactions to rubber. Allergy 42:46, 1987.

Baker S, Brooks SC, and Walker DM: The release of residual monomeric methyl methacrylate from acrylic appliances in the human mouth: An assay for monomer in saliva. J Dent Res 67:1295, 1988.

Bergenholtz G: Relationship between bacterial contamination of dentin and restorative success. In: Rowe N (ed): Reaction to Restorative Materials in the Presence or Absence of Infection: Proceedings of Symposium on Dental Pulp. Ann Arbor, University of Michigan, 1982, pp 93–107.

Bergman G: Microscopic demonstration of liquid flow through human dental enamel. Arch Oral Biol 8:233, 1963.

Blinkhorn AS, and Leggate EM: An allergic reaction to rubber dam. Br Dent J 156:402, 1984.

Blosser RL, and Bowen RL: Effects of purified ferric oxalate/nitric acid solutions as a pretreatment for the NTA-GMA and PMDM bonding system. Dent Mater 5:255, 1988.

Bowen RL, and Cobb EN: A method for bonding to dentin and enamel. J Am Dent Assoc 107:734, 1983.

Bowen RL, Cobb EN, and Misra DN: Adhesive bonding by surface initiation of polymerization Industrial Engineering Chemical Products Research Division 23:78, 1984. *Part 28 of a series on adhesive bonding of various materials to hard tooth tissues.*

Bowen RL, Cobb EN, and Rapson JE: Adhesive bonding of various materials to hard tooth tissues: Improvement in bond strength to dentin. J Dent Res 61:1070, 1982.

Bowen RL, Rupp NW, Eichmiller FC, and Stanley HR: Clinical biocompatibility of an experimental dentine-enamel adhesive for composites. Int Dent J 39:247, 1989.

Brännstrom M: Dentin and Pulp in Restorative Dentistry. Nacka, Sweden, Dental Therapeutics AB, 1981.

Brännstrom M, and Johnson G: Effects of various conditioners and cleaning agents on prepared dentin surfaces. J Prosthet Dent 36:422, 1974.

Brännstrom M, and Nordenvall KJ: The effect of acid etching on enamel, dentin, and the inner surface of the resin restoration: A scanning electron microscopic investigation. J Dent Res 56:917, 1977.

Brännstrom M, and Nyborg H: The presence of bacteria in cavities filled with silicate cement and composite resin materials. Swed Dent J 64:149, 1971.

Bratel J, and Jontell M: Effect of selective replacement of amalgam fillings on lichenoid reactions [Abstract]. J Dent Res 73:127, 1994.

Council on Dental Materials, Instruments, and Equipment; Council on Dental Therapeutics; and Council on Dental Research: Reactions to latex in the health care setting: Dealing with patient/worker concerns. J Am Dent Assoc 124:91, 1993.

Dorland's Illustrated Medical Dictionary, 28th ed. Philadelphia, WB Saunders, 1994, p 198.

Field EA, and King CM: Skin problems associated with routine wearing of protective gloves in dental practice. Br Dent J 169:281, 1990.

Grossman LI: Endodontic Practice, 10th ed. Philadelphia, Lea & Febiger, 1982, p. 297.

Halse A: Metals in dentinal tubules beneath amalgam fillings in human teeth. Arch Oral Biol 20:87, 1975.

Hamlin P, Lynch E, and Samarawickrama D: Effect of a new conditioning agent on dentin. Am J Dent 3:119, 1990.

Hermann BW: Calciumhydroxyd als mittel zum behandeln und fullen von wurzelkanalen [Dissertation]. Wurzberg, Germany, 1920.

Ingle JI, and Bakland LK: Endodontics, 4th ed. Baltimore, Williams & Wilkins, 1994, pp 208; 228–235, 240–246, 290, 439.

International Organization for Standardization/Technical Committee (ISO/DIS): Preclinical Evaluation of Biocompatibility of Medical Devices Used in Dentistry Test Methods, No. 7405. International Organization for Standardization, January, 1995.

Kakehashi S, Stanley HR, and Fitzgerald RJ: The effects of surgical exposures of dental pulps in germ-free and conventional laboratory rats. Oral Surg Oral Med Oral Pathol 20:340, 1965.

Kurosaki N, and Fusayama T: Penetration of elements from amalgam into dentin. J Dent Res 52:309, 1973.

Laeijendecker R, and van Joost T: Oral manifestations of gold allergy. JAMA 271:818, 1994.

Mackert JR Jr, Fairhurst CW, and Rueggeberg FA: Dental Materials—DPS 531. Augusta, GA, Medical College of Georgia, 1988.

Malten KE, Nater JP, and Van Ketal WG. Patch Testing Guidelines. Nijmegen, The Netherlands, Dekker & van de Vegt, 1976, p 63.

March PJ: An allergic reaction to latex rubber gloves. J Am Dent Assoc 117:590, 1988.

Mejare I, Mejare B, and Edwardsson S: Effect of a tight seal on survival of bacteria in saliva-contaminated cavities filled with composite resin. Endodont Dent Traumatol 3:6, 1987.

Meryon SD: The model cavity method incorporating dentine. Int Endodont J 21:79, 1988.

Mount GJ: Glass ionomer cements: Clinical considerations. In: Hardin JF (ed): Clark's Clinical Dentistry, Vol 4, 2nd ed. Hagerstown, MD, Harper & Row, 1990, pp 1–24.

Nordenvall KJ, Brännstrom M, and Torstensson B: Pulp reactions and micro-organisms under ASPA and Concise composite fillings. J Dent Child 46:449, 1979.

Pameijer CH, and Stanley HR: Primate response to anhydrous Chembond [Abstract]. J Dent Res 63:171, 1984.

Pameijer CH, and Stanley HR: Pulp reactions to resin cements. Am J Dent 5:81, 1992.

Pameijer CH, Stanley HR, and Ecker G: Biocompatibility of a glass ionomer luting agent. II. Crown cementation. Am J Dent 4:134, 1991.

Pashley DH: Clinical considerations of microleakage. J Endodont 16:70, 1990.

Podshadley AG: Gingival response to pontics. J Prosthet Dent 19:51, 1969.

Powell LV, Gordon GE, and Johnson GH: Sensitivity restored of class V abrasion/erosion lesions. J Am Dent Assoc 121:694, 1990.

Powell LV, and Johnson GH: Personal communication, 1991.

Rankin KV, Jones DL, and Rees TD: Latex reactions in an adult dental population. Am J Dent 6:274, 1993.

Slavin RG, and Ducomb DF: Allergic contact dermatitis. Hosp Pract 24:39, 1989.

Smith DC, and Ruse ND: Acidity of glass ionomer cements during setting and its relation to pulp sensitivity. J Am Dent Assoc 112:654, 1986.

Snyder HA, and Settle S: The rise in latex allergy: Implications for the dentist. J Am Dent Assoc 125:1089, 1994.

Soremark R, Wing K, Olsson K, and Goldin J: Penetration of metallic ions from restorations in teeth. J Prosthet Dent 20:531, 1968.

Stanley HR, and Lundy T: Dycal therapy for pulp exposures. Oral Surg Oral Med Oral Pathol 34:818, 1972.

Stanley HR, Bowen RL, and Cobb EN: Pulp responses to a dentin and enamel adhesive bonding procedure. Oper Dent 13:107, 1988.

Stanley HR, Pereira JC, Spiegel E, et al: The detection and prevalence of reactive and physiologic sclerotic dentin, reparative dentin, and dead tracts beneath various types of dental lesions according to root surface and age. J Oral Pathol 12:257, 1983.

Stephen HY, and Ingram MJ: Analyses of the amalgam-tooth interface using the electron microprobe. J Dent Res 48:317, 1969.

Swerdlow H, and Stanley HR: Response of the human pulp to amalgam restoration. Oral Surg Oral Med Oral Pathol 15:499, 1962.

US Food and Drug Administration: Allergic reactions to latex-containing medical devices. FDA Medical Alert, MDA91-1, March 29, 1991.

van der Linden LWJ, and van Aken J: The origin of localized increased radiopacity in the dentin. Oral Surg Oral Med Oral Pathol 35:862, 1973.

Vojinovic O, Nyborg H, and Brännstrom M: Acid treatment of cavities under resin fillings: Bacterial growth in dentinal tubules and pulpal reactions. J Dent Res 52:1189, 1973.

6 *Hydrocolloid Impression Materials*

- Purpose and Requirements of Impression Materials
- Classification of Impression Materials
- Colloids
- General Characteristics of Gels
- Agar (Reversible Hydrocolloid)
- Manipulation of Agar Impression Materials
- Accuracy of Agar Impression Material
- Alginate (Irreversible Hydrocolloid)
- Manipulation of Alginate Impression Material
- Additional Applications of Hydrocolloids
- Care and Handling of Hydrocolloid Impressions

TERMINOLOGY

Aerosol–colloidal sol composed of liquid or solid in air

Agar (reversible hydrocolloid)–an aqueous impression material used for recording maximum detail, such as that required to produce dies for fixed restorations

Alginate (irreversible hydrocolloid)–an aqueous impression material used for recording minimal detail, such as that required to produce study models

Aqueous elastomers–agar or alginate hydrocolloid

Cast–a dimensionally accurate reproduction of a portion of the oral cavity and extraoral facial structures produced in a durable hard material and used as a base for construction of orthodontic and prosthetic appliances

Colloid–suspension of two phases

Dispersed phase, dispersed particle–particles in a solution

Dispersion phase, dispersed medium–solution suspending the particles

Elastomer–lightly cross-linked impression material with elastic properties

Evaporation–conversion of water from the liquid state to the vapor state

Gel–network of fibrils that form a weak, slightly elastic brush-heap structure

Gelation–transformation from sol to gel

Hydrocolloid–colloid that contains water as the dispersion phase

Hydrophilic–strong affinity for water

Hydrophobic–lack of affinity for water

Imbibition–absorption of water

Irreversible hydrocolloid–alginate impression material

Lyophilic–strong affinity between dispersed and continuous phase in a colloid

Lyosol–colloidal sol of gas, liquids, or solids in liquid

Model–a positive full-scale replica of the dentition and surrounding or adjoining structures used as a diagnostic aid

Reversible hydrocolloid–agar impression material

Syneresis–fluid exuded when gel structures reconfigure to achieve equilibrium through stress relaxation

Thermoplastic–reversible "setting" based on a physical effect produced by a temperature change—warm/sol $\rightleftharpoons$ cold/gel

Thermosetting–"setting" reaction that involves a chemical change that is not easily reversible

Undercuts–recessed areas on oral structures including teeth, edentulous ridges, appliances, and restorations

PURPOSE AND REQUIREMENTS OF IMPRESSION MATERIALS

Constructing a cast or model is an important step in numerous dental procedures. Various types of casts and models can be made from gypsum products using an impression or negative likeness as a mold for the gypsum. It is on the gypsum cast that the dentist designs and constructs both removable and fixed prostheses. Thus, the cast must be an accurate representation of the oral structures.

To produce an accurate impression, the materials used to produce replicas of intraoral and some extraoral tissues should fulfill the following criteria. First, they should be fluid enough to adapt to the oral tissue and viscous enough to remain contained in the tray that delivers the impression to the mouth. Second, while in the mouth, they should transform (set) into a rubbery solid in a reasonable amount of time; ideally, the total setting time should be less than 7 minutes. Finally, the set impression should not distort or tear when removed from the mouth, and the materials should remain dimensionally stable so the cast can be poured.

Environmental conditions and the characteristics of the tissue often dictate the choice of materials, the quality of the impression, and the quality of the cast. This chapter and the following two chapters discuss the unique properties of the currently used impression materials and how these characteristics affect the quality of an impression and therefore of a cast or model constructed from the impression.

CLASSIFICATION OF IMPRESSION MATERIALS

The impression materials can be classified as *reversible* or *irreversible,* according to the manner in which the material sets (or hardens). The term *irreversible* implies that chemical reactions have occurred; thus, the material cannot be reverted to its preset state in the dental office. For example, alginate hydrocolloid, zinc oxide–eugenol (ZOE) impression paste, and plaster of Paris harden by chemical reactions, and elastomeric impression materials set by polymerization.

On the other hand, *reversible* means the materials soften under heat and solidify when they are cooled, with no chemical change taking place. Reversible hydrocolloid and impression compounds belong to this category. Impression compounds are mixtures of resin and wax and are classified as *thermoplastic* substances.

Another way of classifying dental impression materials is according to their use. Some impression materials become rigid and cannot be removed past undercuts without fracturing or distorting the impression. These inelastic impression materials were used for all impressions before the advent of agar. Although they are obsolete for dentate patients, the inelastic materials have some advantages for making impressions of edentulous patients. In fact, ZOE impression paste and plaster of Paris are called *mucostatic impression materials* because they do not compress the tissue during seating of the impression. Before the recent development of the very fluid light-body elastomeric impression materials, impression paste and plaster of Paris were often the materials of choice to record the oral structures for complete denture prostheses. The other material classified as inelastic is impression compound.

Elastic impression materials define the second usage category. These materials are capable of accurately reproducing both the hard and soft structures of the mouth, including the undercuts and interproximal spaces. Although these materials can be employed for edentulous impressions, they are used most extensively to prepare casts for fixed and removable partial dentures as well as for single restorative units.

Table 6–1 shows the classification of the various dental impression materials based on setting mechanism, dental application, and mechanical deformation behavior.

COLLOIDS

Colloids are often classified as a fourth state of matter, the *colloidal state*, because of their differences in structure, constitution, and reactions. How does a colloid differ from a solid and a liquid? Let us first examine a solution of sugar in water. The sugar molecules (or solute) are assumed to be dispersed uniformly in the water (or solvent). There is no visible, physical separation between the solute and the solvent molecules. If the sugar molecules are replaced with larger, visible, nonsoluble particles, such as sand (in water), the system is termed a *suspension*. If these particles become liquids, like vegetable oil in water, the system is then called an *emulsion*. These suspended particles or liquid droplets

TABLE 6–1. Classification of Dental Impression Materials

By Setting Mechanism	By Application or Mechanical Properties	
	Rigid or Inelastic (edentulous ridge)	*Elastic (tooth form)*
Chemical reaction (irreversible)	Plaster of Paris Zinc oxide–eugenol	Alginate hydrocolloid Nonaqueous elastomers Polysulfides Polyethers Condensation silicones Addition silicones
Temperature changes (reversible)	Compound (preliminary impression) Wax	Agar hydrocolloid

do not readily diffuse and tend to fall out of the suspending medium unless mechanically or chemically held in place. Somewhere between the extremes of the very small molecules in solution and the very large particles in suspension is the colloidal solution, or *sol.*

True solutions exist as a single phase. However, both the colloid and the suspension have two phases: *dispersed* and *dispersion.* In the colloid, the particles in the dispersed phase consist of molecules that are held together either by primary or secondary forces. The sizes of the colloid particles range from 1 to 200 nm.

The two phases are either compatible or incompatible. Thus, the dispersed phase may or may not stay suspended in the dispersion medium. In addition to particle size, factors common to any two-phase system, for example, surface energy, surface charge, and wettability, determine the stability of the colloid.

Types of Colloids. Colloidal substances may be combinations of any states of matter, with the exception of gaseous states. For example, liquids or solids in air are called *aerosols*; gases, liquids, or solids in a liquid are called *lyosols*; gases, liquids, and solids in a solid are called *foams, solid emulsions*, and *solid suspensions*, respectively. All colloidal dispersions are termed *sols,* regardless of the type of dispersion phase. When a liquid is used as the dispersion phase, the colloid is called *lyophilic* for liquid-preferring dispersed species or *lyophobic* for liquid-avoiding dispersed species. The colloidal materials used for making impressions are either agar or algin dissolved in water, hence the name *hydrocolloids.*

Sol-Gel Transformation. If the concentration of the dispersed phase in the hydrocolloid is sufficient, the sol may be changed to a semisolid material known as a *gel*. In the gel state, the dispersed phase agglomerates, forming chains or fibrils, called *micelles*. The fibrils may branch and intermesh to form a brush-heap structure, which can be imagined to resemble the intermeshing of twigs in a brush pile. The dispersion medium is held in the interstices between the fibrils by capillary attraction or adhesion.

For agar, the fibrils are held together by secondary molecular forces. These bonds are very weak; they break at slightly elevated temperatures and become re-established as the hydrocolloid cools to room temperature. The temperature at which this change occurs is the *gelation temperature* and is about 37° C or slightly higher for agar. The process is reversible. Thus, the agar is also called a *reversible hydrocolloid.*

For alginate, the fibrils are formed by chemical action. In this instance, the transformation is not reversible, hence the name *irreversible hydrocolloid.*

GENERAL CHARACTERISTICS OF GELS

Gel Strength. The gel can support considerable stress, particularly shear stress, without flow, provided the stress is applied rapidly. The stiffness and strength of the gel are directly related to the brush-heap density or concentration. For example, in a reversible gel, the greater the concentration of the dispersed phase in the sol, the greater the number of fibrils formed on gelation. However, if the stresses are sustained, the material will flow, possibly as a result of disturbing the network relation between the dispersion medium and the fibrillar structure.

For the reversible gel, the lower the temperature, the stronger the gel, and vice versa. When the gel is heated, the kinetic energy of the fibrils increases, resulting in greater interfibrillar distances and reduction of their cohesion. The temperature increase also favors formation of the sol. As the temperature continues to rise, more of the fibrils revert until finally more fibrils are reverting than are forming. At this temperature, the liquefaction to the sol occurs. The strength of the irreversible gel is not as greatly affected by normal temperature changes, because the fibrils are formed by chemical action and do not revert to the sol condition on heating.

The strength of both gels can be increased by the addition of certain modifiers such as fillers and chemicals. The fillers usually consist of fine powders of an inert substance. The powder particles are trapped in the micelle network in such a manner that the brush heap is rendered more rigid with less flexibility.

Dimensional Effects. As might be expected from the structure of the hydrocolloids, a large part of the gel volume is occupied by water. If the water content of the gel is reduced, the gel will shrink, and if the gel takes up water, it will expand or swell. These changes in dimension are of considerable importance in dentistry because any change in dimension that occurs after the impressions are removed from the mouth leads to an inaccurate cast.

The gel may lose water by *evaporation* from its surface or by exudation of fluid onto the surface by a process known as *syneresis*. This is one of the characteristic properties of a gel. The exudate that appears on the surface of the gel during and after syneresis is not pure water. It may be either alkaline or acid, depending on the composition of the gel. In any event, whenever water or fluid is removed from the micelles of the gel by evaporation or syneresis, the gel shrinks.

If a gel is placed in water, it will absorb water by a process known as *imbibition*. The gel swells during imbibition, thereby altering the original dimensions. Imbibition can cause just as much distortion as syneresis and evaporation. The effects of syneresis, evaporation, and imbibition must be limited to ensure the proper dimensions of the impression. Although the dentist has no control over syneresis, the amount of distortion can be reduced by pouring cast or model material into the impression immediately. Fabricating the gypsum cast immediately also limits the effects of evaporation. If it is not possible to pour it up immediately, then the impression should be wrapped in a moist paper towel. This creates a 100% humidity environment that slows the evaporation process. The covering should not be too wet or imbibition may occur.

AGAR (REVERSIBLE HYDROCOLLOID)

Composition. The basic constituent of the hydrocolloid impression materials is agar, but it is by no means the main constituent by weight (Table 6–2). Agar is an organic hydrophilic colloid (polysaccharide) extracted from certain types of seaweed. It is a sulfuric ester of a linear polymer of galactose. It is present in a concentration of 8% to 15%, depending on the desired properties of the material. The principal ingredient by weight is water (>80%). Modifiers present in minor amounts exert a considerable influence on the properties of the material. A small percentage of borax is added to strengthen the gel. It is probable that a borate is formed that increases the strength or density of the micelle framework in the gel. Almost any soluble borate, either organic or inorganic, produces the same effect. Unfortunately, borax also is an excellent retarder for the setting of gypsum. Its presence in the hydrocolloid impression materials is detrimental because it retards the setting of the plaster or stone cast that is poured into the agar impression. The water content of the hydrocolloid impressions also inhibits the

TABLE 6–2. Composition of Commercial Reversible Hydrocolloid Impression Materials

Component	Function	Composition (%)
Agar	Brush-heap structure	13–17
Borates	Strength	0.2–0.5
Sulfates	Gypsum hardener	1.0–2.0
Wax, hard	Filler	0.5–1.0
Thixotropic materials	Thickeners	0.3–0.5
Water	Reaction medium	Balance

Courtesy of K. H. Strader.

setting of the gypsum. Consequently, the incorporation of the borax further retards the setting of gypsum.

To counteract the effects of water and borax, potassium sulfate is added because it accelerates the setting of gypsum. Some commercial products contain a certain amount of filler for the control of strength, viscosity, and rigidity, as previously discussed. Some of the fillers used are diatomaceous earth, clay, silica, wax, rubber, and similar inert powders. Other ingredients, such as thymol and glycerin, may also be added as a bactericide and plasticizer, respectively. Pigments and flavors are usually included.

Gelation Process. The setting of a reversible hydrocolloid, often called *gelation*, is a solidification process. The reaction can be expressed as

$$Sol \rightleftarrows Gel$$

The physical change from the sol to gel, and vice versa, is induced by a temperature change. However, the hydrocolloid gel does not return to the sol at the same temperature at which it solidified. The gel must be heated to a higher temperature, known as the *liquefaction temperature* (70° to 100° C), to return it to the sol condition. When cooled, the material remains a sol far below the liquefaction temperature. It transforms into a gel between 37° and 50° C. The exact gelation temperature depends on several factors, including the molecular weight, the purity of the agar, and the ratio of agar to other ingredients. The gelation temperature is critical. If the gelation temperature is too high, the heat from the sol may injure the oral tissues, or if the surface of the sol transforms to a gel as soon as it contacts the tissues, a high surface stress may develop. Conversely, if the gelation temperature is too far below the oral temperature, it will be difficult or even impossible to chill the material sufficiently to obtain a firm gel adjacent to oral tissues.

The temperature lag between the gelation temperature and the liquefaction temperature of the gel makes it possible to use agar as a dental impression material. The dentist can liquefy the gel, place it in the impression tray, temper it to lower the temperature to one that the patient can tolerate, and maintain it in its fluid state to capture the details of the oral structures. Once in the mouth, the material is cooled below mouth temperature to ensure gelation. There are concerns in getting the gel too cold because the chilling sensation may be uncomfortable to the patient and the impression undergoes thermal expansion as it warms up to room temperature.

MANIPULATION OF AGAR IMPRESSION MATERIALS

Using reversible hydrocolloid impression material involves a three-step process: (1) advanced preparation of the material; (2) preparation immediately before making the impression; and (3) the making of the impression. For a brief overview of the process, we begin with the fact that material is supplied in tubes and exists as a gel at room temperature. The first step in using the material is to liquefy it and store it as a sol. Immediately before an impression is made, the sol is placed in an impression tray and tempered or conditioned so that the temperature is tolerable to the oral tissues. Then, the third step occurs once the impression is seated against the oral tissues. At this point, the material must be chilled so that gelation occurs rapidly. Water is circulated through the impression tray until the material has gelled. The tray is then removed and the impression is poured in dental stone. The process of using reversible hydrocolloid impression materials is somewhat complex, which is an initial drawback that is quickly overcome once the technique is learned.

Preparation of the Material. Proper equipment for liquefying and storing the agar impression material is essential. Various types of conditioning units for preparation and storage of this hydrocolloid are available, such as the one shown in Figure 6–1.

The hydrocolloid is usually supplied in two forms: syringe and tray materials. Tubes to fill the water-cooled trays and cartridges for use in the syringes are shown in Figure 6–2. The only difference between the syringe and tray material is the color and a greater fluidity of the syringe material.

The first step is to reverse the hydrocolloid gel to the sol state. Boiling water is a convenient way of liquefying the material. The material must be held at this temperature for a minimum of 10 minutes. At high altitudes, such as in Denver, Colorado, the boiling point of water is too low to liquefy the gel. Propylene glycol can be added to the water to obtain a temperature of 100° C. Otherwise, materials that have been formulated specifically to liquefy at lower temperatures should be used.

It is possible to reliquefy a portion of an unused tube. However, after previous use, it is more difficult to break down the agar brush-heap structure, so an

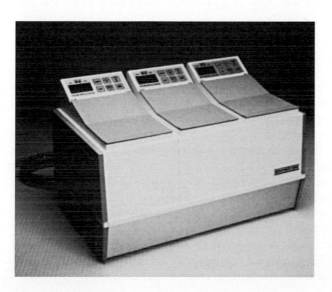

Figure 6–1. Conditioning unit for the agar hydrocolloid impression materials. The three compartments are used for liquefying the material, for storage after boiling, and for tempering the tray hydrocolloid. (Courtesy of Van R Dental Products, Inc., Los Angeles, CA.)

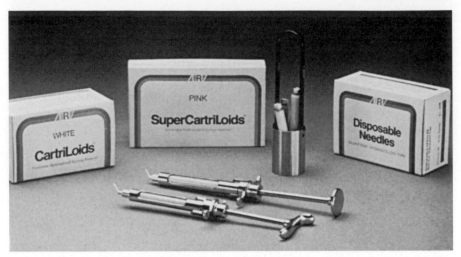

Figure 6–2. Cartridges of agar hydrocolloid and syringes used for injecting into the prepared cavity. Also seen is the holder for carrying the agar hydrocolloid into the conditioning unit.

additional 3 minutes of boiling time should be allowed each time the material is reliquefied. Theoretically, the material that was used to make the impression can be reused. Because disinfection is a major problem and the material is inexpensive, only unused portions should be recycled.

After it has been liquefied, the material may be stored in the sol condition until it is needed for injection into the cavity preparation or for filling the tray. Because the liquefaction process takes some time and the material can be stored for several days, it is a general practice to prepare a number of tubes and syringes for use throughout the week. The material is kept at the storage temperature so it is ready for quick use. Lower temperatures may result in a higher viscosity material that is incapable of accurately reproducing fine detail. Usually, there are at least three compartments in the conditioning unit, making it possible to simultaneously liquefy, store, and temper the reversible hydrocolloid material (see Fig. 6–1). Temperatures required in each of the steps of preparing the hydrocolloid are critical. Check the temperatures in the conditioning unit weekly.

Conditioning or Tempering. Because 55° C is the maximum tolerable temperature, the storage temperature of 65° C would be too hot for the oral tissues, especially given the bulk of the tray material. Therefore, the material that is used to fill the tray must be cooled or *tempered*. For the immediate preparation step, a tube of hydrocolloid sol is removed from the storage bath, the tray is filled, a gauze pad is placed over the top of the tray material, and the tray is placed in the tempering section (approximately 45° C) of the conditioning unit. The tempering time is brief (3 to 10 minutes), just sufficient to ensure that all the material has reached a lower temperature (≤55° C).

Because the rate of gelation is influenced by the temperature at which the hydrocolloid is held, various combinations of tempering temperatures and times may be employed to produce a satisfactory result. The time may be varied for the particular batch or brand of hydrocolloid and for the fluidity preferred by the dentist. For example, impressions for partial dentures require less body. Therefore, a shorter tempering time is indicated. At any rate, the lower the temperature, the shorter should be the storage time in the tempering compartment. Regardless, the loaded tray should never be left in this bath for more than 10 minutes, because gelation may have proceeded too far, thereby making the material unusable.

Eliminating the effects of imbibition is the purpose of placing the gauze pad over the tempering tray materials. When the tray material is placed into the tempering bath, it will begin to absorb water and also a rubbery film forms over the surface. The gauze cannot prevent these events; however, when the tray is removed from the tempering bath, the gauze is removed, and the contaminated surface layer of material clings to the gauze and is removed as well. This fresh surface more readily adheres to the syringed material that was injected over the prepared teeth.

In addition to lowering the temperature, tempering also increases the viscosity of the hydrocolloid material so that it does not flow out of the tray. Although this is an advantage for the tray material, increasing the viscosity of the syringe material would be undesirable. Thus, this material is *never* tempered. The effect of extruding the material out the small opening of the syringe lowers the temperature of the syringe material sufficiently such that it is comfortable for the patient.

Making the Impression. Just before the tempering process of the tray material is completed, the syringe material is taken directly from the storage compartment and applied to the prepared cavities. It is first applied to the base of the preparation, and then the remainder of the prepared tooth is covered. The point of the syringe is held close to the tooth, beneath the surface of the syringe material, to prevent entrapment of air bubbles.

In a standardized procedure, by the time the cavity preparations and adjoining teeth have been covered, the tray material has been properly tempered and is now ready to be placed immediately in the mouth to form the bulk of the impression. The water-soaked outer layer of tray hydrocolloid is removed with the gauze that was covering the tray impression material. If the outer surface of the tempered tray hydrocolloid is not removed, it may not firmly bond with the syringe hydrocolloid. The tray is immediately brought into position and seated with light pressure and held in place passively. Too much pressure may displace the sol on the tooth.

Gelation is accelerated by circulating cool water, approximately 18° to 21° C through the tray for 3 to 5 minutes (Fig. 6–3). During the gelation process, it is

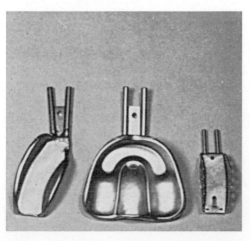

Figure 6–3. Water-cooled trays are used to carry the bulk material into the mouth.

important that the tray be held in the mouth until the gelation has proceeded to a point at which the gel strength is sufficient to resist deformation or fracture. Waiting an extra minute greatly increases the strength and tear resistance. Also, the lower the temperature, the more rapidly gelation occurs, and to a certain extent, the stronger the material becomes.

Even though the material sets last against the teeth (because they are at a higher temperature), care must be exercised to prevent any movement of the tray as the gel forms. The brush-heap structure of the gel is more likely to resist distortion or fracture if the force is applied quickly rather than slowly. Consequently, when the impression is removed, it is necessary to remove it suddenly, with a jerk, rather than to tease it out. However, any twisting or torquing should be avoided. Properly done, the resulting impression (Fig. 6–4) accurately reproduces the dimensions and details of hard and soft tissues.

Wet Field Technique. The aqueous elastomers are the only true hydrophilic impression materials. Recently, a technique for making impressions in a wet field has become popular. It differs in that the tooth surfaces and tissue are purposely left wet. The areas are actually flooded with warm water, then the syringe material is introduced quickly, liberally, and in bulk to cover the occlusal and incisal areas only. The tray material is seated over the syringe material in the same fashion as previously described. It is postulated that the hydraulic pressure of the viscous tray material forces the fluid syringe hydrocolloid into the areas to be restored. This motion displaces the syringe material, blood, and debris with the stronger tray material throughout the sulcus. Theoretically, there is less chance that this material will tear when the impression is removed from the mouth.

ACCURACY OF AGAR IMPRESSION MATERIAL

Reversible hydrocolloids are among the most accurate of the impression materials. This material has a long history of successful use for single units and for

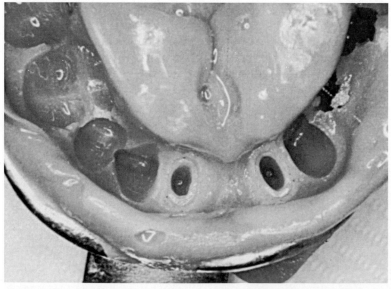

Figure 6–4. The final agar hydrocolloid impression made for the cavity preparations and teeth.

fixed partial denture applications. To demonstrate the accuracy of an impression material, studies are conducted that involve fabricating castings to fit standardized dies, as shown in Figure 6–5. These standard preparations simulate an inlay, an onlay, and a full-coverage crown. Because of their blunt 90-degree angles and 1% to 2% taper, they represent a more exacting situation than most clinical cavity preparations. Therefore, any impression that accurately reproduces these dies more than satisfies the conventional clinical requirements. To achieve that accuracy, care must be taken to ensure that the following variables related to the properties are optimal.

Viscosity of the Sol. The viscosity of the sol is of considerable importance in the successful manipulation of the material. After the material has been liquefied, it must be sufficiently viscous so that it does not flow out of the tray if the tray is inverted, such as when a mandibular impression is made. On the other hand, its viscosity must not be so great that it does not readily penetrate every detail of the teeth and soft tissues.

Even when the material has sufficient viscosity to be stabilized in the tray, it does not offer much resistance to seating. It is easy for the patient to "bite through" the impression material. For this reason, the triple-tray is commonly used with reversible hydrocolloids. With a triple-tray technique, one impression records the oral structures of both the maxillary and mandibular arches as well as the occlusal relationship. The procedure is somewhat technique sensitive because the dentist must guide the patient into centric occlusion as the patient "bites" into the impression material. For this type of impression, the material must not resist the patient's efforts to "articulate the teeth together." Most hydrocolloids have just the right consistency to allow this technique to be used successfully.

Viscoelastic Properties. The stress-strain relationship of the hydrocolloid impression materials changes as the rate of loading changes. This is a characteristic of *viscoelastic* behavior, which also occurs with nonaqueous elastomeric impression

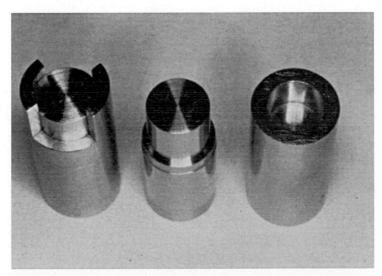

Figure 6–5. Steel dies used for determining accuracy in techniques that involve impression materials and castings. They represent a mesial-occlusal-distal *(left)*, full-crown *(center)*, and one-surface inlay *(right)*.

materials as discussed in Chapter 7. As the name implies, viscoelastic behavior is intermediate between that of an elastic solid and a viscous liquid. An elastic solid can be viewed as a spring, which deforms instantly to a certain extent when one applies a definite amount of load. The amount of deformation will recover completely when the load is removed. On the other hand, a viscous liquid is like an oil dashpot, that does not respond instantly to any sudden external force or load but will exhibit deformation when the force acts over time. The dashpot will continue to deform until the force or load is removed. Contrary to the behavior of an elastic solid, the amount of deformation exhibited by the dashpot is permanent, which will not recover by itself when the force is removed. We can demonstrate the viscoelastic behavior by considering a simple mechanical model of springs and dashpots in a certain fashion.

The simplest model is a Maxwell-Voigt model (Fig. 6–6A), which consists of a spring (S1) and a dashpot (D1) in series, and a second set (S2 and D2) in parallel. When one applies a force (either tension or compression) shown by the arrow, spring S1 responds instantaneously with a definite amount of strain (deformation). At that instant, dashpot D1 will not show any deformation and dashpot D2 prevents spring S2 from deforming because of dashpot inertia (Fig. 6–6B). If the same force remains exerted on the model, both dashpots start and continue to deform as long as the loading is applied (Fig. 6–6C). Meanwhile, spring S1 maintains the same magnitude of strain. At the moment the load is removed, the deformation exhibited by spring S1 recovers while the rest remains unchanged (Fig. 6–6D). As the time passes, spring S2 will slowly overcome the inertia of dashpot D2 and recover along with it (Fig. 6–6E). The process usually takes time and may not recover completely. The deformation of dashpot D1 never recovers.

This viscoelastic behavior has considerable clinical importance. It demonstrates the necessity of deforming the impression rapidly when it is removed

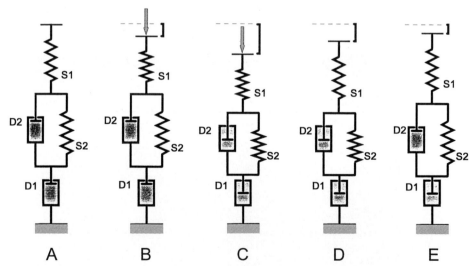

Figure 6–6. A mechanical model showing the response of a viscoelastic material to external loading and unloading. *A,* A Maxwell-Voigt viscoelastic model in the stress-free state. *B,* At the instant of loading, only S1 responds. *C,* When the loading continues, all elements deform depending on the duration of loading. No change in S1 is expected. *D,* When the load is released, S1 recovers instantly while the rest remains unchanged. *E,* As time passes, S2 and D2 will recover the majority of deformation while D1 will remain deformed. The right-hand bracket on the top of each model denotes the degree of deformation.

from the mouth, which reduces the amount of permanent deformation (or distortion) attributed to dashpot D1. The impression should never be removed by a teasing or weaving method, but rather it should be removed suddenly in a direction as nearly parallel as possible to the long axes of the teeth. A slow removal of the impression is a common cause of distortion and tearing.

As discussed earlier, regardless of the type of loading, the elastic recovery of the hydrocolloid is never complete, and it does not return entirely to its original dimension after deformation. However, the amount of permanent deformation is clinically negligible, provided that (1) the material has adequately gelled, (2) the impression has been removed rapidly, and (3) the undercuts present in the cavity preparation are minimal.

Distortion during Gelation. Certain stresses are always introduced during gelation. Some contraction occurs because of the physical change in the hydrocolloid transformation from a sol to a gel. If the material is held rigidly to the tray, then the impression material shrinks toward the center of its mass, thereby creating larger dies. Because the sol is a poor thermal conductor, rapid cooling may cause a concentration of stress near the tray where the gelation first takes place. Consequently, water at approximately 20° C is more suitable for cooling the impression than is ice water.

Reproducibility. This property represents the ability to make duplicate dies from sequential impressions. With some impression materials it is possible to pour up the impression more than once and produce duplicate dies using this procedure. Although reversible hydrocolloids are accurate, they cannot be poured up more than once—one can use a pin-indexing technique or a two-impression double-die technique. With the double-die technique, one impression is made and cut apart into individual dies of the prepared teeth. The second impression is made in a triple tray so that both arches and the occlusal relationship are recorded. Both maxillary and mandibular impressions are poured at the same time and attached to a simple hinge articulator. The wax patterns are fabricated on the individual dies and then transferred to the intact casts to adjust occlusal and interproximal contacts. For most impressions made from thermosetting impression materials (set by polymerization), it would not be possible to transfer the wax patterns between dies made from two separate impressions. Thus, to use the double-die technique, the clinician would need to pour up two casts from the same impression. However, when agar impression material is handled correctly, the dies from different impressions are interchangeable.

ALGINATE (IRREVERSIBLE HYDROCOLLOID)

At the end of the last century, a chemist from Scotland noticed that certain brown seaweed (algae) yielded a peculiar mucous extraction. He named it *algin*. This natural substance was later identified as a linear polymer with numerous carboxyl acid groups and named *anhydro-β-d-mannuronic acid* (also called *alginic acid*), with the structural formula shown in Figure 6–7. Alginic acid and most of the inorganic salts are insoluble in water, but the salts obtained with sodium, potassium, and ammonium are soluble in water.

When the agar impression material became scarce because of World War II (Japan was a prime source of agar), research was accelerated to find a suitable substitute. The result was, of course, the present irreversible hydrocolloid, or

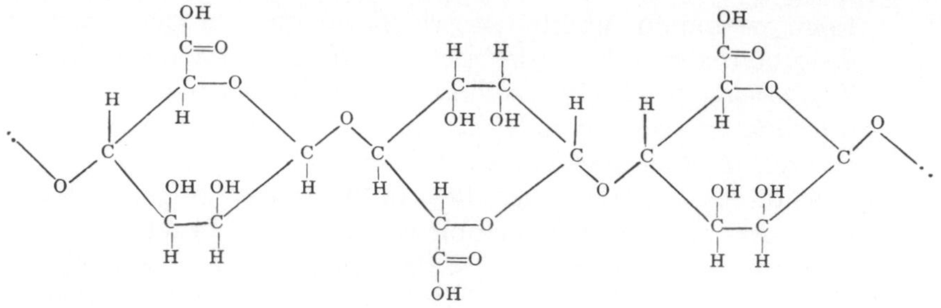

Figure 6–7. Structural formula of alginic acid.

alginate impression material. The general use of irreversible hydrocolloid far exceeds that of other impression materials available. The principal factors responsible for the success of this type of impression material are that it is (1) easy to manipulate; (2) comfortable for the patient; and (3) relatively inexpensive because it does not require elaborate equipment.

Composition. The chief active ingredient of the irreversible hydrocolloid impression materials is one of the soluble alginates, such as sodium, potassium, or triethanolamine alginates. When the soluble alginates are mixed with water, they form a sol. The sols are quite viscous even in low concentrations, but the soluble alginates form sols quite readily if the alginate powder and water are mixed vigorously. The molecular weight of the alginate compounds may vary widely, depending on the manufacturing treatment. The greater the molecular weight, the more viscous the sol. The manufacturer-supplied alginate powder contains a number of components. Table 6–3 shows a formula for the powder component of an alginate impression material with the function of each component.

The exact proportion of each chemical to be used varies with the type of raw material. The purpose of the diatomaceous earth is to act as a filler. If the filler is added in proper amounts, it can increase the strength and stiffness of the alginate gel, produce a smooth texture, and ensure a firm gel surface that is not tacky. It also aids in forming the sol by dispersing the alginate powder particles in the water. Without a filler, the gel formed lacks firmness and exhibits a sticky surface covered with an exudate produced by syneresis. Zinc oxide also acts as a filler and has some influence on the physical properties and setting time of the gel.

Any type of calcium sulfate can be used as the reactor. The dihydrate form is generally used, but under certain circumstances, the hemihydrate produces an increased shelf life of the powder and a more satisfactory dimensional stability of the gel. A fluoride, such as potassium titanium fluoride, is added as an

TABLE 6–3. Formula for the Powder Component of an Alginate Impression Material

Component	Function	Weight Percentage
Potassium alginate	Soluble alginate	15
Calcium sulfate	Reactor	16
Zinc oxide	Filler particles	4
Potassium titanium fluoride	Accelerator	3
Diatomaceous earth	Filler particles	60
Sodium phosphate	Retarder	2

accelerator for the setting of the stone to ensure that a hard, dense stone cast surface is produced against the impression.

Shelf Life. Storage temperature and moisture contamination from the ambient air are the two major factors that affect the shelf life of alginate impression materials. Materials stored for 1 month at 65° C are unsuitable for dental use, either failing to set at all or setting much too rapidly. Even at 54° C there is evidence of deterioration, probably because alginate depolymerizes.

The alginate impression material is dispensed in individually sealed pouches, with sufficient powder preweighed for an individual impression, or in bulk form in a can. The individual pouches are preferred because there is less chance for contamination during storage. In addition, the correct water:powder ratio is ensured, because plastic cups are provided for the measurement of the water. However, the bulk form of packing is less expensive. If a bulk package is employed, the lid should be firmly replaced on the container as soon as possible after each use so that a minimal amount of moisture contamination occurs.

An expiration date for a stated condition of storage should be clearly identified by the manufacturer on each package delivered to dental offices. In any event, it is better not to stock more than one year's supply in the dental office and to store the material in a cool, dry environment.

Modified Alginates. As can be seen, the traditional alginate is used as a two-component system, a powder and water. There is no reaction until the water is added to the powder to initiate the reaction.

However, the alginate can also be purchased in the form of a sol containing the water but no source of calcium ions. A reactor of plaster of Paris can then be added to the sol. In this instance, the second component is the reactor, not the water.

There is yet another form that is available. The two-component system may be in the form of two pastes: one contains the alginate sol and the other contains the calcium reactor. Impression materials of this type may also contain silicone and may be supplied both in a tray viscosity and in a syringe viscosity.

Gelation Process. The typical sol-gel reaction can be described simply as a reaction of soluble alginate with calcium sulfate and the formation of an insoluble calcium alginate gel. Calcium sulfate reacts rapidly to produce the insoluble calcium alginate from the potassium or sodium alginate in an aqueous solution. The production of the calcium alginate is so rapid that it does not allow sufficient working time. Thus, a third water-soluble salt, such as trisodium phosphate, is added to the solution to prolong the working time. The strategy is that the calcium sulfate will react with the other salt in preference to the soluble alginate. Thus, the reaction between the calcium sulfate and the soluble alginate is prevented as long as there is unreacted trisodium phosphate. For example, if suitable amounts of calcium sulfate, potassium alginate, and trisodium phosphate are mixed and partially or totally dissolved in proper proportions in water, the following reaction will first take place:

$$2Na_3PO_4 + 3CaSO_4 \rightarrow Ca_3(PO_4)_2 + 3Na_2SO_4$$

When the supply of trisodium phosphate is exhausted, the calcium ions begin to react with the potassium alginate to produce calcium alginate as follows:

$$K_{2n}Alg + n\,CaSO_4 \rightarrow n\,K_2SO_4 + Ca_nAlg$$

The added salt is known as a *retarder*. There are a number of soluble salts that can be used, such as sodium or potassium phosphate, potassium oxalate, or potassium carbonate, trisodium phosphate, sodium tripolyphosphate, and tetrasodium pyrophosphate. The latter two are now the most common. The amount of retarder (sodium phosphate) must be adjusted carefully to provide the proper gelation time. In general, if approximately 15 g of the powder is mixed with 40 mL of water, gelation will occur in about 3 to 4 minutes at room temperature.

Gel Structure. In a sodium or potassium alginate, the cation is attached at a carboxyl group to form an ester or a salt. When the insoluble salt formed by the reaction of the sodium alginate in solution reacts with the calcium salt, the calcium ions may replace the sodium ions in two adjacent molecules to produce a crosslinking between the two molecules. As the reaction progresses, a crosslinked molecular complex or polymer network forms. Such a network can constitute the brush-heap structure of the gel.

The crosslinking of hydrocolloid is diagrammed in Figure 6–8. The base molecules represent the sodium salt of alginic acid, where H atoms of the carboxyl group are replaced by sodium atoms. With the exception of the polar groups, all the side chains have been omitted for simplification. Some of the sodium ions have not reacted as yet, but they may be replaced by a calcium ion as indicated in the other polar groups. Thus, the individual sodium alginate molecules may be linked to form larger molecules or, theoretically, one large molecule. The reaction may be classified as a form of polymerization because crosslinking occurs.

If a soluble salt such as calcium chloride is used as the reactor, the crosslinkage is virtually complete in a few seconds, and the entire sol is converted to

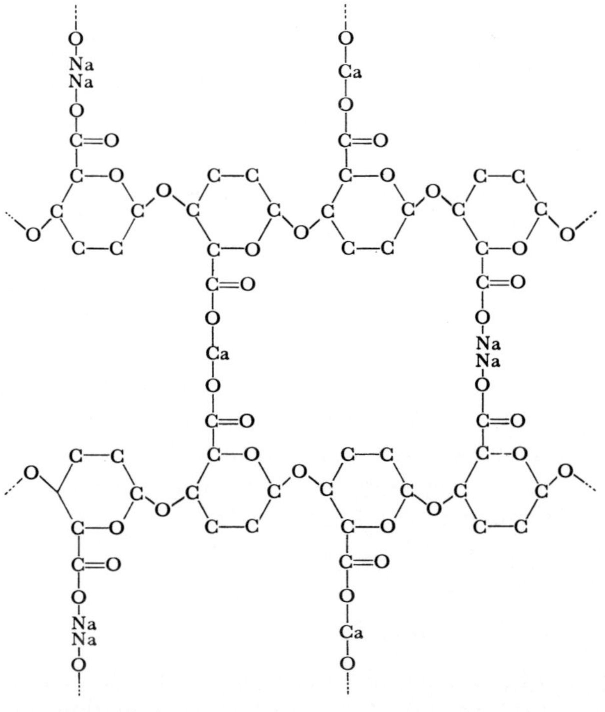

Figure 6–8. Schematic representation of crosslinking of sodium alginate molecules to form calcium alginate. Note that only some of the molecules have been crosslinked.

insoluble calcium alginate instantly, thereby producing a useless mass. Calcium sulfate, which is less soluble than calcium chloride, supplies calcium ions at a slower rate so that only a fraction of the alginate molecules become crosslinked. The remaining sol becomes encapsulated in a sheath of the insoluble calcium alginate. As a result, the reaction does not continue to completion. The final structure can be envisioned as a brush heap of a calcium alginate fibril network enclosing unreacted sodium alginate sol, excess water, filler particles, and reaction by-products, such as sodium sulfate and calcium phosphate.

Controlling Gelation Time. The gelation time, measured from the beginning of mixing until gelation occurs, must allow sufficient time for the dentist to mix the material, load the tray, and place it in the patient's mouth. Once gelation starts, the impression material must not be disturbed because the growing fibrils will fracture and the impression would be significantly weakened.

The practical method of determining gelation time for the dental practitioner is to observe the time from the start of mixing until the material is no longer tacky or sticky when it is touched with a clean, dry, gloved finger tip. Probably the optimal gelation time is between 3 and 4 minutes at room temperature (20° C). Normally, the manufacturers make both fast setting (1 to 2 minutes) and normal setting alginate (2.5 to 4 minutes) to provide clinicians the opportunity to choose the materials that best suit their working style.

In the clinical setting, it is tempting to alter the gelation time by changing the water:powder ratio or the mixing time. This slight modification can have marked effects on the properties of the gel, impairing the tear strength and the elasticity. Thus, the gelation time is best regulated by the amount of retarder added during manufacturing.

Another way the clinician can safely influence the gelation time is to alter the temperature of the water. The effect of the water temperature on the gelation time of an alginate impression material is shown in Figure 6–9. It is evident that the higher the temperature, the shorter the gelation time. In hot weather, special precautions should be taken to provide cool water for mixing so that premature gelation does not occur. It may even be necessary to precool the mixing bowl and spatula, especially when small amounts of impression material are to be mixed. In any event, it is better to err by having the mix too cool rather than too warm.

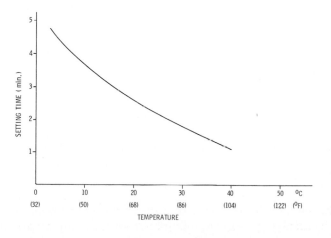

Figure 6–9. The effect of water temperature on the setting time of an alginate impression material. (Courtesy of J. Cresson.)

Materials exhibit different degrees of sensitivity to temperature changes. For example, Figure 6–9 shows 1 minute of reduction in gelation time for each 10° C of temperature increase. Some commercial materials have exhibited as much as a 20-second change in gelation time for every degree Celsius change in temperature. In such a case, the temperature of the mixing water should be controlled carefully within 1 or 2 degrees of a standard temperature, usually 20° C, so that a constant and reliable gelation time can be obtained. If the desired setting time cannot be achieved by varying the water temperature within reasonable limits, it is better to select another product having the desired setting time and less sensitivity to temperature change rather than to resort to other modifications in the manipulation technique.

MANIPULATION OF ALGINATE IMPRESSION MATERIAL

Alginate impression materials are easy to use. The materials are hydrophilic, so moist tissue surfaces are not a problem. Generally, alginates are used as a preliminary impression to construct a custom tray for a more accurate second impression or to make study models to help with treatment planning and discussions with the patient. Unlike many of the other impression materials, alginates do not feature a range of different viscosities.

Because only one mix of alginate is made, the bulk of the material is placed in the tray. The clinician may take a small amount on a gloved finger and flow the material into the central pits and fossae and into the fissures of the occlusal surfaces. This technique reduces the chance of trapping air bubbles when the tray is seated in the mouth. Because it is clean and sets quickly, this impression material is easily tolerated by patients. Orthodontists use alginate frequently to make impressions of young patients. For this market, the manufacturers have "flavored" the material to smell like bubble gum or cinnamon. Another product is designed to undergo color changes as it gels, indicating the end of mixing, the time to seat the tray, and the time to remove the impression.

Preparing the Mix. The measured powder is sifted into premeasured water that has been placed in a clean rubber bowl. The powder is incorporated into the water by careful mixing with a metal spatula. Care should be taken to avoid whipping air into the mix. Many prosthodontists use a vacuum mixer to avoid this problem. Improper mixing of alginate materials can impair the quality of the final impression. A vigorous figure-eight motion is best, with the mix being swiped or stropped against the sides of the rubber mixing bowl with intermittent rotations (180 degrees) of the spatula to press out air bubbles, as demonstrated in Figure 6–10. This is effective in working out most of the air bubbles, and it promotes complete dissolution. It is important to get all the powder dis-solved—if residual powder remains, a good gel cannot form and the properties are compromised.

The mixing time is particularly important. For example, the strength of the gel can be reduced as much as 50% if the mixing is not complete. A mixing time of 45 seconds to 1 minute is generally sufficient, depending on the brand and type of alginate. The result should be a smooth, creamy mixture that does not drip off the spatula when it is raised from the bowl. With superior commercial products, a smooth creamy mixture can be expected. A variety of mechanical devices are also available for spatulating the alginate materials. Their principal benefit is convenience, speed, and elimination of the human variable.

Clean equipment is important because many of the problems and related

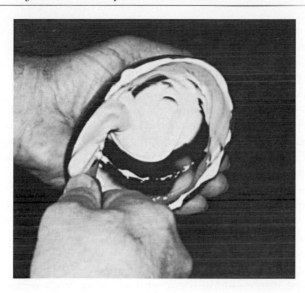

Figure 6–10. The mix of an alginate impression material is made by a vigorous "stropping" of the material against the side of the mixing bowl.

failures are attributed to dirty or contaminated mixing or handling devices. Contamination during mixing may result in too rapid a set, inadequate fluidity, or even rupture of the impression on removal from the mouth. For example, small amounts of gypsum left in the bowl from a previous mix of plaster or stone contaminate the impression material and accelerate the set. It is desirable to use separate bowls for mixing the alginate and stone.

Ideally, the powder should be weighed and not measured volumetrically by means of a scoop, as many manufacturers suggest. However, unless one uses a grossly incorrect method of scooping the powder, it is improbable that the variation in powder weight per scoop is greater than 0.2 to 0.4 g. Such variations in individual mixes would have no measurable effect on the physical properties.

Nonetheless, if reasonable care is not exerted in following the manufacturer's directions precisely, the handling characteristics of the alginate mix will be affected adversely. For example, a variation of only 15% from the recommended powder:liquid ratio markedly affects the setting time and consistency.

If the powder in the can is fluffed before measuring, it is important to avoid breathing the dust, which will rise from the can when the lid is removed. Some of the silica particles in the dust are of such a size and shape as to be a possible health hazard. In an effort to reduce the dusting encountered after tumbling, manufacturers have incorporated glycerin into the alginate powder to agglomerate the particles. This causes the powder to become more dense than in the uncoated state. After tumbling, the powders no longer have a tendency to release dust, as evidenced by the reduction in airborne particles as the canister lid is removed. One of these products is sold as "dustless alginate."

Making the Impression. Before seating the impression, the material should have developed sufficient body so that it does not flow out of the tray and choke the patient. Clinicians must learn to recognize the viscosity changes so that they seat the impression during the critical interval between the running stage and the nonrunning stage.

The mixture is placed in a suitable tray, which is carried into place in the mouth. It is imperative that the impression adhere to the tray so that the impression can be withdrawn from around the teeth. Therefore, a perforated tray is generally used. If a plastic tray or a metal rim-lock tray is selected, a thin layer of tray adhesive should be applied and allowed to dry completely before mixing and loading the alginate in the tray. Thin layers of alginate are weak; therefore, the tray must fit the patient's arch so that there is a sufficient bulk of material. The thickness of the alginate impression between the tray and the tissues should be at least 3 mm.

The strength of the alginate gel increases for several minutes after the initial gelation. As noted in Table 6–4, the gel strength in this case actually doubled during the first 4 minutes after gelation, but it did not increase appreciably after the first 4-minute period. Most alginate materials improve in elasticity over time, which minimizes distortion of the material during impression removal, thereby permitting superior reproduction of undercut areas. Such data clearly indicate that the alginate impression should not be removed from the mouth for at least 2 to 3 minutes after gelation has occurred, which is approximately the time at which the material loses its tackiness.

Although the tendency is to remove the impression prematurely, it is possible to leave an alginate impression in the mouth too long. With certain alginates, it has been shown that if the impression is held for 6 to 7 minutes, rather than 2 to 3 minutes after gelation, significant distortion results.

Strength. Maximum gel strength is required to prevent fracture and to ensure elastic recovery of the impression on its removal from the mouth. All manipulative factors that are under the control of the clinician affect the gel strength. For example, if too much or too little water is used in mixing, the final gel will be weakened, making it less elastic. The proper water:powder ratio should be employed as specified by the manufacturer. Insufficient spatulation results in failure of the ingredients to dissolve sufficiently so that the chemical reactions can proceed uniformly throughout the mass. Overmixing breaks up the calcium alginate gel network as it is forming and reduces its strength. The directions supplied with the product should be followed in all respects.

Viscoelasticity. Hydrocolloids are strain-rate dependent. Thus, the tear strength is increased when the impression is removed with a snap. The speed of removal must be a compromise between a rapid movement and the comfort of the patient. Usually, an alginate impression does not adhere to the oral tissues as strongly as some of the nonaqueous elastomers, so it is easier to remove the alginate impression rapidly. However, it is always best to avoid torquing or twisting the impression in an effort to remove it quickly.

Accuracy. Most alginate impression materials are not capable of reproducing the finer details that are observed in impressions with other elastomeric impression materials. Manufacturers have attempted to increase the concentration of algi-

TABLE 6–4. Compressive Strength of an Alginate Gel as a Function of Gelation Time

Time from Gelation (min)	Compressive Strength (MPa)
0	0.33
4	0.77
8	0.81
12	0.71
16	0.74

nate to make the material more accurate. However, this does not increase the dimensional stability of the material. The roughness of the impression surface is sufficient to cause distortion at the margins of prepared teeth. Surfactants can be used to produce a smooth surface, but addition of a layer of solution over the surface of the impression also obscures the accuracy. To ensure that the alginate material provides a realistic representation for study casts, the impression must be handled correctly.

ADDITIONAL APPLICATIONS OF HYDROCOLLOIDS

Laminate Technique. A recent modification to the traditional agar procedure is the combined agar-alginate technique. The tray hydrocolloid is replaced with a mix of chilled alginate that bonds to the syringe agar. The alginate gels by a chemical reaction, whereas the agar gels by means of contact with the cool alginate rather than the water circulating through the tray. Because the hydrocolloid, not the alginate, is in contact with the prepared teeth, maximum detail is reproduced. The advantages are that the cost of the equipment is lower because only the syringe material needs to be heated. Also, there is less preparation time for the same reason. The main disadvantages of this technique are as follows: (1) the bond between the agar and the alginate is not always strong; (2) the higher viscosity alginate displaces the agar during seating; and (3) the dimensional inaccuracy of the alginate limits the use to single units. This laminate technique is the most cost-effective way of producing an impression with adequate detail. Recent reports indicate that careful selection of the materials is necessary to obtain reproducible results.

Duplicating Materials. Both types of hydrocolloid are used in the dental laboratory to duplicate dental casts or models. The duplicated cast is used in the construction of prosthetic appliances and for orthodontic models. Reversible hydrocolloid is the most popular because it can be used many times. Also, with intermittent stirring, it can be kept in liquid form for 1 or 2 weeks at a constant pouring temperature, and its price is reasonable.

The hydrocolloid-type duplicating materials have the same composition as the impression materials, but their water content is higher. Consequently, the agar or alginate content is lower, which influences their compressive strength and percent set. These property requirements are identified in American Dental Association Specification No. 20.

CARE AND HANDLING OF HYDROCOLLOID IMPRESSIONS

Disinfection. The need to disinfect impressions is well established. Because the hydrocolloid impression must be poured within a short time after removal from the mouth, the disinfection procedure should be relatively rapid to prevent dimensional change.

Most manufacturers recommend a specific disinfectant, and it should be prepared according to their directions. The agent may be iodophor, bleach, or glutaraldehyde. The distortion is minimal if the recommended immersion time is followed and if the impression is poured promptly.

The irreversible hydrocolloids may be disinfected by 10-minute immersion in, or spraying with, an antimicrobial agent such as sodium hypochlorite and glutaraldehyde without significant dimensional changes. However, certain disinfectants may result in gypsum casts that have a lower surface hardness or diminished surface detail.

The current protocol for disinfecting hydrocolloid impressions recommended by the Centers for Disease Control and Prevention is to use household bleach (1-to-10 dilution), iodophors, or synthetic phenols as disinfectants. After the impression is thoroughly rinsed, the disinfectant is sprayed liberally on the exposed surface. The impression should not be submerged or soaked in the disinfectant solution. Immediately wrap the impression in a disinfectant-soaked paper towel and place it in a sealed plastic bag for 10 minutes. Finally, remove the wrapped impression from the bag, unwrap, rinse thoroughly, shake off the excess water, and pour the model with the stone of your choice.

Dimensional Stability. As previously noted, gels are invariably subject to changes in dimension by syneresis, evaporation, and imbibition. Once the impression is removed from the mouth and exposed to the air at room temperature, some shrinkage that is associated with syneresis and evaporation is bound to occur. Conversely, if the impression is immersed in water, swelling will occur as a result of imbibition. A typical example of the dimensional change that can occur during syneresis and imbibition of a hydrocolloid impression material is shown in Figure 6–11. This graph illustrates that the material has shrunk in air. During subsequent imbibition, there was an overexpansion because of swelling with the absorbed water.

It is clear that the impression should be exposed to air for as short a time as possible if the best results are to be obtained. The importance of immediately constructing the stone cast is clearly illustrated in Figure 6–12 where part *A* shows an accurate fit of a casting on the die and part *B* shows an unacceptable fit caused by dimensional change of the impression.

Various storage media, such as 2% potassium sulfate or 100% relative humidity, are suggested to reduce the dimensional change of agar impressions. Results obtained for impressions made from one dental agar hydrocolloid in several media are shown in Figure 6–13. These results are typical, and they indicate that 100% relative humidity is the best storage environment to preserve the normal water content of the impression.

The gels are also subject to stresses in localized areas. One cause for production of such stresses is exertion of pressure on the tray during the gelation period. The relaxation of the internal stresses causes syneresis and corresponding dimensional changes.

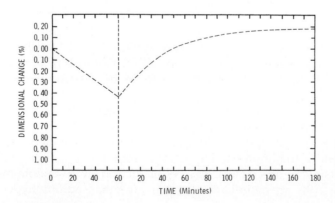

Figure 6–11. Linear contraction of a representative reversible hydrocolloid in air (31% to 42% relative humidity) and subsequent expansion in water.

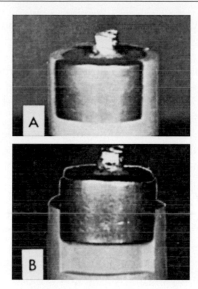

Figure 6–12. *A,* Fit of a master casting on a stone die constructed immediately after the agar hydrocolloid impression was removed from a master steel die. *B,* Fit of same casting when the stone die was constructed 1 hour after the impression was removed.

Thermal changes also contribute to dimensional change. With alginates, impressions shrink slightly because of the thermal differential between mouth temperature (35° C) and room temperature (23° C). The agar hydrocolloid impression materials experience a temperature shift in the opposite direction, from the chilled water-cooled tray (15° C) to the warmer room temperature. Even this slight change can cause the impression to expand and distort.

If pouring of the impression must be delayed, it should be rinsed in tap water and wrapped in a paper towel, saturated with water, and placed in a closed container to create a 100% humid environment. The container, such as a plastic

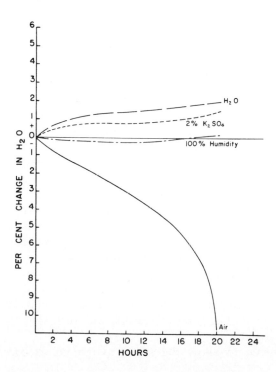

Figure 6–13. Percentage of change in water content by weight of an agar hydrocolloid impression material in various storage media.

bag or a humidor, should be kept closed until time is available to pour the die. Do not leave unattended in the storage solution.

Compatibility with Gypsum. Some form of gypsum is used as the cast or die material for a hydrocolloid impression. However, gypsum casts are not compatible with both types of hydrocolloid impressions and the surface of the gypsum cast may be too soft for some applications.

Every precaution must be taken to ensure maximum surface hardness of the gypsum cast. It has been shown that the surface of a gypsum cast prepared from a hydrocolloid impression may be too soft for waxing procedures. This disadvantage can be overcome in two ways: (1) by immersing the impression in a solution containing an accelerator for the setting of the gypsum product, before pouring the impression with the gypsum; or (2) by incorporating a plaster hardener or accelerator in the material by the manufacturer. The sulfates in the formula given in Table 6–2 serve the latter purpose. The hardening solution may increase the hardness of the stone in a number of ways. It may act as an accelerator for the set of the gypsum product to overcome the retarding action of the gel surface on the setting of the dental stone. Also, it may react with the gel to produce a surface layer that reduces or prevents syneresis and eliminates the retarding action of the gel.

Improvements in some commercial reversible hydrocolloid materials have made it possible to obtain a satisfactory surface on stone casts without using a hardening solution. Still some clinicians prefer to use this method to further increase the surface hardness of the stone. The impression is immersed in the hardening solution before the stone is poured. Various chemicals have been employed, such as potassium sulfate, zinc sulfate, manganese sulfate, and potash alum. The most effective, however, is a 2% potassium sulfate solution.

Similar additives have been used for the alginate impression materials. For example, titanium fluoride is a hardener that is added to the material. In general, a hardening solution is not required unless specifically indicated by the manufacturer. For an effective infection control practice, the impression should be disinfected before the cast is poured.

After the impression is removed from the mouth, it is immediately rinsed under running water to remove oral fluid from the surface. A rough stone surface results if excess rinse water has collected on the surface of the impression at the time the stone mixture is poured. However, the surface of the impression should not be dried completely; otherwise, the gel adheres to the surface of the cast on its removal. Undue dehydration also results in syneresis and a distortion of the impression. The surface of the impression should be shiny but with no visible water film or droplets at the time the cast is constructed.

The pouring of stone mixture to fill the impression should start from one end of the arch. After the impression has been filled with stone, it may be placed in either a humidor or a 2% potassium sulfate solution while the stone hardens. Slightly superior stone surfaces are obtained if the stone hardens in an atmosphere of approximately 100% relative humidity. In any event, the filled impression should never be immersed in water while the stone sets.

The stone cast, or die, should be kept in contact with the impression, preferably for 60 minutes or for a minimum of 30 minutes before the impression is separated from the cast. The setting time of the stone in contact with the impression material will probably be increased, and sufficient time should be allowed for the stone to set.

It is possible, however, to allow the stone to remain in contact with the hydrocolloid gel for too long. On occasion, if the cast is allowed to remain in contact with the hydrocolloid impression overnight, a chalky stone surface may be produced. For this reason, it is wise to separate the cast within a reasonable period. Waiting too long allows the surface of the impression material and the surface of the stone to interact. With prolonged contact, the set stone absorbs water from the water-filled impression. The result is a chalky surface with poor detail. Reproduction of surface detail may also vary, depending on the particular impression material–stone combination used. Some combinations are more compatible than others.

Effects of Mishandling. Common causes for failures encountered with both reversible and irreversible hydrocolloid impression materials are summarized in Table 6 5.

TABLE 6–5. Common Causes for Remaking of Hydrocolloid Impressions

	Cause	
Effect	*Agar*	*Alginate*
1. Grainy material	a. Inadequate boiling b. Storage temperature too low c. Storage time too long	a. Improper mixing b. Prolonged mixing c. Undue gelation d. Water:powder ratio too low
2. Separation of tray and syringe material	a. Water-soaked layer of tray material not removed b. Premature gelation of either syringe or tray material	Not applicable
3. Tearing	a. Inadequate bulk b. Premature removal from mouth c. Syringe material partially gelled when tray seated	a. Inadequate bulk b. Moisture contamination c. Premature removal from mouth d. Prolonged mixing
4. External bubbles	a. Gelation of syringe material, preventing flow	a. Undue gelation, preventing flow b. Air incorporated during mixing
5. Irregularly shaped voids	a. Material too cool or grainy	a. Moisture or debris on tissue
6. Rough or chalky stone model	a. Inadequate cleansing of impression b. Excess water or potassium sulfate solution left in impression c. Premature removal of die d. Improper manipulation of stone e. Air-drying the impression before pouring	a. Inadequate cleaning of impression b. Excess water left in impression c. Premature removal of model d. Leaving model in impression too long e. Improper manipulation of stone
7. Distortion	a. Impression not poured immediately b. Movement of tray during gelation c. Premature removal from mouth d. Improper removal from mouth e. Use of ice water during initial stages of gelation	a. Impression not poured immediately b. Movement of tray during gelation c. Premature removal from mouth d. Improper removal from mouth e. Tray held in mouth too long (only with certain brands)

SELECTED READING

Cook W: Alginate dental impression materials: Chemistry, structure, and properties. J Biomed Mater Res 20:1, 1986.
The viscosity, calcium ion activity, shear modulus, and compressive modulus were monitored during the setting reaction. Bond rupture appears to be the primary cause of a permanent set. An increase in alginate concentration reduces bond rupture and increases tear energy.

Fusayama T, Kurosaki N, Node H, and Nakamura M: A laminated hydrocolloid impression for indirect inlays. J Prosthet Dent 47:171, 1982.
Presents a description of the laminate hydrocolloid-alginate method for impressions.

Heisler WH: Accuracy and bond strength of reversible with irreversible hydrocolloid impression systems. J Prosthet Dent 68:578, 1992.
The accuracy was acceptable for a three-unit fixed partial denture. A recommendation is made to use the matched materials prepared by one manufacturer.

Johnson GH, and Craig RC: Accuracy and bond strength of combination agar-alginate hydrocolloid impression materials. J Prosthet Dent 55:1, 1986.
Bond strength between the reversible and irreversible hydrocolloid combinations varied considerably. When both bond strength and accuracy were considered, one alginate in combination with either of two agar hydrocolloids produced the most desirable results.

Jones ML, Newcombe RG, Bellis H, and Bottomley J: The dimensional stability of self-disinfecting alginate impressions compared to various immersion regimens. Angle Orthod 60:123, 1990.
The small differences in the interarch–intraarch linear measurements were not statistically significant.

Lepe A, Sandrik JL, and Land MF: Bond strength and accuracy of combined reversible-irreversible hydrocolloid impression systems. J Prosthet Dent 67:621, 1992.
Variability in the tensile bond strength of different brands of the combined impression material systems is described.

Lewinstein I, and Craig RG: Accuracy of impression materials measured with a vertical height gauge. J Oral Rehabil 17:303, 1990.
Vertical and horizontal changes were greatest for the combined agar-alginate impressions.

Merchant VA, Radcliffe RM, Herrera SP, and Stroster GT: Dimensional stability of reversible hydrocolloid impressions immersed in selected disinfectant solutions. J Am Dent Assoc 119:533, 1989.
Immersion of hydrocolloid impressions in three different disinfectant solutions did not adversely affect dimensional stability.

Murakami H, Takehana S, Abe T, et al: Correlation between the degree of deformation of the stone die and the amount of the master die undercut. Aichi-Gakuin Dent Sci 2:57, 1989.
Alginate impression produced results with very wide variations in the dimensional distortion.

Olsson S, Bergman B, and Bergman M: Agar impression materials, dimensional stability, and surface detail sharpness following treatment with disinfectant solutions. Swed Dent J 11:169, 1987.
Spray disinfectants did not affect the surface detail of reversible hydrocolloid impressions.

Petters MC, and Tieleman A: Accuracy and dimensional stability of a combined hydrocolloid impression system. J Prosthet Dent 67:873, 1992.
The accuracy of these systems is judged to be adequate.

Reed HV: Reversible agar-agar hydrocolloid. Quintessence Int 21:225, 1990.
A review of the history and success of this cost-effective impression material.

Rice CD, Dykstra MA, and Feil PH: Microbial contamination in two antimicrobial and four control brands of alginate impression materials. J Prosthet Dent 67:535, 1992.
Alginate materials that contain antimicrobial agents were found to have fewer viable organisms on samples incubated on agar medium than conventional alginate specimens.

Rosen M, and Touyz LZ: Influence of mixing disinfectant solutions into alginate on working time and accuracy. J Dent 19:186, 1991.
Disinfectant solutions used in place of water do not modify the working time beyond acceptable limits, and they have no effect on the dimensional stability. A 0.12% solution of chlorhexidine gluconate is recommended.

Rueggeberg FA, Beall FE, Kelly MT, and Schuster GS: Sodium hypochlorite disinfection of irreversible hydrocolloid impression material. J Prosthet Dent 67:628, 1992.
Alginate is susceptible to dimensional change during immersion disinfection but not spray disinfection. Both methods decreased the surface detail. Antimicrobial effects of spray disinfection were similar to immersion disinfection.

Schutt RW: Bactericidal effect of a disinfectant dental stone on irreversible hydrocolloid impressions and stone casts. J Prosthet Dent 62: 605, 1989.
The disinfectant dental stone containing chloramine-T was effective in eliminating bacterial contamination of both the irreversible hydrocolloid impression and the stone cast.

Setcos JC, Ping L, and Palenik CJ: The effect of disinfection procedures on an alginate impression material. J Dent Res 63:235, 1984.
Certain disinfectants can lower the surface hardness of gypsum casts.

Steas A: A new method for making casts from irreversible hydrocolloid impressions. J Prosthet Dent 65:454, 1991.
To minimize distortion, the stone is mixed with an accelerator and is painted over the entire surface. Then a base is added after this first layer sets.

Tan HK, Hooper PM, Buttar IA, and Wolfaardt JF: Effects of disinfecting irreversible hydrocolloid impressions on the resultant gypsum casts. I. Surface quality. III. Dimensional changes. J Prosthet Dent 69:250, and 70:532, 1993.

Only iodophor solution did not produce a difference in the surface quality as a function of time in solution. Disinfecting for a short period did not result in significant dimensional changes

Teteruck WR, Johnson LN, Mills AR, and Downar-Zapolski B: Surface quality of gypsum when poured against alginates. Can Dent Assoc J 55:545, 1989.

In this study, 16 gypsum products were poured against 32 different alginate surfaces, producing 512 gypsum surfaces. Certain gypsum-alginate combinations had surfaces with superior hardness and smoothness.

Thomas CJ: Impression material consistency and peripheral tissue. Aust Dent J 35:134, 1990.

Facial tissue applies sufficient force to restrain the buccal border of alginate impressions, but the lingual tissues are less capable of handling materials with low viscosity.

Tobias RS, Browne RM, and Wilson CA: An *in vitro* study of the antibacterial and antifungal properties of an irreversible hydrocolloid impression material impregnated with disinfectant. J Prosthet Dent 62:601, 1989.

It is not known whether the limited antibacterial and antifungal effects demonstrated in this study are sufficient to prevent bacterial and fungal colonization of the impression surface in the mouth during clinical practice.

Wanis TM, Combe EC, and Grant AA: Measurement of the viscosity of irreversible hydrocolloids. J Oral Rehabil 20:379, 1993.

Three different measurement techniques were used to analyze these impression materials.

7 Nonaqueous Elastomeric Impression Materials

- Background on Development of Elastomers
- Overview of Elastomeric Impression Materials
- Polysulfide Impression Material
- Condensation Silicone Impression Material
- Addition Reaction Silicone (Vinyl Polysiloxane) Impression Material
- Polyether Impression Material
- Techniques for Measuring Properties
- New Advances in Impression Materials
- Effects of Mishandling

TERMINOLOGY

Accelerator–a component of the polymerization reaction that is similar to the catalyst but also speeds up the reaction.

Addition reaction–a polymerization reaction in which each polymer chain grows to a maximum length in sequence and there is no reaction by-product.

Base–the main component of the chemical reaction.

Bench cure–the continuing polymerization reaction of an impression material during short-term storage. This term is often used inappropriately to describe the recovery over time of a distorted impression to its original shape.

Catalyst–a component of a reaction that facilitates the reaction and usually does not become part of the final product.

Compression set–a property that describes the amount of deformation that a set elastomer can withstand without experiencing permanent deformation.

Condensation reaction–a polymerization reaction in which the polymer chains all grow simultaneously and a reaction by-product is formed.

Cross-linking–the reaction that links or joins polymer chains to form a network structure called a *gel*. The amount of cross-linking affects stiffness and elasticity.

Cure–a term used to describe the reaction process that takes place both during and after the setting of the polymer.

Curing rate–the rate of the reaction of the setting polymer.

Dashpots–the model components that describe the viscous response of a cross-linked polymer.

Elastomer–a term that refers to the nonaqueous elastomeric impression materials.

Gel–the solid network structure that defines the cross-linked polymer.

Initiator–the component that starts the chemical reaction. Types include photo-initiators, chemical-initiators, and heat-initiators.

Monophase–*see Single-phase.*

One-step–*see Single-phase.*

Permanent deformation–the irreversible shape changes that occur when the polymer responds as a viscous liquid and the distortion is permanent.

Polymerization–the chemical reaction that transforms small molecules into large polymer chains.

Pseudoplastic–the characteristic of a polymer that allows the material to appear to be less viscous when the shearing rate is increased.

Rheology–the science that explains the fluid or flow characteristic of materials such as viscoelasticity, viscosity, and pseudoplasticity.

Shear thinning–*see Pseudoplastic.*

Set–the state of being sufficiently rigid or elastic to be removed from the mouth.

Single-phase–a single-component material with sufficient shearing potential that it can be used as the syringe material and the tray material.

Springs–a model that describes the elastic behavior of cross-linked polymers.

Strain-rate dependent–*see Pseudoplastic.*

Thixotropic–the time-dependent pseudoplastic flow of polymers that is characterized by the gradual decrease of viscosity under a constant applied shear rate.

Undercuts–that portion of the tooth that lies indented from the largest circumference of the tooth; generally, it is within the gingival half of a tooth.

Viscoelastic–a characteristic of polymers that behave as elastic solids (springs) and as viscous liquids (dashpots).

Vulcanization–the process of heating natural rubber with sulfur to produce cross-linking. This term is commonly used to describe the cross-linking of polymer chains to form an elastomer.

BACKGROUND ON DEVELOPMENT OF ELASTOMERS

In addition to the hydrocolloid gels, there is a group of rubberlike elastic impression materials known as *elastomers*. These materials are classified as synthetic rubbers; they were developed to mimic natural rubber when it became difficult to obtain during World War II. Initially called *rubber impression materials,* these synthetic materials are currently referred to as *elastomers* or *elastomeric impression materials*. The American Dental Association (ADA) Specification No. 19 identifies these materials as "nonaqueous elastomeric dental impression materials."

An elastomeric material consists of large molecules or polymers that are joined by a small amount of cross-linking. The cross-linking ties the coiled polymer chains together at certain points to form a three-dimensional network that is often referred to as a *gel*. In an ideal case, stretching causes the polymer chains to uncoil only to a specific amount that is recoverable; that is, the chains snap back to their relaxed entangled state when the stress is removed. The amount of cross-linking determines the stiffness and the elastic behavior of the material.

The first synthetic rubberlike materials were produced by a process known as *vulcanization* or *curing*. Vulcanization is a cross-linking process that involves sulfur mercaptan groups, the component that gives polysulfide impression material its characteristic odor. These first dental elastomers, polysulfides, were sometime referred to (1) by the type of material, such as rubber-base impression materials; (2) by the processing terminology, such as vulcanizing impression materials; (3) by chemistry, such as mercaptan impression materials; or (4) by the name of one of the first manufacturers, such as the Thiokol Corporation. More detailed information on the properties of the elastomeric polymers can be found in the descriptions of specific elastomers. Basic information on this type of material is given in Chapter 4.

The current ADA specification considers three types of elastomeric impression materials. The type of classification is based on selected elastic properties and the dimensional change of the set materials rather than on their chemistry. However, each type is further divided into four viscosity classes: (1) light body, (2) medium or regular body, (3) heavy body, and (4) putty. Viscosity is a material property that controls the flow characteristics of a material. An estimate of the viscosity can be determined using the consistency test, that is, measuring how much a specific amount of material flows under a given weight.

OVERVIEW OF ELASTOMERIC IMPRESSION MATERIALS

Description. Chemically, there are four kinds of dental elastomers used as impression materials: *polysulfide, condensation polymerizing silicone, addition polymerizing silicone,* and *polyether.* Representative products are seen in Figure 7–1. Each of these materials replicate the oral structures with sufficient accuracy to be used in the fabrication of fixed or removable prosthetic restorations. Most impression materials are two-component systems supplied in paste form. The different colored pastes are dispensed in equal lengths on a mixing pad and spatulated to a homogeneous color. Setting occurs through a combination of

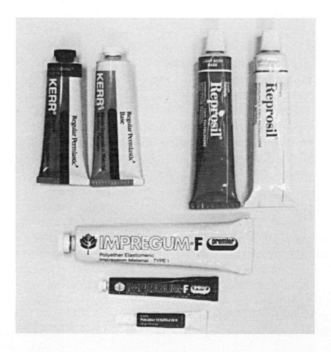

Figure 7–1. Representative commercially available impression materials.

chain-lengthening polymerization or cross-linking or both by either condensation or addition reactions.

During the curing process, it is important to determine how long the impression material remains fluid enough to place in the mouth and when the impression material is sufficiently cured so that it can be removed from the mouth. These stages—the end of the working time and the end of the setting time—are difficult to define. Clinically, the material is past the usable stage when it becomes too thick or viscous to flow and to record the detail of the teeth and soft tissues. Fully set materials rebound completely from a thumbnail indentation. Dental practitioners develop their own methods to identify these characteristic stages of the material.

Handling. The measurement of working time begins with the start of mixing and ends just before the impression material has developed elastic properties. The working time of an acceptable material must exceed the time required for mixing, filling the syringe and tray, injecting the material onto preparations, and seating the tray. Setting time can be described as the time elapsing from the beginning of mixing until the curing has advanced sufficiently that the impression can be removed from the mouth with negligible distortion. Removing the impression too soon is a common cause of impression distortion. If the material is not adequately set, the materials will not have sufficient elastic properties to respond to the strain of removing it from the mouth. Most setting times recommended by the manufacturers are too short. Waiting an extra minute before removing the impression can ensure success. The setting time does not correspond to the curing time. Actually, curing may continue for a considerable time after setting and is referred to as *residual polymerization.*

Characteristics. The rheologic properties of the elastomeric impression materials play a major role in their successful application as high-accuracy impression materials. These materials are introduced into the mouth as a viscous liquid with carefully adjusted flow properties. The setting reaction then converts them into a viscoelastic solid. The flow behavior of the solid form is also quite important if an accurate impression is to be obtained. Even the viscosity and flow behavior of the unmixed components are important, because these control ease of mixing, the amount of air trapped during mixing, and the tendency for the trapped air to escape before the impression is made.

The ideal impression material accurately records the oral structures, releases from the mouth undistorted, and remains dimensionally stable on the laboratory bench or when poured up in stone. Actually, current impression materials accurately record the necessary detail if handled correctly. The distortion on removal is minimal if the clinician remembers that a fast strain rate yields less permanent deformation. Impressions should only be removed rapidly. This rapid removal also maximizes the tear resistance of the impression. However, this should be done preferably after the air seal has been broken. Otherwise, the patient may experience discomfort during a single-motion attempt to break the air seal and to "snap" the tray away from the teeth. Another reason for breaking the air seal first is to minimize the risk of irreversible distortion that is induced when excessive torque is applied on the tray handle when attempting to "break the suction." A better method is to tease the borders of the tray parallel to the path of insertion until the air leaks into the tray. Then the handle can be used to remove the tray rapidly and with minimal torque.

Both distortion and tear energy are related to the strain-rate sensitivity or

TABLE 7–1. Working and Setting Times of Nonaqueous Elastomeric Impression Materials

Impression Material	Mean Working Time (min)		Mean Setting Time (min)	
	23° C	37° C	23° C	37° C
Polysulfide	6.0	4.3	16.0	12.5
Condensation silicone	3.3	2.5	11.0	8.9
Addition silicone	3.1	1.8	8.9	5.9
Polyether	3.3	2.3	9.0	8.3

Fom Harcourt JK: A review of modern impression materials. Aust Dent J 23:178, 1978.

viscoelastic properties of polymers. The set material appears to be stronger if the stress is applied quickly. In addition to an apparent increase in strength, the deformation is mostly elastic and thus recoverable, which minimizes the distortion. Using a slow, steady strain to remove the impression from the mouth can cause plastic or permanent deformation because the chains uncoil beyond a recoverable distance and are unable to snap back.

Once it is removed from the mouth, the impression must maintain its dimensional accuracy. Thermal changes affect the dimensional stability along with residual polymerization, loss of reaction by-product, and distortion caused by the imposed loads, such as the weight of the stone or plaster used to make the cast. The material's compatibility with gypsum can influence the quality of the stone cast. Also, some disinfection procedures can alter the impression material sufficiently to affect the accuracy of the resultant cast. Other important parameters, such as biocompatibility, handling characteristics, and shelf life, are discussed as they pertain to each specific impression material.

The choice of a rubber impression material is governed by the particular characteristics preferred by the operator. In general, the silicone and polyether materials have the advantage of superior color and little or no odor. They are also cleaner to handle. On the other hand, the silicones are inferior to the polysulfide and the polyether impression materials from the standpoint of shelf life. Impressions of similar accuracy can be obtained with all the elastomers if the proper technique is employed. Some of the characteristics of the four different impression materials are summarized in Table 7–1; the data are intended to serve only as a general guideline. There is a noticeable variation among individual products. Likewise, dentists differ greatly in their working habits and skills in handling a given type of material and making impressions.

POLYSULFIDE IMPRESSION MATERIAL

Chemistry. The basic ingredient of the polymer paste is a polyfunctional mercaptan or polysulfide polymer with the general structural formula given in Figure 7–2.

This linear polymer contains approximately 1 mol% of branches to provide enough pendant mercaptan groups as chain cross-linking sites. This polymer is usually cross-linked with an oxidizing agent such as lead dioxide. It is the lead dioxide that gives polysulfide its characteristic brown color. During the condensation reaction of the lead dioxide with the SH groups of the polysulfide polymer, two phenomena occur: (1) chain-lengthening polymerization from the reaction with the terminal —SH groups, and (2) cross-linking from the reaction with the pendant —SH groups (see Fig. 7–2).

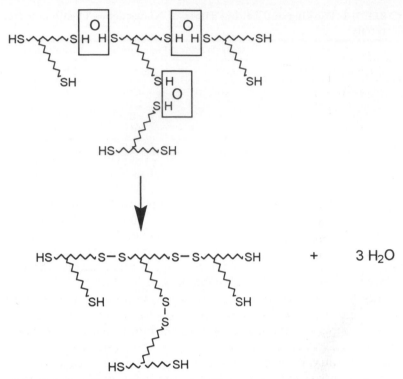

Figure 7–2. Top drawing shows how the SH groups interact with oxygen from the lead peroxide. The lower drawing shows the completion of the condensation reaction that results in the release of three water molecules.

Because the pendant groups compose only a small percentage of the available–SH groups, initially, the polymerization reactions result in chain lengthening, which causes the viscosity to increase. The subsequent cross-linking reactions tie the chains together, forming a three-dimensional network that confers elastic properties to the material. The initial increase in viscosity affects the working time of the material and is a change the dentist becomes accustomed to when handling this material.

The curing reaction starts at the beginning of mixing and reaches its maximum rate soon after the spatulation is complete, at which stage a resilient network has started to build. During the final set, a material of adequate elasticity and strength is formed that can be removed over undercuts quite readily.

The polymerization reaction of polysulfide polymers is exothermic; the amount of heat generated depends on the amount of total material and the concentration of initiators. Moisture and temperature exert a significant effect on the course of reaction. In particular, hot, humid conditions accelerate the setting of polysulfide impression material. The condensation reaction by-product is water. Loss of even this small molecule from the set material has a significant effect on the dimensional stability of the impression.

A representative commercial product is LP-2 (Thiokol Corporation), and its technology is well known. Dental polysulfide polymers use this technology with modifications appropriate for dental use.

Composition. The *base paste* contains (1) the polysulfide polymer; (2) a suitable filler (e.g., lithopone and titanium dioxide) to provide the required strength; (3) a plasticizer (e.g., dibutyl phthalate) to confer the appropriate viscosity to the paste; and (4) a small quantity of sulfur, approximately 0.5%, to enhance the reaction.

The so-called catalyst or accelerator paste contains the lead dioxide that produces the characteristic dark-brown color. However, the terms *catalyst* and *accelerator* are really misnomers. The term *reactor* is more appropriate for the polysulfide reaction. In addition, the same plasticizer as is used in the base paste, as well as a quantity of the same filler, is included in the reactor paste along with oleic or stearic acid, both retarders, which are added to control the rate of setting.

Each paste is supplied in a tube with appropriate openings so that dispensing equal lengths of each paste gives the correct ratio of polymer to cross-linking agent. Because the composition of the material in the tube is balanced with that of the accelerator, the same matched tubes originally supplied by the manufacturer should always be used. For certain products, some flexibility in working and setting times can be obtained by changing proportions. This must be done with caution, because mechanical properties such as tear strength and elasticity may be adversely affected.

Manipulation. With the proper lengths of the two pastes squeezed onto a mixing pad or glass slab, the catalyst paste is first collected on a stainless steel spatula and then distributed over the base, and the mixture is spread out over the mixing pad. The mass is then scraped up with the spatula blade and again smoothed out. The process is continued until the mixed paste is of uniform color, with no streaks of the base or catalyst appearing in the mixture. If the mixture is not homogeneous, curing will not be uniform, and a distorted impression will result. Adherence to the manufacturer's instructions is always advisable.

Just as the set material is strain-rate dependent, so is the unset material. Medium-body and heavy-body polysulfide impression pastes are extremely viscous and sticky. Consequently, they are difficult to mix. However, if sufficient force is applied and spatulation is performed rapidly, the material will seem thinner and easier to handle. This phenomenon is known as *pseudoplasticity*.

Working and Setting Times. Working and setting times for the various kinds of elastomeric materials, as measured by an oscillating rheometer, are shown in Table 7–1. An increase in temperature accelerates the curing rate of all these elastomeric impression materials and thus decreases both setting and working times. Cooling is a practical method of increasing the working time of most polysulfide impression materials. This can be accomplished by storing the materials at a low room temperature or by mixing on a chilled, dry glass slab. Then, when the impression material is carried to the mouth, setting time is decreased by the higher oral temperature.

As mentioned in the previous section on composition, oleic acid is also an effective retarder for the lead dioxide–cured polysulfide materials. Conversely, adding a drop of water accelerates the curing rate. The curing rate of some, but not all, of the polysulfide impression materials is sensitive to alterations in the base:accelerator ratio. However, mechanical properties can be adversely affected when marked changes in the base:accelerator ratio occur. Altering the base:accelerator ratio to change the working or setting time is not economical, because a portion of the paste is not used. Moreover, because the accelerator paste contains a retarder as well as a reactor, increasing the base:accelerator ratio may not produce a predictable change in the polymerization rate.

Elasticity. As might be expected, the elastic properties of these rubber impression materials improve with curing time. In other words, the longer the impression can remain in the mouth before removal, the greater the accuracy. As mentioned earlier, the impression material must undergo some distortion as it is removed from the mouth, but the elastic properties of the impression material help minimize this distortion. Such distortion is more likely to occur when the tray is torqued or removed or both at a significant angle to the path of insertion of the tray.

The setting times as stated by a manufacturer, or as determined by a rheometer, are not always adequate for the development of sufficient elasticity to prevent permanent deformation on removal of the impression, especially with the polysulfide impression materials. For example, the setting times as measured by a rheometer are 1 or 2 minutes less than those required to produce an acceptable level of elasticity before removal of the impression.

Recovery of elastic deformation after strain is less rapid for the polysulfides than for the other three kinds of materials. Also, polysulfides exhibit the most permanent deformation following strain in compression compared with the other materials. Polysulfides also sustain more distortion when the strain rate is slow.

Despite the possibility of a large dimensional change occurring when the polysulfide impression is removed from the mouth, there is no advantage to "bench cure" the materials. If the polymer chains have been stretched past their elastic limit, no amount of waiting will enable them to return to their original shape. Although the distortion is permanent, the chains may relax, but they have no "memory," so the relaxed state probably will not resemble the undistorted shape no matter how long the impression is allowed to bench cure.

Rheology. Polysulfide ranks as one of the least stiff of the elastomeric impression materials. This flexibility allows the set material to release from undercut areas and be removed from the mouth with a minimum of stress. Despite the lack of stiffness, the unset material has a high level of viscosity. This thick consistency of the uncured material helps displace any unwanted fluid present while seating the impression. Also, the excess material extruded from the tray does not flow easily because of the high viscosity, reducing the potential discomfort to the patient during seating of a tray.

Tear Energy. Polysulfides have the highest resistance to tearing. Thin sections of polysulfide impression material are less likely to tear than similar thicknesses of polyether or silicone impression materials. However, because of its susceptibility to distortion, it is possible that the polysulfide impressions may distort rather than tear. This presents a dilemma because tearing can be seen immediately by carefully checking the impression, whereas distortion caused by stretching is almost impossible to detect. This distortion can result in a casting that does not seat on the model die. Again, strain rate influences the tear resistance and permanent deformation. To minimize the negative effects of both, the impression should be strained rapidly for as brief a time as possible.

Dimensional Stability. The stone cast should be poured up immediately because the impression is the most accurate immediately after removing it from the mouth. The following are sources of dimensional change:

1. During setting most polymers contract slightly during cross-linking, be-

cause tied together, the chains occupy less volume, and there is a reduction in bond length.

2. After setting, the by-product (water) of the condensation reaction is lost, which causes shrinkage.

3. Although polysulfide impression materials are water repellent, the materials can absorb fluids if exposed to water, a disinfectant, or a high-humidity environment over time.

4. After setting, there is incomplete recovery of deformation because of the viscoelastic properties.

The rubber materials are much more stable dimensionally when they are stored in air than are the hydrocolloid impression materials (Figure 7–3). However, it is evident that all materials change dimensionally over time and that such a change is greater in magnitude for the polysulfide rubber materials than for the polyether and addition polymerizing silicone elastomers.

If maximal accuracy is to be maintained, the stone die or cast should be constructed within the first 30 minutes after the removal of the impression from the mouth whenever a polysulfide material is used.

Spherical indentations sometimes appear on the surface of an impression obtained with a polysulfide rubber material. Such indentations appear on the surface of the stone die as convexities, or nodules. Presumably, this effect is caused by the collapse of a void near the surface. Such voids are probably the result of air bubbles trapped during mixing. However, because such imperfections usually do not appear for a number of hours after the impression is removed from the mouth, they should not be troublesome if the stone die is constructed within the first 30 minutes, as recommended.

Biocompatibility. The ADA specification for testing biocompatibility includes dental impression materials, despite the fact that the probability of allergic or toxic reactions from impression materials or their components is small. Comparisons of cell cytotoxicity for different impression materials show that polysulfide resulted in the lowest cell death count (Fig. 7–4). Multiple exposure tests, simulating what might occur in a dental school setting when a student remakes an impression several times, indicate that polysulfide has little effect on cell viability. Perhaps the most likely elastomer-induced biocompatibility problem occurs when a piece of the impression material is left in the gingival sulcus. The irritation can range from minor to severe. The radiopacity of the lead-containing polysulfide materials is an advantage in these situations, as is the material's resistance to tearing.

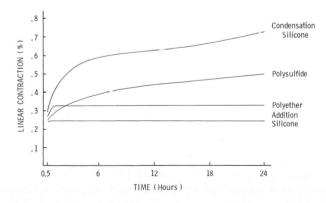

Figure 7–3. Contraction of four elastomeric impression materials.

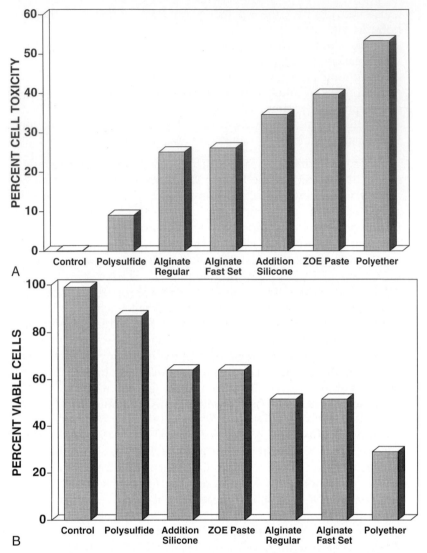

Figure 7–4. The graph of cell cytotoxicity *(A)* shows that after 3 days of incubation with Vero cells all the impression materials were cytotoxic to varying degrees. The relative cytotoxicity of each material is shown relative to the control. The graph of cell viability *(B)* gives the relative percent of viable cells after being exposed to the impression materials. (*A* and *B* from Sydiskis RK, and Gerhardt DE: Cytotoxicity of impression materials. J Prosthet Dent 69:431, 1993.)

Handling of the Tray. One way to minimize the effects of polymerization shrinkage, loss of reaction by-product, and deformation associated with distortion is to minimize the amount of material that is used to make the impression. The most accurate polysulfide impressions are made by using a custom acrylic tray. Although stock impression trays are available that can be contoured closely to the oral tissues, constructing a custom tray with a plastic material ensures a uniform thickness of impression material. To fabricate a custom tray, an impression is obtained of the teeth and adjacent tissues using any convenient impression material. A stone cast is constructed. The important parts of the cast, such as the prepared teeth, are covered with one or two thicknesses of base plate wax and tin foil to act as a spacer for the impression material. Chemical-curing or light-curing resin (described in a subsequent chapter) is placed over the tin foil to form the tray. After curing, the resin "custom" tray is separated from the cast, and the wax and tin foil are removed. The impression material is placed in the space previously occupied by the wax. Because the base plate wax forms a uniform space, a uniform thickness of material is produced when the impression is made. This uniformity minimizes the dimensional changes that might distort an impression if a bulk of material is used.

Although perforated trays, similar to those used for hydrocolloid impressions, would be satisfactory from this standpoint, they are not as convenient or practical as the custom-built resin tray just described. Adhesion can be obtained by the application of a minimal, uniform thickness of adhesive to the plastic tray, before the insertion of the impression material. The adhesive then forms a tenacious bond between the rubber material and the tray.

The adhesive cements furnished with the various types of rubber impression materials *are not interchangeable.* Adhesives employed with the polysulfide rubber impression materials include butyl rubber or styrene-acrylonitrile dissolved in a suitable volatile solvent such as chloroform or a ketone. Note that a slightly roughened surface on the tray increases the adhesion.

Handling Technique. A polysulfide impression of a number of teeth can be obtained at one time with the use of syringe and tray materials. To provide a less viscous material for use with the syringe, most manufacturers have provided impression materials with at least two consistencies: one for use with the tray and a thinner one for use with the syringe. The syringe type may also have longer working and setting times. In addition, the syringe material contains less filler particles, so it has greater polymerization shrinkage and more thermal contraction. For these reasons, it is not advisable to use the syringe material alone.

The method of using both the syringe and the tray materials is often referred to as the *multiple mix* technique because two separate mixtures are required with two separate mixing pads and spatulas. With the elastomeric impression materials, the mix thickens as it begins to set. Although the consistency may be acceptable for the tray material, it may be too thick to be extruded from the syringe. Thus, it is advisable to mix the tray material first and fill the tray with a uniform thickness of material and set it aside, while a second person begins mixing and filling the syringe. The material is injected from the filled syringe within and around the prepared teeth. The filled tray is then carried to place and seated over the syringe material. The two materials should cure together. Timing the procedure is critical because if the tray or the syringe material becomes too set, they may not cohere. If either material has progressed past its working time when the two are brought together, the bond between them will not be strong. The clinician may or may not realize the materials have separated when the tray is removed; however, the distortion in the final casting will be apparent. Polysulfide has a long working time, which can be beneficial for the student who is just learning to make an impression, for the advanced student who is making an impression of several teeth prepared for a fixed partial denture (bridge), or for the dentist who must work without an assistant.

Under no circumstance should the impression material be allowed to develop elastic properties before the tray is seated. If a partially set material is seated, the elastic component will be compressed. Once removed, the impression "springs back" or relaxes, and the dies from this impression will be too narrow and too short, as illustrated in Figure 7–5.

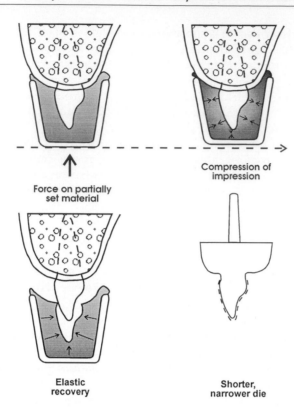

Force on partially set material

Compression of impression

Elastic recovery

Shorter, narrower die

Figure 7–5. Diagram illustrating the distortion that can occur if excessive pressure is applied to an elastomeric impression material after some inital elasticity has developed. (Artwork prepared by Dr. Nicola Richards.)

For much the same reason, it is difficult to repair a polysulfide impression by adding more material and then reseating the impression. The added material is cushioned by the induction of compressive stress in the already cured impression. When the impression is removed, the stresses are released. Therefore, a small die or cast results. If such a repair is attempted, it is essential to relieve the first impression. This is usually done by cutting away the interproximal and gingival areas of the impression. Even with proper relief of the initial impression, reseating the tray is difficult. For polysulfide, the surface must be roughened to ensure that the new material bonds to the set impression. The safest method is to obtain a new impression when bubbles or similar defects appear.

Disinfection of Impressions. Polysulfide can be disinfected by most of the various antimicrobial solutions without adverse dimensional changes, provided the disinfection time is short. Prolonged immersion may produce minimal distortion. However, the surface hardness of the gypsum cast may be affected by the type of disinfection agent used. Although polysulfide was not affected, there is evidence that disinfecting the custom tray can interfere with the bond of some impression materials to the custom tray. One recommended procedure is a 10-minute immersion in a 10% solution of hypochlorite.

Handling of the Stone Cast. It is possible to construct successive stone dies or casts from polysulfide impressions when duplicate stone dies are needed. The successive dies are less accurate than the first die constructed from the material. The distortion that occurs is primarily caused by the normal dimensional change that takes place with the polysulfide impression material and only partly because

TABLE 7–2. Advantages and Disadvantages of Polysulfide Materials

Advantages	Disadvantages
Long working time	Requires a custom tray
Proven accuracy	Must be poured in stone immediately
High tear resistance	Potential for significant distortion
Less hydrophobic	Odor offends patients
Inexpensive to use	Messy and stains clothes
Long shelf life	Second pour is less accurate

of the process of pouring or removing the stone dies. Thus, for polysulfide, the time interval between impression pours should not be longer than 30 minutes.

Shelf Life. A properly compounded polysulfide impression material does not deteriorate appreciably in the tubes when it is stored under normal environmental conditions. To maximize the shelf life, always keep the tubes tightly closed when they are not in use. Storage in a cool environment is also advisable. ADA Specification No. 19 requires that after storage of the base and accelerator for 7 days at $60 \pm 2°$ C $(140 + 3.6°$ F), the material must still meet the test for permanent deformation. If the shelf life is exceeded, the components of the pastes may separate. Poor elastic behavior exhibited as high "set" values (low recovery) is another indication that the material has exceeded its shelf life.

Pros and Cons of Polysulfide Impression Materials. Although many clinicians have achieved consistently good results over many years of use, there is never a guarantee that any material will yield a 100% accurate impression every time. There are other factors that may not lead to an inaccurate result but nevertheless may contribute to an unsatisfactory experience for the patient and the dentist during the impression-making procedure. The positive and negative features of polysulfide materials are summarized in Table 7–2.

Modifications. The lead dioxide reactor contributes to some of the disadvantages of polysulfide impression material. Several alternatives have been tried. Organic hydroperoxide can be used (e.g., *t*-butyl hydroperoxide), but these compounds have poor dimensional stability because of the hydroperoxide volatility. The inorganic hydroxides, such as copper, are used as the cross-linking system in dental polysulfides. Their chemical mechanism is obscure. Although copper hydroxide–cured materials are a viable alternative to traditional polysulfides, these materials have not been popular mainly because they were introduced at the same time that polyether and addition silicones were developed. As addition reaction materials, the latter have several advantages over even an improved condensation reaction material.

CONDENSATION SILICONE IMPRESSION MATERIAL

Chemistry. The polymer consists of an α-ω-hydroxy-terminated polydimethyl siloxane (Fig. 7–6A).

The condensation polymerization of this material involves a reaction with trifunctional and tetrafunctional alkyl silicates, commonly tetraethyl orthosilicate, in the presence of stannous octoate $(Sn[C_7H_{15}COO]_2)$. These reactions can take place at ambient temperatures; thus, the materials are often called *room temperature vulcanization* (RTV) silicones. The average RTV polymer chain con-

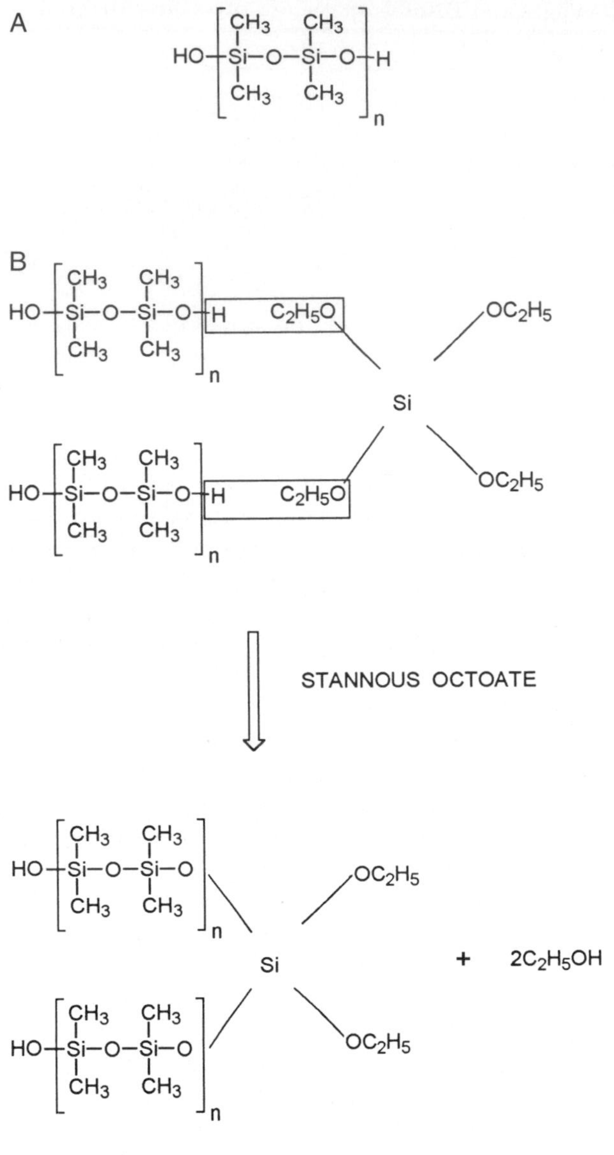

A

$$HO \left[\begin{array}{cc} CH_3 & CH_3 \\ | & | \\ Si-O-Si-O \\ | & | \\ CH_3 & CH_3 \end{array} \right]_n H$$

B

STANNOUS OCTOATE

$+ \quad 2C_2H_5OH$

Figure 7–6. A, Structural formula of the molecule, α-ω hydroxy-terminated poly(dimethyl siloxane). *B,* Condensation reaction between the OH end groups of the α-ω hydroxy-terminated poly(dimethyl siloxane) and tetraethyl orthosilicate in the presence of stannous octoate. The reaction results in the release of two ethanol molecules.

sists of about 1000 units. The formation of the elastomer occurs through a cross-linking between terminal groups of the silicone polymers and the alkyl silicate to form a three-dimensional network (Fig. 7–6B).

Ethyl alcohol is a by-product of the condensation setting reaction. Its subsequent evaporation probably accounts for much of the contraction that takes place in a set silicone rubber. Improvements in the chemistry of the cross-linking reactions have resulted in addition reaction silicones that are discussed in a subsequent section. The advantages of the newer silicones resulted in a significant drop in the use of the condensation silicones. However, the information in this section on these original silicone impression materials is useful since it sets the stage for the discussion of the addition reaction materials.

Composition. The condensation silicone impression materials are supplied as a base paste and a low-viscosity liquid or catalyst paste. Because the silicone polymer is a liquid, colloidal silica or microsized metal oxide is added as a filler to form a paste. The selection and pretreatment of the filler are of extreme importance because silicones have a low cohesive energy level and, therefore, a weaker intermolecular interaction. Frequently, the filler particles separate from the polymer, and the dispensed material appears as two components.

The influence of the filler on the strength of a silicone elastomer is much more critical than for any of the other impression materials, as discussed in the subsequent section on dimensional stability. The particle size should be within the optimum range of 5 to 10 μm. Smaller particles tend to aggregate, but larger ones do not contribute to reinforcement. The particles are often surface treated to provide better compatibility with, and reinforcement of, the silicone rubber.

A high-viscosity material, commonly referred to as a "putty," was developed to overcome the large polymerization shrinkage of the condensation silicone impression materials. These putties are highly filled so there is less polymer present; hence, there is less polymerization shrinkage. Because the material has such a large concentration of filler particles, the properties of the impression material are influenced by properties of the filler, a phenomenon known as the *law of mixtures.* Therefore, the overall thermal expansion is less than that of the polymer because the filler particle has a smaller coefficient of thermal expansion. This effect of the law of mixtures holds true for all multicomponent materials. It is more pronounced when the amount of the additional component is high, as with putty materials. Putty is used as the tray material in conjunction with a low-viscosity silicone. This technique and details on the properties of these elastomers are discussed later in this chapter.

These polymers do not have a characteristic color, such as the brown color of the lead dioxide used in polysulfides. Condensation silicone paste materials and putty can be made in a variety of colors. Pastel pinks, blues, greens, and purples are common. Each manufacturer supplies the material in several different colors corresponding to the viscosity. Several types of organic dyes or pigments are used to produce the colors. The choice of the material product depends on the system, the properties desired, and the manufacturer.

Manipulation. Condensation silicones are supplied as a base paste and a liquid catalyst or reactor. A length of the base is dispensed from the tube onto a graduated mixing pad. Then, one drop of the liquid catalyst is added for each unit length of base. These materials are somewhat difficult to mix because of the disparity in the viscosity of the two components. However, the color difference of the two components provides a visual clue as to how completely the two are blended; for example, a homogeneous mix has a uniform color.

The putty material is supplied as a very thick paste and a liquid accelerator. Because the putty is so viscous, it is packaged in a jar rather than a tube and dispensed by volume using a scoop. The manufacturer's directions indicate the number of drops of accelerator needed for each scoop. Again, producing a well-mixed material is not easy when putty and an oily liquid are mixed, so some manufacturers have formulated a two-paste putty system. With either system, the best mixing technique is to knead the material with the fingers. Wearing gloves adds another complication, because some latex gloves contain a sulfur component that inhibits the setting of the putty. For the same reasons, some latex rubber dam materials inhibit the setting of these impression materials.

Working and Setting Times. A comparison of the working and setting times is given in Table 7–1. As the times in the table indicate, temperature has a significant influence on the rate of curing for condensation silicone impression materials. Chilling the material or mixing on a cool slab slows the reaction rate. Altering the base:catalyst ratio is another effective and practical method of changing the curing rate of these impression materials. When the base:catalyst ratio is modified, it is wise to test the setting time for the new ratio before it is used for a patient. There is no greater mess to clean off the teeth than an impression that did not set properly.

Elasticity. Condensation silicone impression materials are more ideally elastic than polysulfides. They exhibit minimal permanent deformation and recover rapidly when strained. Like polysulfides, these materials are not very stiff, which means it is not difficult to remove them from undercuts without distortion.

Rheology. The viscoelastic characteristics of these materials suggest that they can respond elastically (snap back like springs) or as viscous liquids that easily sustain permanent deformation (never return to the exact same spot, like dashpots). The material is more likely to respond as an elastic if it is strained rapidly; hence, impressions must be removed quickly so that the deformation is elastic and recoverable. Prolonging the strain by removing the impression slowly increases the chance for the permanent deformation to occur because the polymer chains respond in a viscous manner.

The most common consistencies of the condensation materials are the putty and the wash material. Putty is at the extreme end of the high-viscosity materials. The wash material is equivalent to the light-body or syringe material. Detailed information is included in the handling section.

Tear Energy. The tear resistance is low for condensation silicone impression materials. Although they do not tear as easily as alginates or agar hydrocolloids, they must be handled carefully to avoid ruining a margin of a crown preparation when it is torn. The strain-rate sensitivity described for polysulfides is also a controlling factor for condensation silicones. Applying a force rapidly ensures the highest tear resistance, so it is important to remove the impression quickly once the air seal is broken.

Dimensional Stability. The excessive polymerization shrinkage of the condensation silicones requires a modification of the impression-making technique to produce accurate impressions. Rather than the custom tray-multiple mix technique recommended for polysulfides, a putty-wash technique is used for condensation silicones. This technique is able to compensate for the poor dimensional stability of these materials. The amount of linear contraction is two to four times greater than for the other impression materials (see Fig. 7–3). In addition to the large setting shrinkage, the dimensional instability is also caused by the loss of the volatile reaction product, ethyl alcohol. Polysulfides undergo condensation polymerization, but the reaction product, water, is a relatively small molecule; thus, this loss has a much smaller effect on the material than the loss of the larger alcohol molecule resulting from the silicone condensation reaction. Because the polymerization reaction continues even after the material is "clinically set," the polymerization shrinkage continues. Once the impression is removed from the mouth, the evaporation of the reaction by-product occurs continuously. Thus, the most accurate model is obtained by pouring up the impression with a gypsum stone slurry immediately after it is removed from the mouth. "Immediately" can be defined as within the first 30 minutes, even when the putty-wash technique is used. The effect of delaying this pouring time is shown in Figure 7–7.

Biocompatibility. Silicone is one of the most biologically inert materials. Thus, it is highly unlikely that condensation silicone impression materials would cause a biocompatibility problem (see Fig. 7–4). The one danger, as discussed with the polysulfides, is the possibility of leaving torn impression material in the gingival sulcus. Because the silicone materials are not radiopaque, it can be difficult to detect the presence of torn material. Often the gingival inflammation that accompanies the presence of this "foreign body" is attributed to irritation from preparing the tooth or cementing the restoration. Careful visual inspection of the impression to check for torn areas is needed to ensure that the necessary detail is recorded. If evidence of tearing is detected during this inspection, the clinician should immediately check the tissue to remove any remnant of the impression.

Shelf Life. The alkyl silicates are slightly unstable, particularly if they are mixed with a tin compound to form a single catalyst liquid. Thus, a limited shelf life may result because of oxidation of the tin component within the catalyst. Shelf-life failure may also occur as a result of degradation of the base or cross-linkage of the base during storage. The goal of the supplier is to achieve a compromise in the conflicting requirements, such as long shelf-life stability, rapid rate of cure, and excellent physical properties.

Handling of the Tray. Because the putty-wash technique is used for making condensation silicone impressions, the custom tray described for polysulfides is not needed. Most clinicians use disposable stock trays to support the putty. Even

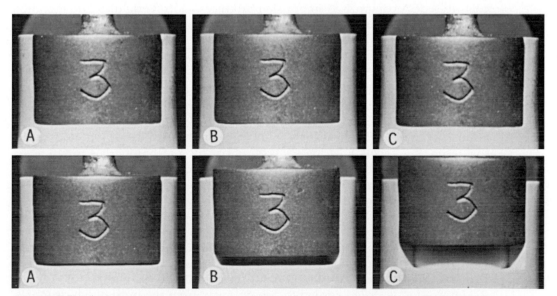

Figure 7–7. Fit of a master casting placed on stone dies constructed from an addition silicone *(top row)* and a condensation silicone *(bottom row)*. Stone poured at 30 minutes *(A)*, 6 hours *(B)*, and 24 hours *(C)*.

with this very stiff material, the tray should be rigid to prevent distortion. To hold the material in place, the tray is painted with the adhesive supplied by the manufacturer. Because the material extends over the edge of the tray, it is advisable to paint the adhesive on the outer borders of the tray to maximize retention. For silicone materials, the adhesive may contain polydimethyl siloxane or other silicone that reacts with the impression material and an ethyl silicate to create a physical bond with the tray.

Handling Technique. As discussed previously, a putty-wash technique is frequently used for making condensation silicone impressions. First, the thick putty material is placed in a stock tray, and a preliminary impression is made. This results in what is essentially an intraoral custom-made tray formed by the putty. Space for the light-bodied "wash" material is provided either by cutting away some of the "tray" putty or by using a thin polyethylene sheet as a spacer between the putty and the prepared teeth. After the spacer is removed, a mix of the thin-consistency wash material is placed into the putty impression, and then the putty wash is seated in the mouth to make the final impression. This method is referred to as the *two-stage putty-wash technique* or the *reline technique.*

For reliable reproduction of sharp angles in cavity preparations, it is often necessary to use a syringe and inject the wash material within and onto the preparations. With certain products, the condensation silicone used for the wash or final impression is the manufacturer's light-bodied or syringe material. An alternative to the two-step procedure is to syringe the wash into place, then seat the unset putty over the light-bodied material. One difficulty with combining the wash and putty steps is that the higher viscosity material may displace the more fluid wash material. If this occurs, critical areas of the preparation may be reproduced in putty rather than in the light-bodied material, but the putty is too thick to replicate the required detail.

As manufacturers made stiffer and stiffer putties to try to avoid the distortion that can occur with disposable stock trays, a different kind of distortion became apparent. If the clinician seats the putty impression with too much force or holds the impression in place with more than a light touch, the impression can be compressed. A compressed impression produces short, wide dies (see Fig. 7–5), and castings made from these dies are not accurate, because they do not seat completely. This phenomenon is similar to the distortion that occurs when attempts are made to reseat a polysulfide impression to "repair" an area with insufficient detail. With the two-stage putty-wash technique, it is obvious that excessive force results in an impression that is not dimensionally accurate. What is not as obvious is that the same distortion can occur in impressions made using the combined technique. As it begins to set, the putty material rapidly builds up viscosity and elasticity (stiffness). Recent studies of the accuracy of this technique versus a syringe-tray (multiple mix) technique has raised some controversy. The stiffness of the material at the time the impression is seated influences the accuracy. If the material has cured to a point when elastic properties have developed, elastic deformation will occur when the impression is seated. On removal from the mouth, that deformation recovers, and a smaller die results. Ideally, each commercial product has an optimal time at which it should be carried to the mouth. Even when seating the putty at the optimal working time, it is possible to elastically compress or deform the material. The frequency of distortions associated with the stiffness of the material at the time the impression is seated has led to a move away from the putty-wash materials.

The mixing of the base and accelerator for the putty-consistency material may

TABLE 7–3. Advantages and Disadvantages of Condensation Silicones Compared with Polysulfide Materials

Advantages	Disadvantages
Adequate working and setting time	Adequate accuracy if poured immediately
Pleasant odor and no staining	Poor dimensional stability
Adequate tear strength	Potential for significant distortion
Better elastic properties on removal	Putty-wash method is technique sensitive
Less distortion on removal	Slightly more expensive
	Poor to adequate shelf life

seem strange at first. Some clinicians prefer to incorporate the liquid accelerator into the putty by first mixing on a pad, then completing the process by kneading with the fingers. Heavy-body tray and light-body syringe materials may be used to make condensation silicone impressions using the multiple-mix technique described for polysulfide.

Pros and Cons of Condensation Silicones Compared with Polysulfides. The advantages and disadvantages of polysulfide impression materials have been described earlier. The condensation silicones are compared and contrasted with polysulfide materials in Table 7–3.

Disinfection of the Impression. Condensation silicone impressions can be immersed in most of the commercial antimicrobial solutions for a short period (less than an hour) and not experience any adverse effects.

Preparation of the Stone Die. As previously noted, the stone die should be constructed shortly after the impression has been removed from the mouth to prevent distortion of the impression. Generally, the condensation silicones are compatible with all gypsum products.

Modifications. As mentioned previously, the major modification of the condensation silicone impression materials is a change in the setting mechanism. This modification has brought about a new family of impression materials, the addition reaction silicones.

ADDITION REACTION SILICONE (VINYL POLYSILOXANE) IMPRESSION MATERIAL

Chemistry. The addition silicones are frequently called *polyvinylsiloxane* or *vinyl polysiloxane* impression materials. In contrast with the condensation silicones, the addition reaction polymer is terminated with vinyl groups and is cross-linked with hydride groups activated by a platinum salt catalyst. Figure 7–8 illustrates the addition reaction.

There are no reaction by-products as long as the correct proportions of vinyl silicone and hydride silicone are maintained and there are no impurities. If the proportions are out of balance or impurities are present, then side reactions will produce hydrogen gas. Both moisture and polymeric impurities such as residual silanol groups react with the hydrides of the base polymer and contribute to the development of hydrogen gas. Although technically not a reaction by-product, the hydrogen gas that evolves from the set material can result in pinpoint voids

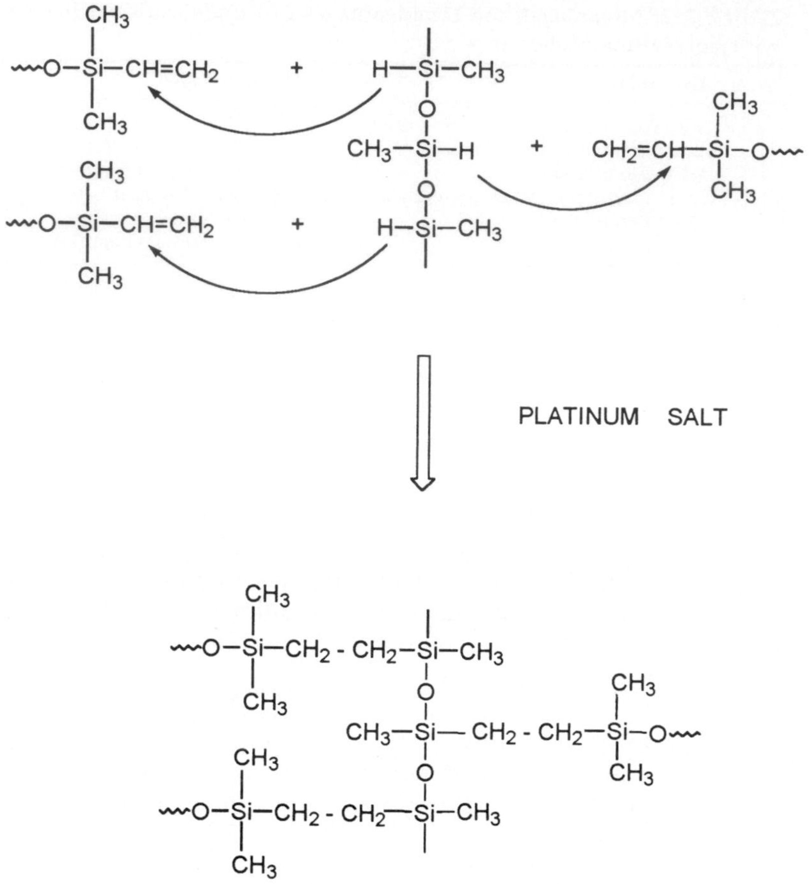

Figure 7–8. Top figure shows how the hydrogen atoms along the backbone structure of the vinyl silicone chain will move to the vinyl groups during addition polymerization. The lower figures show the final structure after the platinum salt has initiated the addition polymerization reaction.

in the stone casts that are poured immediately after removing the impression from the mouth. Manufacturers often add a noble metal, such as platinum or palladium, to act as a scavenger for the released hydrogen gas. Another way to compensate for the hydrogen gas is to wait an hour or longer before pouring up the impression. This delay does not cause any clinically detectable dimensional change.

Composition. Both base and catalyst pastes contain a form of the vinyl silicone. The base paste contains polymethyl hydrogen siloxane, as well as other siloxane prepolymers. The catalyst paste contains divinyl polydimethyl siloxane and other siloxane prepolymers. If the "catalyst" paste contains the platinum salt activator, then the paste labeled *base* must contain the hybrid silicone. Retarders may also be present in the paste that contains the platinum catalyst. Both pastes contain fillers.

One of the disadvantages of the silicone impression materials is their inherent hydrophobicity. To compensate for this serious drawback, manufacturers have made the addition silicones more hydrophilic ("water loving"). To render the surface of the impression hydrophilic, a surfactant is added to the paste. This surfactant then allows the impression material to wet soft tissue better and to be poured in stone more effectively. These materials still require a dry field, but they reproduce the surface of soft tissue better. Pouring of the set impression is easier, because the wet stone has a greater affinity for the hydrophilic surface. This may be the biggest benefit of the hydrophilic additives being placed in the vinyl polysiloxanes.

Previously, it was believed that the chemicals used for soft tissue management and on teeth adjacent to the preparation were retarding the polymerization of the hydrophilic vinyl polysiloxanes, especially if the chemical contained sulfur (such as aluminum sulfate). New research indicates that these chemicals, which are used to control bleeding and widen the sulcus, do not retard the set of the vinyl polysiloxane impression. Any distortion or fuzziness at the margins of the impression is probably caused by undetected moisture present in the area to be replicated.

Sulfur contamination from natural latex gloves inhibits the setting of the addition silicone impression materials. Some vinyl gloves may have the same effect because of the sulfur-containing stabilizer used in the manufacturing process of certain gloves. The contamination is so pervasive that touching the tooth with the glove before seating the impression can inhibit the setting of the critical surface next to the tooth. This inhibition produces a major distortion.

Manipulation. The light-body and medium-body vinyl polysiloxanes are supplied as two pastes, and the putty is supplied as two jars of high-viscosity base and catalyst materials. Because both the base and catalyst contain similar materials, they also have nearly equivalent viscosities. Thus, they are much easier to mix than the condensation silicones.

The similarity of the paste consistencies and the shear-thinning behavior of these impression materials made the vinyl polysiloxanes suitable for an automatic dispensing and mixing device. An example of the device is shown in Figure 7–9. It is generally used for light-viscosity and medium-viscosity materials, but heavy-body and putty materials have been modified to accommodate the automatic mixing device. This apparatus has certain advantages compared with hand dispensing and spatulation. With the mechanical device, there is greater uniformity in proportioning and in mixing, less air is incorporated into the mix, and the mixing time is reduced. Also, there are fewer possibilities for contamination of the material.

The mixed impression material is ejected directly into the adhesive-coated tray or onto the prepared teeth if the syringe tip (not shown in Fig. 7–9) is in place.

The basic automatic mixers sold by various manufacturers are interchangeable, but the double-spiral mixing tips are not. The tips vary in diameter, in length, and perhaps more importantly, in the number of spiral units within the tip. More units provide more thorough mixing. Thus, an impression material that is uniformly mixed in a 13-spiral unit may be inadequately mixed in an 11-spiral tip.

One caution in using these automatic mixing devices is to make sure that the openings of the tubes that dispense the pastes remain unclogged. Often the color difference of the two pastes is so slight that it is difficult to determine visually if the proper amounts of base and catalyst pastes have been mixed together. Problems can be avoided if a small amount is extruded from the cartridge of materials before the mixing tip is attached. The lack of color difference also makes it difficult to ensure that the mix is homogeneous. However, investigation

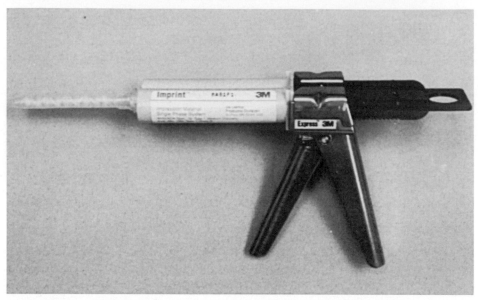

Figure 7–9. Automixer and dispenser for addition polymerization silicone impression materials. When the trigger is pulled, the plunger is driven forward (to the left) so that the base and accelerator pastes are forced from the two cartridges into the mixing tip (extreme left) containing the spiral mixer. The pastes pass down the bore, over and through the spiral, which has sections rotated 180 degrees to one another. It then exits at the muzzle as a uniformly mixed paste.

of the automatic mixing devices has demonstrated that the mix is adequate if the device is used properly.

As previously mentioned, some putties can be automatically mixed, and some are supplied in a jar with the proper quantity measured by volume. Initially, the putty-wash application of the vinyl polysiloxanes was extremely popular; however, current trends do not favor this impression technique. The single-viscosity or monophase impression materials are becoming more popular. These materials are supplied as two components: a base and a catalyst. The difference is that one mix of the materials is used for both the syringe material and the tray material. When used in conjunction with the automatic mixing devices, the monophase material is the most convenient for the practitioner.

Working and Setting Times. In contrast with the condensation silicones, the curing rate of the addition silicones appears to be even more sensitive to ambient temperature than are the polysulfides (see Table 7–1). Working and setting times can be extended (up to 100%) by the addition of a retarder as supplied by the respective manufacturer and by cooling the mixing slab. The addition silicone can also be refrigerated before use. This cooling has little effect on viscosity. Once the impression material is in the mouth, it warms rapidly, and the setting time is not extended as much as when a chemical retarder is used. Retarders are impractical with the automatic mixing devices. However, because the automatic mixers speed up the preparation step, the net effect is a longer working time without slowing down the setting time. The ease and speed of transferring the material into the mouth have created a demand for a shorter setting time. Several manufacturers sell a fast-setting material along with the regular-setting vinyl polysiloxanes. Tests of the properties indicated little difference between the accelerated setting material and the material that sets more slowly.

Elasticity. The vinyl polysiloxane impression materials are the most ideally elastic of the currently available materials. Distortion on removal from undercuts is virtually nonexistent, because these materials exhibit the lowest strain-in-compression values (permanent distortion). The excellent elastic properties present a problem in that the heavy-body putty material begins to build up elastic response while still in the working stage. If the material is compressed elastically during the seating of the impression, then distortion can occur when the material elastically rebounds. For most of these materials, the stiffness is proportional to the consistency of the material; for example, putties are stiff, but light-bodied materials are quite flexible. The exceptions are the newer hydrophilic one-step materials that are extremely stiff and handle like the traditional polyether impression materials.

Rheology. As one of the most pseudoplastic impression materials, the effect of increased strain rate on the unset material is quite pronounced for vinyl polysiloxane. This large discrepancy between the flow properties of the material under strong force, such as during syringing, and light force, such as during seating the tray, has allowed manufacturers to market the one-step material. One mix of this medium viscosity material can be used for capturing the fine detail and recording the bulk of the oral structures. When syringed, it flows readily and yet holds its shape when placed in an impression tray. With these "single-phase" materials intended for both injection and tray use, the primary consideration is viscosity.

Some investigators confuse this pseudoplastic phenomenon with another rheologic property referred to as *thixotropism.* Ketchup is an example of a thixotropic material; it does not flow until sufficient energy is supplied (by shaking the bottle numerous times) to overcome the yield stress. Beyond this point, the material is very fluid (all the ketchup comes out at once). Manufacturers have developed impression materials with thixotropic properties so they remain in place, both the material syringed into the mouth and the material loaded in the tray. This is an important characteristic, but it is different from the shear-thinning pseudoplastic behavior of elastomers.

Tear Energy. The resistance to tearing is adequate, similar to that of the condensation silicones. If not handled correctly, these materials will tear rather than stretch like the polysulfides. The materials are highly viscoelastic, so using a rapid strain rate produces an elastic response, and the vinyl polysiloxane is less likely to tear. Only a few materials, such as Express and Rapid, have been modified by the manufacturer to make them less radiolucent and more detectable radiographically.

Dimensional Stability. Vinyl polysiloxane impression materials are the most dimensionally stable of all the existing materials. No volatile reaction by-product is released to cause the material to shrink. (Note that the hydrogen gas is not a true reaction by-product.) The clinically set material is close to being completely cured, so there is little residual polymerization to contribute to the dimensional change. The primary dimensional change comes from thermal shrinkage as the material cools from mouth temperature to room temperature (see Fig. 7–3).

This unusual stability means that the impression does not have to be poured in stone immediately. In fact, these impressions are often sent to the laboratory to be poured. Research has shown that a cast poured between 24 hours and 1 week was as accurate as a cast made the first hour, assuming that there was no problem with the hydrogen bubbles (see Fig. 7–7).

The combination of excellent dimensional stability and superior elasticity means that multiple casts that are made from the same impression all have the same degree of accuracy. This would not be true for a material such as polysulfide because the act of removing the first cast from the impression can cause some distortion, and after several casts are removed, the impression is no longer accurate.

Biocompatibility. As discussed in the section on condensation silicones, these materials are highly biocompatible (see Fig. 7–4). The danger of leaving a piece of material during the removal of the impression can be avoided by proper handling of the material and a thorough inspection of the margins in the impression to ensure there are no torn areas. A foreign body of impression material can cause severe gingival inflammation and may be misdiagnosed at a subsequent appointment.

Handling of the Tray. The popularity of a stock tray rather than a custom tray may be associated with the increased use of the putty reline technique. The primary putty impression actually serves as a custom tray for the wash or reline material. This technique is described in detail in the handling section for the condensation silicone impression materials.

In general, the tray adhesives for polysulfide, polyether, and condensation silicones are quite satisfactory. Some of the materials used with the addition silicones were formerly less effective but have been improved in recent years. Certain putty-type silicones require mechanical retention in the tray, because the adhesive is ineffective.

Handling Technique. The putty-wash technique has been popular for the vinyl polysiloxane impression materials. When the putty-wash technique is properly used, it can produce impressions with accuracy comparable to that of the multiple-mix procedure. Theoretically, the putty-wash procedure is more convenient, and the bulk of the impression is formed by the highly filled putty material, which has relatively low polymerization shrinkage and a low thermal contraction coefficient.

However, with the addition silicone materials, the putty-wash system can, and frequently does, produce a grossly inaccurate impression. This occurs if the putty impression is held under pressure. Problems can occur because of the pressure applied to the setting putty when the simultaneous technique is used, and they can also occur with the set putty that is used in the two-stage technique. Removing the impression from the mouth releases the pressure; the putty recovers but the recovery is excessive since the elastic precompression is recovered in addition to elastic deformation recovery from undercut areas. The distortion that is produced with the stiff, compressible putty results in shorter and narrower dies (see Fig. 7–5). In addition to excessive pressure, some of the distortion in putty-wash impressions may be attributable to inadequate spacing for the wash material.

The extremely high viscosity of the putty means that it is incapable of adequately recording the detail required in an impression for fixed prosthodontics. Stops within the tray should be used to avoid pushing through the wash or syringe material when the putty is seated. If the putty material is visible in an area of the impression, especially in contact with a prepared tooth, then the accuracy of the impression is highly suspect.

The addition silicones are supplied in a wide variety of viscosities, including the single-phase or monophase viscosity. Although these materials have become popular, there is some controversy about the accuracy of impressions for multiunit fixed prosthetic restorations. Some investigators claim greater distortion in the interpreparation distance with the single-viscosity impression technique when using a stock tray. They used regular and reinforced stock trays to rule out distortion caused by the tray. One possible explanation is that a bulk amount of the single-viscosity material may have more polymerization shrinkage than a bulk amount of the putty or the heavy-body material that have higher filler contents. It is expected that the lower-viscosity materials do not have the dimensional stability that is associated with the higher-viscosity materials. Even the "less" dimensionally stable monophase materials are considerably more accurate and dimensionally stable than the polysulfides or the condensation silicones. Currently, there are several brands of the single-viscosity materials to select. The best results are probably obtained from the stiffer, higher-viscosity versions of these monophase materials.

A comparison of the different techniques shows that using a custom tray is the most accurate technique. However, if the material is used correctly, results that are clinically acceptable can be produced with any of these impression material techniques.

Disinfection. Vinyl impression materials are easily disinfected by immersing in 10% hypochlorite or 2% glutaraldehyde solutions. Usually, a 10- to 15-minute immersion is sufficient. One drawback of a longer immersion is that the surfactant component, which makes the materials more hydrophilic and easier to pour in stone, tends to leach out during the disinfection procedure. The net result is that the "hydrophilic" materials become "hydrophobic."

Preparation of Stone Casts and Dies. The hydrophobic characteristics of these vinyl polysiloxane impression materials make it difficult to wet the surface, so it is difficult to pour a bubble-free stone cast from an addition silicone impression material. The physical properties of the hydrophobic and hydrophilic vinyl polysiloxanes are comparable. The only property that is different is the contact angle. The hydrophobic materials have a water contact angle of approximately 95 degrees, whereas that of the hydrophilic materials ranges from approximately 30 to 35 degrees.

There are a number of surfactant sprays on the market (Hydrosystem, manufactured by Zhermack and sold by B & H Technical Services, Belleview, WA) that reduce the surface tension so that the stone wets the surface of the impression. Pooling of the spray liquid or a thick layer of the wetting agent can affect the dimensional accuracy of the impression and can also cause the surface of the stone to be soft and porous. A dilute solution of soap is an effective surfactant, but the taste is rather offensive, so the commercially available wetting agents may be preferable if the intent is to improve the intraoral flow characteristics of the impression material.

Other than the difficulty of pouring the stone, most of the vinyl polysiloxane impression materials are compatible with the available gypsum products. The minimal interaction between the surface of the stone and the surface of the impression material is probably a contributing factor to the success of multiple pours from the same impression. This impression material is also compatible with epoxy resins used for more accurate casts and dies. These replica materials can be poured repeatedly into the same impression, as can also be done with gypsum products.

TABLE 7–4. Advantages and Disadvantages of Addition Silicones Compared with Polysulfide Materials

Advantages	Disadvantages
Shorter setting time	Hydrogen gas evolution in some materials
Easy to mix—automatic mixing devices	Hydrophilic materials still need careful
Adequate tear strength	handling and a very dry field
Extremely high accuracy	More expensive, especially with automatic
Undetectable distortion on removal	mixing device
Dimensionally stable even after 1 week	
Less distortion on removal	
If hydrophilic, good compatibility with gypsum	

Shelf Life. Manufacturers claim that the vinyl polysiloxanes have a 2-year shelf life, which is considerably longer than that of the condensation silicones. The silicone material tubes or containers must remain tightly closed because air hastens their deterioration. The shelf life can be prolonged by storing the material in a cool, dry environment. The viscosity of these materials is not affected by temperature; however, the curing rate is reduced.

Advantages and Disadvantages of Addition Silicones Relative to Polysulfides. The positive and negative features of addition silicone impression materials are listed in Table 7–4.

Modifications. The major changes in the development of vinyl polysiloxane impression materials have been focused on making the materials easier to use. This includes adding a palladium scavenger to tie up any hydrogen gas, making the materials less hydrophobic, formulating a material that can be used with a one-step technique and developing the automatic mixing device. The most recent changes are the improvements in the automatic mixing devices. The gun, or holding device, is smaller, the cartridges containing the material are smaller, and the mixing tubes are smaller. The size reduction makes the device easier to manipulate, especially if a clinician wants to syringe material directly into the mouth. The smaller mixing tubes are designed to reduce waste and thus reduce material costs.

POLYETHER IMPRESSION MATERIAL

Chemistry. This type of elastomeric impression material was introduced in Germany in the late 1960s. It is a polyether-based polymer that is cured by the reaction between aziridine rings (Fig. 7–10*A*), which are at the end of branched polyether molecules (Fig. 7–10*B*).

The main chain is probably a copolymer of ethylene oxide and tetrahydrofuran. Cross-linking, and thus setting, is brought about by an aromatic sulfonate ester of the type (Fig. 7–10*C*), where R is an alkyl group. This produces cross-linking by cationic polymerization via the imine end groups (Fig. 7–10*D*).

This material was the first elastomer to be developed primarily to function as an impression material. All the other materials were adapted from other uses.

Composition. The polyether rubbers are supplied as two pastes. The base contains the polyether polymer, a colloidal silica as a filler, and a plasticizer such as a glycolether or phthalate. The accelerator paste contains the alkyl-aromatic sulfonate in addition to the aforementioned filler and plasticizer.

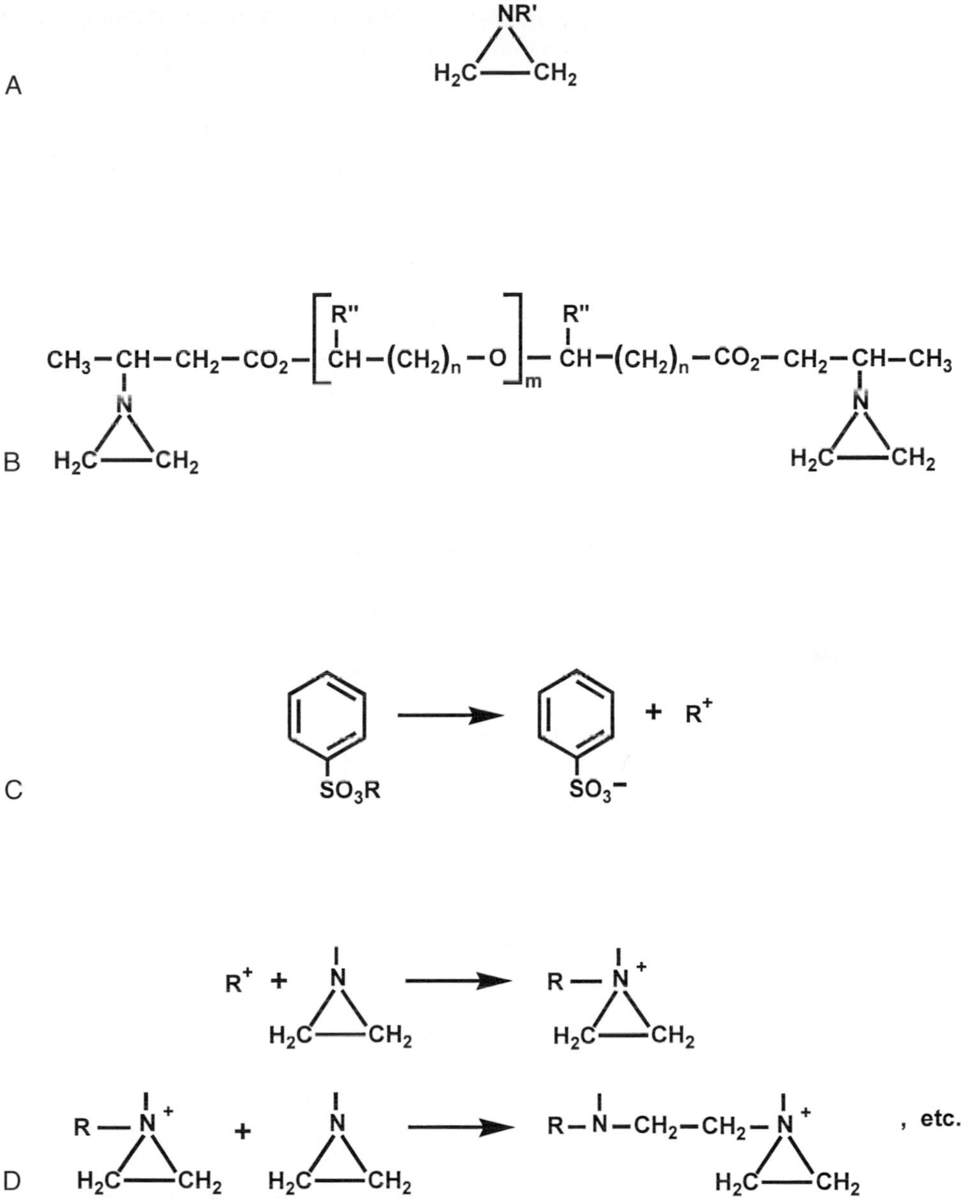

A

B

C

D

Figure 7–10. A, Structure of the aziridine ring. *B,* Copolymer of ethylene oxide and tetrahydrofuran. *C,* Structure of the aromatic sulfonate ester acting as an initiator by releasing a cation, R$^+$. *D,* Cross-linking occurs by cationic polymerization via the imine end groups.

Manipulation. Originally, polyethers were only supplied in one viscosity. The pseudoplasticity of the materials allowed one mix to be used for both syringe and tray material. Subsequently, manufacturers supplied an additional paste that could be used to produce a thinner mix. The volume differences between the base and catalyst pastes are evident in the bottom of Figure 7–1. The component materials required a reformulation to adapt the material to use with the automatic mixing devices. Although this device is successful, most polyethers are still mixed by hand. In addition, to compete with the addition silicones, the manufacturers realized that clinicians preferred the multiple viscosities of the vinyl polysiloxanes. Thus, polyether was changed so that it could be supplied in several viscosities. As a consequence, the stiffness of the polyether also was reduced.

Working and Setting Times. The curing rate of the polyethers is less sensitive to temperature change than that of the addition silicones (see Table 7–1). Some modification in base:accelerator ratio can be used to extend working time. Use of the thinner also extends working time with only a slight increase in setting time. In addition to reducing the viscosity of the unset material, the thinner alters the properties of the set materials. The elastic modulus or stiffness of the set material is reduced without increasing the permanent deformation, or flow. Also available for use with polyethers is a retarder that can extend working time without reducing the elastic properties or increasing polymerization shrinkage.

Elasticity. The polyethers have always been considered the stiffest of the impression materials, excluding the high-viscosity putties. The original material was extremely difficult to remove from undercut areas because of the high modulus of elasticity. Some of the new formulations of regular or medium-bodied materials are actually less stiff than the one-step hydrophilic vinyl polysiloxane impression materials. Results of compression set testing indicate that the polyethers are slightly less elastic than the vinyl polysiloxanes.

Rheology. The rheologic properties of the polyethers play a major role in their successful application as highly accurate impression materials. The pseudoplastic characteristics allowed the original single-viscosity materials to be used as both syringe and tray materials. The thinner component was used mostly to reduce the stiffness of the set material.

Tear Energy. Tear resistance is better than that of the condensation silicone impression materials and most of the addition silicone impression materials. However, polyether is more prone to tearing than polysulfide. Because it is also the most radiolucent impression material, the margins should be carefully inspected immediately after removing the impression to avoid leaving a thin fragment of impression material in the gingival sulcus.

Dimensional Stability. The dimensional change of the polyether impression materials is small, as shown in Figure 7–3. Like the addition silicones, polyethers have no reaction by-product. Although the residual polymerization continues beyond the clinical set time, it is for a much shorter period than for the polysulfide impression materials. Theoretically, the ring-opening reaction should produce a setting expansion rather than a setting shrinkage. However, it is difficult to measure the individual parameters that contribute to the dimensional change. It is possible that the thermal shrinkage more than offsets any polymerization expansion, if it occurs.

   The stiffness of the material means that the force needed to remove the impression is greater for polyether impressions than for the other types of materials. Yet, the recovery is nearly complete because of the excellent elastic properties of the polyether. Thus, the polyether impressions can be poured immediately, after several hours, or after several days and the resulting casts will have the same accuracy. The time interval is not nearly as critical for the addition silicones and polyethers as it is for the condensation silicones and the polysulfides (see Fig. 7–3). The polyethers exhibit the least amount of distortion from the loads imposed on the set material. Thus, pouring up the impression and removing the cast several times does not alter the dimensional stability of the polyether, even though a fairly substantial force is needed each time the cast is removed from the impression.

One property that has a negative effect on the materials is the absorption of water or fluids and the simultaneous leaching of the water-soluble plasticizer. Thus, the stored impressions must be kept in a dry, cool environment to maintain their accuracy.

Biocompatibility. Originally, there was some concern about hypersensitivity to the polyether catalyst system. Contact dermatitis from the polyether, especially to the dental assistant, has been reported. However, recent studies indicate no cytotoxic effects associated with the imine catalyst. The set polyether impression material did produce the highest cell cytotoxicity scores and the lowest viable cell count after multiple exposures (see Fig. 7–4).

Perhaps the most likely elastomer-induced problem for the patient arises from pieces of the impression material being left in the sulcus. The irritation can range from minor to severe.

Handling of the Tray. The need for custom trays for polyether impressions can be argued convincingly from two points of view. Those in favor of custom trays suggest that a thinner, uniform layer (approximately 2 mm) of the very stiff polyether material makes it easier to remove the impression from the mouth. Conversely, those arguing against custom trays do so because the extremely stiff material does not need the support of a custom tray to avoid distortion. Both sides are convincing. Regardless of what type of tray is used, it is important to use an adequate amount of adhesive so that the stress during removal does not dislodge the material from the tray.

Handling Technique. Most clinicians continue to use the monophase or single-viscosity material despite the fact that polyether is supplied in several viscosities and with an automatic mixing device. With a single-viscosity material, only one mix is made and part of the material is placed in the tray and another portion is put in the syringe for injecting into the cavity preparation. The stiffness and good elastic properties prevent distortion of the impressions made from the single-viscosity polyethers. The fast setting of this material requires the clinician to work rapidly, especially if several teeth are prepared. This is possible because the material flows and easily wets the tooth surfaces. Despite the availability of rapid curing materials, one manufacturer makes a fast-setting version of the polyether—this material is for the truly impatient dentist who does not want to use agar, the only accurate impression material that sets faster than polyether.

Disinfection. The elastomers can generally be disinfected by various antimicrobial solutions without adverse dimensional changes, provided that the disinfection time is brief. Prolonged immersion may produce measurable distortion, and certain agents may reduce the surface hardness of poured gypsum casts. In particular, the polyethers are susceptible to dimensional change if the immersion time is longer than 10 minutes, because of their pronounced hydrophilic nature. Two percent glutaraldehyde is a satisfactory solution for most elastomers.

As has been noted earlier in the text, the impression material itself may contain a disinfectant, which may be present in some dental stones.

TABLE 7–5. Advantages and Disadvantages of Polyethers Compared with Polysulfides

Advantages	Disadvantages
Fast working and setting times	Adequate accuracy if poured immediately
Proven accuracy	Poor dimensional stability
Adequate tear strength	Clean but tastes bad
Less hydrophobic—better wetting	Stiffness requires blocking undercuts
Less distortion on removal	Slightly more expensive
Long shelf life	Multiple casts can be poured
Good dimensional stability	

Handling of the Stone Cast. Pouring the stone cast in a polyether impression is much easier than in one made from silicone materials. In addition, there is little evidence of any negative surface interactions between polyether impressions and gypsum products. For polyether impressions, it is not a good idea to "shorten" the setting time of the stone by trying to remove the cast early. The stiffness of polyether makes it difficult to remove the stone cast from the impression. A weak stone cast may fracture during removal.

Shelf Life of Polyethers. A properly compounded polyether impression material does not deteriorate appreciably in the tubes when it is stored under normal environmental conditions. Storing in a cool, dry environment prolongs the shelf life. However, chilled polyether impression material becomes rigid and cannot be mixed. Thus, it is necessary to allow the material to reach room temperature before using.

Advantages and Disadvantages of Polyethers Compared with Polysulfides. The positive and negative features of polyethers compared with polysulfides are listed in Table 7–5.

Modifications. Reducing the stiffness and producing polyether in low and heavy viscosities have been the major changes for this type of impression material. The low viscosity is supplied with an automatic mixing device. Some clinicians who liked the original polyether because of its stiffness are less satisfied with the lower stiffness materials.

TECHNIQUES FOR MEASURING PROPERTIES

Reproduction of Oral Detail. The necessity for the impression material to reproduce the finest detail of the oral cavity is, of course, self-evident. Various tests have been employed by investigators to evaluate the ability of impression materials to reproduce surface detail. A surface reproduction test is a part of the specification for the elastic impression materials. There is no doubt that these elastomers and the reversible hydrocolloids record detail to a fine degree. When dental stone is poured over such test impressions, the finest detail is not always reproduced. In other words, the rubber impression materials are capable of reproducing detail more accurately than can be transferred to the stone die or cast.

The clinical significance of the surface reproduction tests is not entirely evident. It is possible that the detail obtained with the rubber impression materials on the *in vitro* test specimen might be greater than that obtained in the mouth because of the hydrophobicity exhibited by some of these materials.

Measurement of Working and Setting Times. Ordinarily, working time is measured at room temperature, whereas setting time is measured at mouth temperature. Penetrometer tests have been used to assess both working and setting times. For example, the end of working time might be defined as the time when a needle of a certain diameter and weight fails to penetrate a volume of impression material to a specified depth. Setting time would not have been reached until another flat-ended needle or other blunt instrument fails to permanently indent the set impression material.

In the British Standards Test, a reciprocating rheometer is used to measure both setting and working times. The property being recorded is more closely related to viscosity and shear properties than it is to elasticity.

In ADA Specification No. 19, working time is determined from an indirect measurement of viscosity. Working time as determined by that method, or by a clinical type test such as probing the material in the mouth with a blunt instrument, tends to be somewhat shorter than that recorded by a rheometer.

Rheologic Properties. The viscosity of single-phase addition silicone materials is critical to their success. It is useful to consider the information presented in Table 7–6 to select a material that has a sufficiently high viscosity so that unnecessary distortion can be avoided. The high viscosity is deemed desirable because viscosity is usually related directly to filler content. The greater the amount of filler, the better is the dimensional stability of the material.

As noted previously, the reason that monophase materials are possible is because of the pseudoplasticity of the material. How long does the shear-thinning effect last? An experiment was designed to find what length of time the viscosity remained low under a shear-thinning force. Comparing hand-mixed and automatic-mixed materials, the investigators found no residual effect of the mixing force on the viscosity of the material. Stated another way, the shear-thinning, pseudoplastic behavior occurs only while the force is applied and does not permanently alter the material.

Complete characterization of the flow properties of impression materials requires measurement of viscosity as a function of shear rate over a wide range of values. Estimates indicate that shear rates up to 1600 s^{-1} may be encountered

TABLE 7–6. Viscosity ($\times 10^4$ cp) of Single-Phase Vinyl Polysiloxanes at 37° C

Material	Base	Catalyst	Mixed at 1 min	Mixed at 1.5 min
Baysilex (Miles)	65.5 (0.6)	70/6 (1.0)	68.9 (2.5)	148.8 (1.2)
Green-Mouse (Parkell)	29.8 (1.3)	25.0 (1.5)	56.7 (2.9)	78.0 (2.8)
Hydrosil (Caulk)	16.1 (0.9)	19.1 (0.8)	129.4 (4.1)	153.5*
Imprint (3M)	42.3 (1.1)	50.0 (0.6)	79.7 (2.2)	146.2 (5.9)
Omnisil (Coe)	35.2 (0.9)	58.5 (2.0)	102.5 (1.9)	153.5†

*Value at 75 s after mixing.
†Value at 77 s after mixing.
From Kim K-N, Craig RG, and Koran A: Viscosity of monophase addition silicones as a function of shear rate. J Prosthet Dent 67:794, 1992.

during mixing, and rates up to 1000 s^{-1} during extrusion from the syringe. These rates are considerably higher than those employed in many of the measurements of viscosity that have been reported.

Future studies of these materials will probably focus on these details, and specifications for these materials may likely include quantitative ranges for viscosity and a characterization of the rheologic behavior for the elastomeric impression materials.

Elasticity. As might be expected, the elastic properties of these rubber impression materials improve with curing time. In other words, the longer the impression can remain in the mouth before removal, the more accurate it will be. Setting time as stated by a manufacturer, or as determined by a rheometer, is not always adequate for the development of sufficient elasticity to prevent permanent deformation on removal of the impression, especially with the polysulfides and addition silicones. For example, the setting times as measured by a rheometer are 1 or 2 minutes less than those required to produce an acceptable level of elasticity before removal of the impression.

In Specification No. 19, the Types I and II elastomers are allowed 2.5% permanent deformation after 12% strain in compression is held for 30 seconds. Type III materials are permitted 5.5% under the same test. With the exception of the putty rubbers, strain should fall between 2% and 20% when the stress is increased from 0.0098 to 0.098 MPa (1.42 to 14.2 psi).

The ranking for permanent deformation following strain in compression, in increasing order, for the four kinds of nonaqueous elastomeric impression materials is (1) addition silicone, (2) condensation silicone, (3) polyether, and (4) polysulfide. Recovery of elastic deformation following strain is less rapid for the polysulfides than for the other three kinds of materials. However, even when strain is prolonged, as when an impression is removed slowly rather than rapidly from the prepared teeth, recovery is sufficiently rapid that pouring of the impression need not be delayed.

Excluding the very high viscosity putty class of rubbers, stiffness of the various kinds increases in the following order: (1) polysulfide, (2) condensation silicone, (3) addition silicone, and (4) polyether.

Removal of the Impression. Under no circumstances should the impression be removed until the curing has progressed sufficiently to provide adequate elasticity so that distortion will not occur. One method for determining the time of removal is to inject some of the syringe material into an interproximal space that is not within the area of operation. As previously noted, this material can be prodded with a blunt instrument from time to time, and when it is firm and returns completely to its original contour, the impression is sufficiently elastic to be removed. When a multiple mix technique is used, it is advisable to test both the syringe and the tray materials in this manner. The curing times may vary for the two different consistencies.

From a practical standpoint, the curing rate of the rubber impression material should not be so slow that the time before removal from the mouth is unduly long. It is estimated that the impression should be ready for removal within at least 10 minutes from the time of mixing, allowing 6 to 8 minutes for the impression to remain in the mouth.

Dimensional Stability. Dimensional changes during curing have been measured directly and indirectly, using confined and free-standing specimens of the elastomers in various geometric shapes. In ADA Specification No. 19 for elastomeric impression materials, a disk of the impression material is placed on a talc-covered glass plate. At the end of 24 hours, the contraction should not exceed 0.50% for Types I and III materials or 1% for a Type II elastomer. Thus, the measurement includes contraction caused by a thermal change (35° C to 23° C), polymerization shrinkage, and loss of volatile components. For example, the linear coefficients of thermal expansion for the elastomeric impression materials range from 150 to 220 $\times$ 10^{-6} per degree centigrade.

Mean values for linear contraction for a number of nonaqueous elastomers, using the method just described, are shown in Figure 7–3. As noted in the discussion on working and setting times, there is considerable variation between brands for the condensation silicone and polysulfide materials.

Effect of Custom Trays. The accuracy of impression materials can be readily determined by the use of master castings constructed on critical steel dies. The better the fit of the casting when it is placed back on the stone dies, the more accurate is the impression material and technique. The fit of the master castings (shown in Figure 7–11) on the stone dies constructed from rubber-base impressions of different thickness illustrates the importance of using a custom tray to minimize the bulk of the impression material. This finding contradicts the recommendation for the hydrocolloid impression that a greater bulk of material does produce better accuracy than does a smaller bulk. Not only should the bulk be less with the rubber impression materials, but also it should be evenly distributed. In general, the optimal thickness of the impression is 2 mm or less.

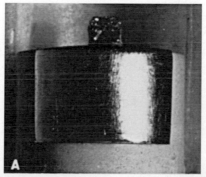

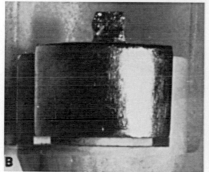
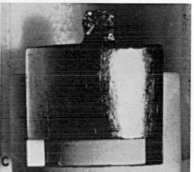

Figure 7–11. The greater the thickness of the wall of the rubber impression from which the above stone dies were constructed, the poorer the fit of the casting. Wall thickness: 0.5 mm *(A)*; 2.0 mm *(B)*; and 4.5 mm *(C)*.

Biologic Properties. In the Western world more stringent legislation is now being applied to dental materials, and this is not limited to those materials that are to be retained permanently in the mouth. The ADA has a specification for testing biocompatibility that includes impression materials.

NEW ADVANCES IN IMPRESSION MATERIALS

Attempts at developing visible light-curing elastomeric impression materials have not been successful. One of these products is the visible light-curable polyether urethane dimethacrylate shown in Figure 7–12. It was based on a polyether urethane dimethacrylate resin with visible light-cure photoinitiators and photoaccelerators. The silicon dioxide filler had a refractive index close to that of the resin to provide the translucency necessary for maximum depth of cure.

New technology is available to overcome one of the major problems of these materials, that is, the ability to set completely against a wet field. With the original light-cured materials, the surface that set against the teeth and gums was tacky, probably because moisture inhibited the setting. The new hydrophilic polymers that have been developed for dentin bonding agents should be useful in overcoming the surface setting problem. That leaves the problem of making the cross-linked material less stiff. The final obstacle is to direct the light to all areas of the mouth so that the material will cure completely and in a reasonable amount of time. With the improvements in the technology of the light-curing

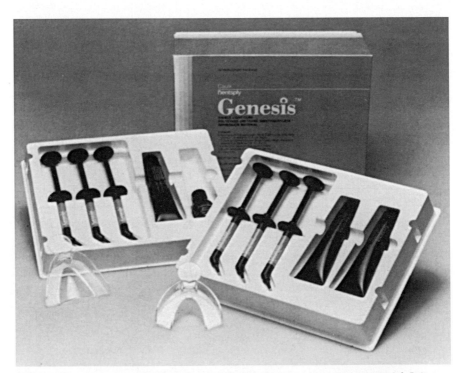

Figure 7–12. A discontinued visible light-activated elastomer impression material. It is a single-component system. The syringes contain the more fluid light body material, while the black tubes contain the tray material. A light used for polymerizing light-activated resin-based composites (to be discussed in Chapters 12 and 13) is employed after the material has been carried to place in the mouth in the transparent tray.

TABLE 7–7. Characteristics of Elastomeric Impression Materials

Generic Type	Brand Names	Advantages	Disadvantages
Polysulfide	Coe-flex (GC-Amer) Neo-plex (Miles) Omiflex (GC-Amer) Permlastic (Kerr)	Long working time High tear resistance Easily read margins Pour up within 1 hr Moderate cost	Requires custom tray Stretching leads to distortion Hydrophobic Messy Obnoxious odor
Condensation silicone (putty-wash)	Accoe (GC-Amer) Cuttersil (Miles) Elasticon (Kerr) Xantopren (Unitek)	Putty for customized tray Clean and pleasant Good working time Easily read margins Moderate cost	High polymerization shrinkage Volatile by-product Low tear strength Hydrophobic Must pour immediately
Vinyl polysiloxane (single-phase or monophase)	Baysilex CD (Miles) Examix (GC-Amer) Hydrosil (Caulk) Imprint (3M)	One material Automatic mixer dispenser Clean and pleasant Easily read margins Ideally elastic Pour repeatedly Stable—delay pour	Hydrophobic Poor flow in moist sulcus Difficult to pour cast High cost

Vinyl polysiloxane (putty-wash/multimix)	Exaflex (GC-Amer)
	Express (3M)
	Extrude (Kerr)
	President (Coltene)
	Reprosil (Caulk)
		Putty for customized tray
		Automatic mixer/
		  dispenser
		Clean and pleasant
		Easily read margins
		Pour repeatedly
		Stable—delay pour
			Hydrophobic
			Putty displaces wash
			Wash has low tear
			  strength
			Putty too stiff
			Putty and wash separate
			Difficult to pour cast
			Very high cost

Polyether	Impregum F (ESPE) Permadyne (ESPE) Polyjel NF (Caulk)	Fast setting Clean but tastes Least hydrophobic Easily read margins Good stability Delay pour Shelf life: 2 yr	Stiff, high modulus Absorbs water Leaches components High cost
Reversible hydrocolloid (agar)	Rubberloid (Van R) Surgident (Lactona)	Moist field OK Accurate and pleasant Hydrophilic Low cost Long shelf life	Requires equipment Thermal discomfort Tears easily Pour immediately Difficult to read
Irreversible hydrocolloid (alginate)	Jeltrate (Caulk) Shurgel (Columbus)	Moist field OK Clean and pleasant Hydrophilic Low cost Long shelf life	Less accurate, rough Tears easily Pour immediately Can retard stone setting

units, it is possible that the one-component light-curable impression materials will be reintroduced in the future.

Unfortunately, clinicians are moving away from the putty-wash technique just as the manufacturers figured out how to put putty in an automatic mixing device. The pseudoplasticity of these mixable putties is exciting; however, the difficulties with the impression technique suggest that this new advance is too little too late.

A summary of the characteristics of the elastomeric impression materials is given in Table 7–7.

TABLE 7–8. Common Failures that Occur with Use of Nonaqueous Elastomeric Impression Materials

Type of Failure	Causes
Rough or uneven surface on impression	Incomplete polymerization caused by premature removal from the mouth; improper ratio or mixing of components, or organic material, such as oil, on the teeth. For addition silicone, agents that contaminate the material and inhibit polymerization Too rapid polymerization caused by high humidity or high temperature Excessively high acclerator:base ratio for condensation silicone
Bubbles	Too rapid polymerization, preventing flow Air incorporated during mixing
Irregularly shaped voids	Moisture or debris on surface of teeth
Rough or chalky stone cast	Inadequate cleaning of impression Excess water left on surface of the impression Excess wetting agent left on impression Premature removal of cast Improper manipulation of stone Failure to wait at least 20 min before pouring
Distortion	Continuing polymerization shrinkage of tray caused by inadequate aging Lack of rubber adhesion to the tray caused by too few coats of adhesive; filling tray with material too soon after applying adhesive; using wrong adhesive Lack of mechanical retention for those materials where adhesive is ineffective Development of elastic properties in the material before tray is seated Excessive bulk of material Insufficient relief for the reline material (if used) Continued pressure against impression material that has developed elastic properties Movement of tray during polymerization Premature removal from mouth Improper removal from mouth Delayed pouring of the polysulfide or condensation silicone impression

EFFECTS OF MISHANDLING

The failure to produce an acceptable die or cast is more likely associated with a technique error rather than a deficiency in the material properties. The common failures that are experienced with impression materials are summarized in Table 7–8. The causes of the failures are also given in the table.

SELECTED READING

Braden M: Characterization of the setting process in dental polysulfide rubbers. J Dent Res 45:1066, 1966.
   The setting reactions in polysulfide impression materials are well described.
Braden M, Causton B, and Clarke RL: A polyether impression rubber. J Dent Res 51:889, 1972.
Chai J, and Pang I-C: A study of the "thixotropic" property of elastomeric impression materials. Int J Prosthodont 7:155, 1994.
   Shear-thinning activities such as mixing or syringing do not have a lasting effect on the viscosity of vinyl polysiloxanes, polyethers, or polysulfides. Once the force is removed, the material's viscosity returns to the presheared value. This study demonstrated that elastomers are not thixotropic.

Chai JY, and Yeung T-C: Wettability of nonaqueous elastomeric impression materials. Int J Prosthodont 4:555, 1991.
Polyether has better hydrophilic characteristics than the vinyl polysiloxanes, especially for wetting "wet" tissue.

Chee WWL, and Donovan TE: Polyvinyl siloxane impression materials: A review of properties and techniques. J Prosthet Dent 68:728, 1992.
This study demonstrated that the resiliency of the putty materials creates undetectable distortion in the impressions and the "simultaneous technique" exhibited the poorest accuracy.

Chew C-L, Chee WWL, and Donovan TE: The influence of temperature on the dimensional stability of poly (vinyl siloxane) impression materials. Int J Prosthodont 6:528, 1993.
Chilling the material had little effect on the properties of two vinyl polysiloxanes.

Council on Dental Materials, Instruments, and Equipment: Infection control recommendations for the dental office and the dental laboratory. J Am Dent Assoc 116:148, 1988.
Disinfection is the focus of only a portion of article. Hydrophobic elastomers can be safely disinfected by immersion in a number of disinfectants listed. Spray disinfection is more suitable for the hydrophilic materials (i.e., polyethers).

Craig RG: Review of dental impression materials. Adv Dent Res 2:51, 1988.
Excellent review that cites 150 publications of all types of impression materials. Includes mechanical mixing systems and disinfection.

Cullen DR, and Sandrik JL: Tensile strength of elastomeric impression materials, adhesive, and cohesive bonding. J Prosthet Dent 62:141, 1989.
The reline technique, consisting of a light-body cured to previously cured heavy-body putty, gave results similar to a simultaneous cure technique. Tested materials exhibited a tensile strength greater than that of the bond strength.

Davis BA, and Powers JM: Effect of immersion disinfection on properties of impression materials. J Prosthodont 3:31, 1994.
Disinfection affects the surface wetting and contact angle making the vinyl polysiloxanes more difficult to wet. The dimensional stability of both vinyl polysiloxanes and polyethers was unchanged.

de Camargo LM, Chee WWL, and Donovan TE: Inhibition of polymerization of polyvinylsiloxanes by medicaments used on gingival retraction cords. J Prosthet Dent 70:114, 1993.
Disproves the theory that sulfur-containing chemical agents used on tissue retraction cord inhibit the setting of addition silicones.

Hung SH, Purk JH, Tira DE, and Eick JD: Accuracy of one-step versus two-step putty wash addition silicone impression technique. J Prosthet Dent 67:583, 1992.
Concludes that the material has more effect than the technique; operators familiar with a particular technique produced the best results.

Johnson GH, and Craig RG: Accuracy of addition silicone as a function of technique. J Prosthet Dent 55:197, 1986.
Both condensation and addition polymerizing silicone impressions lead to dies larger in diameter and shorter in height than the prepared tooth. Custom tray did not produce dies more accurate than those produced in a stock tray.

Kim K-N, Craig RG, and Koran A: Viscosity of monophase addition silicones as a function of shear rate. J Prosthet Dent 67:794, 1992.
Comparison of viscosity values for the unset components and the set materials shows significant differences between the single viscosity addition silicones.

Klooster J, Logan GI, and Tjan AHL: Effects of strain rate on the behavior of elastomeric impressions. J Prosthet Dent 66:292, 1991.
Good comparison of standard information on permanent deformation, strength, elastic recovery of polysulfide, condensation silicone, and vinyl polysiloxane materials.

Lewinstein I: The ratio between vertical and horizontal changes of impressions. J Oral Rehabil 20:107, 1993.
Measured the dies produced with different impression materials and compared them to the master die; for polysulfides the dies were much wider (five times) and much shorter (six times); for condensation silicone the dies were slightly longer and thinner; for vinyl polysiloxane the dies were fatter and shorter.

Lim K-C, Chong Y-H, and Soh G: Effect of operator variability on void formation in impressions made with an automixed addition silicone. Aust Dent J 37:35, 1992.
Impressions made by handmixing had an order of magnitude more bubbles than impressions made by automatic mixing. Submerged bubbles can affect the accuracy of the impression and subsequent cast; therefore, the cost-saving in handmixing could be offset by the expense of redoing a crown.

McCabe JF, and Carrick TE: Rheological properties of elastomers during setting. J Dent Res 68:1218, 1989.
Suggests that for some elastomers, the rate of increase in viscosity or rigidity cannot be used to indicate the rate at which elasticity develops. Once the mix has been made, the material should be used as soon as possible.

McCormick JT, Antony SJ, Dial ML, et al: Wettability of elastomeric impression materials: Effect of selected surfactants. Int J Prosthodont 2:413, 1989.
Contact angle of die stone on seven types of impression materials was measured after treatment of the impression with water and two surfactants. Compared with water, the surfactants significantly reduced the contact angle, thus improving wetting.

Munoz CA, Goodacre CJ, Schnell RJ, and Harris RK: Laboratory and clinical study of a visible-light polymerized elastomeric impression material. Int J Prosthodont 1:59, 1988.
A visible light-activated elastomer was compared with an addition reaction silicone in a series of clinical and laboratory tests. Although handling characteristics were quite different, properties were similar.

Parissis N, Iakovidis D, Chirakis S, and Tsirlis A: Radiopacity of elastomeric impression materials. Aust Dent J 39:3, 1994.
Comparison of the optical density and radiolucency of 28 impression materials showed that polyethers and most silicones were least radiopaque.

Pratten DH, and Novetsky M: Detail reproduction of soft tissue: A comparison of impression materials. J Prosthet Dent 65:188, 1991.
The polyethers were much better at recording soft tissue and had less wetting problems than the vinyl polysiloxanes.

Robinson PB, Dunne SM, and Millar BJ: An *in vitro* study of a surface wetting agent for addition reaction silicone impressions. J Prosthet Dent 71:390, 1994.
Topical surfactant reduced the number of air bubbles in casts poured from vinyl polysiloxanes and enhanced the wetting of the impression material on the tooth.

Salem NS, Combe EC, and Watts DC: Mechanical properties of elastomeric impression materials. J Oral Rehabil 15:125, 1988.
The types studied included addition and condensation silicones, polysulfides, and a polyether. The polysulfides had the greatest resistance to tearing; their elastic modulus and tensile strength were less than those of the silicones.

Stackhouse JA Jr: The accuracy of stone dies made from rubber impression materials. J Prosthet Dent 24:377, 1970.
One of the first papers that measured accuracy of certain elastomeric impression materials and a number of variables associated with their use. An increase in diameter and decrease in height occurred in successively poured stone dies.

Sy JT, Munoz CA, Schnell RJ, et al: Some effects of cooling and chemical retarders on five elastomeric impression materials. Int J Prosthodont 1:252, 1988.
The effect of chemical retardation and cooling on the polymerization rate, dimensional change, and several elastic properties of four addition silicones and one polyether was determined. Both methods of retardation increased working and setting times.

Sydiskis RK, and Gerhardt DE: Cytotoxicity of impression materials. J Prosthet Dent 69:431, 1993.
Comparison of cell cytotoxicity and cell viability for seven different types of impression materials showed that the polyethers and the zinc oxide eugenol materials exhibited the most adverse effects.

Takahashi H, and Finger WJ: Effects of the setting stage on the accuracy of double-mix impressions made with addition-curing silicone. J Prosthet Dent 72:78, 1994.
Most inaccuracies can probably be attributed to the development of elastic characteristics before the impression is seated.

Thompson GA, Vermilyea SG, and Agar JR: Effect of disinfection of custom tray materials on adhesive properties of several impression material systems.
Disinfection treatments affected the retention of polyether in autopolymerizing resin trays. Other materials were affected to lesser amounts.

Tjan AHL: Effect of contaminants on the adhesion of light-bodied silicones to putty silicones in putty-wash impression technique. J Prosthet Dent 59:562, 1988.
Salivary contamination or chemical residues from an acrylic resin used in a temporary restoration weakens the bond strength of a light-body silicone to a putty silicone.

Tjan AHL, Nemetz H, Nguyen LTP, and Contino R: Effect of tray space on the accuracy of monophasic polyvinyl siloxane impressions. J Prosthet Dent 68:19, 1992.
Rigid stock trays could be used with the monophasic vinyl polysiloxanes, but the interpreparation dimensions may not be accurate enough for multiple-unit fixed prosthodontics.

Wassell RW, and Ibbetson RJ: The accuracy of polyvinyl siloxane impressions made with standard and reinforced stock trays. J Prosthet Dent 645:748, 1992.
Using stock trays, the heavy-body/light-body combination was superior to the putty-wash impressions made with addition silicones.

Wilson HJ: Impression materials. Br Dent J 164:221, 1988.
A number of properties of the nonaqueous elastomers are discussed. The testing methods are also described.

8

Inelastic Impression Materials

- Impression Compound
- Zinc Oxide–Eugenol Impression Paste
- Physical and Mechanical Properties of Zinc Oxide–Eugenol Impression Paste
- Noneugenol Paste
- Other Dental Applications of Zinc Oxide–Eugenol Paste

Inelastic impression materials represent a group of materials that exhibit an insignificant amount of elastic deformation when subjected to bending or tensile stresses. In addition, they tend to fracture without exhibiting any plastic deformation if the applied pressure exceeds their tensile, shear, or compressive strength. These materials include plaster of Paris, impression compound, and zinc oxide–eugenol (ZOE) impression paste. Because of their inability to sustain a substantial amount of elastic deformation without fracture, their use in dental impression making is limited. However, they have also been used in other relevant dental applications. The use of plaster of Paris as an impression material is described in Chapter 9. The remainder of this chapter focuses on impression compound and ZOE paste.

IMPRESSION COMPOUND

Compound, also called *modeling plastic,* is softened by heat, inserted in an impression tray, and pressed against tissue before it hardens. Its primary indication for use has been for making an impression of the edentulous ridge. Occasionally, compound is used in operative dentistry to obtain an impression of a single-tooth preparation or to stabilize matrix bands or other operative devices. For single-tooth impressions, a cylindrical copper band (called a *matrix band*) is filled with the softened compound. The filled band is then pressed over the tooth, forcing the compound to adapt to the preparation. Such an impression is sometimes referred to as a *tube impression.* After the compound has been cooled, the impression is withdrawn, and a cast, or die, is constructed in the impression.

A somewhat more viscous compound, called *tray compound,* can be used to form a tray for the construction of dentures. An impression of the soft tissue is obtained with tray compound, as was described. This impression is referred to as the *primary impression.* It is then used as a tray to support a thin layer of a second impression material, which is to be placed against the tissues. This impression is known as the *secondary impression*. Secondary impressions may also be made with a ZOE paste, a hydrocolloid, or a nonaqueous elastomer.

The other common application of compound is for border molding of an acrylic custom tray during fitting of the tray. Figure 8–1 shows two basic forms of impression compounds, a cake form and a stick form.

Composition. In general, compounds are composed of a mixture of waxes, thermoplastic resins, a filler, and a coloring agent. One of the first substances used as an impression material was beeswax. Because such waxes are brittle, substances such as shellac, stearic acid, and gutta-percha are added to improve plasticity and workability. When these substances are used in this manner, they are referred to as *plasticizers*. Synthetic resins are being used increasingly, usually in conjunction with the natural resins.

Fillers. Many materials are strengthened or otherwise changed in physical properties by the addition of small particles of usually inert materials, known as *fillers*, which are chemically distinct from the principal ingredient or ingredients.

The waxes or resins in the impression compound are the principal ingredients and comprise the *matrix*. This structure is too fluid to handle and imparts a low strength even at room temperature. Consequently, a filler must be added. The fillers increase the viscosity at temperatures above that of the mouth and increase the rigidity of the compound at room temperature.

The structure of impression compound is somewhat like that of a *composite*. The concept of composite is used extensively in the production of dental materials and is discussed in greater detail in Chapter 12.

Thermal Properties. Softening by heat is a prerequisite for the use of compounds. Their usefulness is dictated by their responses to the temperature change in the surrounding environment.

Fusion Temperature. The practical significance of the fusion temperature is that it indicates a definite reduction in plasticity of the material during cooling. Above this temperature, the softened material remains plastic while the impression is being obtained. Thus, every detail of oral tissues is more likely to be reproduced. Once the impression tray is seated, it should be held firmly in position until the impression cools below the fusion temperature. Under no

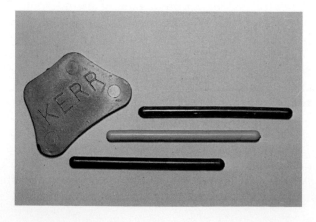

Figure 8–1. Typical cake and stick configurations of commercial impression compound.

circumstances should the impression be disturbed or removed until it reaches oral temperature.

Thermal Conductivity and Contraction. As might be expected, the thermal conductivity of these materials is low, indicating the need for extended time to achieve thorough cooling and heating of the compound. It is important that the material be uniformly soft at the time it is placed in the tray and thoroughly cooled in the tray before the impression is withdrawn from the mouth. Usually cold water can be sprayed on the tray while it is in the mouth until the compound is thoroughly hardened throughout before the impression is withdrawn. Failure to attain a complete hardening of the material before withdrawing the impression can result in a severe distortion of the impression.

The average linear contraction of impression compounds on cooling from mouth temperature to room temperature of 25° C varies between 0.3% and 0.4%. The resulting error from this magnitude of contraction is unavoidable, and it is inherent in the technique.

Softening of Impression Compound. Compound may be softened in an oven or over a flame. When a direct flame is used, the compound should not be allowed to boil or ignite so that the constituents are volatilized.

When a large amount of compound, such as that required for an entire arch, is to be softened, immersion in a water bath is recommended. Prolonged immersion or overheating in the water bath is not indicated; the compound may become brittle and grainy if some of the low-molecular-weight ingredients are leached out of the material.

Softening of the compound is the only way to remove the cast from a compound impression after the stone sets. The recommended method is to immerse the impression in *warm* water until the compound softens sufficiently to permit easy separation from the cast.

Flow. After the compound has softened, and during the period it is impressed against the tissues, the material should flow easily to conform to the tissues so that every detail and landmark are recorded accurately. On the other hand, if the amount of flow at mouth temperature is too great, distortion can occur when the impression is withdrawn from the mouth.

Distortion. Relaxation can occur quite readily either during a comparatively brief time or with an increase in temperature. The result is warpage or distortion of the impression. To minimize the distortion, the safest procedures are to allow thorough cooling of the impression before removal from the mouth and to construct the cast or die as soon as possible after the impression has been obtained—at least within the first hour.

ZINC OXIDE–EUGENOL IMPRESSION PASTE

Under the proper conditions, the reaction between zinc oxide and eugenol yields a relatively hard mass that possesses certain medicinal advantages as well as mechanical benefits in certain dental operations. This type of material has been applied to a wide range of applications in dentistry, including its use as an impression material for edentulous arches, a surgical dressing, a bite registration paste, a temporary filling material, a root canal filling, a cementing medium, and as a temporary relining material for dentures.

Impression pastes for edentulous mouths can be classified as rigid or inelastic impression materials that harden by chemical action.

Chemistry. It is fairly well established that the setting mechanism for ZOE materials consists of zinc oxide hydrolysis and a subsequent reaction between zinc hydroxide and eugenol to form a chelate. The reactions are represented by the following:

$$ZnO + H_2O \rightleftharpoons Zn(OH)_2$$

$$\underset{Base}{Zn(OH)_2} + \underset{\substack{Acid \\ (eugenol)}}{2HE} \rightleftharpoons \underset{\substack{Salt \\ (zinc\ eugenolate)}}{ZnE_2} + 2H_2O$$

Water is needed to initiate the reaction and it is also a by-product of the reaction. This type of reaction is often called *autocatalytic*. This is the reason why the reaction proceeds more rapidly in a humid environment. The setting reaction is accelerated by the presence of zinc acetate dihydrate, which is more soluble than zinc hydroxide and which can supply zinc ions more rapidly. Acetic acid is a more active catalyst for the setting reaction than is water, because it increases the formation rate of zinc hydroxide. High atmospheric temperature also accelerates the setting reaction.

The free eugenol content of the set cement is probably extremely low. It appears to be much higher than it actually is, because the chelate hydrolyzes readily, forming free eugenol and zinc ions.

Composition. Most modern impression materials are dispensed as two separate pastes. A typical formula is shown in Table 8–1. One tube contains zinc oxide and fixed vegetable or mineral oil and the other contains eugenol and rosin. The fixed vegetable or mineral oil acts as a plasticizer and aids in offsetting the action of the eugenol as an irritant.

The zinc oxide used should be finely divided and it should contain only a slight amount of water for the reason described earlier. Oil of cloves, which contains 70% to 85% eugenol, is sometimes used in preference to eugenol because it reduces the burning sensation experienced by patients when it contacts the soft tissues.

The addition of rosin to the paste in the second tube apparently facilitates the speed of the reaction, and it yields a smoother, more homogeneous product. Canada balsam and Peru balsam are often used to increase flow and improve

TABLE 8–1. Composition of a Zinc Oxide–Eugenol Impression Paste

Components	Percentage
Tube No. 1 (base)	
Zinc oxide (French processed or U.S.P.)	87
Fixed vegetable or mineral oil	13
Tube No. 2 (accelerator)	
Oil of cloves or eugenol	12
Gum or polymerized rosin	50
Filler (silica type)	20
Lanolin	3
Resinous balsam	10
Accelerator solution (CaCl$_2$) and color	5

Courtesy of E. J. Molnar.

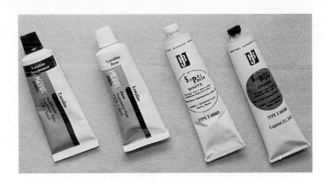

Figure 8–2. Representative commercial products of zinc oxide–eugenol impression paste.

mixing properties. If the mixed paste is too thin or lacks body before it sets, a filler (such as a wax) or an inert powder (such as kaolin, talc, and diatomaceous earth) may be added to one or both of the original pastes.

There are many soluble salts that may act as accelerators. Chemicals commonly used are zinc acetate, calcium chloride, primary alcohols, and glacial acetic acid. The accelerator can be incorporated in either one or both pastes. Examples of two ZOE impression materials are shown in Figure 8–2.

Manipulation. The mixing of the two pastes is generally accomplished on an oil-impervious paper, although a glass mixing slab can be used as well. The proper proportion of the two pastes is generally obtained by squeezing two strips of paste of the same length, one from each tube, onto the mixing slab. A flexible stainless steel spatula is satisfactory for the mixing. The two strips are combined with the first sweep of the spatula, and the mixing is continued for approximately 1 minute (or as directed by the manufacturer) until a uniform color is observed.

Setting Time. The initial and final setting times are defined by the American Dental Association Specification No. 16 for dental impression pastes. The initial setting time, like working time, includes the time for mixing, filling the tray, and seating the impression in the mouth properly. It may vary between 3 and 6 minutes. The final setting time is defined as the time at which the material is hard enough to resist penetration under a load. It should occur within 10 minutes for Type I pastes (hard) and 15 minutes for Type II pastes (soft). When the final set occurs, the impression can be withdrawn from the mouth. The actual time is shorter when the setting occurs in the mouth.

Control of the Setting Time. Most factors are solely under the control of the manufacturer. The following, however, are methods by which the operator may control the setting time:

1. Adding a small amount of an accelerator, such as zinc acetate, or a drop of water to the eugenol paste before blending the two pastes can shorten the setting time. Water should be added cautiously, however, because the effect may be unpredictable.

2. Cooling the spatula and mixing slab may help increase the setting time, provided the temperature is not lower than the dew point.

3. Adding certain inert oils and waxes during mixing, such as olive oil, mineral oil, and petrolatum, can prolong setting time. However, such a practice can reduce the rigidity of the set material and yield an inhomogeneous mix.

4. Altering the ratio of the two pastes can result in retardation or acceleration, depending on which paste contains the accelerator. However, the result may be unpredictable if both pastes contain an accelerator.

5. Extended mixing time affects the setting time to a limited extent. With most pastes, the longer the mixing time (within limits), the shorter the setting time.

General Considerations. The impression paste can be spread over a compound preliminary impression or a secondary resin tray fabricated to fit the gypsum cast of an edentulous ridge. The mixture is carried into the mouth in the usual manner, thus constituting the second or final *wash impression.*

The impression should be held firmly in position until it has thoroughly hardened. The accelerating action of body temperature and saliva on the surface of the tissues may cause the adjacent surface of the impression to harden first. Any disturbance of the impression at this stage results in warpage. Only when the material has completely hardened should the impression be removed from the mouth. The cast can be constructed in the usual manner. As with impression compound, no separating medium is necessary.

PHYSICAL AND MECHANICAL PROPERTIES OF ZINC OXIDE–EUGENOL IMPRESSION PASTE

A paste of a thick consistency or high viscosity can compress the tissues, whereas a thin, fluid material results in an impression that captures a negative replica of the tissues in a relaxed condition with little or no compression. In any event, the impression paste should be homogeneous. Pastes of varying consistencies are commercially available from which the dentist may choose. The heavier consistency material yields a greater strength.

Flow. For testing purposes the flow of a particular paste in a specified time is expressed in terms of the spread of the disk in millimeters or the increase in diameter at the various times of load application. The flow of the freshly mixed paste varies as it is related to the time before setting.

Generally, there is a correlation between flow and setting time. Those materials that show a decrease in flow at various time intervals also have a shorter setting time and a shorter time interval between the initial and final set.

Rigidity and Strength. As is the case for impressions obtained with compound, the paste impression should be unyielding when it is removed from the mouth and should resist fracture. Impression paste can be compounded to increase resistance to flow at mouth temperature such that it is comparable or superior to that of compound.

Dimensional Stability. The dimensional stability of the impression pastes is quite satisfactory. A negligible shrinkage (<0.1%) may occur during hardening. No significant dimensional change subsequent to hardening should occur with high-quality commercial products. The impressions can be preserved indefinitely without a change in shape that can result from relaxation or other causes of warpage. Such a statement assumes that the tray material is dimensionally stable.

NONEUGENOL PASTE

One of the chief disadvantages of the ZOE pastes is the possible stinging or burning sensation caused by eugenol when it contacts soft tissues. Furthermore, as previously noted, the ZOE reaction is never completed, with the result that the free eugenol may leach out. Some patients find the taste of eugenol extremely disagreeable, and in patients who wear a surgical pack for several weeks, a chronic gastric disturbance may result.

A material similar to the ZOE reaction product can be formed by a saponification reaction to produce an insoluble "soap" if the zinc oxide is reacted with a carboxylic acid. The reaction is

$$ZnO + 2RCOOH \rightarrow (RCOO)_2Zn + H_2O$$

Almost any carboxylic acid reacts with zinc oxide, but only a few such acids provide compounds of dental interest. Orthoethoxybenzoic acid, commonly abbreviated as EBA, is valuable in this regard. The carboxylic acid is not necessarily a liquid. Powdered acids can be dissolved or dispersed in a liquid-carrying agent, such as ethyl alcohol. The reaction is well understood, and it is not greatly affected by temperature or humidity. Bactericides and other medicaments can be incorporated without interfering with the reaction.

OTHER DENTAL APPLICATIONS OF ZINC OXIDE–EUGENOL PASTE

Surgical Pastes. After a gingivoplasty (the surgical removal of hyperplastic gingival tissues and for creation of physiologic gingival contour), a ZOE paste may be placed over the wound to aid in the retention of a medicament and to promote healing.

The ingredients of the surgical pastes are essentially the same as those of the impression pastes. However, these pastes are generally softer and slower setting in comparison with impression pastes. The mixture should be capable of being formed into a rope that is packed into the gingival wounds and the interproximal spaces to provide retention of the dressing. The final product should be strong enough to resist displacement during mastication but not so brittle that it shears readily under localized stresses.

Bite Registration Pastes. The materials that are used for recording the occlusal relationships between natural or artificial teeth include impression plaster, compound, wax, resin, and metallic oxide paste. ZOE pastes are often used as recording materials in the construction of complete dentures and fixed or removable partial dentures. Plasticizers such as petrolatum are often added to reduce the tendency of the paste to adhere to oral tissues.

In contrast with wax, the ZOE impression paste offers almost no resistance to closing of the mandible, thus allowing a more accurate interocclusal relationship record to be formed. Also, the ZOE interocclusal record is more stable than one made of wax.

SELECTED READING

Batchelor RF, and Wilson AD: Zinc oxide–eugenol cements. I. The effect of atmospheric conditions on rheological properties. J Dent Res 48:883, 1969.

The precise effects of temperature and humidity on the setting reaction of zinc oxide–eugenol are studied. Both accelerate the set.

Braden M, and Clark RL: Dielectric properties of zinc oxide–eugenol–type cements. J Dent Res 53:1263, 1974.

Water formed in the setting reaction of zinc oxide–eugenol binds the individual chelate units together.

Crisp S, Ambersley M, and Wilson AD: Zinc oxide–eugenol cements. V. Instrumental studies of the catalysis and acceleration of the setting reaction. J Dent Res 59:44, 1980.

A chelate (zinc eugenolate) is formed in the acid-base reaction of zinc oxide and eugenol.

Molnar EJ: Residual eugenol from zinc oxide–eugenol compounds. J Dent Res 46:645, 1967.

This study identified the time at which free eugenol remains in the ZOE mixture. The use of an accelerator does not alter that time.

Smith DC: A materialistic look at periodontal packs. Dent Pract 20:263, 1970.

Two studies showing the chemistry of formulating a noneugenol paste.

9 *Gypsum Products*

Chemistry of Setting, Basic Principles, and Technical Considerations

- **Uses of Gypsum in Dentistry**
- **Dental Plaster and Stone**
- **Setting of Gypsum Products**
- **Tests for Working, Setting, and Final Setting Times**
- **Control of the Setting Time**
- **Setting Expansion**
- **Accelerators and Retarders: Practice and Theory**
- **Hygroscopic Setting Expansion**
- **Strength**
- **Types of Gypsum Products**
- **Proportioning, Mixing, and Caring for Products**
- **Infection Control Concerns**

USES OF GYPSUM IN DENTISTRY

Gypsum is a mineral that is mined in various parts of the world. It is also a by-product of some chemical-processing operations. Chemically, the gypsum that is produced for dental purposes is nearly pure *calcium sulfate dihydrate* ($CaSO_4 \cdot 2H_2O$). Different forms of gypsum have been used for many centuries for construction purposes. It is assumed that the alabaster used in the building of King Solomon's temple of biblical fame was a form of gypsum. Products made from gypsum are widely used in industry, and practically all homes and buildings have walls of plaster.

Gypsum products are used in dentistry for the preparation of study models for oral and maxillofacial structures and as important adjuncts to dental laboratory operations that are involved in the production of dental prostheses. Various types of plaster are used to form molds and casts on which dental prostheses and restorations are constructed. When the plaster is mixed with silica, it is known as *dental investment*. Such dental investments are used to form molds for the casting of dental restorations with molten metal, and they are discussed at length in Chapter 22. The present discussion is confined to the relatively pure gypsum products, such as plaster, that harden when mixed with water.

The use of gypsum in dentistry is widespread. Its use can be demonstrated in the preparation of a cast for a denture. A mixture of plaster of Paris and water is placed in an *impression tray* and pressed against the tissues of the jaw, for example. The plaster is allowed to harden, or *set*, and then the impression is withdrawn. The dentist now has a *negative* form of these tissues that was made within the oral cavity. If another variety of plaster known as *dental stone* is now mixed with water, poured into the impression, and allowed to set, the hardened plaster impression serves as a mold to form a positive model, or master cast. It is on this cast that the denture is constructed, without the patient being present.

DENTAL PLASTER AND STONE

Production of Calcium Sulfate Hemihydrate. These materials are the results of the calcining of calcium sulfate dihydrate, or gypsum. Commercially, the gypsum is ground and subjected to temperatures of 110° to 120° C (230° to 250° F) to drive off part of the water of crystallization. This corresponds to the first step in reaction (1). As the temperature is further raised, the remaining water of crystallization is removed, and products are formed as indicated.

$$
(1) \quad \underset{\substack{\text{Gypsum} \\ \text{(calcium sulfate} \\ \text{dihydrate)}}}{CaSO_4 \cdot 2H_2O} \xrightarrow{110\text{--}130°C} \underset{\substack{\text{Plaster or stone} \\ \text{(calcium sulfate} \\ \text{hemihydrate)}}}{CaSO_4 \cdot \tfrac{1}{2}H_2O} \xrightarrow{130\text{--}200°C} \underset{\substack{\text{Hexagonal} \\ \text{anhydrite}}}{CaSO_4} \xrightarrow{200\text{--}1000°C} \underset{\substack{\text{Orthorhombic} \\ \text{anhydrite}}}{CaSO_4}
$$

The principal constituent of the dental plasters and stones is the calcium sulfate hemihydrate $(CaSO_4)_2 \cdot H_2O$ (or $CaSO_4 \cdot \tfrac{1}{2} H_2O$). Depending on the method of calcination, different forms of the hemihydrate can be obtained. These forms are referred to as α-hemihydrate or β-hemihydrate. The use of α and β prefixes suggests two phases from the point of view of the phase rule, but this is not the case. Although the α and β designations are continued in this edition because of tradition and convenience, it should not be inferred that there are mineralogic differences between them. The differences between α- and β-hemihydrates are a result of differences in crystal size, surface area, and degree of lattice perfection. In reality, the β form is a fibrous aggregate of fine crystals with capillary pores, whereas the α form consists of cleavage fragments and crystals in the form of rods or prisms.

If gypsum is heated to the temperatures indicated in the first part of reaction 1 in a kettle, vat, or rotary kiln open to the air, a crystalline form of the hemihydrate is produced. As can be seen in Figure 9–1, the β-hemihydrate crystals are characterized by their "sponginess" and irregular shape. In contrast the α-hemihydrate (stone) crystals, the α-hemihydrate (stone) crystals are more dense and have a prismatic shape. Powder particles of dental stone (α-hemihydrate) are shown in Figure 9–2.

Different procedures can be employed to obtain the hemihydrate. The product of these processes is the principal constituent of the dental stones from which casts and models are made. When the α-hemihydrate is mixed with water, reaction 1 is reversed, as described in the next section, and the product obtained is one much stronger and harder than that resulting from β-hemihydrate. The chief reason for this difference is that the α-hemihydrate powder requires much

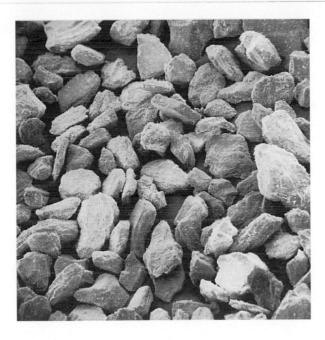

Figure 9–1. Powder particles of plaster of Paris (β-hemihydrate). Crystals are spongy and irregular in shape. ×400. (Courtesy of B. Giammara and R. Neiman.)

less water when it is mixed than does the β-hemihydrate. The β-hemihydrate requires more water to float its powder particles so that they can be stirred, because the crystals are more irregular in shape and are porous in character.

Although particle size and the total surface area are the chief factors in determining the amount of gauging water, the particle size distribution also plays an important role. The grinding of the particles after the preparation of the hemihydrate can eliminate needlelike crystals and provide better packing characteristics, hence lowering the amount of mixing water required.

Adhesion between the particles of hemihydrate is also a factor in determining

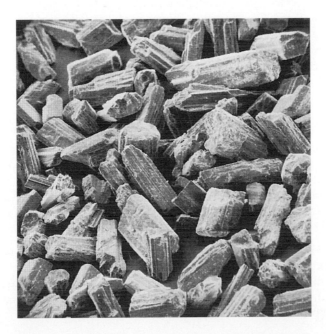

Figure 9–2. Powder particles of dental stone (α-hemihydrate). Crystals are prismatic and more regular in shape than those of plaster. The very fine particles that are normally present have been removed, as was done for the plaster particles in Figure 9–1. ×400. (Courtesy of B. Giammara and R. Neiman.)

the amount of water required to produce a product that can be poured. Small amounts of some surface-active materials, such as gum arabic plus lime, added to the hemihydrate can reduce markedly the water requirements of both plaster and dental stone.

From the preceding description, it is clear that various gypsum products require different amounts of water and that these differences are accounted for principally by shape and compactness of the crystals. These factors are regulated by the manufacturer and are dependent on the type of process used, dehydration temperatures, particle size of the gypsum to be calcined, length of calcination, time of grinding of finished product, and addition of surface active ingredients to the final product.

Commercial Gypsum Products. The various plasters and stones that are available commercially consist of one of the forms of hemihydrate. Because they are processed products, however, they contain additional small amounts of impurities, unconverted hexagonal or orthorhombic anhydrites. Additional gypsum and other salts may also be added to control the setting time and expansion, as discussed in later sections.

SETTING OF GYPSUM PRODUCTS

Reaction 1 described the sequence for calcining calcium sulfate dihydrate to form calcium sulfate hemihydrate, the starting material used for production of gypsum casts, models, certain casting investments, and impression plasters. This reaction can be reversed as follows:

(2) $$(CaSO_4)_2 \cdot \tfrac{1}{2} H_2O + 3H_2O \longrightarrow 2CaSO_4 \cdot 2H_2O + \text{Heat}$$

The product of the reaction is gypsum, and the heat evolved in the exothermic reaction is equivalent to the heat used originally in calcination.

The products formed during calcination all react with water to form gypsum, but at different rates. For example, hexagonal anhydrite reacts very rapidly, whereas the reaction may require hours when orthorhombic anhydrite is mixed with water. This is caused by the fact that the orthorhombic anhydrite has a more stable and closely packed crystal lattice.

Setting Reactions. Nature has provided us with a unique material in gypsum. The various hydrates have a relatively low solubility with a distinct difference in the solubility of the hemihydrate and the dihydrate. The dihydrate is too soluble for use in structures exposed to the atmosphere, which is probably fortunate, because such usage would long ago have exhausted our natural supply of gypsum.

In Figure 9–3 it can be seen that the hemihydrate is four times more soluble in water than is the dihydrate near room temperature (20° C). Thus, the setting reactions can be understood as follows:

1. When the hemihydrate is mixed with water, a suspension is formed that is fluid and workable.
2. The hemihydrate dissolves until it forms a saturated solution.
3. This saturated hemihydrate solution is supersaturated with dihydrate, so the latter precipitates out.

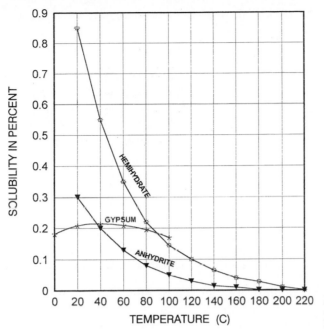

Figure 9–3. Equilibrium diagram of calcium sulfate and water between 0° and 220° C.

4. As the dihydrate precipitates, the solution is no longer saturated with the hemihydrate, so it continues to dissolve. Thus, the process continues, that is, dissolution of the hemihydrate and precipitation of the dihydrate occur as either new crystals form or further growth occurs on those already present. The reaction is continuous and proceeds until no further dihydrate precipitates out of solution. The anhydrite is not formed in aqueous media.

The curves from a plot of heat rise (or temperature) during setting as a function of time are similar in shape to those shown in Figure 9–9 (discussed later) for compressive strength as a function of time. The peak is reached earlier or later, depending on the setting time. The mass will begin to cool in 5 to 15 minutes, but the reaction and strengthening process may continue slowly for hours.

The effect of varying the water:powder (W:P) ratio is best illustrated by measuring the crushing (compressive) strength that develops. Figure 9–4 shows a plot of the strength values that have been measured for the five different types of gypsum products as a function of the W:P ratio. The products represented in Figure 9–4 cover the wide range of gypsum products that are used in dentistry. The figure includes data from many of the products on the market that meet American Dental Association (ADA) Specification No. 25 for dental gypsum products and the strength values represent the *wet strength* at 1 hour. The strength values increase as the specimens dry and may double in a week.

As the amount of gypsum increases during the setting period, the mass thickens because of the formation of needlelike crystals as shown in Figure 9–5. When a lower W:P ratio is used, the crystals become broader and, through intergrowth, they form a strong, solid mass. At a W:P ratio near the theoretical limit of 0.18, some of the hemihydrate crystals do not fully dissolve, but they hydrate and still tend to harden the structure.

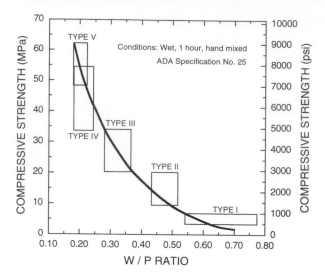

Figure 9–4. Compressive strength as a function of W:P ratio for the five types of gypsum products.

W:P Ratio. The amounts of water and hemihydrate should be gauged accurately by weight. The ratio of the water to the hemihydrate powder is usually expressed as the water:powder ratio, or the quotient obtained when the weight (or volume) of the water is divided by the weight of the powder. The ratio is usually abbreviated as W:P. For example, if 100 g of plaster is mixed with 60 mL of water, the W:P ratio is 0.6; if 100 g of dental stone is mixed with 28 mL of water, the W:P ratio is 0.28. The W:P ratio is an important factor in determining the physical and chemical properties of the final gypsum product. For example, the higher the W:P ratio, the longer the setting time and the weaker is the gypsum product. Although the W:P ratio varies for the particular brand of plaster or stone, the following are some typical recommended ranges: Type II plaster, 0.45 to 0.50; Type III stone, 0.28 to 0.30; and Type IV stone, 0.22 to 0.24.

TESTS FOR WORKING, SETTING, AND FINAL SETTING TIMES

Mixing Time. This is the time from the addition of the powder to the water until mixing is completed. Mechanical mixing of stones and plasters is usually

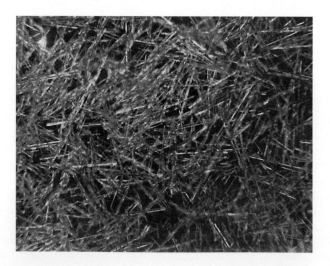

Figure 9–5. Dark-field photomicrograph of set plaster mixed with excess water to prevent the field from becoming opaque. ×200.

completed in 20 to 30 seconds. Hand spatulation generally requires at least a minute to obtain a smooth mix.

Working Time. This is the time available to use a workable mix, one that maintains an even consistency that may be manipulated to perform one or more tasks. For example, sufficient working time might be needed to pour an impression, pour a spare impression, and clean the equipment before the gypsum fully sets. Generally, a 3-minute working time is adequate.

Setting Time. Reaction 2 requires a definite time for completion. The powder is mixed with water, and the time that elapses from the beginning of mixing until the material hardens is known as the *setting time*. This is usually measured by some type of penetration test, using the instruments in Figure 9–6. One normally thinks of this as a certain time in minutes as stated on the package label. Actually, there are a number of stages in the setting of a gypsum product, as described by use of an actual strength test on a dental model plaster (Fig. 9–7). In Figure 9–7, 1 minute is indicated for mixing (MT), with an additional 3 minutes for working (WT), that is, pouring into an impression.

Loss of Gloss Test for Initial Set. As the reaction proceeds, some of the excess water is taken up in forming the dihydrate so that the mix loses its gloss (LG). In the example shown, this occurred at approximately 9 minutes, and the mass

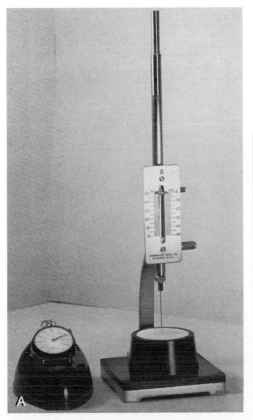
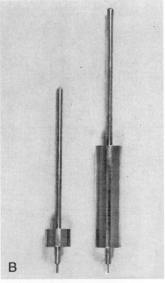

Figure 9–6. A, Vicat needle being used to measure the setting time of a gypsum product. The setting time is the elapsed time from the start of mix until the needle no longer penetrates to the bottom. *B,* Set of Gillmore needles.

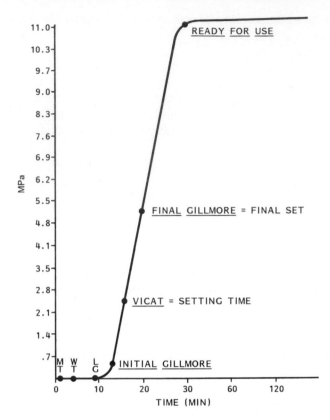

Figure 9–7. Compressive strength of a Type-II model plaster during setting. The W:P ratio was 0.50. The various stages in the setting reaction are indicated by the particular instruments used in measuring the hardening of the mix. MT, mixing time; WT, working time; and LG, loss of gloss from the surface of the mix.

still had no measurable compressive strength. Therefore, it could not be safely removed from the mold.

Initial Gillmore Test for Initial Set. At the right of Figure 9–6 are shown two Gillmore needles. The smaller one is most frequently used for testing the setting time of dental cements, but it is sometimes used on gypsum products. The mixture is spread out. The needle is lowered onto the surface, and the time at which it no longer leaves an impression is called the *initial set*, noted at Initial Gillmore on the curve in Figure 9–7. This time is marked by a definite increase in strength. The initial set in the example seen in Figure 9–7 is 13 minutes.

Vicat Test for Setting Time. Another instrument is used to determine the next stage in the reaction, the Vicat penetrometer seen on the left in Figure 9–6. The needle with a weighted plunger rod is supported and is held just in contact with the mix. Soon after the gloss is lost, the plunger is released. The time elapsed until the needle no longer penetrates to the bottom of the mix is known as the *setting time*. In some cases, the Vicat and Initial Gillmore measurements occur at the same time, whereas in others there is a small difference, as shown.

Gillmore Test for Final Setting Time. The next stage in the setting process may be measured by the use of the heavier Gillmore needle. The elapsed time when it leaves only a barely perceptible mark on the surface is called the *final setting time*. It is rarely used as an indication of the ready-for-use stage.

Ready-for-Use Criterion. This is a subjective measure of the time at which the set material may be safely handled in the usual manner. There is no designated test, but the ability to judge readiness improves with experience. Technically, it may be considered as the time when the compressive strength is at least 80% of that attained at 1 hour. Most modern products reach the ready-for-use state in 30 minutes (see Fig. 9–7).

The preceding illustrates the stages in the setting of gypsum products. The figures are for one typical model plaster, but they vary, depending on each product, the W:P ratio, and the time of mixing. Only the Vicat setting time is listed under tables of physical properties. Although manufacturers have developed their own tests for working time, the Vicat test is useful in batch control.

CONTROL OF THE SETTING TIME

As previously noted, it is necessary to control the setting time. Theoretically, there are at least three methods by which such control can be effected.

1. The solubility of the hemihydrate can be increased or decreased. For example, if the solubility of the hemihydrate is increased, supersaturation of the calcium sulfate will be greater. The rate of crystalline deposition is thus increased.

2. The number of nuclei of crystallization can be increased or decreased. The greater the number of nuclei of crystallization, the faster the gypsum crystals form and the sooner the hardening of the mass will occur because of crystalline intermeshing.

3. If the rate of crystal growth can be increased or decreased, the setting time can be accelerated or retarded, respectively.

In practice, these methods have been incorporated into the commercial products available. Then the operator can vary the setting time within reason by the W:P ratio and mixing time.

Impurities. If the calcination is not complete so that gypsum particles remain, or if the manufacturer adds gypsum, the setting time will be shortened because of the increase in potential nuclei of crystallization. If orthorhombic anhydrite is present, the induction period will be increased; it will be decreased if hexagonal anhydrite is present.

Fineness. The finer the particle size of the hemihydrate, the faster the mix hardens, particularly if the product has been ground during manufacture. Not only is the rate of the solution of the hemihydrate increased but also the gypsum nuclei are more numerous and, therefore, a more rapid rate of crystallization occurs.

W:P Ratio. The more water that is used for mixing, the fewer nuclei there are per unit volume. Consequently, the setting time is prolonged. This effect is evidenced by the results presented in Table 9–1.

Mixing. Within practical limits, the longer and the more rapidly the plaster is mixed, the shorter is the setting time. Some gypsum crystals form immediately when the plaster or stone is brought into contact with the water. As the mixing begins, the formation of these crystals increases; at the same time the crystals are broken up by the mixing spatula and are distributed throughout the mixture,

TABLE 9–1. Effect of the Water:Powder (W:P) Ratio and the Mixing Time on the Setting Time of Plaster of Paris

W:P Ratio	Mixing Time (min)	Setting Time (min)
0.45	0.5	5.25
0.45	1.0	3.25
0.60	1.0	7.25
0.60	2.0	4.50
0.80	1.0	10.50
0.80	2.0	7.75
0.80	3.0	5.75

From Gibson CS, and Johnson RN: J Soc Chem Ind 51:25T, 1932.

with the resulting formation of more nuclei of crystallization. Thus, the setting time is decreased, as indicated in Table 9–1.

Temperature. Although the effect of temperature on the setting time is likely to be erratic and may vary from one plaster (or stone) to another, little change occurs between 0° C (32° F) and 50° C (120° F); but if the temperature of the plaster-water mixture exceeds approximately 50° C (120° F), a gradually increasing retardation occurs. As the temperature approaches 100° C (212° F), no reaction takes place. At the higher temperatures, reaction 2 is reversed, with the tendency for any gypsum crystals formed to be changed to the hemihydrate form.

Retarders and Accelerators. Probably the most effective and practical method for the control of the setting time is the addition of certain chemical modifiers to the mixture of plaster or dental stone. If the chemical added decreases the setting time, it is known as an *accelerator*; if it increases the setting time, it is known as a *retarder*.

Retarders generally act by forming an adsorbed layer on the hemihydrate to reduce its solubility and on the gypsum crystals present to inhibit growth. Organic materials, such as glue, gelatin, and some gums, behave in this manner. Another type of retarder consists of salts that form a layer of a calcium salt that is less soluble than is the sulfate. In small concentrations, many inorganic salts act as accelerators, but when the concentration is increased they can become retarders. Because the action of these chemical additions also affects other properties such as setting expansion, the behavior of accelerators and retarders is discussed at greater length in a subsequent section.

SETTING EXPANSION

Regardless of the type of gypsum product employed, an expansion of the mass can be detected during the change from the hemihydrate to the dihydrate. Depending on the composition of the gypsum product, this observed linear expansion may be as low as 0.06% to as high as 0.5%.

On the other hand, if equivalent volumes of the hemihydrate, water, and the reaction product (dihydrate) are compared, the volume of the dihydrate formed will be less than the equivalent volumes of the hemihydrate and water. The calculations are as follows:

(3)
$$(CaSO_4)_2 \cdot H_2O + 3H_2O \longrightarrow 2CaSO_4 \cdot 2H_2O$$

Molecular mass	290.284	54.048	344.332
Density (g/cm³)	2.75	0.997	2.32
Equivalent volume	105.556	54.211	148.405
Total volume	159.767		148.405

(4)
$$\text{Change in volume} = \left(\frac{148.405 - 159.767}{159.767}\right) 100 = -7.11\%$$

This represents a linear change in the gypsum object of -2.37%. Thus, according to these calculations, a volumetric contraction should occur during the setting reaction. However, a setting expansion is actually observed, and this phenomenon can be rationalized on the basis of the crystallization mechanism.

As previously noted, the crystallization process is pictured as an outgrowth of crystals from nuclei of crystallization. On the basis of the entanglement of the dihydrate crystals, as indicated in Figure 9–5, one can see that crystals growing from the nuclei can intermesh with and obstruct the growth of adjacent crystals.

If this process is repeated by thousands of the crystals during growth, an outward stress or thrust develops that produces an expansion of the entire mass. Thus, a setting expansion can take place even though the *true volume* of the crystals alone may be less as calculated. This crystal impingement and movement result in the production of micropores.

Because the product of the setting reaction for gypsum (reaction 2) in practice is greater in external volume but less in *crystalline* volume, it follows that the set material must be porous.

The structure immediately after setting is, therefore, composed of interlocking crystals, between which are micropores and pores containing the excess water required for mixing, as previously described. On drying, the excess water is lost, and the void space is increased.

As far as the technician or dentist is concerned, only the setting expansion that occurs after the initial set is of interest. Any expansion or contraction that occurs before this time can be overcome by friction between the mold surface onto which the plaster is poured and the fluid plaster. At the time of initial set, the crystalline framework is sufficiently rigid that it can overcome, for the most part, such frictional retention. However, it cannot always overcome any confinement by the mold boundaries. Furthermore, any initial contraction that occurs during the induction period does not affect the accuracy, because the mix is fluid at this stage and the contraction occurs at the free surface.

If a mixture of plaster and water is spread on a glass surface, the distance between any two surface reference points will not change appreciably during the induction period. The adhesion of the water-powder mix to the glass can prevent the linear contraction that is theoretically expected. Only when the crystalline framework is sufficiently rigid (after the initial set) is a visible setting expansion evident.

On the other hand, if the frictional factor is reduced by spreading the mixture on a frictionless surface such as liquid mercury, for example, the setting expansion curve shown in Figure 9–8 might result. The initial contraction is evident. When sufficient crystals form to produce the outward thrust by impingement, the setting expansion follows. The initial setting time occurs approximately at the minimal point of the curve, the point at which the expansion begins. According to

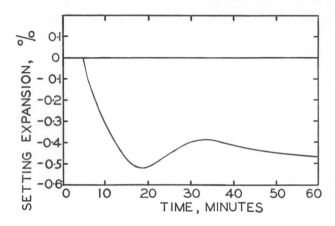

Figure 9–8. Dimensional changes that occur during the setting of a gypsum product. (Courtesy of A. R. Docking.)

the graph, the stone actually has shrunk during setting and it has not recovered its original dimensions. On the other hand, in the previous experiment on the glass plate, a setting expansion of approximately 0.12% would have been reported.

Control of Setting Expansion. As discussed in subsequent chapters, sometimes a setting expansion is advantageous in a dental operation and sometimes it is disadvantageous, because it may be a source of error. Consequently, it is necessary to control it to obtain the desired accuracy in dental applications.

As can be noted from the results presented in Table 9–2, the less the W:P ratio and the longer the mixing time within practical limits, the greater is the setting expansion. The effect of the W:P ratio on the setting expansion is to be expected on theoretical grounds. With the higher W:P ratios, fewer nuclei of crystallization per unit volume are present than with the thicker mixes, and because it can be assumed that the space between the nuclei is greater in such a case, it follows that there is less growth interaction of the dihydrate crystals and less outward thrust. However, the most effective method for the control of the setting expansion is the addition of chemicals.

ACCELERATORS AND RETARDERS: PRACTICE AND THEORY

Why are accelerators and retarders used? In industry, the gypsum product requires a gradual set or hardening so that the object may be formed or shaped over time. However, its use in dentistry generally involves pouring or vibrating the mix into a mold with any shaping requiring only a few minutes. At that

TABLE 9–2. Effect of the Water:Powder (W:P) Ratio and Mixing Time on the Setting Expansion of Plaster of Paris

W:P	Mixing Time (min)	Setting Expansion (per cent)
0.45	0.6	0.41
0.45	1.0	0.51
0.60	1.0	0.29
0.60	2.0	0.41
0.80	1.0	0.24

From Gibson CS, and Johnson RN: J Soc Chem Ind 51:25T, 1932.

time, the material should harden rapidly and will be ready for use within 30 minutes or less.

Figure 9–9 illustrates in a practical way the need for, and the interplay of, accelerators and retarders on the strength (in MPa units) of plaster. The same effects hold true for other gypsum products, including investments. The curve at the right shows the rate of hardening of a natural plaster, that is, a pure β-hemihydrate. It has only a few minutes of working time and then hardens gradually, usually too slowly for dental use. The addition of an accelerator (the curve at the left) produces a set that makes it possible to use the plaster within 30 minutes. However, the working time has been seriously reduced. Therefore, to make a usable plaster, it is necessary to also add a retarder (the curve in the middle). This increases the latent initial setting period so that the mix retains a reasonable plastic state that permits handling or working it into a useful shape. Then the mass hardens in time for use.

Not only do the chemical accelerators and retarders regulate the setting time of the gypsum products but also they generally reduce the setting expansion. The theory of such effects is still obscure.

Accelerators. Because the rate of setting is influenced by the rate of solution of the hemihydrate, it is logical to assume that materials that increase the rate of solution accelerate the reaction. However, it must be remembered that the rate of precipitation of the dihydrate is also important. Therefore, the accelerator must increase the solubility of the hemihydrate without also increasing the solubility of the dihydrate. Thus, the acceleration caused by an additive depends on the *amount* and *rate* of solubility of the hemihydrate versus the same effect on the dihydrate.

To further complicate matters, although inorganic salts are often accelerators, they can also become retarders when more than a certain amount is added. Sodium chloride is an accelerator up to about 2% of the hemihydrate, but at a

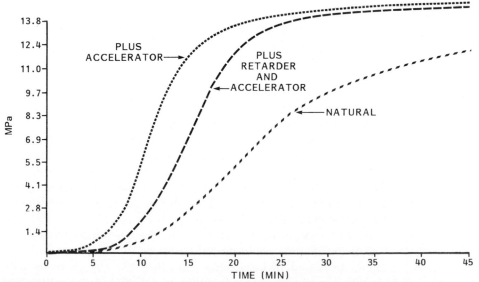

Figure 9–9. Compressive strength of a model plaster plotted against time when accelerators and retarders are added to the plaster. The gain in strength is a measure of the rate of hardening or setting.

higher concentration, it acts as a retarder. Sodium sulfate has its maximum acceleration effect at approximately 3.4%; at greater concentrations, it becomes a retarder.

The most commonly used accelerator is potassium sulfate. It is particularly effective in concentrations higher than 2%, since the reaction product, which seems to be syngenite ($K_2Ca[SO_4]_2 \cdot H_2O$), crystallizes rapidly. Many soluble sulfates act as accelerators, whereas powdered gypsum (calcium sulfate dihydrate) accelerates the setting, because the particles act as nuclei of crystallization. A slurry of ground gypsum casts acts in this way, although the clear saturated liquid is hardly effective. It takes the crystals themselves to accelerate the setting. Another way of accomplishing this effect is to increase either or both the time and the speed of mixing, because they increase the formation of more nuclei and thus accelerates the mix. Decreasing the mixing time or adding more water slightly retards the mix.

Retarders. The behavior of retarders is even more complicated. The common belief is that certain chemicals form a coating on the hemihydrate particles and thus prevent the hemihydrate from going into solution in the normal manner.

The citrates, acetates, and borates generally retard the reaction. For a given anion, the particular cation employed appears to affect the retardation markedly. For example, with the acetates, the order of retardation in terms of the cation employed appears to be $Ca^+ < K^+ < H^+$, whereas potassium tartrate has a marked accelerating effect in contrast with the calcium salt, which has little effect on setting. The behavior of citrates is more complex.

Because the manufacturer has already added accelerators and retarders and other control agents, it is not wise to add other ingredients as they may counteract the effects already incorporated into the product.

HYGROSCOPIC SETTING EXPANSION

It has been assumed in the discussion thus far that the plaster or stone is allowed to set in air. If the setting process is allowed to occur under water, the setting expansion may be more than doubled in magnitude. The reason for the increased expansion when the hemihydrate is allowed to react under water is related to the additional crystal growth permitted and not to any differences in chemical reaction 2.

The theory is illustrated diagrammatically in Figure 9–10. In Stage I, shown at the top of the figure, the initial mix is represented by the three round particles of hemihydrate surrounded by water.

In Stage II, the reaction has started and the crystals of the dihydrate are beginning to form. In the diagram on the left, the water around the particles is reduced by the hydration and the particles are drawn more closely together by the surface tension action of the water. In the right diagram, because the setting is taking place under water, the water of hydration is replaced and the distance between the particles remains the same.

As the crystals of dihydrate grow, they contact each other, and the setting expansion begins. As indicated in Stage III, the water around the particles is again decreased in the example on the left. The particles with their attached crystals tend to be drawn together as before, but the contraction is opposed by the outward thrust of the growing crystals. On the other hand, the crystals in the right diagram are not so inhibited, because the water is again replenished

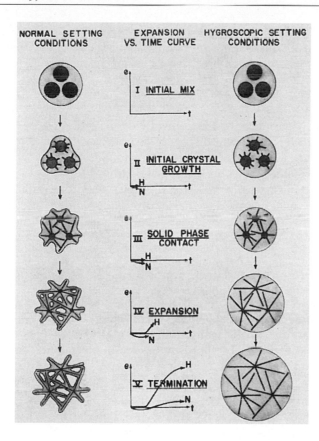

Figure 9–10. Diagrammatic representation of the setting expansion of plaster. In the left column, the crystal growth is inhibited by the lack of excess water. As shown in the right column, water added during setting provides more room for longer crystal growth. θ, expansion; t, time; H, hygroscopic setting expansion; N, normal setting expansion. (From Mahler DB, and Ady AB: Explanation for the hygroscopic setting expansion of dental gypsum products. J Dent Res 39:578, 1960.)

from the outside. In fact, the original particles are now separated further as the crystals grow, and the setting expansion is definitely evident.

In Stages IV and V, the effect becomes more marked. The crystals being inhibited on the left become intermeshed and entangled much sooner than those on the right, which grow much more freely during the early stages before the intermeshing finally prevents further expansion. Consequently, the observed setting expansion that occurs when the gypsum product sets under water may be greater than that which occurs during the setting in air.

It follows, therefore, that the basic mechanism of crystal growth is the same in both instances, and both phenomena are true setting expansions. To distinguish between them, the setting expansion without water immersion is often termed the *normal setting expansion* (N in Fig. 9–10), whereas the expansion that occurs under water is known as *hygroscopic setting expansion* (H in Fig. 9–10). The hygroscopic setting expansion is physical and is not caused by a chemical reaction any more than is the *normal setting expansion*. The reduction in the W:P ratio increases the hygroscopic setting expansion and the normal setting expansion in the same manner. Increased spatulation results in increased hygroscopic expansion as well.

The hygroscopic expansion obtained during the setting of dental stone or plaster is generally small in magnitude. For example, a dental stone used in making casts may exhibit a normal linear setting expansion of 0.15%, with a maximum hygroscopic expansion of not more than 0.30%. Nevertheless, this difference may be sufficient to cause the misfit of a denture or similar device made on the cast.

On the other hand, as explained in a subsequent chapter, the greater hygroscopic setting expansion of gypsum-bonded investments is sometimes used in the fabrication of cast restorations.

STRENGTH

The strength of gypsum products is generally expressed in terms of compressive strength, although tensile strength should also be considered if one is to secure a satisfactory guide to the total strength characteristics.

As might be expected from the theory of setting, the strength of a plaster or stone increases rapidly as the material hardens after the initial setting time. However, the free water content of the set product definitely affects its strength. For this reason, two strengths of the gypsum product are recognized: the *wet strength* (also known as *green strength*) and the *dry strength*. The wet strength is the strength obtained when the water in excess of that required for the hydration of the hemihydrate is left in that test specimen. When the specimen has been dried of the excess water, the strength obtained is the dry strength. The dry strength may be two or more times the wet strength. Consequently, the distinction between the two is of considerable importance.

The effect of drying on the compressive strength of set plaster is shown in Table 9–3. Note the relatively slight gains in strength that occurred after 16 hours. Between an 8-hour and 24-hour period, only 0.6% of the excess water was lost, yet the strength doubled. A somewhat similar change in surface hardness takes place during the drying process.

A good explanation of this effect is the fact that as the last traces of water leave, fine crystals of gypsum precipitate. These anchor the larger crystals. Then if water is added, or if excess water is present, these small crystals are the first to dissolve, and thus the reinforcing anchors are lost.

As previously noted, the set plaster or stone is porous in nature, and the greater the W:P ratio, the greater will be the porosity. As might be expected on such a basis, the greater the W:P ratio, the less is the dry strength of the set material, as shown by the data in Table 9–4, because the greater the porosity, the fewer crystals are available per unit volume for a given weight of hemihydrate.

The tensile strength of plaster or stone is less affected by variations in the W:P ratio than is the compressive strength. However, the materials mixed at a high W:P ratio have tensile strengths as high as 25% of the corresponding compressive strength. When materials are mixed at low W:P ratios, the tensile strength is less than 10% of the corresponding compressive strength.

As shown in Table 9–4, the spatulation time also affects the strength of the

TABLE 9–3. Effect of Drying on the Strength of Plaster of Paris

Drying Period (h)	Compressive Strength		Loss in Weight (per cent)
	MPa	*psi*	
2	9.6	1400	5.1
4	11.7	1700	11.9
8	11.7	1700	17.4
16	13.0	1900	—
24	23.3	3400	18.0
48	23.3	3400	18.0
72	23.3	3400	—

From Gibson CS, and Johnson RN: J Soc Chem Ind 51:25T, 1932.

TABLE 9–4. Effect of the Water:Powder (W:P) Ratio and Mixing Time on the Strength of Plaster of Paris

W:P	Mixing Time (min)	Compressive Strength (Dry)	
		MPa	psi
0.45	0.5	23.4	3400
0.45	1.0	26.2	3800
0.60	1.0	17.9	2600
0.60	2.0	13.8	2000
0.80	1.0	11.0	1600

From Gibson CS, and Johnson, RN: J Soc Chem Ind 51:25T, 1932.

plaster. In general, with an increase in mixing time, the strength is increased to a limit that is approximately equivalent to that of a normal hand mixing for 1 minute. If the mixture is overmixed, the gypsum crystals formed are broken up, and less crystalline interlocking results in the final product.

The incorporation of an accelerator or retarder lowers both the wet and the dry strengths of the gypsum product. Such a decrease in strength can be partially attributed to the salt added as an adulterant and to the reduction in intercrystalline cohesion.

When relatively pure raw hemihydrate is mixed with minimal amounts of water, the working time is short and the setting expansion is unduly high. However, as just noted, dental gypsum products contain additives that reduce the setting expansion, increase the working time, and provide a rapid final set. The addition of more chemicals can upset the delicate balance of these properties. Thus, if a change is desired in the setting time it should be done by modest alterations in either or both the W:P ratio and the spatulation time.

TYPES OF GYPSUM PRODUCTS

Having discussed the basic principles of gypsum products, we turn our attention to the various types of dental gypsum and practical considerations in their use.

The criteria for selection of any particular gypsum product depend on its use and the physical properties necessary for that particular use. For example, a dental stone is a poor material for use as an impression material because if teeth are present it is impossible to remove the impression over the undercuts in the teeth without injury, because of the high strength of the stone (α-hemihydrate).

On the other hand, if a strong cast is required on which to build a denture, one would not choose to employ a weak plaster (β-hemihydrate). In other words, there is no all-purpose dental gypsum product.

The various types of gypsum products can be seen in Table 9–5. Listed are the five types identified by ADA Specification No. 25, and the properties required for each.

Impression Plaster (Type I). These impression materials are composed of plaster of Paris to which modifiers have been added to regulate the setting time and the setting expansion. Impression plaster is rarely used anymore for dental impressions, because it has been replaced by less rigid materials such as the hydrocolloids and elastomers (discussed earlier in Chapters 6 and 7). Plaster is primarily restricted to a final, or *wash*, impression in the construction of full dentures.

TABLE 9–5. Types of Gypsum Products*

Type	Setting Time (min)	Fineness		Setting Expansion at 2 Hours		Compressive Strength at 1 Hour§		W:P Ratio
		Passes 150 μm (%)	Sieves 75 μm (%)	Min (%)	Max (%)	kg/cm²	psi	
I. Plaster, impression	4 ± 1	98	85	0.00	0.15	40 ± 20	580 ± 290	0.50–0.75
II. Plaster, model	12 ± 4	98	90	0.00	0.30	90	1300	0.45–0.50
III. Dental stone†	12 ± 4	98	90	0.00	0.20	210	3000	0.28–0.30
IV. Dental stone,‡ high strength	12 ± 4	98	90	0.00	0.10	350	5000	0.22–0.24
V. Dental stone, high strength, high expansion	12 ± 4	98	90	0.10	0.30	490	7000	0.18–0.22

*Properties required in the 5 gypsum products covered by American Dental Association Specification No. 25. Typical water:powder (W:P) ratios are added at the right, and the traditional terminology for Types III and IV is seen at the bottom.
†III Dental stone, sometimes designated as Class I stone or Hydrocal.
‡III Dental stone, high strength, sometimes designated as Class II stone, densite, or improved stone.
‡IV Dental stone, high strength, sometimes designated as Class II stone, densite, or improved stone.
§Minimum values.

Model Plaster (Type II). This model plaster or laboratory Type II plaster is now used principally to fill a flask in denture construction when setting expansion is not critical and the strength is adequate, according to the limits cited in the specification. It is usually marketed in the natural white color, thus contrasting with stones that are generally colored.

Dental Stone (Type III). In 1930 a major milestone was established when α-gypsum was discovered and introduced within dentistry. Combined with the advent of hydrocolloid impression material, the improved hardness of α-gypsum made stone dies workable and the indirect pattern became possible.

Dentistry shared in the greatest improvement in plaster that has been made in all of history. A researcher at U.S. Gypsum Corporation learned that the plaster mold used for forming rubber denture bases in a vulcanizer under steam pressure became unusually hard overnight. Examination showed that the set gypsum, calcined under steam pressure, formed a much better quality of crystallized calcium sulfate hemihydrate. Because of this improvement, it was soon thereafter patented as α-gypsum. Since this discovery, this process has been performed commercially in an autoclave.

Type III stone has a minimum 1-hour compressive strength of 20.7 MPa (3000 psi), but it does not exceed 34.5 MPa (5000 psi). It is intended for construction of *casts* in the fabrication of full dentures that fit soft tissues. Stone *dies* are reproductions of prepared teeth on or within which prostheses are constructed. Because of the severe wear conditions that occur at the margins during carving of wax patterns and because of the higher stresses induced in stone dies during try-in and adjustments, greater strength and hardness are required of die materials. This type of stone is discussed in the following sections. In addition, a slight setting expansion can be tolerated in casts that reproduce soft tissues but not when a tooth is involved. Type III stones are preferred for casts used to process dentures because the stone has adequate strength for that purpose and the denture is easier to remove after processing.

Regardless of the type of stone used, there are at least two methods for the construction of the cast. In one method, a mold for the cast is constructed by wrapping strips of soft wax around the impression so that they extend approximately 12 mm beyond the tissue side of the impression. A base for the cast is formed in this region. This process is called *boxing*. The mixture of stone and water is then poured into the impression under vibration. The mixture is allowed to flow slowly in a controlled pathway along the impression, so that it pushes the air ahead of itself as it fills all tooth impressions without entrapment of air bubbles.

Another method is to fill the impression first as described. The remainder of the stone-water mixture is poured on a glass plate. The filled impression is then inverted over the mound of stone, and the base is shaped with the spatula, before the stone sets. Such a procedure is not indicated if an impression material that is easily deformed has been used or if the stone is "runny." The cast should not be separated from the impression until it has initially hardened. The minimum time to be allowed for setting will vary from 30 to 60 minutes, depending on the rate of setting of the stone or plaster and the type of impression material used.

Dental Stone, High Strength (Type IV). The principal requisites for a die material stone are strength, hardness, and minimum setting expansion. To obtain these properties, an α-hemihydrate of the "Densite" type is used. The cuboidal-shaped particles (Fig. 9–11) and the reduced surface area produce such properties without undue thickening of the mix. Summarized in Table 9–5 are some of the physical properties of Type IV stones compared with those of Type III stones.

A hard surface is necessary for a die stone, because the cavity preparation is filled with wax and carved flush with the margins of the die. A sharp instrument is used for this purpose; therefore, the stone must be resistant to abrasion. Gypsum hardening solutions and other methods of increasing the abrasion resistance are discussed in Chapter 23. It is fortunate that the surface hardness increases more rapidly than does the compressive strength, because the surface dries more rapidly. This is a real advantage in that the surface resists abrasion, whereas the core of the die is tough and less subject to accidental breakage. The average dry surface hardness of the Type IV stones ("die stones") is approximately 92 (Rockwell Hardness); that of Type III stone is 82. Even though the surface is harder, care should be observed when the pattern is being carved.

Dental Stone, High Strength, High Expansion (Type V). This is a recent gypsum product, having an even higher compressive strength than the Type IV dental stone. The improved strength is attained by making it possible to lower the W:P ratio even further. In addition, the setting expansion has been increased from a maximum of 0.10% to 0.30% (see Table 9–5). The rationale for the increase in setting expansion limits is that certain newer alloys, such as base metal, have a greater casting shrinkage than do the traditional noble metal alloys. Thus, higher expansion is required in the stone used for the die to aid in compensating for the alloy solidification shrinkage. Additional information on the use of Type IV and V stones is provided in the discussion of die materials in Chapter 23.

Synthetic Gypsum. It is also possible to make the α-hemihydrates and β-hemihydrates from the by-products or waste products of the manufacture of phosphoric acid. The synthetic product is usually much more expensive than that made from natural gypsum, but when the product is properly made, its

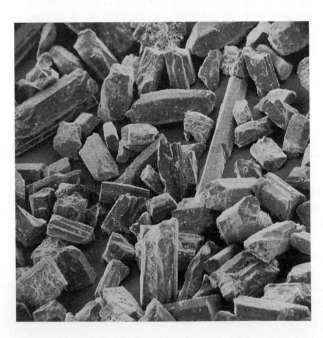

Figure 9–11. Powder particles of Type IV and V stones. ×400. (Courtesy of B. Giammara and R. Neiman.)

properties are equal to or exceed those of the latter. The processing problems are considerable, and few have succeeded. The methods employed are trade secrets, and no further discussion is appropriate. For our purpose, the source of the hemihydrate is not as important as the nature and use of the final product, which is essentially the same regardless of the origin.

PROPORTIONING, MIXING, AND CARING FOR PRODUCTS

Proportioning. Because the strength of a stone is indirectly proportional to the W:P ratio, it is most important to keep the amount of water as low as possible. However, it should not be so low that the mix will not flow into every detail of the impression. Once the optimum W:P is determined, using the manufacturer's suggested W:P as a guide, the same proportions should be adhered to subsequently. The water and powder should be measured by using an accurate graduated cylinder for the water volume and a weighing balance for the powder. The powder should not be measured by volume (use of a scoop), as it does not pack uniformly. It may vary from product to product and will pack harder as the container remains unused. If the container is shaken, then the volume will increase as a result of entrapment of air. Preweighed envelopes have become popular, because they promote accuracy, reduce waste, and save time.

Mixing. If mixing by hand, the bowl should be parabolic in shape, smooth, and resistant to abrasion. The spatula should have a stiff blade and handle that is convenient to hold. Entrapment of air in the mix must be avoided to avoid porosity leading to weak spots and surface inaccuracies, as illustrated in Figure 9–12. The use of an automatic vibrator, of high frequency and of low amplitude, is helpful. A measured amount of water is placed in the bowl, and the weighed powder is sifted in. The mixture is then vigorously stirred, with the periodic wiping of the inside of the bowl with the spatula to ensure the wetting of all of the powder and breaking up of any agglomerates, or lumps. The mixing should continue until a smooth mix is obtained, usually within a minute. A longer spatulation time drastically reduces the working time (see Table 9–1), particularly for pouring models.

The guesswork of repeatedly adding water and powder to achieve the proper consistency must be avoided. It yields an uneven set within the mass, resulting in low strength and distortion, one of the main causes of inaccuracy in the use of gypsum products.

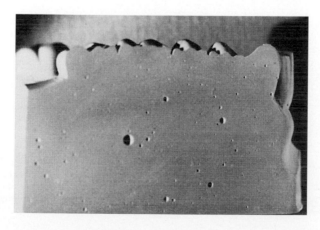

Figure 9–12. Section through a cast of a set stone that was improperly mixed. Air voids weaken the stone and impair its appearance.

The preferred method of mixing is to add the measured water first, followed by gradual addition of the preweighed powder. The powder is incorporated during approximately 15 seconds of mixing with a hand spatula, followed by 20 to 30 seconds of mechanical mixing under vacuum by a mixer. In this way, a properly mixed stone results in a solid cast (Fig. 9–13). The strength and hardness obtained in such mechanical vacuum mixing usually exceed that obtained by 1 minute of hand mixing.

Caring for the Cast. If the surface of the cast is not hard and smooth when it is removed from the impression, its accuracy is questionable. The cast is supposedly an accurate reproduction of the oral tissues, and any departure from the expected accuracy will probably result in a poorly fitting prosthesis. The cast should, therefore, be handled carefully. Once the setting reactions in the cast have been completed, its dimensions will be relatively constant thereafter under ordinary conditions of room temperature and humidity. As later outlined, however, it is sometimes necessary to soak the gypsum cast in water, in preparation for other techniques. The gypsum of which the cast is composed is slightly soluble in water. When a dry cast is immersed in water, there may be a negligible expansion, provided that the water is saturated with calcium sulfate. If it is not so saturated, gypsum may be dissolved. If the stone cast is immersed in running water, its linear dimension may decrease approximately 0.1% for every 20 minutes of such immersion. The safest method for soaking the cast is to place it in a water bath made for the purpose, in which plaster debris is allowed to remain constantly on the bottom of the container to provide a saturated solution of calcium sulfate.

As previously noted, storage of either set plaster or stone at room temperature produces no significant dimensional change. However, if the storage temperature is raised to between 90° and 110° C (194° to 230° F), a shrinkage occurs as the water of crystallization is removed and the dihydrate reverts to the hemihydrate. The contraction of the plaster at high temperature is greater than that of the stone, and it also loses strength.

Such contractions may occur during storage in air above room temperature, as when a stone cast is dried. Probably it is not safe to store or heat a stone cast in air at a temperature higher than 55° C (130° F).

Special Gypsum Products. In addition to the standardized gypsum materials just described, there are some that have been characterized for special purposes. For example, the orthodontist prefers a white stone or plaster for study models

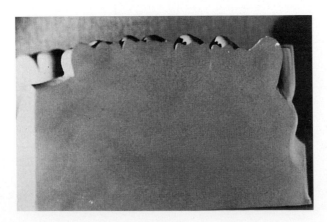

Figure 9–13. Section through a cast of a set stone that was properly proportioned and mixed.

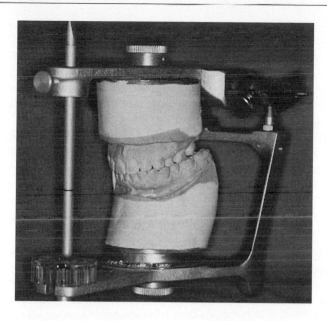

Figure 9–14. Dental articulator, a device that incorporates artificial temporomandibular joints. This permits orientation of casts in a manner that simulates various positions of the mandible. (Courtesy of C. Munoz.)

and may even treat the surface with soap for an added sheen. These products generally have a longer working time for ease of trimming.

The use of an articulator makes it necessary to mount the casts with a gypsum product, as shown in Figure 9–14. These materials are referred to as "mounting" stones or plasters. They are fast setting and have low setting expansion. In the case of the mounting plaster, it has low strength to permit easy trimming and to separate the cast readily from the articulator mounting plates.

Since 1991, a plethora of new dental stones have appeared, mostly as time savers. One type is extremely fast setting and ready to use in 5 minutes, but it has little working time. Another product changes color to help denote when it is ready for use. Most recently, the trend is to add a small amount of plastic or resin that reduces the brittleness and improves the resistance to scratching during the carving of wax patterns.

Usually, when one feature is improved, another feature is sacrificed. A faster set is accepted in return for less working time. An improved resistance to carving is accepted in return for a greater difficulty in incorporation, the need to box the impression because of excessive runniness, and decreased detail reproduction. Improvements in materials and testing equipment have made it possible to use silicone-stone combinations that can reproduce spacings between lines as fine as 10 μm or less. Current specifications require an accuracy of only 50 μm.

Currently, there is a wide choice of gypsum products available to suit almost any desired individual requirements or combinations thereof.

Caring for Gypsum Products. Gypsum products are somewhat sensitive to changes in the relative humidity of their environment. Even the surface hardness of plaster and stone casts may fluctuate slightly with the relative humidity of the atmosphere. Gypsum surfaces made with thinner mixes appear to be affected more than those with a low W:P ratio.

The hemihydrate of gypsum takes up water from the air readily. For example, if the relative humidity exceeds 70%, the plaster takes up sufficient water vapor to start a setting reaction. The first hydration probably produces a few crystals of gypsum on the surface of the hemihydrate crystal. These crystals act as nuclei of crystallization, and the first manifestation of the plaster deterioration is a decrease in the setting time.

As the hygroscopic action continues, more crystals of gypsum form until the entire hemihydrate crystal is covered. Under these conditions, the water penetrates the dihydrate coating with difficulty, and the setting time is unduly prolonged. It is, therefore, important that all types of gypsum products be stored in a dry atmosphere. The best means of storage is to seal the product in a moisture-proof metal container. When gypsum products are stored in closed containers, generally the setting time is retarded only slightly, approximately 1 or 2 minutes per year. This may be counteracted by a slight increase in the mixing time if necessary.

INFECTION CONTROL CONCERNS

As noted elsewhere in this text, there is increased interest in expanding infection control measures to the dental laboratory. Concern over possible cross-contamination to dental office personnel by micro-organisms, including hepatitis B virus and human immunodeficiency virus, via dental impressions has prompted study of the effect of spray and immersion disinfecting techniques on impression materials, as discussed in Chapter 7. The effect of such agents on the surface quality and accuracy of the resulting gypsum casts is an important consideration.

If an impression were not disinfected, or if the laboratory has no assurance that an appropriate disinfection protocol was followed, it is prudent to disinfect the stone cast. Disinfecting solutions can be used that do not adversely affect the quality of the gypsum cast. Alternatively, a dental stone containing a disinfectant may also be employed. Although the addition of a disinfectant may have a slight effect on some of the physical properties of certain products, the disinfected stones apparently compare favorably with the nondisinfected controls.

The widespread availability of a spectrum of disinfecting dental stones (Types II to V) with proven efficacy and unimpaired physical properties would undoubtedly strengthen the barrier system of infection control in the dental laboratory. When patients with known cases of infection are being treated, overnight gas sterilization is an option. However, the procedure is impractical for routine use by practitioners and dental laboratory personnel.

In the United States, the incorporation of disinfectants in dental stones has been delayed by failure to obtain approval of the U.S. Food and Drug Administration.

SELECTED READING

Bailey JH, Donovan TE, and Preston JD: The dimensional accuracy of improved dental stone, silver-plated, and epoxy resin die materials. J Prosthet Dent 59:307, 1988.
Silver-plated and epoxy resin die systems were found to be acceptable alternative systems to the improved dental stones.

Dilts WE, Duncanson MG Jr, and Collard EW: Comparative stability of cast mounting materials. J Okla Dent Assoc 68:11, 1978.
Certain properties of mounting gypsum products are cited, particularly their low-setting expansion.

Donovan T, and Chee WWL: Preliminary investigation of a disinfected gypsum die stone. Int J Prosthodont 2:245, 1989.
Two such die materials were found comparable with existing products in almost all physical properties tested. One of the new materials was weaker in compressive and tensile strength and deficient in detail reproduction.

Jørgensen KD: Studies on the setting of plaster of Paris. Odont T 61:305, 1953.
Porosity of set gypsum was calculated, as influenced by the W:P ratio. The higher the ratio, the greater the porosity.

Kuntze RA: The Chemistry and Technology of Gypsum. Philadelphia, American Society for Testing and Materials, STP 861, 1984.

Excellent reference on the basic chemistry and technologic aspects of gypsum.

Mahler DB, and Ady AB: Explanation for the hygroscopic setting expansion of dental gypsum products. J Dent Res 39:578, 1960.

This is a classic study that best defines the mechanics of hygroscopic expansion.

Schelb E, Cavozos E, Kaiser DA, and Troendle K: Compatibility of Type IV dental stones with polyether impression materials. J Prosthet Dent 60:540, 1988.

A further study on impression material–stone compatibility using polyethers. A plea again is made to manufacturers to identify stones that are compatible with their impression materials.

Schelb E, Mazzocco CV, Jones JD, and Prihoda T: Compatibility of Type IV dental stones with polyvinyl siloxane impression materials. J Prosthet Dent 58:19, 1987.

Before using a dental stone with an impression material, the compatibility of the two components should be determined. Differences in surface reproduction were noted between various combinations.

10 *Chemistry of Synthetic Resins*

CLASSIFICATION OF RESINS

Synthetic resins are often called *plastics*. A plastic material is a substance that, although dimensionally stable in normal use, was plastic at some stage of manufacture. Plastics are usually polymers that are *thermoplastic* if they soften again when reheated and *thermosetting* if they are resistant to change after further application of heat.

Synthetic resins are composed of very large molecules. The particular form and morphology of the molecule determine whether the plastic is a fiber, a hard, rigid resin, or a rubberlike product. Plastics have had an enormous impact on dentistry, and they are now used as sealants (prophylactic material used to seal fissures against the ingress of cariogenic bacteria), bonding materials, restorative materials, veneering materials, dentures, and impression materials.

The popularity of plastics relates to their ability to be formed into complex shapes, often by the application of heat and pressure. Based on their thermal behavior they can be divided into *thermoplastic* and *thermosetting* resins. Thermoplastic resins, such as impression compounds and acrylics, soften when heated above their glass transition temperatures (T_g). They can then be shaped and, on cooling, will harden in this form. However, on reheating they soften again and they can be reshaped if required before hardening as the temperature decreases.

This cycle can be carried out repeatedly. Thermoplastic resins are fusible, and they are usually soluble in organic solvents. Most plastics used in dentistry belong to the thermoplastic group.

The thermosetting resins become permanently hard when heated above a critical temperature, and they do not soften again on reheating. They are usually cross-linked in this state. Thermosetting resins are generally insoluble and infusible. The thermosetting plastics generally have superior abrasion resistance and dimensional stability compared with that of thermoplastic resins, which have better flexural and impact properties.

A third group of polymeric materials are the *elastomers*. The modern elastomer industry was founded on the naturally occurring latex isolated from the *Hevea brasiliensis* tree. Since the early twentieth century, chemists have been attempting to synthesize materials whose properties duplicate or at least simulate those of natural rubber, and this has led to the production of a wide variety of synthetic elastomers. Some of these elastomers are used in dentistry as impression materials. Elastomers readily undergo deformation and exhibit extensive reversible elongation under small applied stresses, that is, they exhibit elasticity.

DENTAL RESINS

The dentist uses thermoplastic resins mainly to restore and replace missing teeth and tooth structure. These resins can be bonded with other resins directly to tooth structure or to other restorative materials. If all teeth are missing, a denture base (the part of the denture that rests on the soft tissues of the mouth) with attached denture teeth can be made to restore chewing ability.

Most resin systems used in dentistry are based on methacrylates, particularly methyl methacrylate. However, because the field is dynamic and new types of resins are being developed on a regular basis, the dentist's knowledge must include basic concepts of resin chemistry so that new developments in the field can be critically evaluated. This chapter provides a brief review of the fundamentals of resin chemistry.

REQUISITES FOR DENTAL RESIN

Methacrylate polymers have earned great popularity in dentistry because they are economical and because they can be processed easily using relatively simple techniques. They represent a main polymer group that is capable of providing essential properties and characteristics needed for use in the oral cavity. These performance features are related to their biologic, physical, aesthetic, and handling characteristics.

Biologic Considerations. The resin should be tasteless, odorless, nontoxic, and nonirritating to the oral tissues. To fulfill these requirements it should be completely insoluble in saliva or in any other fluids taken into the mouth, and it should be impermeable to oral fluids to the extent that it does not become unsanitary or disagreeable in taste or odor. If the resin is used as a filling material or cement, it should bond to tooth structure to prevent microbial ingrowth along the tooth-restoration interface.

Physical Properties. The resin should possess adequate strength and resilience and resist biting or chewing forces, impact forces, and excessive wear that can occur in the oral cavity. It should also be dimensionally stable under all conditions of service, including thermal changes and variations in loading. When used as a denture base for maxillary dentures, its specific gravity should be low.

Aesthetic Properties. The material should exhibit sufficient translucency or transparency such that it can be made to match the appearance of the oral tissues it is to replace. It should be capable of being tinted or pigmented, and there should be no change in color or appearance of the material subsequent to its fabrication.

Handling Characteristics. The material should not produce toxic fumes or dust during handling and manipulation. It should be easy to mix, insert, shape and cure, and it must be insensitive to variations in these handling procedures. Clinical complications, such as oxygen inhibition, saliva contamination, and blood contamination, should have little or no effect on the final outcome. In addition, the final product should be easy to polish, and in case of unavoidable breakage, it should also be possible to repair the resin easily and efficiently.

Economic Considerations. The cost of the resin and its processing method should be low, and processing should not require complex and expensive equipment.

Overall Performance of Methacrylates. Although the methacrylates fulfill these requirements reasonably well, no resin has yet met all of the requirements just discussed. The conditions in the mouth are most demanding, and only the most chemically stable and inert materials can withstand such conditions without deterioration.

POLYMERIZATION

Dental resins solidify when they polymerize. Polymerization occurs through a series of chemical reactions by which the macromolecule, or the *polymer*, is formed from large numbers of molecules known as *monomers*.

The most significant features of polymers are that they consist of very large molecules and that their molecular structure is capable of virtually limitless configurations and conformations. The polymer is made up of one or several simple, recurring structural units, consisting of the individual monomer structure. These monomer units are connected to each other along the polymer chain by covalent bonds. Polymerization is a repetitive intermolecular reaction that is functionally capable of proceeding indefinitely. Because any chemical compound possessing a molecular weight in excess of 5000 is considered to be a macromolecule, most polymer molecules can be described as macromolecules. In some instances, the molecular weight of the polymer molecule can be as high as 50 million.

In addition to the traditional polymers, macromolecules can also consist of inorganic polymers such as the silicon dioxide network found in different fillers and ceramics used in dentistry. The discussion in this chapter is limited to organic polymers.

Synthetic resins polymerize randomly from local sites that have been activated. Thus, depending on the ability of the chains to grow from their local activation sites, the molecules within a polymeric material consist of molecular species that vary in degree of polymerization. In addition, the molecular weight distribution does not always follow a normal distribution curve. Because of the molecular weight distribution, the term *molecular weight* of a polymer can be defined differently. The *number average molecular weight* is given by $\overline{M}_n = M_0 \overline{x}_n$ and the *weight average molecular weight* by $\overline{M}_w = M_0 \overline{x}_w$ where M_0 is the molecular weight of the structural unit, $\overline{x}_n$ is the number average degree of polymerization, and $\overline{x}_w$ is the weight average degree of polymerization. The number average degree of polymerization is determined by dividing the total number of monomer units by the total number of molecules, whereas the weight average degree of polymerization represents the weight of the sample divided by the number of moles it contains.

The number average molecular weight for various commercial dental denture polymers varies from 8000 to 39,000, but molecular weights as high as 600,000 have been reported. Cross-linked resin denture teeth may have an even higher molecular weight.

Biologically, it is important to realize that polymerization seldom is entirely complete and that residual monomer molecules can be leached from polymeric materials. These low-molecular-weight compounds sometimes cause adverse reactions, mainly allergic reactions. The residual monomer also has a pronounced effect on the molecular weight of the polymer. For example, 0.9% of residual monomer in a polymer that could theoretically have a number average molecular weight of 22,400 if completely cured, reduces the molecular weight of the polymer to approximately 7300.

Considering the aspects just discussed, the ratio $\overline{M}_w:\overline{M}_n$ (called the *polydispersity*) is a useful measure of the range of the polymer molecule size distribution. Larger values of $\overline{M}_w:\overline{M}_n$ indicate a very wide range, with substantial amounts of materials at both extremes. When $\overline{M}_w:\overline{M}_n$ equals 1, all polymeric molecules have the same molecular weight and there is no distribution of molecular sizes.

POLYMERIZATION MECHANISMS

Polymerization can occur either by a series of localized reactions that often, but not always, produce a by-product, or by simple addition reactions. If the polymerization occurs by the first mechanism, the process is known as a *step-growth* or *condensation polymerization*. If the polymerization is brought about by an addition reaction, *addition polymerization* takes place.

Step-growth Polymerization. The reactions producing step-growth polymerization progress by the same mechanism as chemical reactions between two or more simple molecules. The primary compounds react, often with the formation of by-products such as water, halogen acids, and ammonia. The formation of these by-products is the reason step-growth polymerization often is called *condensation polymerization*. The structure of the monomers is such that the process can repeat itself and build macromolecules. This mechanism is also the one used in biologic tissues to produce macromolecules.

In step-growth polymerization, a linear chain of monomer residues is obtained by the stepwise intermolecular condensation or addition of the reactive groups in bifunctional monomers. These reactions are analogous to those in which monofunctional units undergo a polyesterification reaction involving a diol and a dibasic acid (Fig. 10–1). If the water is removed as it is formed, no equilibrium is established and the first step in the reaction is the formation of a dimer that is also bifunctional (see Fig. 10–1). As the reaction proceeds, longer chains, including trimers and tetramers, form through other esterification reactions, all

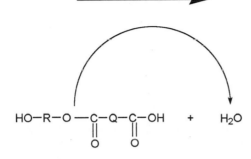

Figure 10–1. Step-growth (or condensation) polymerization between diols and dibasic acids. R and Q symbolize the backbone structures of the two molecules. As seen from the reaction, a condensation product (in this instance, water) is formed.

essentially identical in rate and mechanism, until ultimately the reaction contains a mixture of polymer chains of large molar masses.

In the past, several condensation resins have been used in dentistry in the construction of denture bases. Today, condensation polymerization is mainly used for polymerization of polysulfide and condensation silicone impression materials. However, because these polymerization reactions yield condensation products such as water (polysulfide) and alcohol (condensation polymerized silicone impressions), these by-products may evaporate and affect the dimensional stability of the impression materials. Attempts to improve dimensional stability have resulted in the development of other impression materials, such as polyether and vinylpolysiloxane, that are not associated with by-product formation during setting and the corresponding shrinkage that occurs during subsequent storage of the impression.

As polymer science has progressed, the classification of condensation polymerized resins has broadened. To minimize classification uncertainties, the term *step-growth polymerization* is the preferred term rather than *condensation polymerization*. Polymers, whose repeating units are joined by functional groups without the formation of a by-product, should be called *step-growth polymerized resins* rather than *condensation polymerized resins*. *Polyurethane* is a polymer of this type. It can be formed by reacting a diol with a di-isocyanate (Fig. 10–2). The urethane linkage (OCONH) is repeated throughout the chain as the dimer continues to grow. In dentistry, when the term *urethane* is used to describe a monomer, methacrylate groups are often attached to the urethane molecule. During polymerization of the dental urethanes with attached methacrylate groups, the reaction occurs via addition polymerization of the methacrylate groups, a mechanism that is described in the section on addition polymerization.

Thus, step-growth polymerized resins are those in which (1) polymerization is accompanied by repeated elimination of small molecules or (2) functional groups are repeated in the polymer chain. The formation of polymers by step-growth is rather slow because one proceeds in a stepwise fashion from monomer to dimer to trimer, and so forth, until large polymer molecules containing many monomer molecules are eventually formed. Such a polymerization process tends

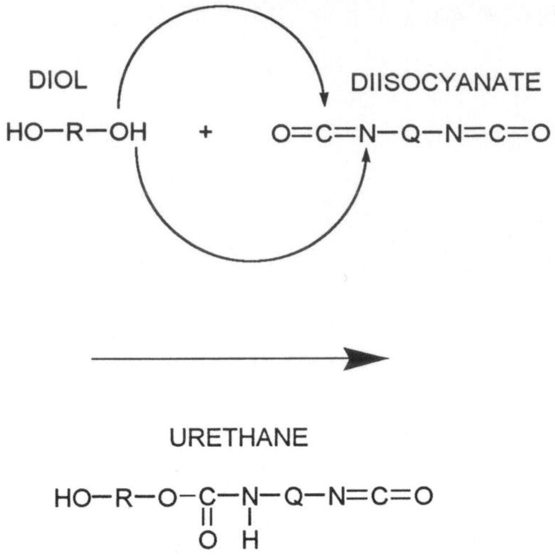

DIOL   DIISOCYANATE

HO—R—OH   +   O=C=N—Q—N=C=O

URETHANE

HO—R—O—C—N—Q—N=C=O
          ‖ |
          O H

Figure 10–2. Step-growth polymerization reaction between diol and diisocyanate. During this reaction no condensation product is formed. Instead, the two molecules are bonded together via a urethane group (—OCONH—).

to stop before the molecules have reached a truly great size because, as the chains grow, they become less mobile and less numerous. Step-growth polymerized polymers such as nylon have acquired their valuable properties when they reach a molecular weight of 10,000 to 20,000. However, polymerizing molecules with molecular weights in the hundreds of thousands or millions by step-growth is difficult.

Currently, step-growth polymerized (condensation polymerized) resins are not employed extensively in dental restorations or prosthetic appliances, whereas the biologic polymers, such as collagen, deoxyribonucleic acid, and ribonucleic acid, are exclusively formed via step-growth polymerization reactions. Examples of two condensation polymerized dental materials that have been widely used in dentistry are the polysulfide and condensation polymerized silicone impression materials. However, considering the fast-growing field of molecular biology and the new advances in polymer chemistry, one can suspect that step-growth polymerized polymers will find new dental applications in the near future.

Addition Polymerization. Most dental resins are polymerized by *addition polymerization.* This type of addition reaction is so common that often the term *polymerization* is generally used to describe the process.

Unlike condensation polymerization, there is no change in composition during addition polymerization. The macromolecules are formed from smaller units, or monomers, without change in composition, because the monomer and the polymer have the same empirical formulas. In other words, the structure of the monomer is repeated many times in the polymer.

Compared with condensation polymerization, the addition method can readily produce giant molecules of almost unlimited size. Starting from an active center, one monomer is added at a time and rapidly forms a chain that theoretically can grow indefinitely, as long as the supply of building blocks is available. The process is simple but not easy to control.

One of the requisites of an addition polymerizable compound is the presence of an unsaturated group, that is, a *double bond.* Ethylene, C_2H_4, the simplest monomer capable of addition polymerization, and a free radical I*, can be used for purposes of illustration:

(1) $\quad\quad\quad\quad\quad\quad I^* + H_2C{=}C_2H \Rightarrow IH_2C{-}CH_2{^*}$

(2) $\quad\quad\quad\quad IH_2C{-}CH_2{^*} + H_2C{=}C_2H \Rightarrow IH_2C{-}CH_2{-}H_2C{-}CH_2{^*}$

Theoretically, I^* can be almost any free radical that one might choose. By definition, a free radical is an atom or group of atoms possessing an odd (unpaired) electron. For example, it can be hydrogen, and the original ethylene gas can be polymerized under heat and pressure to form polyethylene. The free radical has an electron withdrawal ability because it possesses an unpaired electron. When the free radical and its unpaired electron approach the monomer molecule, they absorb one of the π electrons from the double bond of the monomer and form a σ bond between the radical and the monomer molecule, leaving the other π electron in an unsaturated electron orbital. Thus, the original free radical bonds to one side of the monomer molecule. The remaining electron from the unsaturated π orbital then acts as a new free radical center when the free radical-monomer complex approaches another monomer molecule to form a *dimer*, which also becomes a free radical. This reactive species can, in turn, add successively to a large number of ethylene molecules so that the polymerization process continues through the propagation of the reactive center. This chain process leads to large polymer molecules within a matter of seconds. The process continues to complete the formation of the desired polymer. The growth of the polymer chain ceases when the reactive center is destroyed by one of a number of possible termination reactions, as discussed later. The entire addition polymerization process can be pictured as a series of chain reactions. The process occurs rapidly, almost instantaneously. The reactions are exothermic, and considerable heat is evolved.

STAGES IN ADDITION POLYMERIZATION

The addition polymerization process occurs in four stages: induction, propagation, termination, and chain transfer.

Induction. To start an addition polymerization process, free radicals must be present. Free radicals can be generated by activation of monomer molecules with ultraviolet light, visible light, heat, or energy transfer from another compound that acts as a free radical.

The free radical chemical that is used to start the polymerization is not a catalyst, because it enters into the chemical reaction and becomes part of the final chemical compound. A more accurate term is an *initiator* as noted earlier. This method of polymerization is dependent on the formation of a compound with an unpaired electron (free radical), usually a fragment of a larger molecule that has been split by heating. The unpaired electron makes the radical very reactive. The conventional symbol, $C{=}C$, represents two pairs of electrons (π orbital). When a free radical approaches a double bond, it may pair with one of the electrons in the extra bond, leaving the other member of the pair free. Thus, the monomer itself then becomes a free radical.

A number of substances capable of generating free radicals are potent initiators for the polymerization of poly(methyl methacrylate) resins.* The most commonly

---

*The nomenclature of *poly(methyl methacrylate)* has been retained throughout this edition. Frequently, it is referred to as *polymethyl methacrylate* or *methyl methacrylate polymer*. However, the present rules of the International Union of Pure and Applied Chemistry state: "A polymer of unspecified chain length is named with the prefix 'poly' followed by, in parentheses or brackets, as appropriate, the name of the smallest repeating unit. The generic name for a single-stranded linear polymer is thus poly(bivalent radical)." (Macromolecules 1:19, 1968)

employed initiator is benzoyl peroxide, which decomposes at relatively low temperatures to release two free radicals per benzoyl peroxide molecule. The decomposition of benzoyl peroxide, also called *activation*, occurs quite rapidly between 50° and 100° C (Fig. 10–3). The induction (or initiation) period is the time during which molecules of the initiator become energized or activated, forming free radicals that interact with the monomer molecules (Fig. 10–4). This period is greatly influenced by the purity of the monomer. Any impurities present that can react with activated groups can increase the length of this period by consuming the activated initiator molecules. However, the higher the temperature, the shorter the length of the induction period.

The polymerization processes useful for dental resins are commonly activated by one of three processes: heat, chemicals, and light. Most denture base resins are polymerized by heat activation. Thus, the free radicals are obtained by heating benzoyl peroxide. During heating, the benzoyl peroxide molecule splits into two free radicals, which then initiate the polymerization of methyl methacrylate monomer.

A second type of induction system is chemically activated at ambient oral temperature. Such a system consists of at least two reactants that, when mixed together, undergo a chemical reaction that generates free radicals. During storage, these components must be separated from each other; hence, chemically induced systems always consist of two or more parts. An example of such a system is the tertiary amine, the *activator*, and benzoyl peroxide, the *initiator*, which are mixed together to initiate the polymerization of self-cured dental resins. When these two components (activator and initiator) are mixed, the amine catalyzes the split of the benzoyl molecule into two free radicals.

A third type of induction system is light activated. In this system, photons activate the initiator to generate free radicals that, in turn, can initiate the polymerization process. Initially, ultraviolet light was used for this process. However, because of concerns about the effect of ultraviolet light on the retina and unpigmented oral tissues, the limited penetration depth, and the reduction in intensity of the ultraviolet light source over time, systems were developed that were activated by visible light. In the visible light–cured dental restorations, camphorquinone and dimethylaminoethylmethacrylate, an amine, generate free radicals when irradiated by visible light. To trigger this reaction, light with a wavelength of about 470 nm is needed. Because no appreciable polymerization takes place at ambient temperature in the dark, such compositions can be one-part systems, provided that they are stored where they are not exposed to light. However, factors such as light intensity and distance from the light source can

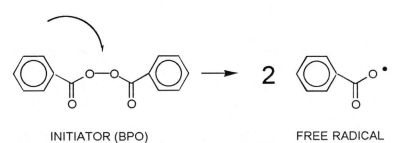

INITIATOR (BPO)   FREE RADICAL

Figure 10–3. Activation (heat or chemical) of benzoyl peroxide (BPO). During activation, the —O—O— bond is broken, and the electron pair is split between the two fragments. The dot adjacent to the oxygen of the free radical symbolizes the unpaired electron.

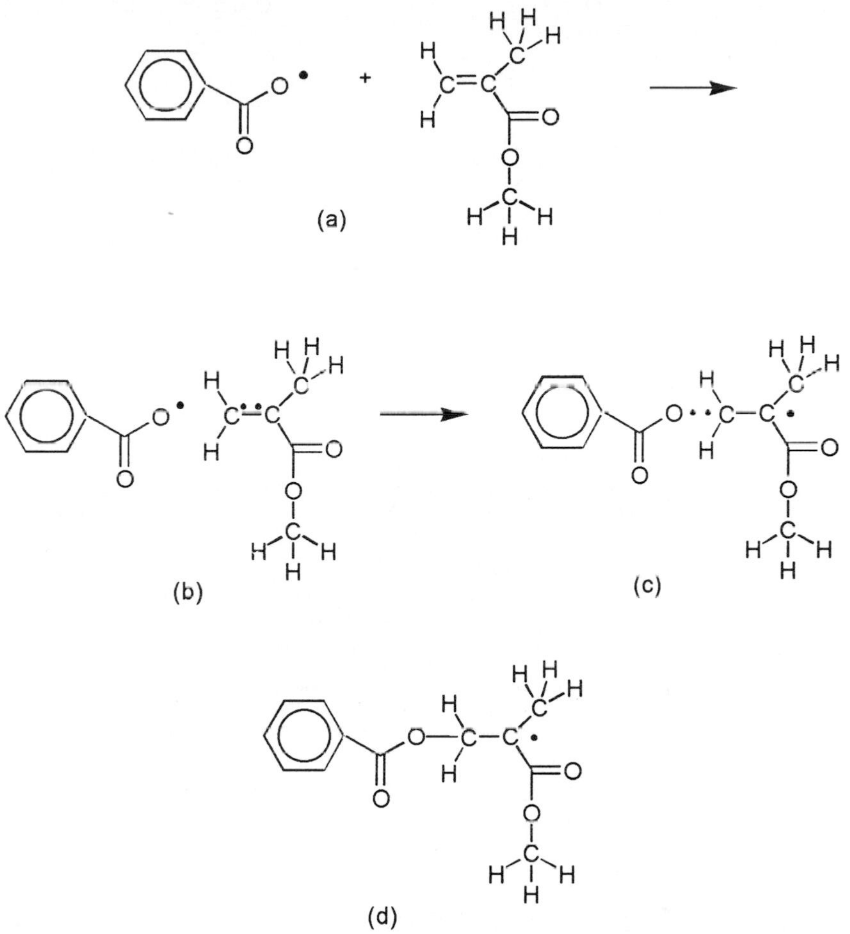

Figure 10–4. Initiation of a methyl methacrylate molecule. As the unpaired electron of the free radical approaches the methyl methacrylate molecule (*a* and *b*), one of the electrons in the double bond is attracted to the free radical to form an electron pair and a covalent bond between the free radical and the monomer molecule (*c* and *d*). When this occurs, the remaining unpaired electron makes the new molecule a free radical (*d*).

significantly affect the number of free radicals that are formed, thereby making this system technique sensitive.

Propagation. The propagation reactions are illustrated in Figure 10–5. Because little energy is required once the growth has started, the process continues with considerable velocity. Theoretically, the chain reactions should continue with the evolution of heat, until all of the monomer has been converted to a polymer. However, the polymerization reaction is never complete.

Termination. The chain reactions can be terminated either by direct coupling or by the exchange of a hydrogen atom from one growing chain to another.

The termination by direct coupling can be illustrated in terms of a diagrammatic reaction. Let $I_I M_m$ represent a polymer of m monomer units and $I_I M_n$ a polymer of n units. Then,

(3) $$I_I M_m{}^* \quad + \quad I_I M_n{}^* \quad \rightarrow \quad I_I M_m M_n I_I$$

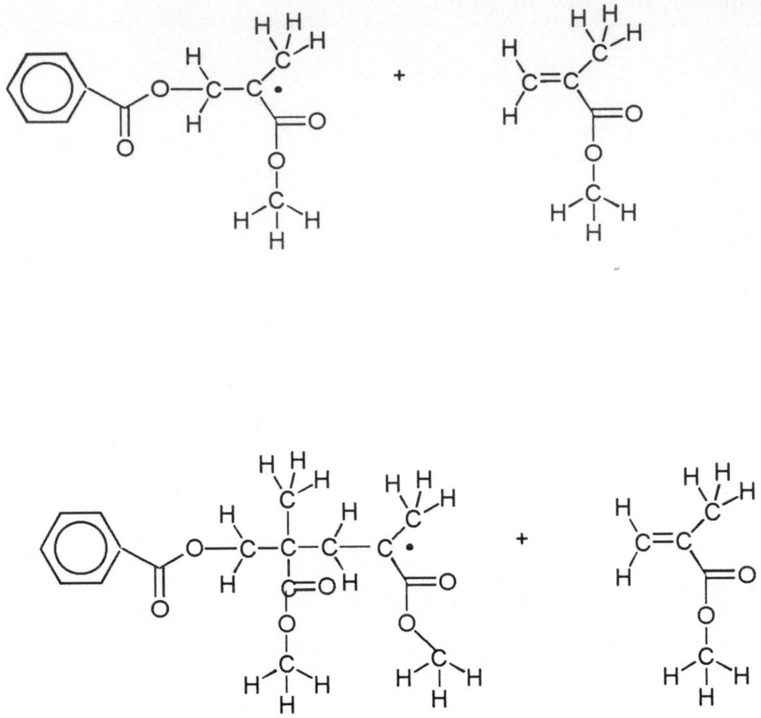

Figure 10–5. Propagation and chain growth. As the initiated molecule approaches other methyl methacrylate molecules, the free electron interacts with the double bond of the methyl methacrylate molecule, and a new, longer free radical is formed.

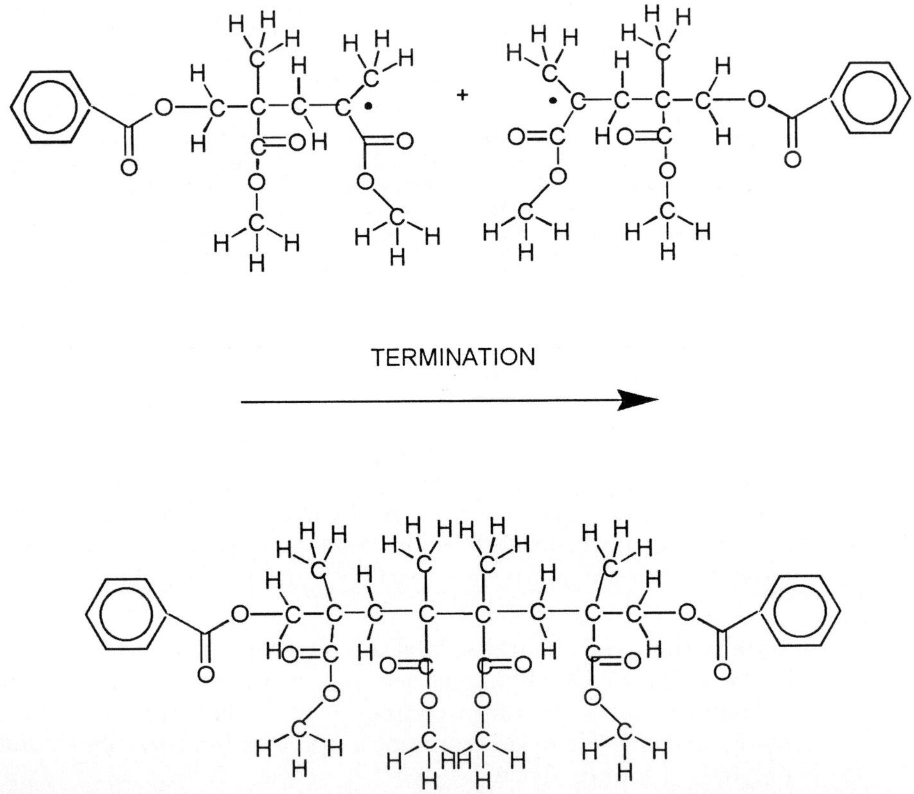

TERMINATION

Figure 10–6. Termination occurs when two free radicals interact and form a covalent bond.

In other words, both molecules combine and become deactivated by an exchange of energy (Fig. 10–6).

Another means by which such an energy exchange can occur is by the transfer of a hydrogen atom from one growing chain to another (Fig. 10–7). However, in the latter case, a double bond is produced when the hydrogen atom is transferred from one chain to the other.

Chain Transfer. Although chain termination can result from *chain transfer*, the process differs from the termination reactions described in that the active state is transferred from an activated radical to an inactive molecule, and a new nucleus for further growth is created. For example, a monomer molecule may be activated by a growing macromolecule in such a manner that termination occurs in the latter (Fig. 10–8). Thus, a new nucleus for growth results.

In the same manner, an already terminated chain might be reactivated by chain transfer, and it will continue to grow (Fig. 10–9).

INHIBITION OF POLYMERIZATION

As noted in the previous section, the polymerization reactions are not likely to result in a complete exhaustion of the monomer, nor do they always form

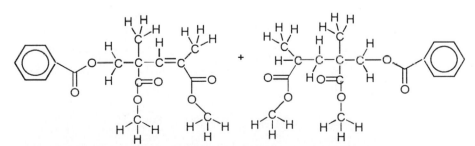

Figure 10–7. When two free radicals approach each other, a new double bond may be formed on the molecule that donates a hydrogen atom to the other free radical.

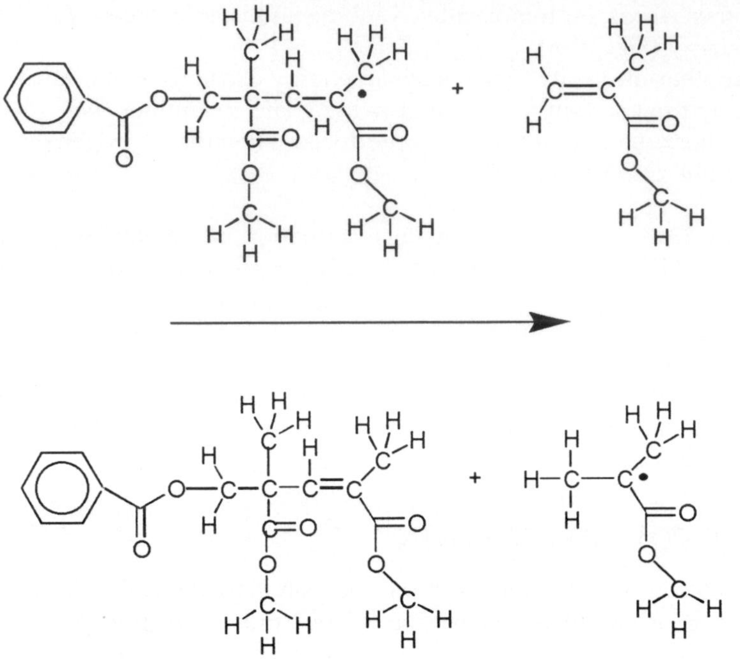

Figure 10–8. Chain transfer occurs when a free radical approaches a methyl methacrylate molecule and donates a hydrogen atom to the methyl methacrylate molecule. When this occurs, the free radical receives a double bond and becomes passive until it reacts again with a free radical. The monomer molecule, though, forms a free radical that participates in a chain propagation reaction.

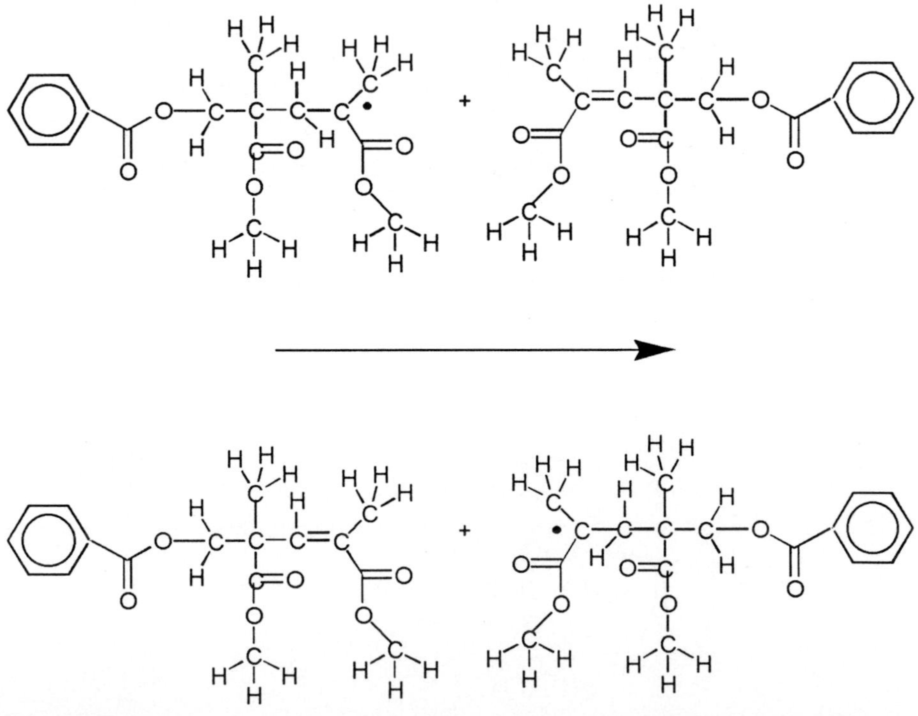

Figure 10–9. Another type of chain transfer can occur when a propagating chain interacts with the passivated segment that was formed in Figure 10–8. During this interaction, the passive segment becomes active, while the active segment becomes passive.

polymers of high molecular weight. Impurities in the monomer often inhibit such reactions.

Any impurity in the monomer that can react with free radicals inhibits or retards the polymerization reaction. It can react with the activated initiator, with any activated nucleus, or with an activated growing chain to prevent further growth. The presence of such inhibitors markedly influences the length of the initiation period as well as the degree of polymerization.

For example, the addition of a small amount of hydroquinone to the monomer inhibits polymerization if no initiator is present, and it retards the polymerization in the presence of an initiator. In other words, an initiator can affect the working time of a dental resin.

The presence of oxygen also causes retardation of the polymerization reaction, because the oxygen reacts with the free radicals. It has been shown, for example, that the reaction velocity and the degree of polymerization are decreased if the polymerization is conducted in open air in comparison with the higher values obtained when the reaction is carried out in a sealed tube. The influence of oxygen on polymerization is governed by many factors, such as its concentration, the temperature, and light intensity. It is important to be aware of the inhibiting effect of oxygen on the polymerization process. Thus, air thinning of bonding resins should be avoided to optimize curing in important regions of a restoration.

It is common commercial practice to add a small amount (approximately 0.006% or less) of an inhibitor such as the methyl ether of hydroquinone to the monomer to aid in the prevention of polymerization during storage.

COPOLYMERIZATION

In the polymerization reactions that have been described, the macromolecule was formed by the polymerization of a single type of structural unit. To custom design the physical properties of a polymer, two or more chemically different monomers, each with some desirable property, can be combined. The polymer thus formed is called a *copolymer*, and its process of formation is known as *copolymerization* (Fig. 10–10). In a copolymer, the relative number and position of the different type units may vary among the individual macromolecules.

Copolymerization is best illustrated with two monomers, although it is possible to incorporate more than two monomers. For example, two monomers (A and B) consisting of ethylene derivatives might possess the following structural formulas:

(4)

$$\begin{array}{ccc} \text{H} & \text{H} & \qquad\qquad \text{H} \quad \text{H} \\ | & | & \qquad\qquad | \quad\; | \\ \text{C}&=&\text{C} \qquad\qquad \text{C}=\text{C} \\ | & | & \qquad\qquad | \quad\; | \\ \text{H} & \text{R}_2 & \qquad\qquad \text{H} \quad \text{R}_3 \end{array}$$

Monomer A Monomer B

in which R_2 and R_3 are two different side groups. It is conceivable that after the polymerization occurs in the usual manner the following copolymer might result:

(5)

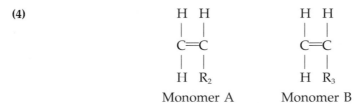

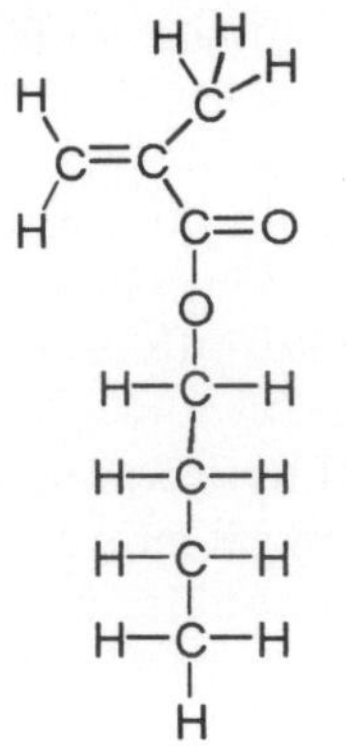

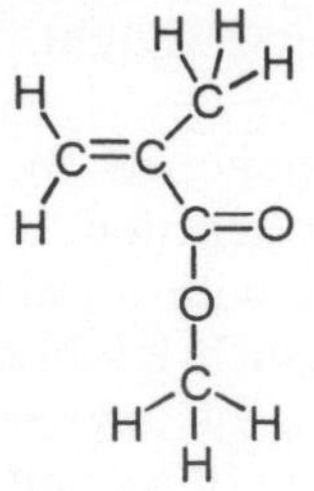

METHYL METHACRYLATE

BUTYL METHACRYLATE

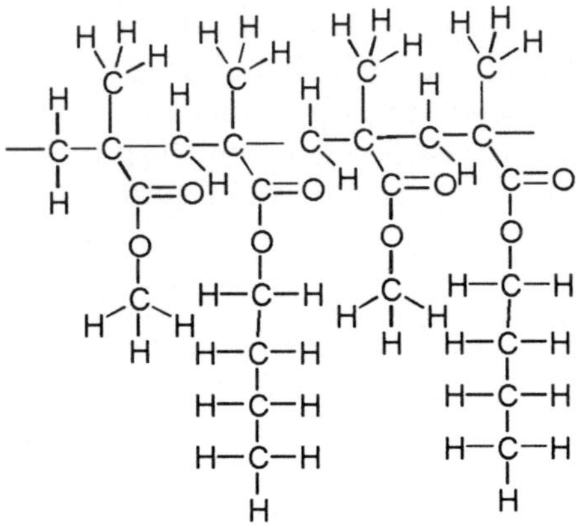

COPOLYMER OF METHYL METHACRYLATE AND BUTYL METHACRYLATE

Figure 10–10. Copolymerization between butyl methacrylate and methyl methacrylate. Because the butyl methacrylate molecules increase the backbone separation of the polymer molecules, the intermolecular interactions decrease, as does the glass transition temperature.

However, this copolymer structure is highly idealized, because the occurrence of alternately placed radicals in the chain would seldom occur. It is more probable that their positions are random—a matter of probability. The composition of the copolymer depends on the relative reactivities of the different molecules and the molecules of the same composition. For example, if the tendency of monomer A to polymerize is so great that it polymerizes independently of B, no copolymerization will occur, and the resulting resin will be formed from a mixture of two polymers. Such a condition seldom, if ever, occurs. On the other hand, A and B may exhibit a greater tendency to polymerize together than to polymerize separately. In such a case, all the monomers present might enter into the copolymer with no independent polymerization taking place. In most instances, the set resin consists of a mixture of polymers and copolymers with varying degrees of polymerization or copolymerization.

Copolymers are of three different types: random, block, and graft. In a *random copolymer*, the different monomer units are randomly distributed along the chain, such as

(6) $\cdots$ M—M—M—Y—M—Y—M—M—Y—Y—M— M$\cdots$

However, if identical monomer units occur in relatively long sequences along the main polymer chain, a *block copolymer* is formed:

(7) $\cdots$ M—M—M$\cdots$ M—M—Y—Y—Y$\cdots$Y—Y—Y—M—M—M— $\cdots$

where —M$\cdots$M— and —Y$\cdots$Y— represent long segments of M and Y molecules, respectively.

In *graft copolymers*, sequences of one of the monomers are grafted onto a "backbone" of the second monomer species, such as the following:

(8) $\cdots$ M—M—M—M—M $\cdots$ M—M—M—M—M $\cdots$
$$\begin{array}{ccc} & | & & | \\ & Y & & Y \\ & | & & | \\ & Y & & Y \end{array}$$

Copolymerization may alter the physical properties of the resulting resin considerably from those of the resins formed individually from the monomers involved. Many useful resins are manufactured by copolymerization. Methyl methacrylate and acrylic and methacrylic esters all copolymerize readily, with little inhibition between monomer pairs. For example, small amounts of ethyl acrylate may be copolymerized with methyl methacrylate to alter the flexibility of a denture.

Grafting of various polymer segments onto a linear chain provides an important mechanism for modifying or tailor-making macromolecules to obtain the required properties for specific uses. For example, block and graft polymers often show improved impact strength. In small quantities, they can modify the adhesive properties of resins as well as their surface characteristics.

MOLECULAR SHAPE

In their simplest forms, both addition and condensation types of polymerization should yield linear macromolecules. Such molecules are seldom realized in practice. In the case of addition polymers, branching side reactions may arise through chain transfer with the monomer or previously formed polymer molecules, a phenomenon that was discussed earlier. Such structural units of the polymer may be connected together in a manner to form a *nonlinear branched* or *cross-linked* polymer. In such cross-linked polymers, some of the structural units must have at least two sites where reactions can occur. A typical branched polymer, in which the branching unit is represented by Y, might be indicated by:

(9)

$$-\overset{\displaystyle \overset{H}{|}}{\underset{\displaystyle \underset{H}{|}}{C}} - \overset{\displaystyle \overset{Y}{|}}{\underset{\displaystyle \underset{H}{|}}{C}} - \overset{\displaystyle \overset{Y}{|}}{\underset{\displaystyle \underset{H}{|}}{C}} - \overset{\displaystyle \overset{H}{|}}{\underset{\displaystyle \underset{H}{|}}{C}} -$$

Highly branched molecular structures may then be formed by further propagation of the branched structure.

CROSS-LINKING

As described in the curing of polysulfide rubber impression materials and in the formation of calcium alginate from sodium alginate, linear polymers may be joined, or bridged, through certain reactive side chains, to form molecular networks (Fig. 10–11).

Cross-linkage provides a sufficient number of bridges between the linear macromolecules to form a three-dimensional network that alters the strength, solubility, and water sorption of the resin. For example, cross-linkage has been used widely in the manufacture of acrylic teeth to increase their resistance to solvents and surface stresses.

The effect of cross-linking on physical properties varies with the composition and concentration of the cross-linking agent and the polymer system. In certain cases, cross-linking of a low-molecular-weight polymer may increase the glass transition temperature (T_g) to that of a high-molecular-weight polymer. Other studies have shown that cross-linking has little influence on tensile strength, transverse strength, or hardness.

PLASTICIZERS

Plasticizers are often added to resins to reduce their softening or fusion temperatures. For example, it is possible to plasticize a resin that is normally hard and stiff at room temperature to a condition in which it is flexible and soft by including a plasticizer in the resin.

The plasticizer acts to partially neutralize secondary bonds or intermolecular forces that normally prevent the resin molecules from slipping past one another when the material is stressed. Its action may be considered analogous to that of a solvent, because it penetrates between the macromolecules and increases the intermolecular spacing. This type of plasticizer is referred to as an *external plasticizer*. It is an insoluble high-boiling compound. Its molecular attraction to the polymer should be extremely high so that it does not volatilize or otherwise leach out during the fabrication or subsequent use of the resin. Such a condition is seldom realized in practice, so this type of plasticizer is used sparingly in dental resins.

Plasticizing of a resin can also be accomplished by copolymerization with a suitable comonomer. In this case the plasticizing agent is a part of the polymer and thus acts as an *internal plasticizer*. For example, when butyl methacrylate is added to methyl methacrylate before polymerization, the polymerized resin is plasticized internally by the butyl methacrylate segments (see Fig. 10–10). The function of the butyl methacrylate molecules is to increase intermolecular spacing via pendant groups.

As expected from theory, plasticizers usually reduce the strength, hardness, and the softening point of the resin.

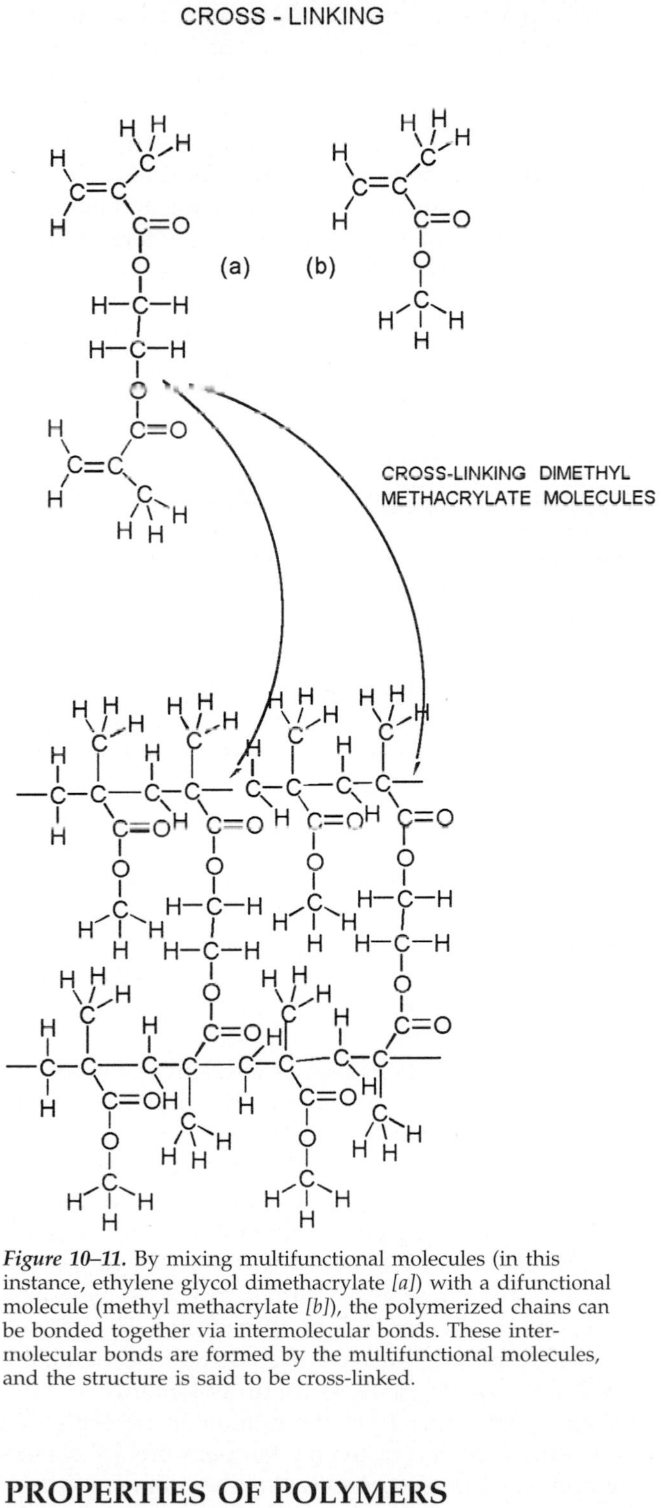

CROSS - LINKING

Figure 10–11. By mixing multifunctional molecules (in this instance, ethylene glycol dimethacrylate [a]) with a difunctional molecule (methyl methacrylate [b]), the polymerized chains can be bonded together via intermolecular bonds. These intermolecular bonds are formed by the multifunctional molecules, and the structure is said to be cross-linked.

PHYSICAL PROPERTIES OF POLYMERS

The physical properties of a polymer are influenced by changes in temperature and environment and by the composition, structure, and molecular weight of the polymer. In general, the higher the temperature, the softer and weaker the polymer becomes.

A temperature of particular interest in polymer science is the so-called T_g. To understand T_g and how it is affected by the polymer structure, one must understand the interatomic bonds that hold the different polymer chains together in a polymer. Along each single-polymer chain, valence electrons continuously move back and forth. Because of these electron movements, varying electron densities exist along the chain at different times and locations. Adjacent chains adapt their electron densities along the chains to balance these differences in charge density. Because of these interactions, interatomic induction forces, called *van der Waals* and *London forces,* are developed between the chains. These forces, as well as hydrogen bonding, form polar bonds between the polymer chains, bonds that are much weaker than the primary bonds along the polymer chains. By heating a polymer to its T_g or to a higher temperature, the weak polar bonds are broken, and the polymer molecular chains can move more freely relative to each other. The increased mobility has a strong impact on many physical properties such as strength, modulus of elasticity, and thermal expansion. Strength and modulus decrease as the temperature approaches T_g, whereas thermal expansion increases.

If two similar polymers consisting of straight-polymer chains are compared, the one which has a higher molecular weight will also have a higher T_g. By increasing the straight-polymer chain length, the probability increases that more polar bond sites will form along that chain. In addition, the increased chain length also increases the chance for chain entanglements. Thus, the increased number of polar bond sites along each chain and their increased chain entanglements explain why polymers with a higher molecular weight need more heat (energy) to reach their T_g.

From a mechanical point of view, chain slippage also decreases as the chain length increases. At a certain chain length, though, the polar bonds and the entanglements are strong enough to resist dislodgment of the individual chain. For this critical chain length, the dislodging force breaks the cohesive bond of the chain. This balance between the strength of the polar bonds and the covalent bond of the chain explains why the physicomechanical properties of the polymer increase with increased molecular weight to a certain point. Subsequently, increased molecular weight becomes less important.

The number average molecular weight is indicative of both T_g and the strength of the polymer. As mentioned previously, the value for the number average molecular weight is lowered markedly by the presence of a relatively few monomer molecules, which lower T_g and weaken the resin considerably.

Although dependent on its type, generally a resin possesses mechanical strength only when its degree of polymerization is relatively high, in the general range of approximately 150 to 200 recurring units. Above this molecular weight, there is not a great change in strength with further polymerization, as explained earlier. Likewise, the molecular-weight distribution of the polymer plays an important role in determining physical properties. In general, a narrow molecular-weight distribution yields the most useful polymers.

Long side chains protruding from the monomer molecule generally produce a weaker resin with a lower softening temperature in comparison with the properties of a polymer that possesses a straight chain structure. This weakened effect is caused by the side chains separating the main chains, thus reducing the effectiveness of the polar bonds along the main chain. However, if the side chains can react with adjacent chains to form a cross-linked polymer, the strength of the polymer is increased.

Based on the above description of a polymer, heat should have a significant impact on the properties. As the temperature increases, the rotation of polymer segments increases. These rotations, coupled with thermal expansion, increase chain separation, break polar bonds, and facilitate chain disentanglement. These factors facilitate chain slippage and explain the thermoplastic behavior of the resin when it reaches T_g. If cross-linkages exist, slippage cannot occur, and the material becomes more difficult to soften.

If a cross-linked resin is softened, it will not easily change shape permanently. The material becomes rubbery in consistency. Thus, an elastomeric dental impression material can be described as a cross-linked polymeric structure with a T_g lower than room temperature. The low T_g implies that the chain segments are thermally agitated at room temperature. In this manner the chains are rendered more flexible. In fact, almost any means can be used to impart elastomeric qualities, by which the polymer molecules are rendered more mobile. Another requisite is that some degree of cross-linking must be present so that any deformation is readily reversible. Such cross-linking must occur only occasionally between the chains. If a high degree of cross-linking is present, a network configuration prevails, and the resin becomes rigid and useless as an impression material. The situation is analogous to that described in the formation of calcium alginate in alginate gels. Such cross-linked bonds cause the polymer to return to its original shape after the load is released, as in the case of the gels.

POLYMER STRUCTURE

Characteristically, the linear dental polymers are disordered or noncrystalline in structure. The polymer chains form in a tangled mass. Their collective structure can be compared with that of cooked spaghetti, with each piece approximately a mile in length. Under such conditions, it is evident that the polymer segments have little chance to diffuse or become mobile in the solid state. As in the case of glass, a short-range ordering results.

However, many polymers have some degree of crystallization, depending on the secondary bonds that can be formed, the structure of the polymer chain, the degree of ordering, and the molecular weight. The conditions for crystallization can be illustrated using ethylene derivatives or vinyl resins, for which the following generalized formula is characteristic:

(10)

$$
\begin{array}{cc}
H & H \\
| & | \\
C & = C \\
| & | \\
H & R
\end{array}
$$

If R is a simple side group such that R is OH, thereby forming polyvinyl alcohol, the polymer chains may form a short-range ordered lattice during polymerization. On the other hand, if the side chain is more complex, a noncrystalline structure results unless the mer units in the polymer chains themselves are arranged symmetrically to each other. In such a case, a crystalline polymer may result, even with a complex side chain. Although polymer crystallinity may increase the tensile strength, it also may reduce the ductility of the resin and increase its molding temperature.

Factors that do not favor crystallinity include the following:

- Long, branched polymers
- Random arrangement of side groups, particularly large side groups that tend to separate the molecules

- Copolymerization, which decreases the regularity of the polymer chains
- Plasticizers, which tend to separate the chains (see previous section)

TYPES OF RESINS

As previously mentioned, for a synthetic resin to be useful in dentistry it must exhibit exceptional qualities regarding its chemical and dimensional stability and yet it must possess properties that render it relatively easy to process. It must be strong and hard but not brittle. A few resins used in dentistry are discussed.

Acrylic Resins. The acrylic resins are derivatives of ethylene and contain a vinyl group

(11)
$$\begin{array}{c} X \\ | \\ H_2C{=}CH \end{array}$$

in their structural formula. There are at least two acrylic resin series that are of dental interest. One series is derived from acrylic acid, $CH_2{=}CHCOOH$, and the other from methacrylic acid, $CH_2{=}C(CH_3)COOH$. Both of these compounds polymerize by addition in the usual manner.

Although the polyacids are hard and transparent, their polarity, related to the carboxyl group, causes them to imbibe water. The water tends to separate the chains and to cause a general softening and loss of strength.

The esters of these polyacids, however, are of considerable dental interest. For example, if R represents any ester radical, the formula for a polymethacrylate will be:

(12)
$$\begin{array}{cccccc} H & H & H & H & H & H \\ | & | & | & | & | & | \\ -C-C-C-C-C-C- \\ | & | & | & | & | & | \\ H & C & H & C & H & C \\ & \| & & \| & & \| \\ O & O & O & O & O & O \\ & | & & | & & | \\ & R & & R & & R \end{array}$$

Because R can be almost any organic or inorganic radical, it is evident that thousands of different acrylic resins are capable of formation. Such a consideration does not include the possibilities of copolymerization, which are even greater.

The effect of esterification on the softening point of a few of the polymethacrylate compounds is shown in Table 10–1. This temperature is always definite for the noncrystalline polymers, such as the polymethacrylates.

For short chain lengths, increasing the length of the side chain lowers the softening point or glass transition temperature. For example, poly(methyl methacrylate) is the hardest resin of the series with the highest softening temperature. Ethyl methacrylate possesses a lower softening point and surface hardness, and *n*-propyl methacrylate has an even lower softening point and hardness. If an

TABLE 10–1. Softening Temperatures of Polymethacrylate Esters

Polymethacrylate	T_g (° C)
Methyl	125
Ethyl	65
n-Propyl	38
Isopropyl	95
n-Butyl	33
Isobutyl	70
sec-Butyl	62
tert-Amyl	76
Phenyl	120

From Powers PO: Synthetic Resins and Rubbers. New York, John Wiley, 1943.

isomer of a straight-chain esterifying agent is used, the softening temperature is increased above that of the normal straight chain compound. For example, the softening temperature of poly(isopropyl methacrylate) is greater than that of poly(ethyl methacrylate), yet the softening temperature of poly(*n*-propyl methacrylate) is only 38° C. As the molecular weight of the straight-chain alkyl groups increases, the softening point continues to decrease until the liquid state is attained at room temperature. For example, poly(dodecyl methacrylate) $(CH_2=C(CH_3)COOC_{12}H_{25})$ is a viscous liquid monomer at room temperature. Some resins, such as addition polymers of isobutylene, may be liquid at temperatures as low as $-70°$ C.

Esterification with an aromatic alcohol increases the softening point, even though the molecular weights of the aromatic and aliphatic esterifying compounds may be nearly the same; this is illustrated by the relatively high softening point of poly(phenyl methacrylate), as given in Table 10–1.

Methyl Methacrylate. Poly(methyl methacrylate) by itself is not used in dentistry to a great extent in molding procedures. Rather, the liquid monomer methyl methacrylate (Fig. 10–12) is mixed with the polymer, which is in the powdered form. The monomer partially dissolves the polymer to form a plastic dough. This dough is packed into the mold, and the monomer is polymerized by one of the methods discussed previously. Consequently, the monomer methyl methacrylate is of considerable importance in dentistry.

Methyl methacrylate is a clear, transparent liquid at room temperature with the following physical properties:

- Melting point = $-48°$ C
- Boiling point = $100.8°$ C
- Density = 0.945 g/mL at 20° C
- Heat of polymerization = 12.9 kcal/mol

It exhibits a high vapor pressure and is an excellent organic solvent. Although the polymerization of methyl methacrylate can be initiated by ultraviolet light, visible light, or heat, it is commonly polymerized in dentistry by the use of a chemical initiator, as described previously.

The conditions for the polymerization of methyl methacrylate are not critical, provided that the reaction is not carried out too rapidly. The degree of polymerization varies with the conditions of polymerization, such as the temperature, method of activation, type of initiator, initiator concentration, purity of chemicals, and similar factors. Because they polymerize readily under the conditions of use, the methacrylate monomers are particularly useful in dentistry. Many

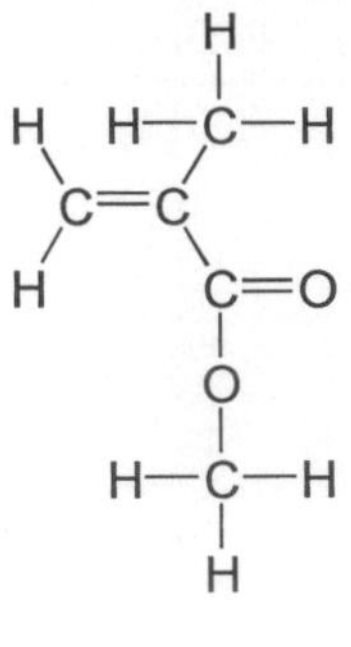

Figure 10–12. Methyl methacrylate molecule.

other resin systems do not polymerize at room temperature in the presence of air. A volume shrinkage of 21% occurs during the polymerization of the pure methyl methacrylate monomer.

Poly(methyl Methacrylate). Poly(methyl methacrylate) is a transparent resin of remarkable clarity; it transmits light in the ultraviolet range to a wavelength of 250 nm. It is a hard resin with a Knoop hardness number of 18 to 20. Its tensile strength is approximately 60 MPa and its density is 1.19 g/cm³. Its modulus of elasticity is approximately 2.4 GPa (2400 MPa).

The resin is extremely stable. It does not discolor in ultraviolet light, and it exhibits remarkable aging properties. It is chemically stable to heat and softens at 125° C, and it can be molded as a thermoplastic material. Between this temperature and 200° C, depolymerization takes place. At approximately 450° C, 90% of the polymer depolymerizes to the monomer. Poly(methyl methacrylate) of high molecular weight degrades to a lower polymer at the same time that it converts to the monomer.

Like all acrylic resins, poly(methyl methacrylate) exhibits a tendency to absorb water by a process of imbibition. Its noncrystalline structure possesses a high internal energy; thus, molecular diffusion can occur into the resin, because less activation energy is required. Furthermore, the polar carboxyl group, even though esterified, can form a hydrogen bridge to a limited extent with water.

Because both absorption and adsorption are involved, the term *sorption* is usually used to describe the total phenomenon. Typical dental methacrylate resins show an increase of approximately 0.5 wt% after 1 week in water. Higher values have been reported for a series of methyl methacrylate polymers. The sorption of water is nearly independent of temperature from 0° to 60° C, but is markedly affected by the molecular weight of the polymer. The greater the molecular weight, the smaller the weight increase. Sorption is reversible if the resin is dried.

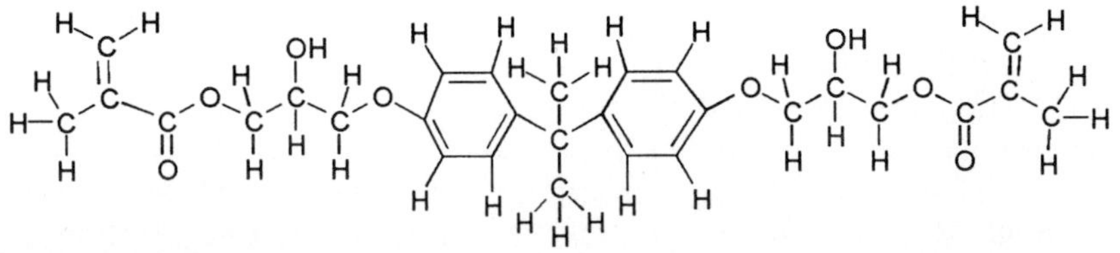

Figure 10–13. Bis-GMA molecule. The central part of the molecule becomes stiff because of restricted rotational ability of the two rings.

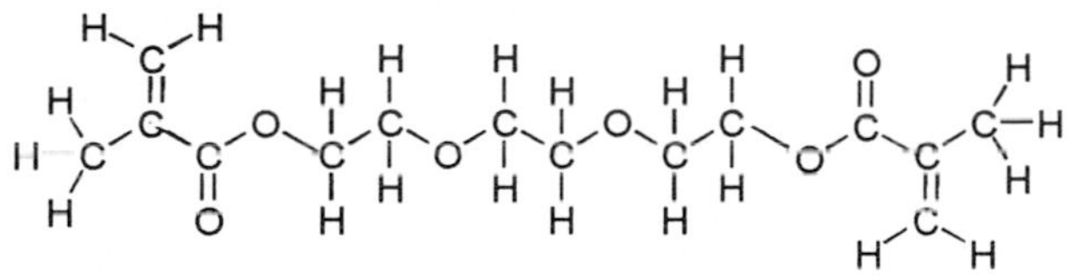

Figure 10–14. TEGDMA molecule. The backbone structure is flexible, which facilitates molecular interaction during polymerization and increases the degree of conversion.

Because poly(methyl methacrylate) is a linear polymer, it should be soluble in a number of organic solvents, such as chloroform and acetone.

Multifunctional Methacrylate and Acrylate Resins. The backbone of the molecule formed in this system can have any shape, but methacrylate groups are found at the ends of the chain or at the end of branching chains. One of the first multifunctional methacrylates used in dentistry was Bowen's resin (or bis-GMA) (Fig. 10–13). The bis-GMA resin can be described as an aromatic ester of a dimethacrylate, synthesized from an epoxy resin (ethylene glycol of *bis*-phenol A) and methyl methacrylate. Because bis-GMA has a rigid central structure (two rings) and two OH- groups, the pure bis-GMA becomes extremely viscous. To reduce the viscosity, a low-viscosity dimethacrylate such as triethyleneglycol dimethacrylate (TEGDMA) (Fig. 10–14) is added.

The rigidity of the bis-GMA molecule reduces its ability to rotate during polymerization and to participate efficiently in the polymerization process. Therefore, one of the methacrylate groups reacts often, whereas the other does not. This process results in a bis-GMA molecule that forms a branch along the polymer chain. Some of these branches cross-link with adjacent chains; some do not. To quantify the efficiency of polymerization and cross-linking, the ratio, R, of unreacted methacrylate groups before and after polymerization can be determined. From the formula

(13) $$(1 - R) \times 100$$

the degree of conversion, expressed in percentage of consumed methyl methacrylate groups, can be determined.

To reduce the viscosity and increase the degree of conversion, different dimethacrylate resin combinations have been explored through the years. One resin group that has shown some promise is *urethane dimethacrylate*. This group can be described as any monomer chain containing one or more urethane groups and two methacrylate end groups (Fig. 10–15).

In addition to the dimethacrylates mentioned earlier, other multifunctional resins have been introduced to dentistry during the last few years. For example,

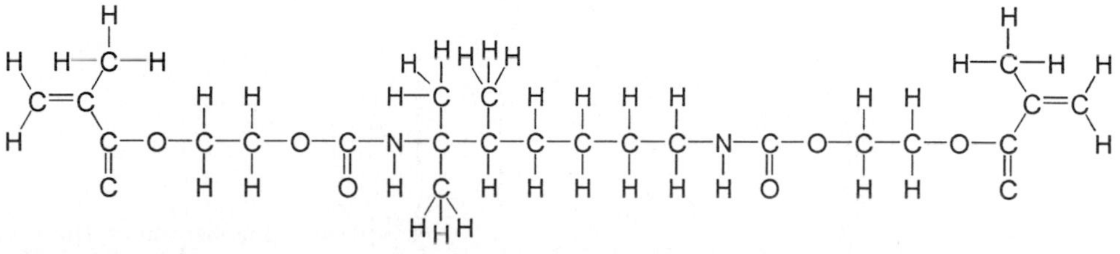

Figure 10–15. UEDMA molecule, which has two urethane groups. Otherwise, the backbone structure is flexible.

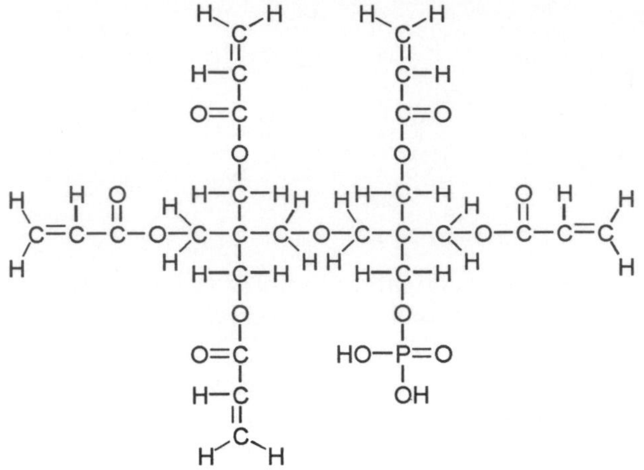

Figure 10–16. PENTA-P molecule. This molecule has a phosphate group and five acrylate groups. The phosphate group can etch enamel and dentin surfaces, whereas the five acrylate groups increase reactivity and cross-linking ability.

in some dentin bonding agents a monomer called dipentaerythiol penta-acrylate monophosphate (PENTA-P) is used (Fig. 10–16). As seen from the PENTA-P formula, this monomer contains as many as five acrylate groups per monomer molecule.

Another multifunctional resin that has gained much popularity during the last few years is polyacrylic acid, to which hydroxyethyl methacrylate (HEMA) has been grafted (Fig. 10–17). Such a modified polyacrylic acid (PAA) is used in light-curable glass ionomer cements. During light exposure, free radical polymerization is initiated, causing the methacrylate groups to react. The reaction that cross-links the PAA molecules constitutes the initial setting reaction. After this reaction, the carboxylate groups continue to react with the glass particles through an acid-base reaction. During this reaction, the PAA releases the hydrogen ions and the PAA chains become negatively charged. These negative charges, though,

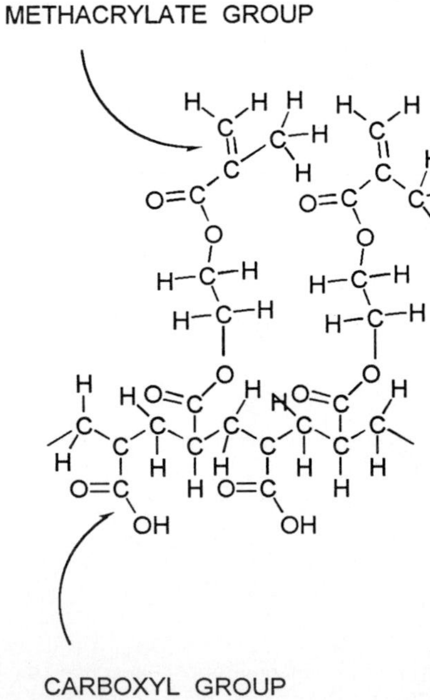

METHACRYLATE GROUP

CARBOXYL GROUP

Figure 10–17. Polyacrylic acid with grafted ethyl methacrylate groups. The carboxyl groups can etch dentin and enamel by giving up their hydrogen ions. When this occurs, the molecule becomes negatively charged and bonds to positive ions, such as calcium, present at the tooth surface. This ionic bond formation can also occur between polyacrylic acid chains, causing the material to set. Another setting mechanism that can be used is addition polymerization. This polymerization reaction can be initiated by light, which causes the methacrylate groups to react.

are balanced by cations leached from the glass. These cations, such as Ca^{2+} and Al^{3+}, form ionic bonds between the chains that now also become ionically cross-linked. In addition, the negatively charged PAA chains also form bonds to tooth tissues containing cations such as Ca^{2+}.

By observing this modified PAA molecule, one can see that as the methacrylate groups increase, the number of carboxylate groups decreases. This is important because fewer carboxylate groups reduce the extent of the acid-base reaction and weaken the enamel-dentin interaction. Thus, a light-cured glass ionomer can be described as a combination of both addition polymerization and acid-base reactivity, yielding a so-called hybrid material. A more meaningful term for this particular class of material is *compomer*, because it combines some of the composite material properties with those of the glass ionomers.

SELECTED READING

Cowie JMG: Polymers: Chemistry and Physics of Modern Materials. Aulesbury, Intertext, 1973.
Provides an excellent introduction to polymer science. It is written so that knowledge is nicely blended with humor.
Morrison RT, and Boyd RN: Organic Chemistry, 5th ed. Boston, Allyn and Bacon, 1987.
A classic textbook in organic chemistry. The book gives the reader a fundamental understanding of the different mechanisms that affect the molecular structure of organic compounds used in different fields of science, including dentistry.
Sun SF: Physical Chemistry of Macromolecules: Basic Principles and Issues. New York, John Wiley, 1994.
Unites biophysical chemistry and physical polymer chemistry. The book offers a good overview of molecular structure, physical properties, and modern experimental techniques.
Ward IM: Mechanical Properties of Solid Polymers, 2nd ed. New York, Wiley-Interscience, 1983.
Follows the approach of first developing the mechanics of the polymer behavior and then discussing molecular and structural phenomena.

11 *Denture Base Resins*

Technical Considerations and Processing Techniques

- Heat-activated Denture Base Resins
- Compression-molding Technique
- Chemically Activated Denture Base Resins
- Light-activated Denture Base Resins
- Physical Properties of Denture Base Resins
- Miscellaneous Resins and Techniques
- Resin Teeth for Prosthodontic Applications
- Materials in Maxillofacial Prosthetics

A *complete denture* may be defined as a removable dental prosthesis intended to replace the masticatory surfaces and associated structures of a maxillary or mandibular dental arch. Such a prosthesis is composed of artificial teeth attached to a denture base. The denture base derives its support through intimate contact with the underlying oral tissues.

Although individual denture bases may be formed from metals or metal alloys, most denture bases are fabricated using common polymers. Such polymers are chosen based on availability, dimensional stability, handling characteristics, color, and compatibility with oral tissues.

A discussion of commonly used denture base polymers is presented in this chapter. Considerable attention is given to individual processing systems and polymerization techniques. In addition, methods for improving the fit and dimensional stability of complete denture prostheses are provided.

General Technique. Several processing techniques are available for the fabrication of denture bases. Each technique requires the fabrication of an accurate impression of the edentulous arch. Using this impression, a dental cast is generated. In turn, a resin record base is fabricated on the cast. Wax is added to the record base, and the teeth are positioned in the wax.

A denture flask is chosen, and the completed tooth arrangement is encased in a suitable investing medium. Subsequently, the denture flask is opened and the wax is eliminated. After a thorough cleansing of the mold, a resin denture base material is introduced into the mold cavity. Subsequently, the denture base resin is polymerized. After polymerization, the denture is recovered and prepared for delivery.

Acrylic Resins. Since the mid-1940s, most denture bases have been fabricated using poly(methyl methacrylate) resins. Such resins are resilient plastics formed by joining multiple methyl methacrylate molecules. The chemical basis for this reaction is described in Chapter 10.

Pure poly(methyl methacrylate) is a colorless, transparent solid. To facilitate its use in dental applications, the polymer may be tinted to provide almost any shade and degree of translucency. Its color and optical properties remain stable under normal intraoral conditions, and its physical properties have proved adequate for dental applications.

One decided advantage of poly(methyl methacrylate) as a denture base material is the relative ease with which it may be processed. Poly(methyl methacrylate) denture base material usually is supplied as a powder-liquid system. The liquid contains unpolymerized methyl methacrylate, and the powder contains prepolymerized poly(methyl methacrylate) resin in the form of small beads. When the liquid and powder are mixed in the correct proportions, a workable mass is formed. Subsequently, the material is introduced into a mold cavity of the desired shape and polymerized. On completion of the polymerization process, the resultant prosthesis is retrieved and prepared for delivery.

HEAT-ACTIVATED DENTURE BASE RESINS

Heat-activated materials are used in the fabrication of nearly all denture bases. Thermal energy required for polymerization of such materials may be provided using a water bath or microwave oven. Because of the prevalence of these resins, emphasis is placed on heat-activated systems.

Composition. As previously noted, most poly(methyl methacrylate) resin systems consist of powder and liquid components (Fig. 11–1). The powder consists of prepolymerized spheres of poly(methyl methacrylate) and a small amount of benzoyl peroxide (the initiator).

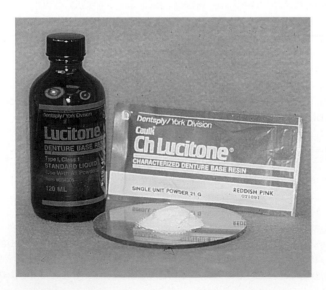

Figure 11–1. A representative heat-activated resin. Most heat-activated resins are supplied as powder-liquid systems.

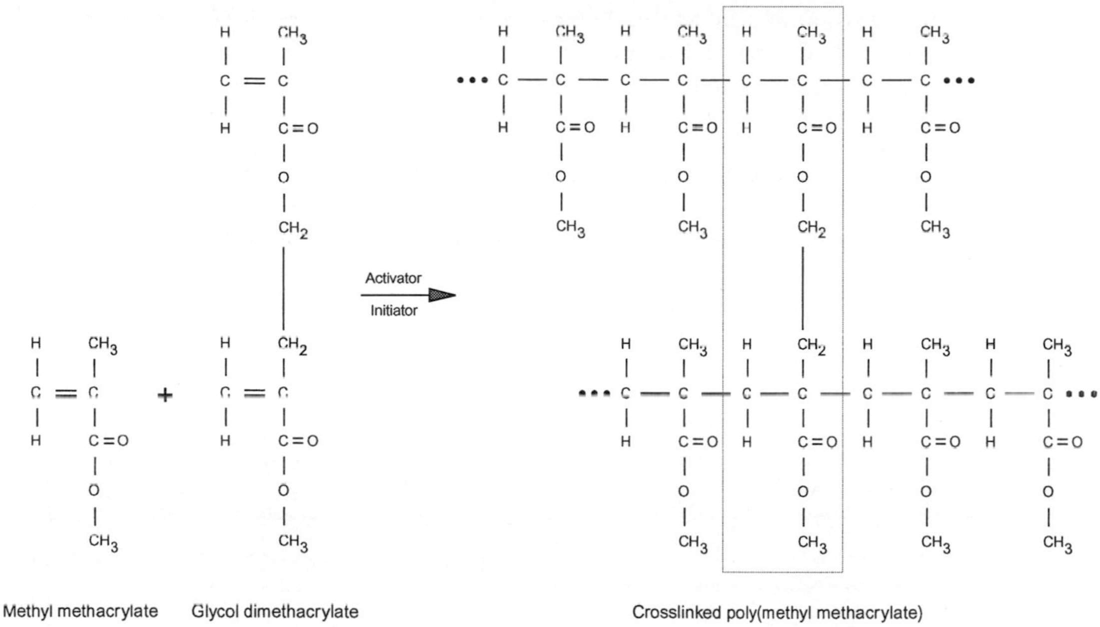

Figure 11–2. Chemical basis for the formation of cross-linked poly(methyl methacrylate). Glycol dimethacrylate is incorporated into poly(methyl methacrylate) chains and may "bridge" or "interconnect" such chains.

The liquid is predominantly unpolymerized methyl methacrylate with small amounts of hydroquinone. Hydroquinone is added as an inhibitor. As such, it prevents undesirable polymerization, or "setting," of the liquid during storage.

A *cross-linking agent* also may be added to the liquid. Glycol dimethacrylate commonly is used as a cross-linking agent in poly(methyl methacrylate) denture base resins. Glycol dimethacrylate is chemically and structurally similar to methyl methacrylate and therefore may be incorporated into growing polymer chains (Fig. 11–2). Although methyl methacrylate possesses one double bond per molecule, glycol dimethacrylate possesses two double bonds per molecule. As a result, an individual molecule of glycol dimethacrylate may serve as a "bridge" or "cross member" that unites two polymer chains. If sufficient glycol dimethacrylate is included in the mixture, several interconnections may be formed. A polymer formed in this manner yields a netlike structure that provides increased resistance to deformation. Cross-linking agents are incorporated into the liquid component at a concentration of 1 to 2 vol%.

Storage. Manufacturers of heat-activated resin systems generally recommend specific temperature and time limits for storage. Strict observance of such recommendations is essential. If recommendations are not followed, components may undergo changes that ultimately can affect working properties of these resins, as well as the chemical and physical properties of processed denture bases.

COMPRESSION-MOLDING TECHNIQUE

As a rule, heat-activated denture base resins are shaped via compression molding. Therefore, the compression-molding technique is described in detail.

Preparation of the Mold. Before mold preparation, prosthetic teeth must be selected and arranged in a manner that fulfills aesthetic and functional requirements. This necessitates absolute accuracy in impression making, cast generating, record base fabricating, articulator mounting, tooth arranging, and wax contouring. When these objectives have been accomplished, the completed tooth arrangement is sealed to the master cast.

Subsequently, the master cast and completed tooth arrangement are removed from the dental articulator (Fig. 11–3A; see also color figure). The master cast is coated with a thin layer of separator to prevent adherence of dental stone during the flasking process. The lower portion of a denture flask is filled with freshly mixed dental stone, and the master cast is placed into this mixture. The dental

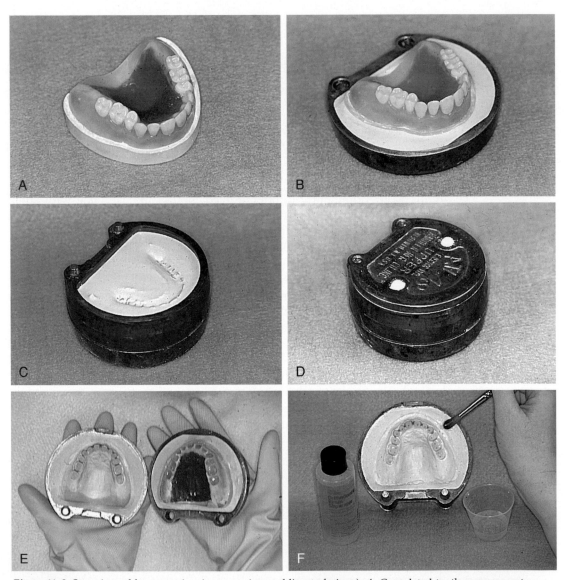

Figure 11–3. Steps in mold preparation (compression-molding technique). *A,* Completed tooth arrangement prepared for the flasking process. *B,* Master cast embedded in properly contoured dental stone. *C,* Occlusal and incisal surfaces of the prosthetic teeth are exposed to facilitate subsequent denture recovery. *D,* Fully flasked maxillary complete denture. *E,* Separation of flask segments during wax elimination process. *F,* Placement of alginate-based separating medium.

stone is contoured to facilitate wax elimination, packing, and deflasking procedures (Fig. 11–3B). On reaching its initial set, the stone is coated with an appropriate separator.

The upper portion of the selected denture flask then is positioned atop the lower portion of the flask. A surface tension–reducing agent is applied to exposed wax surfaces, and a second mix of dental stone is prepared. The dental stone is poured into the denture flask. Care is taken to ensure that the investing stone achieves intimate contact with all external surfaces. The investing stone is added until all surfaces of the tooth arrangement and denture base are completely covered. Incisal and occlusal surfaces are minimally exposed to facilitate subsequent deflasking procedures (Fig. 11–3C). The stone is permitted to set and subsequently is coated with separator.

At this point, an additional increment of dental stone is mixed, and the remainder of the flask is filled. The lid of the flask is gently tapped into place, and the stone is allowed to set (Fig. 11–3D).

On completion of the setting process, the record base and wax must be removed from the mold. To accomplish this, the denture flask is immersed in boiling water for 4 minutes. The flask then is removed from the water, and the appropriate segments are separated. The record base and softened wax remain in the lower portion of the denture flask, while the prosthetic teeth remain firmly embedded in the investing stone of the remaining segment (Fig. 11–3E). The record base and softened wax are carefully removed from the surface of the mold. Residual wax is removed from the mold cavity using wax solvent. The mold cavity subsequently is cleaned with a mild detergent solution and rinsed with boiling water.

Selection and Application of a Separating Medium. The next step in denture base fabrication involves the application of an appropriate separating medium onto the walls of the mold cavity. This medium must prevent direct contact between the denture base resin and the mold surface, that is, the dental stone. Failure to place an appropriate separating medium may cause two major difficulties: (1) if water is permitted to pass from the mold surface into the denture base resin, it may affect the polymerization rate as well as the optical and physical properties of the processed resin; and (2) if dissolved polymer or free monomer is permitted to soak into the mold surface, portions of the investing medium may become fused to the denture base. These difficulties often lead to compromises in the physical and aesthetic properties of processed denture bases. Hence, the importance of selecting an appropriate separating medium should not be overlooked.

One of the first widely accepted methods for protecting denture base materials was to line molds with thin sheets of tin foil. Unfortunately, placement of tin foil sheets was time and labor intensive; therefore, practical substitutes were sought. A variety of paint-on separating media were introduced during subsequent years. The aforementioned materials included cellulose lacquers, as well as solutions containing alginate compounds, soaps, and starches. Because these separating media were used in lieu of tin foil liners, they were termed *tin foil substitutes.*

Currently, the most popular separating agents are water-soluble alginate solutions. When applied to dental stone surfaces, such solutions produce thin, relatively insoluble calcium alginate films. These films prevent direct contact of denture base resins and the surrounding dental stone. Therefore, undesirable interactions between denture base resins and dental stones are eliminated. The physical properties of denture base resins polymerized against calcium alginate films are not significantly different from those of resins polymerized against tin foil liners.

Placement of an alginate-based separating medium is relatively uncomplicated. A small amount of separator is dispensed into a disposable container. A fine brush subsequently is used to spread the separating medium onto the exposed surfaces of a warm, clean stone mold (Fig. 11–3F). The separating medium is carefully guided into interdental regions. Separator should not be permitted to contact exposed portions of acrylic resin teeth, because its presence interferes with chemical bonding between acrylic resin teeth and denture base resins. The mold is inspected to ensure that a thin, even coating of separating medium is evident on all stone surfaces. Afterward, the mold sections are oriented to prevent "pooling" of separator, and the solution is permitted to dry.

Polymer:Monomer Ratio. A proper polymer:monomer ratio is of considerable importance in the fabrication of well-fitting denture bases with desirable physical properties. Unfortunately, most discussions of polymer:monomer ratio are vague and provide little practical information for dental personnel. Furthermore, these discussions do not address the relationships between molecular events and gross handling characteristics of denture base resins. The following paragraphs are intended to provide such information in an understandable manner.

Clinically, the polymerization of denture base resins produces volumetric and linear shrinkage. This is understandable when one considers the molecular events that occur during the polymerization process.

Envision two methyl methacrylate molecules. Each molecule possesses an electrical field that repels nearby molecules. Consequently, the distance between molecules is significantly greater than the length of a representative carbon-to-carbon bond. Now, consider the effects of chemically joining the methyl methacrylate molecules. When the molecules are chemically bonded, a new carbon-to-carbon linkage is formed. This produces a net decrease in the space occupied by the components.

Research indicates the polymerization of methyl methacrylate to form poly-(methyl methacrylate) yields a 21% decrease in the volume of material. As might be expected, volumetric shrinkage of 21% would create significant difficulties in denture base fabrication and service. To minimize dimensional changes, resin manufacturers prepolymerize a significant fraction of the denture base material. This may be thought of as "preshrinking" the selected resin fraction. The prepolymerized material may be mixed with compatible monomer, and the resultant mass is then polymerized.

As previously noted, most denture base resin systems are composed of powder and liquid components. The *powder* consists of prepolymerized poly(methyl methacrylate) beads, commonly referred to as a *polymer*. The *liquid* contains unpolymerized methyl methacrylate and therefore is termed a *monomer*. When the powder and liquid components are mixed in the proper proportions, a doughlike mass results. The accepted polymer:monomer ratio is 3:1 by volume. This provides sufficient monomer to thoroughly wet the polymer particles but does not contribute excess monomer that would lead to increased polymerization shrinkage. Using a 3:1 ratio, the volumetric shrinkage may be limited to approximately 6% (0.5% linear shrinkage).

Polymer-Monomer Interaction. When monomer and polymer are mixed in the proper proportions, a workable mass is produced. On standing, the resultant mass passes through five distinct stages: (1) sandy; (2) stringy; (3) doughlike; (4) rubbery or elastic; and (5) stiff.

During the *sandy* stage, little or no interaction occurs on a molecular level. Polymer beads remain unaltered, and the consistency of the mixture may be described as "coarse" or "grainy." Later, the mixture enters a *stringy* stage. During this stage, the monomer attacks the surfaces of individual polymer beads. Some polymer chains are dispersed in the liquid monomer. These polymer chains uncoil, thereby increasing the viscosity of the mix. This stage is characterized by "stringiness" or "stickiness" when the material is touched or drawn apart.

Subsequently, the mass enters a *doughlike* stage. On a molecular level, an increased number of polymer chains enter solution. Hence, a sea of monomer and dissolved polymer is formed. A large quantity of undissolved polymer also remains. Clinically, the mass behaves as a pliable dough. It is no longer tacky and does not adhere to the surfaces of the mixing vessel or spatula. The physical and chemical characteristics exhibited during the latter phases of this stage are ideal for compression molding. Hence, the material should be packed into the mold cavity during the latter phases of the doughlike stage.

After the doughlike stage, the mixture enters a *rubbery* or *elastic* stage. Monomer is dissipated by evaporation and by further penetration into remaining polymer beads. Clinically, the mass rebounds when compressed or stretched. Because the mass no longer flows freely to assume the shape of its container, it cannot be molded by conventional compression techniques.

On standing for an extended period, the mixture becomes *stiff*. This may be attributed to the evaporation of free monomer. Clinically, the mixture appears very dry and is resistant to mechanical deformation.

Dough-forming Time. The time required for the resin mixture to reach a doughlike stage is termed the *dough-forming time*. American Dental Association (ADA) Specification No. 12 for denture base resins requires that this consistency be attained in less than 40 minutes from the start of the mixing process. Clinically, most resins reach a doughlike consistency in less than 10 minutes.

Working Time. Working time may be defined as the time that a denture base material remains in the doughlike stage. This period is critical to the compression-molding process. ADA Specification No. 12 requires the dough to remain moldable for at least 5 minutes.

As might be expected, working time is affected by the ambient temperature. Hence, the working time of a denture resin may be extended via refrigeration. A significant drawback associated with this technique is that moisture may condense on the resin when it is removed from the refrigerator. The presence of moisture may degrade the physical and aesthetic properties of a processed resin. Moisture contamination may be avoided by storing the resin in an airtight container. After removal from the refrigerator, the container should not be opened until it reaches room temperature.

Packing. Introduction of denture base resin into the mold cavity is termed *packing*. This process represents one of the most critical steps in denture base fabrication. It is essential that the mold cavity be properly filled at the time of polymerization. The introduction of too much material, termed *overpacking*, leads to a denture base that exhibits excessive thickness and resultant malpositioning of prosthetic teeth. Conversely, the introduction of too little material, called "underpacking," leads to noticeable denture base porosity. To minimize the likelihood of overpacking or underpacking, the mold cavity is packed in several steps.

As previously stated, the packing process should be performed while the denture base resin is in a doughlike state. The resin is removed from its mixing container and rolled into a ropelike form. Subsequently, the resin form is bent into a horseshoe shape and placed into the portion of the flask that houses the prosthetic teeth (Fig. 11–4*A*; see also color figure). A polyethylene sheet is placed over the resin, and the flask is reassembled.

The flask assembly is placed into a specially designed press, and pressure is applied incrementally (Fig. 11–4*B*; see also color figure). Slow application of pressure permits the resin dough to flow evenly throughout the mold space.

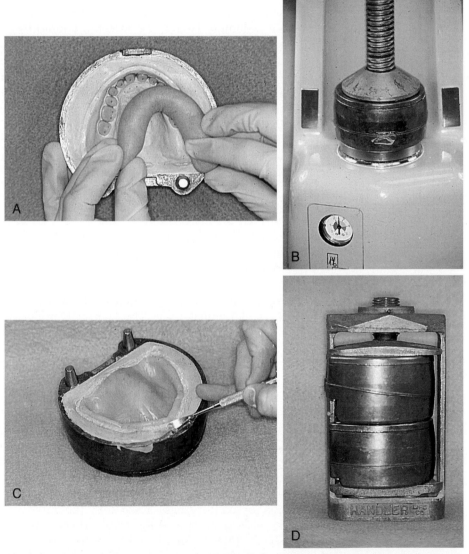

Figure 11–4. Steps in resin packing (compression-molding technique). *A*, Properly mixed resin is bent in a horseshoe shape and placed into the mold cavity. *B*, The flask assembly is placed into a flask press, and pressure is applied. *C*, Excess material is carefully removed from the flask. *D*, The flask is transferred to a flask carrier that maintains pressure on the assembly during processing.

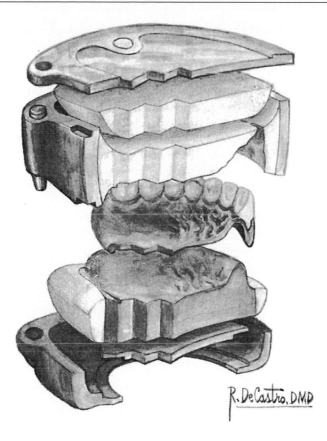

R. DeCastro, DMD

Figure 11–5. Cross-sectional representation of the denture flask and its contents.

Excess material is displaced eccentrically. The application of pressure is continued until the major portions of the flask closely approximate one another. The major flask portions subsequently are separated, and the polyethylene packing sheet is removed from the surface of the resin with a rapid, continuous tug.

Excess resin is found on the relatively flat areas surrounding the mold cavity. This excess resin is called *flash*. Using a gently rounded instrument, the flash is carefully teased away from the body of resin that occupies the mold cavity (Fig. 11–4C). Care is taken not to chip the stone surfaces of the mold. Pieces of stone that have become dislodged must be removed so that they are not incorporated into the processed denture base.

A fresh polyethylene sheet is placed between the major portions of the flask, and the flask assembly is once again placed in the press. Another trial closure is made. In most instances, the flask can be closed entirely during the second trial closure. Nonetheless, care should be taken not to apply excessive force to effect closure. Trial closures are repeated until no flash is observed.

When flash is no longer apparent, definitive closure of the mold may be accomplished. During the final closure process, no polyethylene sheet is interposed between the major mold sections. The mold sections are properly oriented and placed in the flask press. Again, pressure is applied incrementally. The flask then is transferred to a flask carrier (Fig. 11–4D). The flask carrier maintains pressure on the flask assembly during denture base processing. A cross-sectional representation of the denture flask and its contents is presented in Figure 11–5.

Injection-molding Technique. In addition to commonly employed compression-molding techniques, denture bases also may be fabricated via injection molding. To accomplish this, a specially designed flask is used. One half of the flask is filled with freshly mixed dental stone, and the master cast is settled into the stone. The dental stone is contoured and permitted to set. Subsequently, sprues are attached to the wax denture base (Fig. 11–6*A*; see also color figure). The remaining portion of the flask is positioned and the investment process is completed (Fig. 11–6*B*; see also color figure). Wax elimination is performed as previously described (Fig. 11–6*C*; see color figure), and the flask is reassembled. Afterward, the flask is placed into a carrier that maintains pressure on the assembly during resin introduction and processing. Resin is injected into the mold cavity (Fig. 11–6*D*; see also color figure). In the case of polystyrene resin, thermoplastic polymer is softened using heat and introduced into the mold while hot. Subsequently, the resin is permitted to cool and solidify. An advantage of this method is the reduced risk of monomer vapor inhalation.

When a powder-liquid mixture is employed, the resin is mixed and introduced into the mold while at room temperature. The flask then is placed into a water bath for polymerization of the denture base resin (Fig. 11–6*D*). As the material polymerizes, additional resin is introduced into the mold cavity. It is believed that this process offsets the effects of polymerization shrinkage. On completion, the denture is recovered, adjusted, finished, and polished.

Some debate exists regarding the comparative accuracy of denture bases fabricated by compression molding and those fabricated by injection molding. Available data and clinical information indicate that denture bases fabricated by injection molding may provide slightly improved clinical accuracy.

Polymerization Procedure. As previously noted, denture base resins generally contain benzoyl peroxide. When heated above 60° C, molecules of benzoyl peroxide decompose to yield electrically neutral species containing unpaired

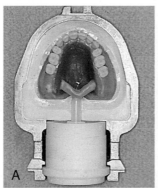
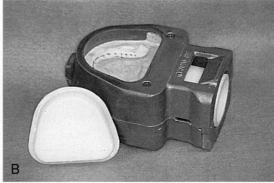
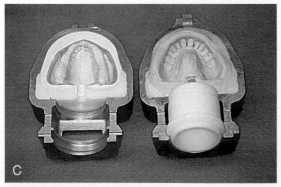
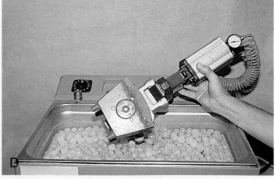

Figure 11–6. Steps in mold preparation (injection-molding technique). *A,* Placement of sprues for introduction of resin. *B,* Occlusal and incisal surfaces of the prosthetic teeth are exposed to facilitate denture recovery. *C,* Separation of flask segments during wax elimination process. *D,* Injection of resin, and placement of assembly into water bath.

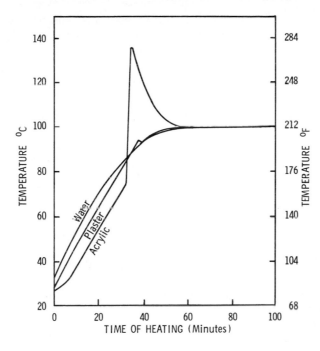

Figure 11–7. Temperature-time heating curves for the water bath, investing plaster, and acrylic resin during the polymerization of a 25.4-mm cube of denture resin. (Modified from Tuckfield WJ, Worner HK, and Guerin BD: Acrylic resins in dentistry. Aust J Dent 47:119–121, 1943.)

electrons. These species are termed *free radicals*. Each free radical rapidly reacts with an available monomer molecule to initiate chain-growth polymerization. Because the reaction product also possesses an unpaired electron, it remains chemically active. Consequently, additional monomer molecules become attached to individual polymer chains. This process occurs rapidly and terminates by (1) coupling of two growing chains (referred to as *combination*) or (2) transfer of a single hydrogen ion from one chain to another (referred to as *disproportionation*).

In the system under discussion, heat is required to cause decomposition of benzoyl peroxide molecules. Therefore, heat is termed the *activator*. Decomposition of benzoyl peroxide molecules yields free radicals that are responsible for the initiation of chain growth. Hence, benzoyl peroxide is termed the *initiator*.

During denture base fabrication, heat is applied to the resin by immersing a denture flask and flask carrier in a water bath. Subsequently, the water is heated to a prescribed temperature and maintained at that temperature for a period suggested by the manufacturer.

Temperature Rise. The polymerization of denture base resins is exothermic, and the amount of heat evolved may affect the properties of the processed denture bases. Representative temperature changes occurring in water, investing stone, and resin are illustrated in Figure 11–7.

As can be seen in Figure 11–7, the temperature profile of the investing gypsum (denoted as *plaster*) closely parallels the temperature of the water. The temperature of the denture base resin lags somewhat during the initial stages of the heating process because the resin occupies a position in the center of the mold and, therefore, heat penetration requires a longer period.

As the denture base resin attains a temperature slightly above 70° C, the temperature of the resin begins to increase rapidly. In turn, the decomposition rate of benzoyl peroxide is significantly increased. This sequence of events leads to an increased rate of polymerization and an accompanying increase in the exothermic heat of reaction. Because the resin and dental stone are relatively poor thermal conductors, the heat of reaction cannot be dissipated. Therefore, the temperature of the resin rises well above the temperatures of the investing stone and surrounding water. The temperature of the resin also exceeds the boiling point of the monomer (100.8° C). As discussed in the following sections, this temperature increase exerts significant effects on the physical characteristics of the processed resin.

Internal Porosity. As we have seen, the polymerization process is exothermic. If the accompanying temperature increase exceeds the boiling point of unreacted monomer or low molecular weight polymers or both, these components may boil.

Clinically, boiling yields porosity within the completed denture base. Experience indicates such porosity usually is *not* seen at the surface of the denture base. Apparently, the heat generated as a result of polymerization can be conducted away from the surface of the resin and into the surrounding dental stone. Consequently, heat is dissipated, and the surface temperature of the resin does not reach the boiling point of the monomer.

As one progresses centrally within a resin mass, thermal characteristics of the system change significantly. Because resin is an extremely poor thermal conductor, heat generated in a thick segment of resin cannot be dissipated. As a result, the peak temperature of this resin may rise well above the boiling point of monomer. In turn, this causes boiling of unreacted monomer and produces porosity within the processed denture base.

Polymerization Cycle. The heating process used to control polymerization is termed the *polymerization cycle* or *curing cycle*. Ideally, this process should be well controlled to avoid the effects of uncontrolled temperature rise, such as boiling of monomer and denture base porosity.

As might be expected, the curing cycle presented in Figure 11–7 is unsatisfactory because of the marked temperature increase during the early stages of polymerization. Fortunately, this process may be controlled by heating the resin more slowly during the polymerization cycle.

The relationship between rate of heating and temperature rise within the denture base resin is illustrated in Figure 11–8. The polymerization cycle repre-

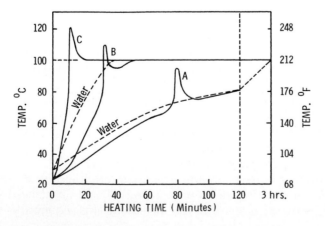

Figure 11–8. Temperature changes in acrylic resin when subjected to various curing schedules. (Modified from Tuckfield WJ, Worner HK, and Guerin BD: Acrylic resins in dentistry. Aust J Dent 47:119–121, 1943.)

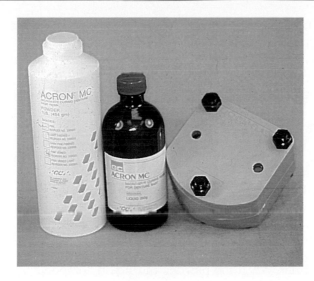

Figure 11–9. Representative microwave resin and nonmetallic microwave flask.

sented by curve C probably would yield porosity in thick portions of the denture, because the temperature of the resin exceeds the boiling point of the monomer (100.8° C). On the other hand, the polymerization cycle represented by curve A probably would result in the presence of unreacted monomer, because the resin temperature fails to reach the boiling temperature of the monomer (100.8° C). Thus, it is logical to assume that an optimum polymerization cycle lies somewhere between curves A and C.

Research has led to the development of certain guidelines for polymerization of denture base resins. Resultant polymerization cycles have proven quite successful for denture bases of various sizes, shapes, and thicknesses. One technique involves processing the denture base resin in a constant-temperature water bath at 74° C (165° F) for 8 hours or longer, with no terminal boiling treatment. A second technique involves processing the resin at 74° C for approximately 2 hours and then increasing the temperature of the water bath to 100° C and processing for 1 hour more.

Following completion of the chosen polymerization cycle, the denture flask should be cooled slowly to room temperature. Rapid cooling may result in warpage of the denture base because of differences in thermal contraction of resin and investing stone. Slow, even cooling of these materials minimizes potential difficulties. Hence, the flask should be removed from the water bath and bench cooled for 30 minutes. Subsequently, the flask should be immersed in cool tap water for 15 minutes. At this time, the denture base may be deflasked and prepared for delivery. To decrease the probability of unfavorable dimensional changes, the denture should be stored in water until it is delivered to the patient.

Polymerization via Microwave Energy. Poly(methyl methacrylate) resin also may be polymerized using microwave energy. This technique employs a specially formulated resin and a nonmetallic flask (Fig. 11–9). A conventional microwave oven is used to supply the thermal energy required for polymerization.

The major advantage of this technique is the speed with which polymerization may be accomplished. Investigations indicate the physical properties of microwave resins are comparable to those described for conventional resins. Furthermore, the fit of denture bases polymerized using microwave energy are comparable with those processed via conventional techniques.

CHEMICALLY ACTIVATED DENTURE BASE RESINS

As discussed, heat and microwave energy may be used to induce denture base polymerization. The application of thermal energy leads to decomposition of benzoyl peroxide and the production of free radicals. The free radicals formed as a result of this process subsequently initiate polymerization.

In addition to the aforementioned methods, *chemical activators* also may be used to induce denture base polymerization. Chemical activation does not require the application of thermal energy and therefore may be completed at room temperature. As a result, chemically activated resins often are referred to as *cold-curing*, *self-curing*, or *autopolymerizing* resins.

In most instances, chemical activation is accomplished through the addition of a tertiary amine, such as dimethyl-*para*-toluidine, to the denture base liquid, that is, the monomer. When the powder and liquid components are mixed, the tertiary amine causes decomposition of benzoyl peroxide. Consequently, free radicals are produced and polymerization is initiated. Polymerization progresses in a manner similar to that described for heat-activated systems.

The fundamental difference between heat-activated resins and chemically activated resins is the method by which benzoyl peroxide is divided to yield free radicals. All other factors in this process remain the same, for example, the initiator and reactants.

As might be expected, denture bases fabricated using chemically activated resins and heat-activated resins are quite similar. Nonetheless, chemically activated resins exhibit certain advantages and disadvantages worthy of discussion.

Generally, the degree of polymerization achieved using chemically activated resins is not as complete as that achieved using heat-activated systems. This indicates there is a greater amount of unreacted monomer in denture bases fabricated via chemical activation. This unreacted monomer creates two major difficulties. First, the residual monomer serves as a potential tissue irritant, thereby compromising the biocompatibility of the denture base. Second, it acts as a plasticizer, which results in decreased transverse strength of the denture resin.

From a physical standpoint, chemically activated resins display slightly less shrinkage than their heat-activated counterparts because of a less complete polymerization. This imparts greater dimensional accuracy to chemically activated resins.

The color stability of chemically activated resins generally is inferior to the color stability of heat-activated resins. This property is related to the presence of tertiary amines within the chemically activated resins. Such amines are susceptible to oxidation and accompanying color changes that may affect the appearance of the resin. Discoloration of these resins may be minimized via the addition of stabilizing agents that prevent such oxidation.

Technical Considerations. Chemically activated denture base resins are most often molded using compression techniques. Therefore, mold preparation and resin packing are essentially the same as those described for heat-activated denture resins.

Polymer and monomer are supplied in the form of a powder and liquid, respectively. These components are mixed according to manufacturer's directions and permitted to attain a doughlike consistency. The working time for chemically activated resins invariably is shorter than for heat-activated materials. Therefore, special attention must be paid to the consistency of the material and rate of polymerization.

A lengthy initiation period is desirable, because this provides adequate time for trial closures. One method for prolonging the initiation period is to decrease the temperature of the resin mass. This may be accomplished by refrigerating the liquid component or mixing vessel prior to the mixing process. When the powder and liquid are mixed, the rate of polymerization process decreases. As a result, the resin mass remains in a doughlike stage for an extended period, and the working time is increased.

Mold preparation and resin packing are accomplished in the same manner described for heat-activated resins. In cases of chemically activated resins with minimal working times, it is doubtful that more than two trial closures can be made. Therefore, extreme care must be taken to ensure that a proper amount of resin is employed and a minimal number of trial closures is required.

Processing Considerations. After final closure of the denture flask, pressure must be maintained throughout the polymerization process. The time required for polymerization varies with the material chosen.

Initial hardening of the resin generally occurs within 30 minutes of final flask closure. Nevertheless, it is doubtful that polymerization will be complete at this point. To ensure sufficient polymerization, the flask should be held under pressure for a minimum of 3 hours.

As previously noted, the polymerization of chemically activated resins is never as complete as the polymerization of heat-activated materials. Resins polymerized via chemical activation generally display 3% to 5% free monomer, whereas heat-activated resins exhibit 0.2% to 0.5% free monomer. Therefore, it is important that the polymerization of chemically activated resins be as complete as possible. Failure to achieve a high degree of polymerization predisposes the denture base to dimensional instability and may lead to soft tissue irritation.

Fluid Resin Technique. The *fluid resin technique* employs a pourable, chemically activated resin for the fabrication of denture bases. The resin is supplied in the form of powder and liquid components. When mixed in the proper proportions, these components yield a low-viscosity resin. Subsequently, this resin is poured into a mold cavity, subjected to increased atmospheric pressure, and allowed to polymerize. Laboratory aspects of the fluid resin technique are described in the following paragraphs.

Tooth arrangement is accomplished using accepted prosthodontic principles. Afterward, the completed tooth arrangement is sealed to the underlying cast and placed in a specially designed flask (Fig. 11–10A; see also color figure). The flask is filled with a reversible hydrocolloid investment medium, and the assembly is cooled. After gelation of the investment medium, the cast with the attached tooth arrangement is removed from the flask (Fig. 11–10B; see also color figure). At this stage, sprues and vents to the mold cavity are cut from the external surface of the flask (Fig. 11–10C; see also color figure).

Wax is eliminated from the cast using hot water. The prosthetic teeth are retrieved and carefully seated in their respective positions within the hydrocolloid investing medium. Subsequently, the cast is returned to its position within the mold (Fig. 11–10D; see also color figure).

The resin is mixed according to manufacturer's directions and poured into the mold via the sprue openings (Fig. 11–10E; see also color figure). The flask then is placed in a pressurized chamber at room temperature, and the resin is permitted to polymerize. According to available information, only 30 to 45

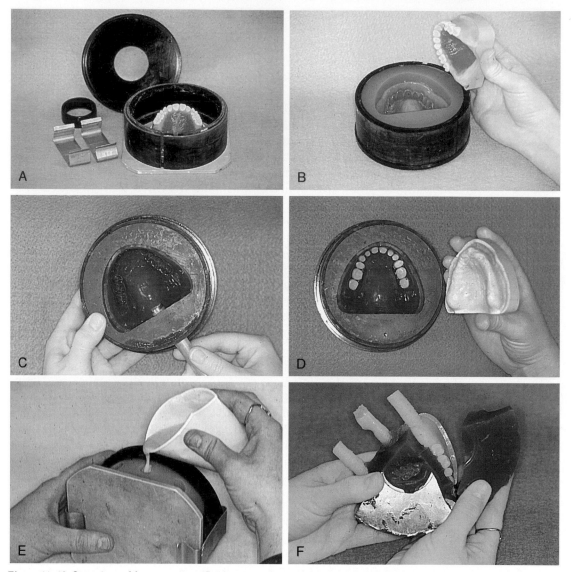

Figure 11–10. Steps in mold preparation (fluid resin technique). *A,* Completed tooth arrangement positioned in a fluid resin flask. *B,* Removal of tooth arrangement from reversible hydrocolloid investment. C, Preparation of sprues and vents for the introduction of resin. *D,* Repositioning of the prosthetic teeth and master cast. *E,* Introduction of pour-type resin. *F,* Recovery of the completed prosthesis.

minutes is required for polymerization. Nevertheless, a longer period is suggested.

Following completion of the polymerization process, the denture is retrieved from the flask (Fig. 11–10*F*; see also color figure), and sprues are removed. The denture-cast assembly is returned to the articulator for correction of processing changes. Subsequently, the denture base is finished and polished.

The advantages claimed for the fluid resin technique include improved adaptation to underlying soft tissues; decreased probability of damage to prosthetic teeth and denture bases during deflasking; reduced material costs; and simplification of the flasking, deflasking, and finishing procedures. The potential disadvantages of the fluid resin technique include noticeable shifting of prosthetic teeth during processing; air entrapment within the denture base material; poor bonding between the denture base material and acrylic resin teeth; and technique sensitivity. Generally, denture bases fabricated in this manner exhibit physical properties that are somewhat inferior to those of conventional heat-processed resins. Nonetheless, clinically acceptable dentures can be obtained using fluid resins.

LIGHT-ACTIVATED DENTURE BASE RESINS

A visible light-activated denture base resin has been available to the dental community for several years. This material has been described as a composite having a matrix of urethane dimethacrylate, microfine silica, and high-molecular-weight acrylic resin monomers. Acrylic resin beads are included as organic filler. *Visible light* is the *activator*, whereas *camphoroquinone* serves as the *initiator* for polymerization. The single-component denture base resin is supplied in sheet and rope forms and is packed in light-proof pouches to prevent inadvertent polymerization (Fig. 11–11A).

As might be expected, denture base fabrication using a light-activated resin is significantly different from the techniques described in previous sections. Opaque investing media prevent the passage of light; therefore, light-activated resins cannot be flasked in a conventional manner. Instead, teeth are arranged

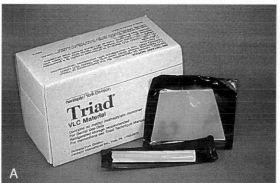

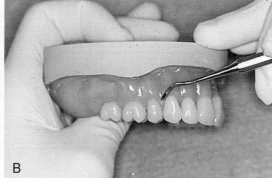

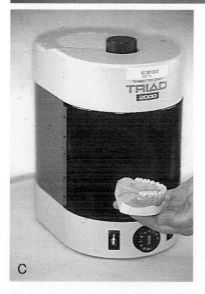

Figure 11–11. Steps in denture fabrication (light-activated denture base resins). *A,* Representative light-activated denture base resin. The sheet and rope forms are supplied in light-proof pouches to prevent inadvertent polymerization. *B,* Teeth are arranged and the denture base is sculpted using light-activated resin. *C,* The denture base is placed into a light chamber and polymerized according to manufacturer's recommendations.

and the denture base is molded on an accurate cast (Fig. 11–11*B*). Subsequently, the denture base is exposed to a high-intensity visible light source for an appropriate period (Fig. 11–11*C*). After polymerization, the denture is removed from the cast, finished, and polished in a conventional manner.

PHYSICAL PROPERTIES OF DENTURE BASE RESINS

The physical properties of denture base resins are critical to the fit and function of removable dental prostheses. Characteristics of interest include polymerization shrinkage, porosity, water absorption, solubility, processing stresses, and crazing. These characteristics are addressed in the following sections.

Polymerization Shrinkage. When methyl methacrylate monomer is polymerized to form poly(methyl methacrylate), the density of the mass changes from 0.94 to 1.19 g/cm^3. This change in density results in a volumetric shrinkage of 21%. When a conventional heat-activated resin is mixed at the suggested powder:liquid ratio, about one third of the resultant mass is liquid. Consequently, the volumetric shrinkage exhibited by the polymerized mass should be approximately 7%. This percentage is in agreement with values observed in laboratory and clinical investigations.

There may be several reasons why materials exhibiting such high volumetric shrinkages can be used to produce clinically satisfactory denture bases. It appears that the shrinkage exhibited by these materials is distributed uniformly to all surfaces. Hence, the adaptation of denture bases to underlying soft tissues is not significantly affected, provided the materials are manipulated properly.

In addition to volumetric shrinkage, one also must consider the effects of linear shrinkage. Linear shrinkage exerts significant effects on denture base adaptation and cuspal interdigitation. By convention, linear shrinkage values are determined by measuring the distance between two predetermined reference points in the second molar regions of a completed tooth arrangement. After polymerization of the denture base resin and removal of the prosthesis from the master cast, the distance between these reference points is measured once again. The difference between prepolymerization and postpolymerization measurements is recorded as linear shrinkage. The greater the linear shrinkage, the greater the discrepancy observed in the initial fit of a denture. Based on an projected volumetric shrinkage of 7%, an acrylic resin denture base should exhibit a linear shrinkage of approximately 2%. In reality, linear shrinkage generally is observed to be less than 1% (Table 11–1).

Examination of the polymerization process indicates that thermal shrinkage of resin is primarily responsible for the linear shrinkage phenomenon in heat-activated systems. During the initial stages of the cooling process, the resin

TABLE 11–1. Polymerization Shrinkage of Maxillary Denture Bases

Material	Linear Shrinkage (%)
High-impact acrylic resin	0.12
Vinyl acrylic resin	0.33
Conventional acrylic resin	0.43
Pour-type acrylic resin	0.48
Rapid heat-cured acrylic resin	0.97

Reprinted from Journal of Dentistry, vol. 8, Stafford GD, Bates JF, Huggett R, Handley RW: A review of the properties of some denture base polymers, p. 292. Copyright 1980, with permission from Elsevier Science Ltd., The Boulevard, Langford Lane, Kidlington 0X5 1GB, UK.

remains relatively soft. Therefore, the pressure maintained on the flask assembly causes the resin to contract at approximately the same rate as the surrounding dental stone.

As cooling proceeds, the soft resin approaches its *glass transition temperature* (T_g). The T_g lies within a thermal range in which the polymerized resin passes from a soft, rubbery state to a rigid, glassy state. Hence, cooling the denture base resin beyond the T_g yields a rigid mass. In turn, this rigid mass contracts at a rate different from the of surrounding dental stone. The shrinkage occurring below the T_g is thermal in nature and varies according to the composition of the resin.

To illustrate the effect of thermal shrinkage, consider the following example. The T_g for poly(methyl methacrylate) is approximately 105° C. Room temperature is 20° C. The generally accepted value for linear coefficient of thermal expansion, α, for poly(methyl methacrylate) is 81×10^{-6} per degrees centigrade. Therefore, as the denture base resin is cooled from the T_g to room temperature, it undergoes a linear shrinkage that may be expressed as:

$$\alpha \Delta T = (81 \times 10^{-6}/° C) (105° C - 20° C) (100\%) = 0.69\%$$

This value is in agreement with linear shrinkages of 0.12% to 0.97% reported for various commercial denture resins.

Complete dentures constructed using chemically activated resins generally display better adaptation than those constructed using heat-activated resins. This phenomenon may be attributed to the negligible thermal shrinkage and more complete cure displayed by chemically activated resins. Processing shrinkage has been measured as 0.26% for a representative chemically activated resin, compared with 0.53% for a representative heat-activated resin.

Given the preceding information regarding polymerization shrinkage and denture base adaptation, chemically activated resins are less biocompatible for laboratory personnel, but they provide significant advantages over heat-activated resins. However, there are several other factors that affect the overall dimensional characteristics of processed denture bases. Such factors include the type of investing medium selected, the method of resin introduction, and the temperature used to activate the polymerization process.

On completion of the polymerization process, individual denture bases and master casts are retrieved and returned to their respective articulators. Subsequently, dimensional changes are assessed with respect to the desired vertical dimension of occlusion.

Fluid resin techniques used in conjunction with hydrocolloid investing media generally yield decreases in overall vertical dimension. Conversely, dentures processed using heat-activated or chemically activated resins in conjunction with compression-molding techniques usually display increases in overall vertical dimension. Minimal increases in vertical dimension are considered desirable, because they permit a return to the proposed vertical dimension of occlusion through occlusal grinding procedures. Dimensional changes occurring in denture bases fabricated from various resins are illustrated in Figure 11–12 (see also color figure).

Porosity. The presence of surface and subsurface voids may compromise the physical, aesthetic, and hygienic properties of a processed denture base. Porosity is likely to develop in thicker portions of a denture base. Such porosity results from the vaporization of unreacted monomer and low-molecular-weight polymers, when the temperature of a resin reaches or surpasses the boiling points of

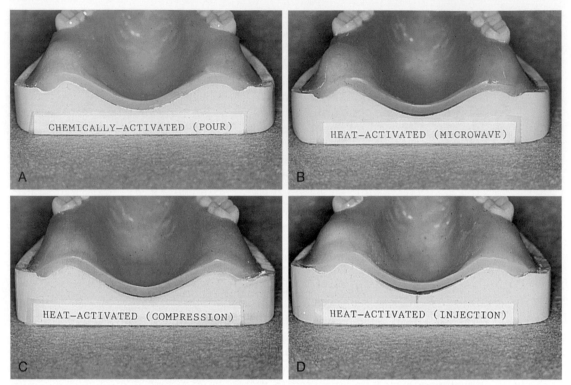

Figure 11–12. Dimensional changes resulting from polymerization. *A,* Chemically activated resin (pour technique). *B,* Microwave resin (compression-molding technique). *C,* Conventional heat-activated resin (compression-molding technique). *D,* Heat-activated resin (injection-molding technique).

these species. Nonetheless, this type of porosity may not occur equally throughout affected resin segments.

To facilitate an understanding of this concept, consider the specimens in Figures 11–13A (with no porosity) and 11–13B (with localized subsurface porosity). Specimens *B* and *C* were flasked in such a manner that the section dis-

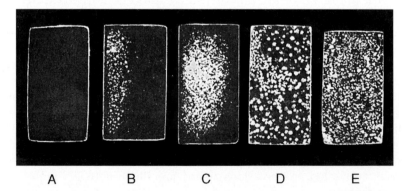

Figure 11–13. Heat-activated denture base resin exhibiting different types and degrees of porosity. *A,* Properly polymerized, no porosity. *B* and *C,* Rapid heating, relatively small subsurface voids. *D,* Insufficient mixing of monomer and polymer, large voids resulting from localized polymerization shrinkage. *E,* Insufficient pressure during polymerization, relatively large, irregular voids. (Modified from Tuckfield WJ, Worner HK, and Guerin BD: Acrylic resins in dentistry. Aust J Dent 47:119–121, 1943.)

playing porosity was nearer the center of the investment mass, whereas the nonporous section was nearer the surface of the metal flask. As might be expected, the metal of the flask conducted heat away from the periphery with sufficient rapidity to prevent substantial temperature rise. Consequently, the low-molecular-weight species did not boil, and porosity did not develop. Conversely, the resin occupying a more central position was surrounded by a larger mass of dental stone. Because this material is a poor thermal conductor, heat was not readily dissipated, low-molecular-weight species were vaporized, and noticeable porosity was produced.

Porosity also may result from inadequate mixing of powder and liquid components. If this occurs, some regions of the resin mass will contain more monomer than others. During polymerization these regions shrink more than adjacent regions, and the localized shrinkage tends to produce voids (Fig. 11–13D).

The occurrence of such porosity can be minimized by ensuring the greatest possible homogeneity of the resin. The use of proper polymer:monomer ratios and well-controlled mixing procedures aids in this connection. Furthermore, because the material is more homogeneous in the doughlike stage, it is wise to delay packing until this consistency has been reached. In evaluating the information presented in Figure 11–13, it should be recognized that such porosities can occur in surface and subsurface locations. Porosities resulting from rapid temperature elevation can be much larger than those presented in Figure 11–13B and C.

A third type of porosity may be caused by inadequate pressure or insufficient material in the mold during polymerization (Fig. 11–13E). Voids produced as a result of these inadequacies are not spherical but assume irregular shapes. These voids may be so abundant that the resultant resin appears significantly lighter and more opaque than its intended color.

A final type of porosity is most often associated with fluid resins. Such porosity appears to be caused by air inclusions incorporated during mixing and pouring procedures. If these inclusions are not removed, sizable voids may be produced in the resultant denture bases. Careful mixing, spruing, and venting seem to help reduce the incidence of air inclusions.

Water Absorption. Poly(methyl methacrylate) absorbs relatively small amounts of water when placed in an aqueous environment. Nevertheless, this water exerts significant effects on the mechanical and dimensional properties of the polymer.

Although absorption is facilitated by the polarity of poly(methyl methacrylate) molecules, the mechanism primarily responsible for the ingress of water is diffusion. Diffusion is the migration of one substance through a space, or within a second substance. In this instance, water molecules penetrate the poly(methyl methacrylate) mass and occupy positions between polymer chains. Consequently, the affected polymer chains are forced apart. The introduction of water molecules within the polymerized mass produces two important effects. First, it causes a slight expansion of the polymerized mass. Second, water molecules interfere with the entanglement of polymer chains and thereby act as plasticizers.

Poly(methyl methacrylate) exhibits a water sorption value of 0.69 mg/cm². Although this amount of water may seem inconsequential, it exerts significant effects on the dimensions of a polymerized denture base. It has been estimated that for each 1% increase in weight produced by water absorption, acrylic resin expands 0.23% linearly. Laboratory trials indicate the linear expansion caused by water absorption is approximately equal to the thermal shrinkage encountered as a result of the polymerization process. Hence, these processes almost offset one another.

As previously noted, water molecules also may interfere with entanglement of polymer chains and thereby change the physical characteristics of the resultant polymer. When this occurs, polymer chains generally become more mobile. This permits the relaxation of stresses incurred during polymerization. As stresses are relieved, polymerized resins may undergo changes in shape. Fortunately, these changes are relatively minor and do not appreciably affect the fit or function of the processed bases.

Because the presence of water exerts significant effects on the physical and dimensional properties of denture base resins, diffusion coefficients also warrant consideration. The diffusion coefficient of water in a typical heat-activated denture acrylic resin is 1.08×10^{-12} m²/s at 37° C. For a representative chemically activated resin, the diffusion coefficient of water is 2.34×10^{-12} m²/s. Because the diffusion coefficients of water in representative denture resins are relatively low, the time required for a denture base to reach saturation can be considerable. This depends on the thickness of the resin, as well as the storage conditions. A typical denture base may require a period of 17 days to become fully saturated with water.

Results of laboratory investigations indicate there is a slight difference in the dimensions of heat-activated and chemically activated denture bases after prolonged storage in water. Compression-molded, heat-activated denture bases are slightly undersized when measured from second molar to second molar. Conversely, compression-molded, chemically activated denture bases are slightly oversized when measured in the same region. The clinical significance of this difference appears negligible.

ADA Specification No. 12 identifies guidelines regarding the testing and acceptance of denture base resins. To test water absorption, a disk of material with specified dimensions is prepared and dried to a constant weight. This weight is recorded as a baseline value. Subsequently, the disk is soaked in distilled water for 7 days. Again, the disk is weighed, and this value is compared with the baseline value. According to the specification, the weight gain following immersion must not be higher than 0.8 mg/cm². Additional information regarding ADA Specification No. 12 is presented in subsequent sections.

Solubility. Although denture base resins are soluble in a variety of solvents and a small amount of monomer may be leached, they are virtually insoluble in the fluids commonly encountered in the oral cavity. ADA Specification No. 12 prescribes a test for resin solubility. This procedure is a continuation of the water sorption test described in the preceding section. After the required water immersion, the test disk is permitted to dry and is reweighed to determine weight loss. According to the specification, weight loss must not be more than 0.04 mg/cm² of specimen surface. Such a loss may seem negligible from a clinical standpoint, but adverse tissue reactions may occur.

Processing Stresses. Whenever a natural dimensional change is inhibited, the affected material contains stresses. If stresses are relaxed, a resultant distortion or warpage of the material may occur. This principle has important ramifications in the fabrication of denture bases, because stresses invariably are induced during processing.

For purposes of this discussion, consider the events that occur during denture base polymerization. As previously stated, a moderate amount of shrinkage occurs as individual monomers are linked to form polymer chains. During this process, it is possible that friction between the mold walls and soft resin may inhibit normal shrinkage of these chains. As a result, the polymer chains are stretched, and the resin contains stresses that are tensile in character.

Stresses also are produced as the result of thermal shrinkage. As a polymerized resin is cooled below its T_g, the resin becomes relatively rigid. Further cooling yields thermal shrinkage. A denture base resin generally is encased in a rigid investing medium, such as dental stone, during this process. Because denture base resins and dental stones contract at markedly different rates, a contraction differential is established. Hence, a disparity in contraction rates also yields stresses within the resin. Additional factors that may contribute to processing stresses include improper mixing and handling of the resin and poorly controlled heating and cooling of the flask assembly.

The release of stresses yields dimensional changes that are cumulative in nature. Fortunately, these dimensional changes are quite small. Total dimensional changes occurring as a result of processing and service are in the range of 0.1 to 0.2 mm (as measured from second molar to second molar). Therefore, it is doubtful such changes would be clinically significant and thus detectable by a patient.

Crazing. Although dimensional changes may occur during relaxation of processing stresses, these changes generally do not cause clinical difficulties. In contrast, stress relaxation may produce small surface flaws that can adversely affect the aesthetic and physical properties of a denture. The production of such flaws, or microcracks, is termed *crazing*.

Clinically, crazing is evidenced by small linear cracks that appear to originate at a denture's surface. Crazing in a transparent resin imparts a "hazy" or "foggy" appearance. In a tinted resin, crazing imparts a whitish cast. In addition, surface cracks predispose a denture base to fracture.

From a physical standpoint, crazing may result from stress application or partial dissolution of a resin. Tensile stresses are most often responsible for crazing in denture base applications. It is believed that crazing is produced by mechanical separation of individual polymer chains on application of tensile stresses.

Crazing generally begins at the surface of a resin and is oriented at right angles to tensile forces. Microcracks formed in this manner subsequently progress internally. An example of crazing is presented in Figure 11–14. This pattern sometimes occurs when porcelain denture teeth are used in conjunction with resin denture bases. During the cooling process that follows polymerization, denture resin shrinks more than dental porcelain. As a result, axial or tangential tensile stresses are generated within the resin. The presence of such stresses leads to the creation of small linear flaws or cracks, as depicted in the figure.

As noted, crazing also may be produced as a result of solvent action. Microcracks produced in this manner are oriented more randomly than those depicted in Figure 11–14. Solvent-induced crazing generally results from prolonged contact with liquids such as ethyl alcohol. The development of improved acrylic resin teeth and cross-linked denture base resins has resulted in a decreased incidence of denture base crazing.

Strength. The strength of an individual denture base resin is dependent on several factors. These factors include composition of the resin, processing technique, and conditions presented by the oral environment.

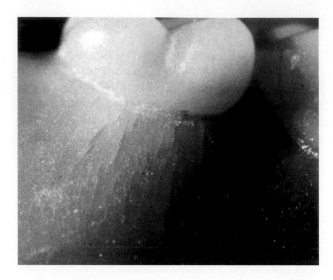

Figure 11–14. Crazing around porcelain teeth.

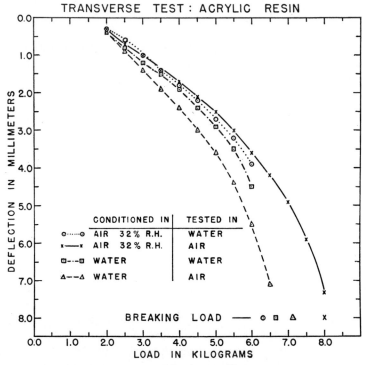

Figure 11–15. Transverse load-deflection curve for a typical denture base resin, showing the influence of different conditioning procedures and testing environments. All specimens were conditioned as indicated for 3 days before testing. (From Swaney AC, Paffenbarger GC, and Caul HJ: American Dental Association Specification No. 12 for denture base resin: Second revision. J Am Dent Assoc 46:54–66, 1953.)

To provide acceptable physical properties, denture base resins must meet or exceed the standards presented in ADA Specification No. 12. A transverse test is used to evaluate the relationship between applied load and resultant deflection in a resin specimen of prescribed dimensions. Typical load-deflection results are presented in Figure 11–15.

Inspection of Figure 11–15 reveals a gentle curvature of the load-deflection plot. Because no straight-line portion is evident, one may assume that plastic deformation, that is, irreversible deformation, occurs during the loading process. Because of the resilient nature of denture base resins, some elastic deformation, that is, recoverable deformation, also occurs. Clinically, this means that load application produces stresses within a resin and a change in the overall shape of the denture base. When the load is released, stresses within the resin are relaxed and the denture base returns to its original shape. Nevertheless, the existence of plastic deformation prevents complete recovery. Therefore, some permanent deformation remains.

Perhaps the most important determinant of overall resin strength is the degree of polymerization exhibited by the material. As the degree of polymerization increases, the strength of the resin also increases. In this regard, the polymerization cycle employed with a heat-activated resin is extremely important. Figure 11–16 reveals the effects that the processing cycle exerts on load-deflection properties. Note that increased duration of the polymerization cycle (bottom to top) appears to yield improved physical properties (reduced deflection).

In comparison with heat-activated resins, the chemically activated resins generally display lower degrees of polymerization. As a result, chemically activated

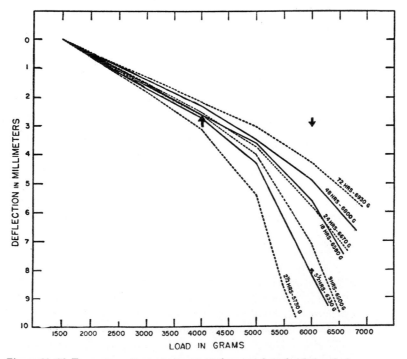

Figure 11–16. Transverse stress-strain curves for samples of poly(methyl methacrylate) polymerized for different periods at 71° C (160° F). Processing times and fracture loads are noted on individual curves. (From Harman IM: Effects of time and temperature on polymerization of a methacrylate resin denture base. J Am Dent Assoc 38:188–203, 1949.)

resins exhibit increased levels of residual monomer and decreased strength and stiffness values. Despite these characteristics, heat-activated and chemically activated resins display similar elastic moduli.

Creep. Denture resins display *viscoelastic behavior*. In other words, these materials act as rubbery solids. When a denture base resin is subjected to a sustained load, the material exhibits an initial deflection or deformation. If this load is not removed, additional deformation may occur over time. This additional deformation is termed *creep*.

The rate at which this progressive deformation occurs is termed the *creep rate*. This rate may be elevated by increases in temperature, applied load, residual monomer, and the presence of plasticizers. Although creep rates for heat-activated and chemically activated resins are similar at low stresses (9.0 MPa), creep rates for chemically activated resins increase more rapidly as stresses are increased.

Miscellaneous Properties. The Charpy impact strength for a heat-activated denture resin may range from 0.98 to 1.27 J, whereas that for a chemically activated resin is somewhat lower (0.78 J). Values for high-impact resins, such as Lucitone 199, can be twice those values reported for conventional poly(methyl methacrylate) resins. These figures are of limited use, because the energy absorbed by an individual specimen is dependent on specimen size and geometry, distance between specimen supports, and the presence or absence of notching.

The Knoop hardness values for heat-activated resins may be as high as 20, whereas chemically activated resins generally display Knoop hardness values of 16 to 18. This information is of academic interest only.

MISCELLANEOUS RESINS AND TECHNIQUES

Repair Resins. Despite the favorable physical characteristics of denture base resins, denture bases sometimes fracture. In most instances, such fractures may be repaired using compatible resins. Repair resins may be light-activated, heat-activated, or chemically activated.

To accurately accomplish repair of a fractured prosthesis, the components must be realigned and luted together using an adherent wax or modeling plastic. When this has been accomplished, a repair cast is generated using dental stone. The denture is removed from the cast, and the luting medium is eliminated. Subsequently, the fracture surfaces are trimmed to provide sufficient room for repair material. The cast is coated with separating medium to prevent adherence of repair resin, and the denture base sections are repositioned and affixed to the cast.

At this point, a repair material is chosen. Chemically activated resins generally are preferred over heat-activated and light-activated resins, despite the fact that chemically activated resins display lower transverse strengths. The principal advantage of chemically activated resins is that they may be polymerized at room temperature. Heat-activated and light-activated repair materials must be placed in water baths and light chambers, respectively. Heat generated by water baths and light chambers often causes stress release and warpage of previously polymerized denture base segments.

The following sequence is employed to accomplish denture base repair using a chemically activated resin. A small amount of monomer is painted onto prepared surfaces of the denture base to facilitate bonding of the repair material.

Increments of monomer and polymer are added to the repair area using a small sable-hair brush or suitable substitute. A slight excess of material is placed at the repair site to account for polymerization shrinkage. Subsequently, the assembly is placed in a pressure chamber and allowed to polymerize. Afterward, the repair site is shaped, finished, and polished using conventional techniques.

The test requirements for chemically activated resins used for repairing denture bases are identified in ADA Specification No. 13.

Relining Resin Denture Bases. Because soft tissue contours change during denture service, it is often necessary to alter tissue surfaces of intraoral prostheses to ensure proper fit and function. In some instances, this may be achieved by selective grinding procedures. In other instances, tissue surfaces must be replaced by *relining* or *rebasing* existing dentures.

Relining involves replacement of tissue surface of an existing denture, whereas rebasing involves replacement of the entire denture base. In both instances, an impression of the soft tissues is obtained using the existing denture as an impression tray. A stone cast is generated in the impression, and the resultant assembly is invested in a denture flask. Subsequently, the flask is opened and prepared for the introduction of resin.

If the denture is to be relined, the impression material is removed from the denture. The tissue surface is cleaned to enhance bonding between the existing resin and the reline material. Following this sequence, an appropriate resin is introduced and shaped using a compression-molding technique.

For relining, a low polymerization temperature is desirable to minimize distortion of the remaining denture base. Hence, a chemically activated resin usually is chosen. The selected material is mixed according to manufacturer's recommendations, placed into the mold, compressed, and permitted to polymerize. The denture subsequently is recovered, finished, and polished.

If a chemically activated resin is selected for relining the existing denture, a specialized mounting assembly, that is, a reline jig, also may be used in lieu of flasking. This assembly maintains the correct vertical and horizontal relationships between the cast and the denture while it eliminates the need to envelop the remaining denture base. This facilitates recovery of the denture at the end of the relining process.

Several manufacturers offer chemically activated resins for relining dentures intraorally. Unfortunately, many of these materials generate sufficient heat to injure oral tissues and monomer can be leached from them to irritate tissues. To receive ADA approval, materials must comply with Specification No. 17, which places limits on the rate of temperature rise and maximum acceptable temperature.

Relining also may be accomplished using resins that are activated by heat, light, or microwave energy. In all of these instances, significant heat may be generated, and distortion of the existing denture base is more likely.

Some materials are manufactured for repair as well as relining purposes. The practitioner should be extremely cautious in using such products. Some of these materials comply with ADA Specification No. 13 for repairs, but fail to meet temperature requirements set forth in Specification No. 17. Other materials comply with Specification No. 17 but fail to meet the requirements of Specification No. 13. Such materials often discolor, harbor micro-organisms, and separate from underlying denture bases.

Similar materials are marketed for home use. Unfortunately, most patients do not possess the knowledge required to manipulate such materials correctly. As a result, the use of such products may result in irreparable damage to the oral tissues. The purchase and use of such products should be discouraged.

Rebasing Resin Dentures. The steps required in denture rebasing are similar to those described for relining. An accurate impression of the soft tissues is obtained using the existing denture as a custom tray. Subsequently, a stone cast is fabricated in the impression. The cast and denture are mounted in a device, the reline jig, designed to maintain the correct vertical and horizontal relationships between the stone cast and surfaces of the prosthetic teeth. The resultant assembly provides indices for the occlusal surfaces of the prosthetic teeth. After these indices have been established, the denture is removed and the teeth are separated from the existing denture base. The teeth are repositioned in their respective indices and held in their original relationships to the cast while they are waxed to a new baseplate.

At this point, the denture base is waxed to the desired form. The completed tooth arrangement is sealed to the cast, and the assembly is invested as previously described. After elimination of the wax and removal of the baseplate, resin is introduced into the mold cavity. The material subsequently is processed. After processing, the denture is recovered, finished, and polished. Hence, the prosthesis consists of a new denture base in conjunction with teeth from the patient's previous denture.

Short-term and Long-term Soft Liners. The purpose of a soft liner is to absorb some of the energy produced by masticatory impact. Hence, a soft liner serves as a "shock absorber" between the occlusal surfaces of a denture and the underlying oral tissues.

The most commonly used liners are *plasticized acrylic resins*. These resins may be heat-activated or chemically activated and are based on familiar chemistries.

Chemically activated soft liners generally employ poly(methyl methacrylate) or poly(ethyl methacrylate) as principal structural components. These polymers are supplied in powder form and subsequently are mixed with liquids containing 60% to 80% of a plasticizer. The *plasticizer* usually is a large molecular species such as *dibutyl phthalate*. The distribution of large plasticizer molecules minimizes entanglement of polymer chains and thereby permits individual chains to "slip" past one another. This slipping motion permits rapid changes in the shape of the soft liner and provides a cushioning effect for the underlying tissues. The liquids used in such applications do not contain acrylic monomers. Consequently, the resultant liners are considered *short-term soft liners* or *tissue conditioners*.

Unlike chemically activated soft liners, heat-activated materials generally are more durable and may be considered *long-term soft liners*. Nonetheless, these materials degrade over time and should not be considered permanent.

A number of heat-activated soft liners are supplied as powder-liquid systems. The powders are composed of acrylic resin polymers and copolymers, whereas the liquids consist of appropriate acrylic monomers and plasticizers. When mixed, these materials form pliable resins exhibiting T_g values lower than mouth temperature.

Although plasticizers impart flexibility, they also present certain difficulties. Plasticizers are not bound within the resin mass and therefore may be "leached out" of soft liners. As this occurs, soft liners become progressively more rigid. Consequently, it is advantageous to use liners that are less prone to leaching phenomena.

As poly(methyl methacrylate) is replaced by higher methacrylates, such as ethyl, n-propyl, and n-butyl, the T_g progressively decreases. As a result, less plasticizer is required and the effects of leaching can be minimized.

Vinyl resins also have been used in soft liner applications. Unfortunately, plasticized poly(vinyl chloride) and poly(vinyl acetate) are subject to leaching and harden during sustained use.

Perhaps the most successful materials for soft liner applications have been the silicone rubbers. These materials are not dependent on leachable plasticizers and therefore retain their elastic properties for prolonged periods. Unfortunately, silicone rubbers may lose adhesion to underlying denture bases.

Silicone rubbers may be chemically or heat activated. Chemically activated silicones are supplied as two-component systems that polymerize via condensation reactions. Hence, these materials are quite similar to condensation silicone impression materials.

Placement of chemically activated soft liners is relatively straightforward. Relief is provided to permit an acceptable thickness of the chosen material. Adhesive is then applied to the surface of the denture base to facilitate bonding of the hard and soft resins. The resilient material is mixed, applied to the denture base via compression molding, and permitted to polymerize. Subsequently, the denture is recovered, finished, and polished.

Heat-activated silicones are one-component systems supplied as pastes or gels. These materials are applied and contoured using compression-molding techniques. Heat-activated silicones may be applied to polymerized denture base resins, or they may be polymerized in conjunction with freshly mixed resins.

To promote adhesion between silicone soft liners and rigid denture base materials, rubber poly(methyl methacrylate) cements often are used. These cements serve as chemical intermediates that bond to both soft liners and denture resins.

At least one silicone liner does not require an adhesive when it is cured in conjunction with an acrylic denture base material. This material actually is a silicone copolymer that contains components capable of bonding to acrylic resins.

Laboratory procedures for heat-activated silicones are similar to those described for chemically activated materials. Individual bases are invested, and mold spaces are prepared as required. Relief is provided to permit acceptable thickness of the chosen materials. Packing, compression molding, and processing are performed in accordance with manufacturer's recommendations. Then, the denture is recovered, finished, and polished.

Other polymers that have been used as soft liners include polyurethane and polyphosphazine. All the described liners display certain shortcomings. For instance, silicone liners are poorly adherent to denture base resins. Silicone liners also undergo significant volume changes with the gain and loss of water.

Many soft liners bond well to denture bases but become progressively more rigid as plasticizers are leached from liner materials. Hardening rates for these liners are associated with initial plasticizer content. As the plasticizer content is increased, the probability for leaching also is increased. Hence, materials displaying high initial plasticizer content tend to harden rather rapidly.

Soft liners also exert significant effects on associated denture bases. As the thickness of a soft liner is increased, the thickness of the accompanying denture base must be decreased. This results in decreased denture base strength. Furthermore, materials used in conjunction with soft liners, such as adhesives and monomers, may cause partial dissolution of the accompanying denture base. The resultant decrease in base strength may result in fracture during clinical service.

Perhaps the greatest difficulty associated with long-term and short-term soft liners is that these materials cannot be cleaned effectively. As a result, patients often report disagreeable tastes and odors related to these materials. Research indicates that the liners themselves do not support mycotic growth, but debris that accumulates in pores of these materials does support such growth. The most common fungal growth is *Candida albicans*.

Several regimens have been used in attempts to improve the hygienic characteristics of soft liners. Unfortunately, these regimens have met with limited success. Both oxygenating- and hypochlorite-type denture cleansers have been employed. These agents cause significant damage to soft liners, especially to the silicone materials.

Mechanical cleaning of soft liners may lead to damage, but such debridement is often necessary. If mechanical cleaning is necessary, a soft brush should be used in conjunction with a mild detergent solution or nonabrasive dentifrice.

Recently, antimycotic agents have been incorporated into soft liners. Although this approach appears promising, the duration of antimycotic activity is questionable. Hence, additional research is necessary.

Based on the preceding information, it appears that none of the existing soft liners may be considered entirely satisfactory. Few of the materials remain soft indefinitely, although some harden more slowly than others. In addition, existing materials accumulate stains and are difficult to clean. For these reasons, available materials should be considered temporary expedients and not permanent clinical agents.

Resin Impression Trays and Tray Materials. Resin trays often are used in dental impression procedures. Unlike stock trays, resin impression trays are fabricated to fit specific arches. As a result, resin impression trays often are called *custom trays*.

The steps in custom tray fabrication may be described as follows: A preliminary impression is made using a stock tray and an appropriate impression material. In turn, a gypsum cast is generated. A suitable spacer is placed on the stone cast to provide the desired relief. Subsequently, a separating medium is painted onto exposed cast surfaces.

A resin dough is formed by mixing an inorganically filled polymer and the appropriate monomer. In most instances, the material of choice is a chemically activated poly(methyl methacrylate) resin. The dough is rolled into a sheet approximately 2-mm thick, adapted to the diagnostic cast, and allowed to polymerize.

A resin impression tray may exhibit noticeable dimensional changes for 24 hours after fabrication and should not be used during this period. At the end of the prescribed period, the fit of the tray is evaluated intraorally, and necessary modifications are made. Subsequently, the spacer is removed and a master impression is made using an appropriate elastomeric impression material.

Recently, light-activated urethane dimethacrylate resins also have been used in tray fabrication. Such resins are supplied in sheet and gel forms. Sheet forms are preferred for custom tray fabrication because of their favorable handling characteristics.

Tray fabrication procedures for urethane dimethacrylate resins are similar to those described in the previous paragraphs. To facilitate tray fabrication, a diagnostic cast is made, and one or more layers of wax relief spacer are placed.

A separating medium is applied to exposed cast surfaces, and a tray is fashioned using urethane dimethacrylate sheet material. The cast and tray are placed in a light chamber, and the resin is polymerized.

Trays fabricated using urethane dimethacrylate resins are dimensionally stable during postpolymerization stages. Nonetheless, these materials are brittle and release fine powder particles during grinding procedures.

Denture Cleansers. Patients use a wide variety of agents for cleaning artificial dentures. In approximate order of preference, these include dentifrices, proprietary denture cleansers, mild detergents, household cleansers, bleaches, and vinegar. Both immersion and brushing techniques are used with these materials.

The most common commercial denture cleansers use immersion techniques. These cleansers are marketed in powder and tablet forms. Immersion agents contain alkaline compounds, detergents, sodium perborate, and flavoring agents. When dissolved in water, sodium perborate decomposes to form an alkaline peroxide solution. This peroxide solution subsequently releases oxygen, which is reported to loosen debris via mechanical means.

Household bleaches (hypochlorites) also are used in denture-cleaning applications. Dilute bleach solutions may be used to remove certain types of stains. Concentrated solutions should be avoided, because prolonged use may affect denture coloration. Bleaches also may discolor soft relining materials, particularly the silicones.

Bleaches and bleach solutions should not be used for cleaning base metal prostheses, such as removable partial denture frameworks. Such solutions produce significant darkening of base metals and may irreparably damage the metal luster and serviceability of affected prostheses.

The effects of abrasive agents on acrylic resin surfaces also have been investigated. Toothbrushes alone exert little effect on resin surfaces. Toothbrushes in conjunction with most commercial dentifrices, mild detergents, and soaps do not appear to be harmful. Conversely, household cleansers, such as kitchen and bathroom abrasives, are definitely contraindicated. Prolonged use of such cleansers may significantly alter the internal and external surfaces of dentures and may adversely affect the function and aesthetics of resin prostheses. As a result, each patient should be educated regarding the care and cleaning of resin prostheses.

Infection Control Procedures. Care should be taken to prevent cross-contamination between patients and dental personnel, including those personnel in the dental laboratory. New appliances should be disinfected before leaving the dental laboratory. Existing prostheses should be disinfected before entering the laboratory and after completion of laboratory procedures. All materials used for finishing and polishing procedures should be dedicated for single disposable use, or sterilized after completion of procedures. Items such as rag wheels should be autoclaved, and materials such as pumice should be used according to unit-dose recommendations.

Allergic Reactions. Possible toxic or allergic reactions to poly(methyl methacrylate) have long been postulated. Theoretically, such reactions could occur after contact with the polymer, residual monomer, benzoyl peroxide, hydroquinone, pigments, or a reaction product between some component of the denture base and its environment.

Clinical experience indicates that true allergic reactions to acrylic resins seldom occur in the oral cavity. Residual monomer is most often cited as an irritant. The residual monomer content of a properly processed denture is less than 1%. However, allergic reactions are dose independent. Furthermore, surface monomer is completely eliminated after 17 hours of storage in water.

Based on the preceding information, reactions to residual monomer should occur shortly after prosthesis delivery. Most patients reporting a denture-induced sore mouth have worn the offending prostheses for months or even years. Clinical evaluation of these cases indicates tissue irritation generally is related to unhygienic conditions or trauma caused by poorly fitting denture bases.

Repeated or prolonged contact with monomer also may result in contact dermatitis. This condition is most commonly experienced by dentists and dental laboratory technicians involved in the manipulation of denture resins. Because of this possibility, dental personnel should refrain from handling such materials with ungloved hands. The high concentration of monomer in freshly mixed resins may produce local irritation and serious sensitization of the fingers.

Finally, inhalation of monomer vapor may be detrimental. Therefore, the use of monomer should be restricted to well-ventilated areas.

Toxicology. There is no indication that commonly used dental resins produce systemic effects in humans. As previously noted, the amount of residual monomer in processed poly(methyl methacrylate) is extremely low. To enter the circulatory system, residual monomer must pass through the oral mucosa and underlying tissues. These structures function as barriers that significantly diminish the volume of monomer reaching the blood stream.

Residual monomer that does reach the blood stream is rapidly hydrolyzed to methacrylic acid and excreted. It is estimated that the half-life of methyl methacrylate in circulating blood is 20 to 40 minutes.

RESIN TEETH FOR PROSTHODONTIC APPLICATIONS

More than 60% of preformed artificial teeth sold in the United States are made of acrylic or vinyl-acrylic resins. As might be expected, most resin teeth are based on poly(methyl methacrylate) chemistries.

Poly(methyl methacrylate) resins used in the fabrication of prosthetic teeth are similar to those used in denture base construction. Nevertheless, the degree of cross-linking within prosthetic teeth is somewhat greater than that within polymerized denture bases. This increase is achieved by elevating the amount of cross-linking agent in the denture base liquid, that is, the monomer. The resultant polymer displays enhanced stability and improved clinical properties.

Cervical portions of prosthetic teeth often exhibit reduced cross-linking. This feature facilitates chemical bonding with denture base resins. Bonding may be further enhanced by removing the glossy "ridge-lap" surfaces of resin teeth.

Chemical bonding between resin teeth and heat-activated denture base materials has proved extremely effective. Nonetheless, bond failures may occur if ridge-lap surfaces are contaminated by residual wax or misplaced separating media. Stone molds must be flushed with hot water, and exposed cervical portions of prosthetic teeth must be thoroughly cleaned with mild detergent solutions. Separating media must be applied to stone mold surfaces but should not be permitted to extend onto the exposed surfaces of resin teeth. As a final measure, ridge-lap surfaces should be wetted with monomer immediately before resin introduction. Adherence to these guidelines facilitates effective chemical interaction and enhanced bonding.

The use of mechanical retention has been the primary means for securing resin teeth to chemically activated denture base materials. Chemical bonding also may be used in joining these resins. To accomplish this, a mixture of equal volumes of methylene chloride and chemically activated methyl methacrylate monomer is applied to the necks of preformed resin teeth for approximately 5 minutes. Excess solution is then removed. This treatment produces softening of the resin and facilitates chemical bonding during denture base polymerization. Resultant bond strengths are similar to those obtained between resin teeth and heat-activated denture base resins.

Despite the current emphasis on resin teeth, prosthetic teeth also may be fabricated using dental porcelains. Hence, a comparison of resin and porcelain teeth is provided for completeness: Resin teeth display greater fracture toughness than porcelain teeth. As a result, resin teeth are less likely to chip or fracture on impact, such as when a denture is dropped. Furthermore, resin teeth are easier to adjust and display greater resistance to thermal shock. In comparison, porcelain teeth display better dimensional stability and increased wear resistance. Unfortunately, porcelain teeth, especially when contacting surfaces have been roughened, often cause significant wear of opposing enamel and gold surfaces. As a result, porcelain teeth should not oppose such surfaces, and if they are used, they should be polished periodically to reduce such abrasive damage.

As a final note, resin teeth are capable of chemical bonding with commonly used denture base resins. Porcelain teeth do not form chemical bonds with denture resins and must be retained by other means, such as mechanical undercuts and silanization.

MATERIALS IN MAXILLOFACIAL PROSTHETICS

For centuries, prostheses have been used to mask maxillofacial defects. Ancient Egyptians and Chinese used waxes and resins to reconstruct missing portions of the craniofacial complex. By the sixteenth century, the French surgeon Ambroise Paré described a variety of simple prostheses used for the cosmetic and functional replacement of maxillofacial structures. During subsequent years, restorative techniques and materials were slowly improved. Casualties in World Wars I and II established a great need for maxillofacial prosthetics, and the dental profession assumed a major role in reconstruction and rehabilitation processes.

Despite improvements in surgical and restorative techniques, the materials used in maxillofacial prosthetics are far from ideal. An ideal material should be inexpensive, biocompatible, strong, and stable. In addition, the material should be skinlike in color and texture. Maxillofacial materials must exhibit resistance to tearing and should be able to withstand moderate thermal and chemical challenges. Currently, no material fulfills all of these requirements. A brief description of maxillofacial materials is included in the following paragraphs.

Latexes. Latexes are soft, inexpensive materials that may be used to create lifelike prostheses. Unfortunately, these materials are weak, degenerate rapidly, exhibit color instability and can cause allergic reactions. Consequently, latexes are infrequently used in the fabrication of maxillofacial prostheses.

A recently developed synthetic latex is a tripolymer of butyl acrylate, methyl methacrylate, and methyl methacrylamide. Superior to natural latex, this material is nearly transparent. Colorants are sprayed onto the reverse or tissue side of the prosthesis, thereby providing enhanced translucency and improved blending. Despite these advantages, technical processes are lengthy, and resultant prostheses last only a few months. As a result, synthetic latexes have limited applications.

Vinyl Plastisols. Plasticized vinyl resins sometimes are used in maxillofacial applications. Plastisols are thick liquids comprising small vinyl particles dispersed in a plasticizer. Colorants are added to these materials to match individual skin tones. Subsequently, vinyl plastisols are heated to impart desired physical characteristics. Unfortunately, vinyl plastisols harden with age because of plasticizer loss. Ultraviolet light also has an adverse effect on these materials. For these reasons, the use of vinyl plastisols is limited.

Silicone Rubbers. Although silicones were introduced in the mid-1940s, only in recent years have they been used in maxillofacial applications. Both heat-vulcanizing and room temperature–vulcanizing silicones are in use today, and both exhibit advantages and disadvantages.

Room temperature–vulcanizing silicones are supplied as single-paste systems that are colored by the addition of dyed rayon fibers, dry earth pigments, and oil paints. Prostheses can be polymerized in artificial stone molds, but more durable molds can be made from epoxy resins or metals. These silicones are not as strong as the heat-vulcanized silicones and generally are monochromatic.

Heat-vulcanizing silicone is supplied as a semi-solid or puttylike material that requires milling, packing under pressure, and a 30-minute heat application cycle at 180° C. Pigments are milled into the material. As a result, intrinsic color can be achieved. Heat-vulcanizing silicone displays better strength and color stability than room temperature-vulcanizing silicones.

The major disadvantage of heat-vulcanizing silicones is the requirement for a milling machine and a press. Furthermore, a metal mold normally is used, and fabrication of the mold is a lengthy procedure. A stone mold within a denture flask may be used, but there is an increased risk of damage to the material during deflasking.

Polyurethane Polymers. Polyurethane is the most recent of the materials used in maxillofacial prosthetics. Fabrication of a polyurethane prosthesis requires accurate proportioning of three components. The material is placed in a stone or metal mold and allowed to polymerize at room temperature. Although a polyurethane prosthesis has a natural feel and appearance, it is susceptible to rapid deterioration.

Additional information may be found in texts that deal with the fabrication of maxillofacial prostheses.

SELECTED READING

Bates JF, Stanford GD, Huggett R, and Handley RW: Current status of pour-type denture base resins. J Dent 5:177, 1977.
The mechanical properties of pour-type denture resins were somewhat lower than those of conventional heat-cured resins, and they were more sensitive to laboratory variables.
Caswell CW, and Norling BK: Comparative study of the bond strengths of three abrasion-resistant plastic denture teeth bonded to a cross-linked and a grafted, cross-linked denture base material. J Prosthet Dent 55:701, 1986.
Based on bond strength measurements of denture base resin to resin teeth, it was found that 83% of fractures occurred within the teeth. Thus, the tensile strength of the tooth is as critical a factor as is the bond strength.
Chaing BKP: Polymers in the service of prosthetic dentistry. J Dent 12:203, 1984.
A comprehensive discussion of polymers used in prosthodontics and a citation of pertinent literature on materials such as denture polymers, soft liners, tissue conditioners, and impression materials.

Chalian VA: Evaluation and comparison of physical properties of materials used in maxillofacial prosthetics [Thesis]. Indiana University School of Dentistry, Indianapolis, Indiana, 1976.
A complete review of the materials used in maxillofacial prostheses, their comparative properties, and characteristics.

Clancy JMS, and Boyer DB: Comparative bond strengths of light-cured, heat-cured, and autopolymerizing denture resins to denture teeth. J Prosthet Dent 61:457, 1989.
Tensile bond strength of heat-cured, autopolymerizing, and light-cured resins to two types of plastic teeth were measured.

Devlin H, and Watts DC: Acrylic "allergy"? Br Dent J 157:272, 1984.
Possible mechanisms of allergy to acrylic resin are described.

Heath JR, Davenport JC, and Jones PA: The abrasion of acrylic resin by cleaning pastes. J Oral Rehabil 10:159, 1983.
A number of abrasive pastes were evaluated for wear on denture resin. The clinical relevance is discussed.

Levin B, Sanders JL, and Reitz PV: The use of microwave energy for processing acrylic resins. J Prosthet Dent 61:381, 1989.
Techniques and equipment for microwave processing are described.

McCabe JF, and Wilson HJ: The use of differential scanning calorimetry for the evaluation of dental materials. II. Denture base materials. J Oral Rehabil 7:235, 1980.
Results of this investigation indicate the glass transition temperature (T_g) for self polymerizing resins is considerably lower than the T_g for heat-cured resins.

Monsenego P, Baszkin A, deLourdes Costa J, and Lejoyeaus J: Complete denture retention: Wettability studies on various acrylic resin denture base materials. J Prosthet Dent 62:308, 1989.
Hydrophilic properties of denture resins were studied. Authors cautiously suggest that air-particle–abraded, heat-polymerized resin provided the best surface for denture retention.

Nyquist G: Study of denture sore mouth: An investigation of traumatic, allergic, and toxic lesions of the oral mucosa arising from the use of full dentures. Acta Odontol Scand 10:154, 1952.
Probably the most comprehensive survey of reported allergic reactions to acrylic resins. The incidence of a true allergy is extremely small.

Sanders JL, Levin B, and Reitz PV: Porosity in denture acrylic resins cured by microwave energy. Quint Int 18:453, 1987.
Microwave polymerization is an effective way of processing acrylic resins. Resultant denture bases appear extremely dense.

Shlosberg SR, Goodacre CJ, Munoz CA, et al: Microwave energy polymerization of poly(methyl methacrylate) denture base resin. Int J Prosthodont 2:453, 1989.
Transverse strength and hardness were comparable with microwave and traditional polymerization techniques. Significant porosity was produced when conventional resins were polymerized using microwave energy.

Smith DC, and Baines MED: Residual methyl methacrylate in the denture base and its relation to denture sore mouth. Br Dent J 98:55, 1955.
Free monomer in a properly polymerized denture leaches out within 17 hours, suggesting that this component is not a likely cause for tissue irritation.

Takamata T, and Setcos JC: Resin denture bases: Review of accuracy and methods of polymerization. Int J Prosthodont 2:555, 1989.
A review of the literature related to modifications in denture base resins, including pourable, microwave, and light-activated systems.

Takamata T, Setcos JC, Phillips RW, and Boone ME: Adaptation of acrylic resin dentures influenced by the activation mode of polymerization. J Am Dent Assoc 118:271, 1989.
Five resins and four processing techniques were evaluated. The two best-fitting groups were prepared from an autopolymerizing resin and the microwave-activated resin.

Tan H-K, Brudvik JS, Nicholls JI, and Smith DE: Adaptation of a visible light-cured denture base material. J Prosthet Dent 61:326, 1989.
Various methods were used to adapt light-polymerizing resin sheets to casts. Vacuum forming produced the best adaptation.

Tulacha GJ, and Moser JB: Evaluation of viscoelastic behavior of a light-cured denture resin. J Prosthet Dent 61:695, 1989.
The viscoelastic properties of a light-polymerizing reline resin (Triad) were compared with those of a rubber-base impression material and a prototype light-polymerizing resin paste.

Vermilyea SG, Powers JM, and Koran A: The rheological properties of fluid denture base resins. J Dent Res 57:227, 1978.
The rheologic properties of six fluid resins were determined. Materials displayed initial non-newtonian behavior and increased viscosity over time.

12 *Restorative Resins*

- Resin-based Restorative Materials
- Composite Restorative Materials
- Curing
- Classification of Resin-based Composites
- Composites for Posterior Restorations
- Prosthodontic Resins
- Biocompatibility of Composites
- Techniques for Insertion of Composites
- Repair of Composites

RESIN-BASED RESTORATIVE MATERIALS

Synthetic resins evolved as restorative materials because they are insoluble, aesthetic, insensitive to dehydration, inexpensive, and relatively easy to manipulate. However, soon after their introduction during the late 1940s and the early 1950s, they were found to be only partially successful in meeting the requirements of a durable aesthetic restorative material for anterior teeth. Certain characteristics, such as a toothlike appearance and insolubility in oral fluids, made them superior to silicate cements, whereas their high polymerization shrinkage and high coefficient of thermal expansion led to clinical deficiencies and premature failures.

To resolve the deficiencies caused by high polymerization shrinkage and a high coefficient of thermal expansion, inert filler particles were added to reduce the volume of the resinous component. The first attempts to improve the performance of composites were not too successful because the filler particles were not chemically bonded to the resin matrix. The incomplete filler resin bond resulted in microscopic defects between the mechanically retained filler particles and the surrounding resin. These defective areas became stained because of fluid leakage, and the surface appearance of restorations was often unacceptable. The poor filler retention also contributed to filler loss and poor wear resistance.

A major advance occurred when Bowen developed a new type of composite material. His main innovations were bisphenol A–glycidyl methacrylate (bis-GMA), a dimethacrylate resin, and the use of a silane to coat filler particles that could bond chemically to the resin. Because bis-GMA has a higher molecular weight than methyl methacrylate, the density of methacrylate double-bond groups is lower in the bis-GMA monomer, a factor that reduces polymerization shrinkage. The use of a dimethacrylate also results in extensive cross-linking and an improvement in the properties of the polymer.

The improved matrix properties and filler-matrix bonding yielded a restorative material that was clearly superior to the unfilled acrylic resins. Since the early 1970s, the composites have virtually replaced the unfilled acrylics for tooth restorations. The resin-based composite systems and their dimethacrylate resins have been used for other dental applications, such as pit and fissure sealants, dentin bonding agents, luting cements for fixed restorations, and veneering materials. The general composition of the various resin-based composites is now discussed in conjunction with their properties, manipulative procedures, and factors that influence clinical behavior.

COMPOSITE RESTORATIVE MATERIALS

The term *composite material* may be defined as a compound of two or more distinctly different materials with properties that are superior or intermediate to those of the individual constituents. Examples of natural composite materials are tooth enamel and dentin. In enamel, enamelin represents the organic matrix, whereas in dentin the matrix consists of collagen. In both of these "composites," the filler particles consist of hydroxyapatite crystals. The difference in the properties of these two tissues is associated in part with differences in the matrix:filler ratios.

Development of modern dental composite restorative materials started in the late 1950s and early 1960s, when Bowen began experiments to reinforce epoxy resins with filler particles. Deficiencies in the epoxy resin system, such as a slow curing rate and a tendency to discolor, stimulated him to work on combining the advantages of epoxies and acrylates. This work culminated in the development of the bis-GMA molecule. It satisfied many of the requirements for the resin matrix of a dental composite. With this breakthrough, the composite materials rapidly replaced silicate cement and acrylic resins for aesthetic restoration of anterior teeth.

Modern composite materials contain a number of components. Major constituents are the resin matrix and the inorganic filler particles. Besides these two constituents, several other components are required to enhance the effectiveness and durability of the material. A coupling agent (silane) is required to provide a bond between the inorganic filler particles and the resin matrix, and an activator-initiator is necessary to polymerize the resin. Small amounts of other additives improve color stability (ultraviolet [UV] light absorbers) and prevent premature polymerization (inhibitors such as hydroquinone). The composite must also contain pigments to achieve an acceptable match to the color of tooth structure.

Resin Matrix. Most dental composite materials use monomers that are aromatic or aliphatic diacrylates. Bis-GMA, urethane dimethacrylate (UEDMA), and triethylene glycol dimethacrylate (TEGDMA) are the most commonly used dimethacrylates in dental composites (Fig. 12–1).

The high-molecular-weight monomers, particularly bis-GMA, are extremely viscous at room temperatures. The use of diluent monomers is essential to attain high filler levels and to produce pastes of clinically usable consistencies. Diluents can be methacrylate monomers but they usually are dimethacrylate monomers, such as TEGDMA. The reduction in viscosity is significant when TEGDMA is added to bis-GMA. A blend of 75 wt% bis-GMA and 25 wt% TEGDMA has a

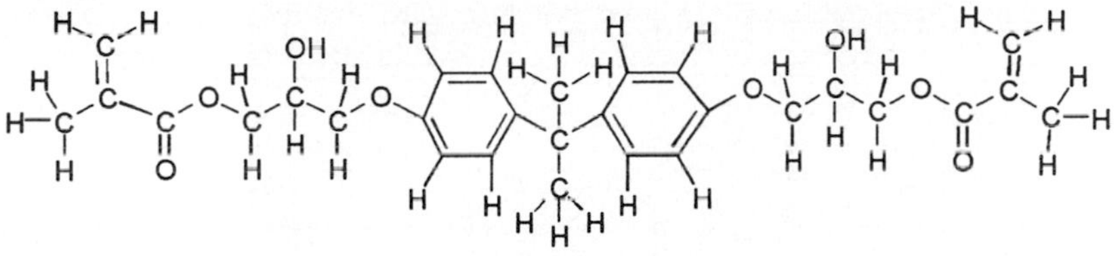

bisGMA

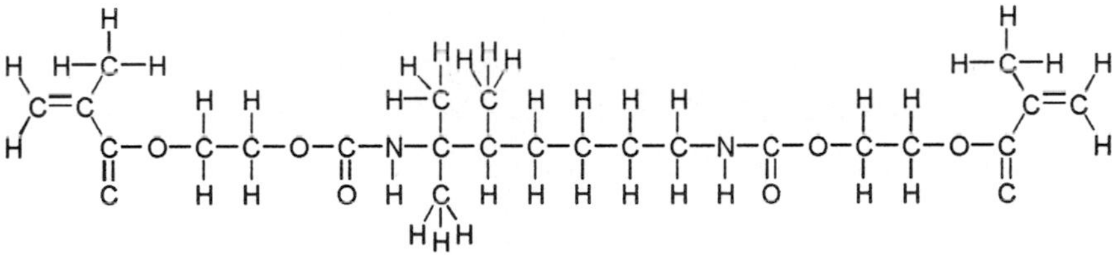

UEDMA

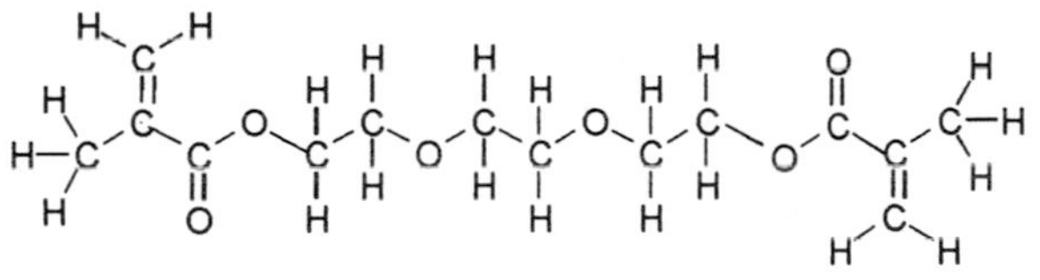

TEGDMA

Figure 12–1. The two resins bis-GMA and UEDMA are used as base resins, whereas TEGDMA is used as a diluent to reduce the viscosity of the base resins, particularly that of bis-GMA.

viscosity of 4300 cP (centiPoise), whereas the viscosity of a 50/50 blend is 200 cP. Unfortunately, the addition of TEGDMA or other low-molecular-weight dimethacrylates increases the polymerization shrinkage, a factor that limits the amount of low-molecular-weight dimethacrylates that can be used in a composite. The dimethacrylate monomers allow extensive cross-linking to occur between chains. This results in a matrix that is more resistant to degradation by solvents.

Although the mechanical properties of the bis-GMA resin are superior to those of acrylic resin, it does not bond to tooth structure more effectively. Thus, the polymerization shrinkage and thermal dimensional change are still important considerations even for filled resins.

In addition to the monomer, other additives are blended within the matrix resin including an activator-initiator system, inhibitors, UV light absorbers, pigments, and opacifiers. These components are present in small concentrations and are discussed in later sections.

Filler Particles. Incorporation of filler particles into a resin matrix significantly improves the properties of the matrix material if the filler particles are well bonded to the matrix. If not, the filler particles can weaken the material. Because

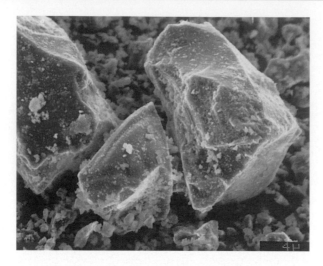

Figure 12–2. Ground quartz particles (with a diameter of 20 to 30 μm) used as filler particles in traditional composites. The smaller particles seen in the background contribute to a broad particle-size distribution.

of the importance of well-bonded filler particles, it is obvious that the use of a filler coupling agent is extremely important to the success of a composite.

Obviously, because less resin is present in a composite, the polymerization shrinkage is reduced, as compared with unfilled resins. Although shrinkage varies from one product to another, it is on the order of 3 vol% at 24 hours. Water sorption and the coefficient of thermal expansion also are less for composites compared with unfilled resins. Mechanical properties such as compressive strength, tensile strength, and modulus of elasticity are improved, as is the abrasion resistance. All these improvements occur with an increase in the volume fraction of filler.

Filler particles are most commonly produced by grinding or milling quartz or glasses to produce particles ranging in size from 0.1 to 100 μm (Fig. 12–2). Silica particles of colloidal size (approximately 0.04 μm), referred to collectively as the *microfiller* or individually as *microfillers*, are obtained by a pyrolytic or precipitation process. During the pyrolytic process, the silicon atoms are present in low-molecular-weight compounds, such as $SiCl_4$, that are typically polymerized by burning $SiCl_4$ in an O_2 and H_2 atmosphere. During this process, macromolecules consisting of SiO_2 are formed, explaining why these particles are called *pyrogenic* (born in fire) *silica particles* (Fig. 12–3). These macromolecules are of a colloidal size and constitute the filler particles (Fig. 12–4).

Composites often are classified on the basis of the average size of the major filler component. In addition to filler volume level, the size, size distribution, index of refraction, radiopacity, and hardness are also important factors in

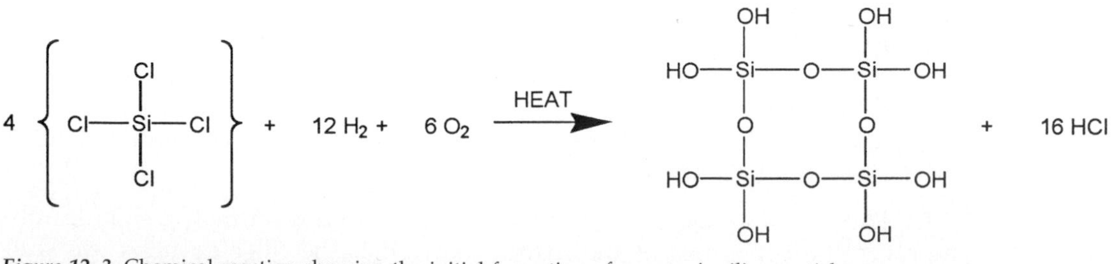

Figure 12–3. Chemical reaction showing the initial formation of pyrogenic silica particles.

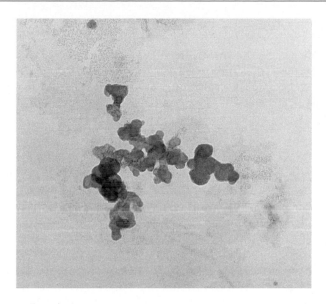

Figure 12–4. Transmission electron microscope image of pyrogenic silica particles (diameter of 0.04 μm).

determining the properties and the clinical application of the resultant composites.

To incorporate a maximum amount of filler into a resin matrix, a distribution of particle sizes is necessary. It is obvious that if a single particle size is used, even with close packing, a space will exist between particles (consider filling a box with marbles). Smaller particles can fill these spaces and, by extending this process, a continuous distribution of particles can afford maximum filler loading. Most composites also contain some colloidal silica. Inorganic filler particles generally account for between 30 and 70 vol% or 50 to 85 wt% of the composite.

The amount of filler that can be incorporated into the resin matrix generally is affected by the relative filler surface area. Colloidal silica particles have large total surface areas ranging from 50 to 300 m²/g. Thus, even small amounts of filler particles have a large total surface area that can form polar bonds with the monomer molecules and thicken the resin. Microfillers, because of their large surface area, are frequently added to composite formulations in amounts of less than 5 wt% to modify the paste viscosity, thereby reducing the risk for sedimentation of the ground particles. The microfillers also enhance filler packing. As discussed for the microfilled composites, colloidal silica is the only inorganic filler.

To ensure acceptable aesthetics of a composite restoration, the translucency of the filler must be similar to that of tooth structure. To ensure acceptable translucency, the index of refraction of the filler must closely match that of the resin. For bis-GMA and TEGDMA, the refractive indices are about 1.55 and 1.46, respectively, and a mixture of the two components in equal proportions by weight yields a refractive index of about 1.5. Most of the glasses and quartz that are used for fillers have refractive indices of approximately 1.5, which is adequate to achieve sufficient translucency.

Quartz has been used extensively as a filler, particularly in the first generation of composites. It has the advantage of being chemically inert but it is also extremely hard, making it difficult to grind into fine particles. Thus, quartz-containing composites are more difficult to polish and may cause more abrasion of opposing teeth or restorations.

The radiopacity of filler materials is provided by a number of glasses and ceramics that contain heavy metals such as barium (Ba), strontium (Sr), and zirconium (Zr). These glasses also have indices of refraction of about 1.5 to match that of the resin. The most commonly used glass filler is barium glass. Although this filler provides radiopacity, it is not as inert as quartz in an aqueous medium. Differences in the composition of storage medium (water vs. saliva) affect the leachability, making it difficult to predict the clinical effects of exposure to saliva.

Coupling Agents. As mentioned earlier, it is important that the filler particles are bonded to the resin matrix. This allows the more flexible polymer matrix to transfer stresses to the stiffer filler particles. The bond between the two phases of the composite is provided by a *coupling agent*. A properly applied coupling agent can impart improved physical and mechanical properties and provide hydrolytic stability by preventing water from penetrating along the filler-resin interface.

Although titanates and zirconates can be used as coupling agents, organosilanes such γ-methacryloxypropyltrimethoxy silane are used most commonly (Fig. 12–5). In its hydrolyzed state, the silane contains silanol groups that can bond with silanols on the filler surface by formation of a siloxane bond (S—O—Si). The methacrylate groups of the organosilane compound form covalent bonds with the resin when it is polymerized, thus completing the coupling process (Fig. 12–6).

The importance of proper coupling by means of the organsilanes is extremely important to the clinical performance of the resin-based composite.

Activator-Initiator System. Methyl methacrylates and dimethyl methacrylate monomers polymerize by the addition polymerization mechanism initiated by free radicals as described earlier. Free radicals can be generated by chemical activation or by external energy activation (heat or light). Because dental composites for direct placement use either chemical or light activation, both systems are discussed.

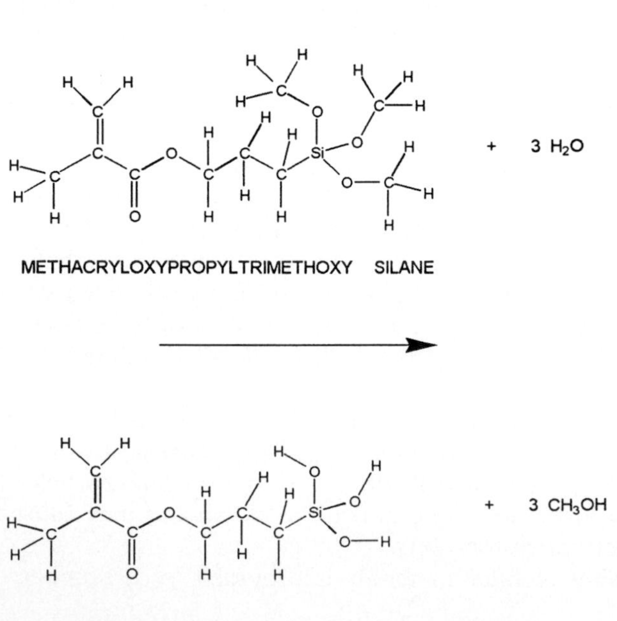

METHACRYLOXYPROPYLTRIMETHOXY SILANE

+   3 H₂O

+   3 CH₃OH

Figure 12–5. Hydrolysis of silane. The chemical formula shows the structure of γ-methacryloxypropyltrimethoxy silane and how this silane is hydrolyzed to form silanol groups.

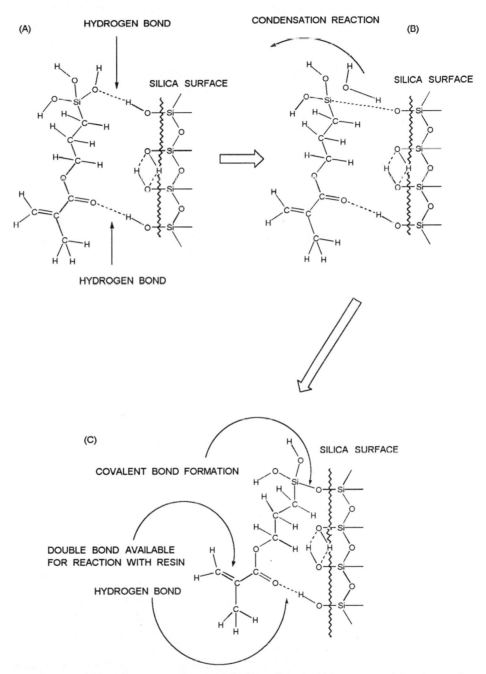

Figure 12–6. *A,* The hydrolyzed silane molecule approaches the OH— groups of the silica surface. When this occurs, hydrogen bonds develop between the silanol groups of the silane and an isolated OH- group of the silica surface. In addition, the carbonyl group of the silane also forms a hydrogen bond to an isolated OH- group of the silica surface. *B,* The interaction between the silanol group of the silane and the OH- group of the silica results in a condensation reaction. This reaction results in a covalent bond formation between the silane molecule and the silica surface during the release of a water molecule. *C,* The remaining hydrogen bond orients the silane molecule parallel to the silica surface. In a real composite, though, the filler is covered with many layers of silane, making the "interphase" much more complex than that represented in this figure. (Adapted from Söderholm K-J, and Shang S-W: Molecular orientation of silane at the surface of colloidal silica. J Dent Res 72:1050, 1993.)

Chemically Activated Resins. Chemically activated materials are supplied as two pastes, one of which contains the benzoyl peroxide initiator and the other a tertiary amine activator (N,N-dimethyl-*p*-toluidine), as previously described for the acrylic resins. When the two pastes are spatulated, the amine reacts with the benzoyl peroxide to form free radicals, and addition polymerization is initiated. These materials are mainly used for restorations and build-ups that are not readily cured with a light source.

Light-Activated Resins. The first light-activated systems used UV light to initiate free radicals. Today, the UV light-cured composites have been replaced by *visible* light-activating systems with a greatly improved ability to polymerize thicker increments up to 2 mm. Also, visible light-activated composites are much more widely used than are chemically activated materials. Light-curable dental composites are supplied as a single paste contained in a syringe. The free radical initiating system, consisting of the photoinitiator molecule and an amine activator, is contained in this paste. When these two components are left unexposed to light, they do not interact. However, exposure to light of the correct wavelength (approximately 468 nm) produces an excited state of the photoinitiator and an interaction with the amine to form free radicals that initiate addition polymerization (Fig. 12–7).

A commonly used photoinitiator is camphoroquinone, which has an absorption range between 400 and 500 nm that is in the blue region of the visible light spectrum. This initiator is present in the paste at levels of approximately 0.2 wt% or less. There are a number of amine accelerators that are suitable for interaction with camphoroquinone such as 0.15 wt% dimethylaminoethyl methacrylate, which is present in the paste.

Inhibitors. To minimize or prevent spontaneous polymerization of monomers, inhibitors are added to the resin systems. These inhibitors have a strong reactivity potential with free radicals. If a free radical has been formed, such as by a brief exposure to light when the material was dispensed, the inhibitor reacts with the free radical and thus inhibits chain propagation by terminating the ability of the free radical to initiate the polymerization process. When all the inhibitors have been consumed, chain propagation will occur. A typical inhibitor is butylated hydroxytoluene that is used in a concentration of 0.01 wt%.

Optical Modifiers. To match the appearance of teeth, dental composites must have visual coloration (shading) and translucency that can simulate tooth structure. Shading is achieved by adding different pigments. These pigments often consist of different metal oxides that are added in minute amounts.

Translucency or opacity is provided to simulate dentin and enamel. For example, if a Class IV incisal area is reconstructed, the translucency of a composite allows too much light to pass through the restoration. As a result, less light is reflected or scattered back to the observer, who perceives that the incisal edge is too dark. By adding an opacifier, this deficiency can be corrected. However, by adding too much opacifier, too much light may be reflected and the observer then perceives that the restoration is "too white," or more correctly, is "too high in value." To increase the opacity, the manufacturer adds titanium dioxide and aluminum oxide in minute amounts (0.001 to 0.007 wt%) to composites because these oxides are effective opacifiers.

All optical modifiers affect the light transmission ability of a composite.

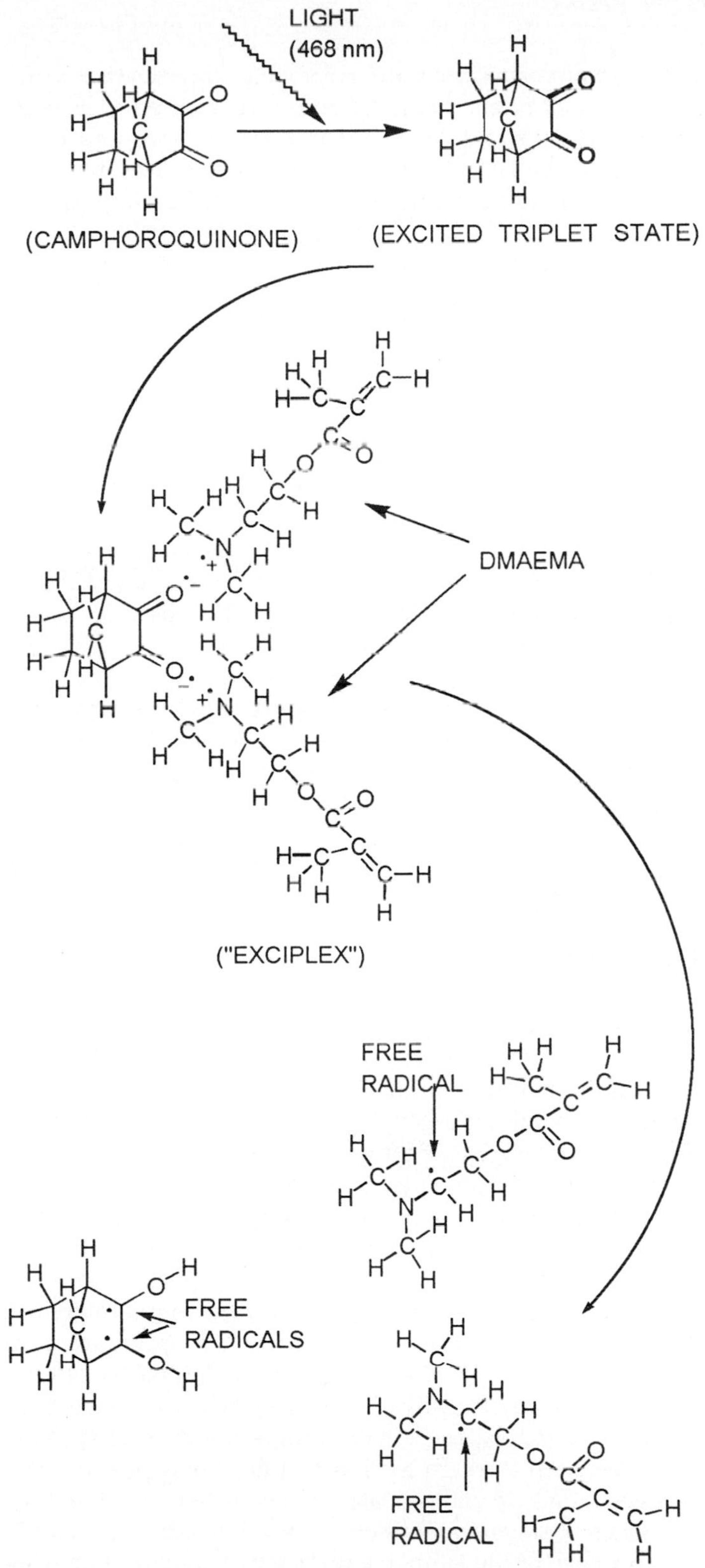

Figure 12–7. Light activation is initiated by energy transfer to the diketone (champhoroquinone). The excited triplets attract DMAEMA molecules and form exciplexes (i.e., excited complexes) that convert both the champhoroquinone and the DMAEMA molecules to free radicals.

281

Because most composites are light cured, this suggests that different shades and opacities have a different depth of cure when cured with light. Studies have confirmed this theory and suggest that darker shades and opacifiers should be placed in thinner layers to optimize polymerization. This consideration is important, because it can also affect the cure of a bonding agent covered with a composite layer.

CURING

The first composites were cured by a chemically activated polymerization process, often referred to as *cold curing* (also called *chemical curing* or *self curing*). Cold curing is initiated by mixing two pastes. During the mixing process it is almost impossible to avoid incorporating air bubbles into the mix. These air bubbles contain oxygen that causes oxygen inhibition during polymerization. Another problem with cold curing is that the operator has no control of the working time after the material has been mixed. Thus, both insertion and contouring must be finished soon after the initiation stage. Thus, the polymerization process is continuously disturbed until the operator has finished the contouring process.

To overcome these problems, materials that required no mixing were developed. This objective was achieved by use of a light source for activation of the initiator system. Considering the drawbacks of the cold-cured resins, it is obvious that the light-cured materials have significant advantages by allowing the operator to complete both insertion and contouring before curing is initiated. Furthermore, when curing is initiated, it takes only 40 seconds of cure time until a 2-mm thick layer has been cured, whereas, for a chemically cured material, setting takes several minutes. Another advantage of the light-curing systems is that they are not as sensitive to oxygen inhibition as the cold-cured systems. However, there are also some limitations with the light-cured composites. First, they have to be placed incrementally when the bulk exceeds a thickness of 2 mm. This means that placing large restorations, such as Class II restorations, can be rather time consuming. Other drawbacks include (1) the tendency to shrink toward the light source, resulting in a pull-back from marginal regions located farther away from the light source, and (2) the complicating factors associated with a light source. Modern light sources are hand-held devices that contain the light source and are equipped with a relatively short, rigid light guide made up of fused optical fibers. The light source is usually a tungsten halogen light bulb. White light generated by the bulb passes through a filter that removes the infrared and visible spectrum for wavelengths greater than 500 nm. There can be a significant difference in the output for various manufactured lights, including the range of wavelengths that they cover. For example, if the light intensity varies by a factor of four, which is not unusual, 80 to 240 seconds might be required for a low-intensity light to achieve the same results as that produced by a 20- to 60-second exposure with a high-intensity light. When attempting to polymerize the resin through tooth structure, the exposure time should be two or three times longer to compensate for the reduction in light intensity.

Light sources also generate different light intensities over time, depending on the quality and age of the lamp, the presence of contamination such as composite material residue on the light tip, and the distance between light tip and restoration. Consequently, the light source should be checked regularly, and the operator should always place the light tip as close as possible to the restorative material. Also, the operator should be aware that light is absorbed when passing through tooth structure, thereby causing incomplete curing in critical regions such as proximal boxes.

Light attenuation coefficients for various composites can also vary considerably from one material to another, depending on the opacity, filler size, filler concentration, and shade of the pigments. The intensity of light can be reduced by a factor of 10 to 100 in a 2-mm-thick layer of composite. Polymerization at any depth relies on attaining a particular concentration of free radicals. This implies that a particular number of photons must be available that is directly related to the light intensity and the time of exposure. Manufacturers recommend curing times for each material and shade, based on a particular curing device.

Because of the potential disadvantages of light-cured materials, there is still a need for chemically cured composites and resins. For example, when a resin cement is needed under metallic restorations, only chemically cured materials can be used with reliable results.

One way to solve the problems associated with light curing is to combine cold-curing and visible light-curing components in the same material. Such materials are commercially available and consist of two light-curable pastes, one of which contains benzoyl peroxide, whereas a tertiary amine is added to the other. When the clinician mixes these two pastes and then exposes them to light, both light curing and cold curing are achieved with the same material. These materials are called *dual-cured materials* and are recommended for cementation of ceramic inlays that may be too thick to allow a sufficient amount of light to radiate through to produce adequate conversion of the monomer.

In addition to chemical and light curing, heat can also be used. For example, a chemically or light-cured composite can be used to produce an inlay on a tooth or a die. That inlay can be cured directly within the tooth or on the die and then transferred to an oven where it receives additional heat curing or light curing. After completion, the inlay is then cemented with a resin-based composite to the tooth.

Degree of Conversion. The degree of conversion is a measure of the percentage of consumed carbon double bonds (Fig. 12–8). In other words, a conversion degree of 50% to 60%, which is typical of bis-GMA–based composites, implies

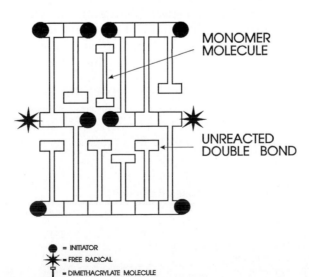

MONOMER MOLECULE

UNREACTED DOUBLE BOND

● = INITIATOR
✳ = FREE RADICAL
I = DIMETHACRYLATE MOLECULE

Figure 12–8. Degree of conversion reflects the percentage of consumed methacrylate double bonds. The figure shows that a dimethacrylate monomer molecule can have one or two unreacted groups. If one group has reacted, the molecule is bonded to the polymer network and will not be released from the polymer as the completely unreacted monomer molecule.

that 50% to 60% of the methacrylate groups have polymerized. This does not imply that 40% to 50% of the monomer molecules are left in the resin, because one of the two methacrylate groups per dimethacrylate molecule may have reacted and be covalently bonded to the polymer structure. Conversion of the monomer to polymer is dependent on several factors, such as the resin composition, the transmission of light through the material, and the amount of activator-initiator and inhibitor that is present. Transmission of light through the material is controlled by absorption and scattering of the light by filler particles and by any tooth structure interposed between the light source and composite.

The total degree of conversion within resins does not differ between chemically activated and light-activated composites containing the same monomer formulations as long as adequate light curing is employed. Degree of conversion values of 50% to 70% are achieved at room temperature for both materials. Likewise, the total polymerization shrinkage of comparable light-activated and chemically activated resins does not differ.

CLASSIFICATION OF RESIN-BASED COMPOSITES

A number of classification systems have been proposed for resin-based composites. One classification system is based on the mean particle size of the major filler (Table 12–1). Subgroups and overlapping may exist for some of these categories, particularly for the *hybrid* category. For instance, a hybrid composite can be one that uses ground filler from either the small or the conventional categories, in combination with microfillers. Actually, resins that contain any combination of ground fillers and microfillers theoretically can be considered as hybrids.

This broad definition is not meaningful, because most modern dental composites that use ground fillers also contain small amounts of microfillers (<5 wt%) that are added to adjust the paste to the desired viscosity and to minimize sedimentation of the larger particles over time. However, the term *hybrid composite* usually refers to materials that contain ground fillers with an average particle size of 0.6 to 1.0 mm in combination with 10 to 15 wt% microfiller. It is within these guidelines that the term hybrid composites are subsequently discussed.

Composition of Traditional Composites. The traditional composites are those that were developed during the 1970s and that have been slightly modified over the years. These composites are also referred to as *conventional* or *macrofilled* composites—the latter because of the relatively large size of the filler particles. Because these materials are no longer the most commonly used materials, the term *conventional* should be replaced with *traditional*. The most commonly used filler for these materials is ground quartz. As can be seen in the photomicrograph of the ground quartz filler in Figure 12–2, there is a wide distribution in particle size. Although the average size is 8 to 12 μm, particles as large as 50 μm may

TABLE 12–1. Classification of Resin-based Composites

Category	Average Particle Size (μm)
Traditional composite	8–12
Small particle–filled composite	1–5
Microfilled composite	0.04–0.4
Hybrid composite	0.6–1.0

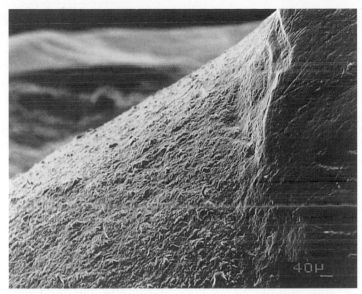

Figure 12–9. Surface of traditional composite (occlusal surface of a posterior composite) that has been in clinical service for 5 years. As shown, the composite has worn (see occlusal margins to the right) and coarse filler particles are being exposed making the surface extremely rough.

also be present. Filler loading generally is 70 to 80 wt% or 60 to 65 vol%. Exposed filler particles, some quite large, are surrounded by appreciable amounts of the resin matrix (Fig. 12–9).

Properties of Traditional Composites. Physical and mechanical properties of traditional composite resins are listed in Table 12–2. Individual products may deviate from these values, but those shown are representative of the properties of the composite categories.

In comparing the properties of traditional composites with those for unfilled acrylic materials, it is obvious that significant improvements have been obtained through a composite structure. The compressive strength of four types of composite materials (see Table 12–2) is substantially improved by 300% to 500%

TABLE 12–2. Properties of Composite Restorative Materials

	Composite Material				
Property	Unfilled Acrylic	Traditional	Microfilled	Small Particle	Hybrid
Inorganic filler					
vol%	0	60–65	20–55	65–77	60–65
wt%	0	70–80	35–60	80–90	75–80
Compressive strength (MPa)	70	250–300	250–350	350–400	300–350
Tensile strength (MPa)	24	50–65	30–50	75–90	70–90
Elastic modulus (GPa)	2.4	8–15	3–6	15–20	7–12
Thermal expansion coefficient ($10^{-6/°}$ C)	92.8	25–35	50–60	19–26	30–40
Water sorption (mg/cm^2)	1.7	0.5–0.7	1.4–1.7	0.5–0.6	0.5–0.7
Knoop hardness number	15	55	5–30	50–60	50–60

through the transfer of stress to the filler particles compared with the strength of unfilled acrylics. Similarly, the elastic modulus is four to six times greater, and the tensile strength is doubled. Likewise, water sorption is reduced, the polymerization shrinkage is approximately 2 vol%, and the thermal expansion is approximately 30×10^{-6} per degree centigrade as compared with 93×10^{-6} per degree centigrade for unfilled acrylic. However, this value is still approximately three times that of tooth structure.

Hardness is considerably greater for composites than for unfilled acrylic resins (approximately 55 Knoop hardness number compared with 15 Knoop hardness number, respectively). The increase is associated with both the filler reinforcement and the cross-linked resin structure. In general, these composites are more resistant to abrasion than are unfilled acrylics. However, they suffer from roughening of the surface as a result of the selective abrasion of the softer resin matrix surrounding the harder filler particles. Composites using quartz as a filler are radiolucent. Their radiopacity is less than that of dentin.

Clinical Considerations of Traditional Composites. A major clinical disadvantage of traditional composites is the rough surface that develops during abrasive wear of the soft-resin matrix that leaves the more wear-resistant filler particles elevated, as diagrammed in Figure 12–9. Finishing of the restoration can produce a roughened surface, as does tooth brushing and masticatory wear over time. These restorations also have a tendency to discolor, in part because of the susceptibility of the rough textured surface to retain stain. Fracture of the conventional composites is not a common problem even when they are employed for stress-bearing restorations such as those in Class IV and II sites.

However, the poor resistance of traditional composites to occlusal wear has been a clinical problem. From this standpoint, they are inferior to materials specifically designated as *posterior composites,* as discussed in a subsequent section. Although polymerization shrinkage and the coefficient of thermal expansion are substantially reduced by the high inorganic filler content compared with unfilled acrylic resins, the resin matrix does not bond chemically to tooth structure. Therefore, techniques of placement must be meticulously carried out, and they must include measures to reduce the effects of these sources of dimensional change.

Composition of Microfilled Composite. In an effort to overcome the problems of surface roughening associated with traditional composites, a class of materials was developed that use colloidal silica particles as the inorganic filler. The individual particles are approximately 0.04 μm in size; thus, they are 200 to 300 times smaller than the average quartz particle in traditional composites. The concept of the *microfilled composite* entails the reinforcement of the resin by means of the filler, yet these composites exhibit a smooth surface similar to that obtained with the unfilled direct-filling acrylic resins.

These tiny colloidal silica particles tend to agglomerate. Agglomerates of raw colloidal silica filler can be seen in Figure 12–10. During mixing, some, but not all, of the agglomerates are broken up. Incidentally, agglomerates account for the 0.04- to 0.4-μm size given in the table used earlier to categorize various types of composites.

It would be ideal if this colloidal silica filler could be added in large amounts directly to the resin matrix. However, this is impossible, as was mentioned earlier, because the large surface area that must be wetted by the matrix resin results in undue thickening even with very small additions of microfillers.

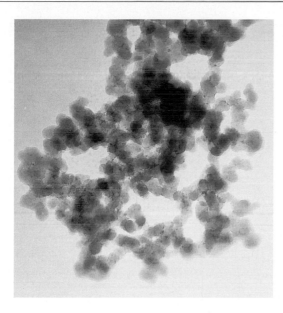

Figure 12–10. The large total surface area of pyrogenic silica used in microfilled composites often causes the pyrogenic silica particles to agglomerate (transmission electron micrograph).

Although several approaches may be used to increase the filler loading, each compromises the idealized concept of a resin filled with dispersed colloidal silica. One approach is to sinter the colloidal silica so that particles several tenths of a micron in size are obtained. This larger agglomerate results in a reduced surface area, allowing more filler to be incorporated with less compromise to the rheology of the material.

The most common method for increasing the filler loading is to make new filler particles from a prepolymerized composite that is highly loaded with colloidal silica particles. Particles of this highly microfilled material are then incorporated in the resin paste to produce a filling material with acceptable handling characteristics.

The preparation of the prepolymerized filler involves adding 60 to 70 wt% (about 50 vol%) of silane-coated colloidal silica to the monomer at a slightly elevated temperature to lower its viscosity. When the filler is thoroughly mixed into the resin, the composite paste is heat cured using the conventional benzoyl peroxide initiator. The degree of conversion of the resin is about 80%. The cured composite is then ground into particles of sizes often larger than the quartz particles used in the traditional composites. The prepolymerized particles are often called *organic fillers,* a term that is not technically correct because they contain a high percentage of inorganic filler. These "composite particles," along with additional silane-coated colloidal silica, are then mixed into the matrix resin to form the composite paste. A diagram representing the structure of microfilled resins of this type is shown in Figure 12–11.

The final inorganic filler content may be only about 50 wt% (or 30 to 40 vol%), but if the composite particles are counted as filler particles, the filler content is closer to 80 wt% (approximately 60 vol%). This is an important consideration for understanding certain properties of these materials, such as the volumetric shrinkage during polymerization. The composite particles do not shrink when the composite is cured. Thus, a microfilled composite, despite having a much lower volume fraction of inorganic filler than a more conventional composite, does not shrink as much as one would expect when one considers the total resin volume. The weakness of these materials is that the bond between the composite

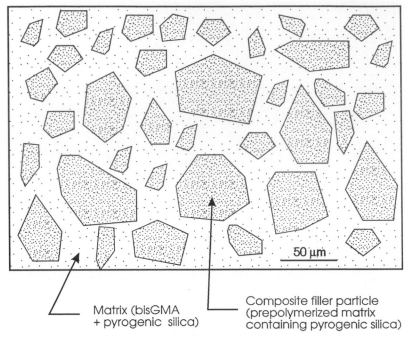

Matrix (bisGMA
+ pyrogenic silica)

Composite filler particle
(prepolymerized matrix
containing pyrogenic silica)

Figure 12–11. Schematic drawing of a microfilled composite. As seen in this drawing, a microfilled composite contains composite filler particles mixed with a curable matrix. The pyrogenic silica particles are present in both the composite filler particles and the curable matrix, but the composite filler particles contain a substantially higher concentration of silica particles.

particles and the curable matrix is weak, facilitating chipping of such restorations (Fig. 12–12). Because of the latter deficiency, most microfilled composites are unsuitable for use as stress-bearing surfaces.

Properties of Microfilled Composite. Microfilled composites have physical and mechanical properties that are inferior to those of traditional composites (see Table 12–2). This is to be expected, because 50 to 70 vol% of the restorative material is made up of resin. The larger amount of resin compared with filler results in greater water sorption, a higher coefficient of thermal expansion, and decreased elastic modulus. In addition, the weak bond of the prepolymerized particles to the resin matrix produces results that are similar to those of the composites that contain unsilanized filler particles. The decreased tensile strength may be related to crack propagation around the poorly bonded filler particles. The microfilled composites are remarkably wear resistant and thus they are comparable in wear resistance to the more highly filled and wear-resistant composites.

However, compared with unfilled acrylic resins, microfilled composites have significantly improved properties, and they provide a smoother surface finish desired for aesthetic restorations than the other composites. Thus, they are often preferred for restoring smooth surface caries lesions (Classes III and V). The inorganic filler particles are smaller than the abrasive particles used for finishing the restoration. Thus, during finishing the silica filler is removed along with the resin in which it is embedded.

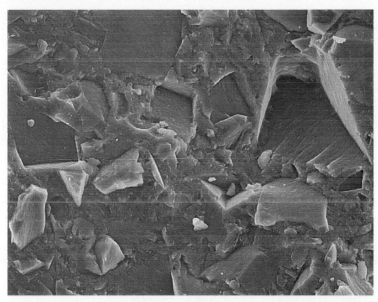

Figure 12–12. Fractured microfilled composite. The fracture surface shows that the composite filler particles are being pulled out, suggesting a poor bond between these particles and the surrounding matrix.

Clinical Considerations of Microfilled Composite. For most applications, the decreased physical properties do not create problems. However, in stress-bearing situations, such as Class I, II, and IV sites, the potential for chipping is greater. The occasional chipping that has been observed at the margins of restorations has been attributed to debonding of the prepolymerized composite filler. To minimize the risk for chipping, diamond burs rather than fluted tungsten-carbide burs are recommended for trimming microfilled composites. Nonetheless, microfilled composites are widely used today. Because of their smooth surface they have become the resin of choice for aesthetic restoration of anterior teeth, particularly in non-stress-bearing situations, and for restoring subgingival areas.

Properties of Small Particle–Filled Composites. Small particle–filled composites were developed in an attempt to achieve the surface smoothness of microfilled composites and yet retain or improve on the physical and mechanical properties of traditional composites. To achieve this goal, the inorganic fillers are ground to a size smaller than those used in traditional composites.

The average filler size of these materials ranges from 1 to 5 μm, but the distribution of sizes is fairly broad, as can be seen in Figure 12–13. This broad particle-size distribution facilitates a high filler loading, and small particle–filled composites generally contain more inorganic filler (80 wt% and 60 to 65 vol%) than traditional composites. This is particularly true of those designated for posterior restorations. The high density of filler particles, compared with that of the matrix resin, is evident in the polished specimen of the small particle–filled composite shown in Figure 12–14.

Some small particle–filled composites use quartz particles as fillers, but most incorporate glasses that contain heavy metals. The matrix resin of these materials is similar to that of traditional and microfilled composite materials. The primary

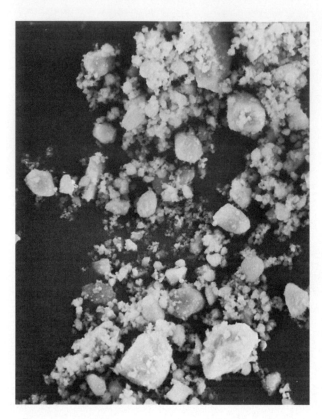

Figure 12–13. Typical particles of a composite filled with small particles. (Courtesy of E. A. Glasspoole and R. Erickson.)

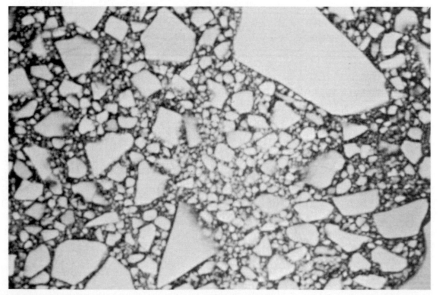

Figure 12–14. Polished surface of a composite filled with small particles. (Courtesy of W. H. Douglas.)

filler consists of silane-coated ground particles. Colloidal silica is usually added in amounts of about 5 wt% to adjust the paste viscosity.

This category of composites exhibits the most superior physical and mechanical properties. With the increased filler content, there is an improvement in virtually all of the relevant properties (see Table 12–2). The compressive strength and elastic modulus of small particle–filled composites exceed those of both traditional and microfilled composites. The tensile strength of small particle–filled composites is double that of the microfilled materials and 1.5 times greater than that of the traditional composites. The coefficient of thermal expansion is less than that of the other composites, although it is still approximately twice that of tooth structure. The surface smoothness of these resins is improved by the use of the small and highly packed filler, as compared with traditional composites. Likewise, the wear resistance is improved. Polymerization shrinkage is comparable to or less than that of traditional resins.

Those materials filled with glass-containing heavy metals are radiopaque. Radiopacity is an important property for materials used for restoration of posterior teeth to facilitate the diagnosis of recurrent caries.

Clinical Considerations of Small Particle–Filled Composites. Because of the improved strength of these composites and higher filler loading, they are indicated for applications in which large stresses and abrasion might be encountered, such as in Class I and II sites. The particle sizes of some small particle–filled composites make it possible to attain reasonably smooth surfaces for anterior applications, but they are not as good as microfilled materials or the more recently developed hybrid composite materials, to be discussed in the following section.

Composition of Hybrid Composites. This category of composite materials was developed in an effort to obtain even better surface smoothness than that provided by the small-particle composites while maintaining the properties of the latter. The hybrid composites are viewed by some as having aesthetic characteristics that are comparable to those of microfilled composites for anterior restorative applications.

As the name implies, there are two kinds of filler particles in the hybrid composites. Most modern hybrid fillers consist of colloidal silica and ground particles of glasses containing heavy metals, constituting a filler content of approximately 75 to 80 wt% (see Table 12–2). The glasses have an average particle size of about 0.6 to 1.0 μm. In a typical size distribution, 75% of the ground particles are smaller than 1.0 μm. Colloidal silica represents 10 to 20 wt% of the total filler content. In this instance, the microfillers also contribute significantly to the properties. The smaller filler particles, as well as the greater amount of microfillers, increase the surface area. Thus, the overall filler loading is not as high as it is for some of the small particle–filled composites.

A polished surface is shown in Figure 12–15. The smaller ground particle size is evident compared with that for the traditional and small particle–filled composites.

Physical and mechanical properties for these systems generally range between those of the traditional and small particle–filled composites. However, as can be seen in Table 12–2, these properties are generally superior to those of the microfilled composites. Because the ground particles contain heavy metal species, they have radiopacities greater than that of enamel.

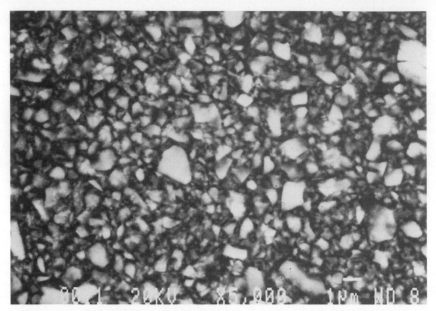

Figure 12–15. Polished surface of a hybrid composite. (Courtesy of R. L. Erickson.)

Clinical Considerations of Hybrid Composites. Because of their surface smoothness and reasonably good strength, these composites are widely used for anterior restorations, including Class IV sites. Although the mechanical properties generally are somewhat inferior to those of small particle–filled composites, the hybrid composites are widely employed for stress-bearing restorations. Because the differences between small particle–filled composites are rather small, these two terms are often used interchangeably to describe the two materials. From a clinical standpoint, this confusion in terminology is not significant as long as filler particle size approaches 1 μm and the volume fraction filler exceeds 60 vol%.

COMPOSITES FOR POSTERIOR RESTORATIONS

Direct Posterior Composites. Amalgam has long been the direct-filling material of choice for restoration of posterior teeth. Its attributes are ease of placement, good mechanical properties, excellent wear resistance, and the unique characteristic of being "self-sealing," that is, of reducing leakage within marginal gaps as the restoration ages. However, with the increasing demand for aesthetic dentistry and the concern about the potential toxicity of mercury, there has been an increased interest in the use of composites for Class I and II restorations. Composites are being employed with greater frequency for this purpose.

During the past 5 to 30 years, materials in each of the four composite categories discussed in this chapter have been employed for posterior restorations. Compared with amalgam, the technique of placement is far more time consuming and demanding. The highly plastic monomeric pastes dictate that the matrix be carefully contoured and wedged to obtain an acceptable proximal contact.

When the gingival margins of the cavity are located in dentin, cementum, or both, and the resin is firmly anchored to the etched enamel at the other margins, the material tends to shrink away from the gingival margins during polymerization. This leads to formation of a gap at that interface. Subsequently, marginal leakage, with its ensuing problems, is enhanced.

Undoubtedly, polymerization shrinkage is one of the greatest problems of composites used for Class II and V restorations. Every measure must be taken to maintain the integrity of the dentin-resin or cementum-resin interfaces (see Chapter 13).

Radiopacity is an important property of any posterior restorative material. Many resin-based composites are radiopaque, so this no longer poses a problem. Clinically, fractures are uncommon causes of failure with most properly formulated products. In addition to the polymerization shrinkage, another frequent clinical problem has been occlusal wear (Fig. 12–16).

The mechanism of occlusal wear is a complex problem that has been the subject of much research. Unfortunately, abrasion and wear resistance can be measured only by a laboratory test that duplicates the particular environmental conditions presented. As yet, no test method has been agreed on as a valid predictor of clinical performance. Until this matter is resolved, one must rely on controlled clinical evaluations. Based on such studies, the best composites designed for posterior restorations still wear more than natural enamel under identical conditions. Although wear rate differences of 10 to 20 μm annually may seem small, posterior composites still wear 0.1 to 0.2 mm more than the enamel over a 10-year period. Because of these wear rates, and the potential implications of wear on occlusion, it is still important to select with caution the clinical cases to be treated with posterior composites.

Germane to this critical property of the posterior composites is the nature of wear mechanics. Two principal mechanisms of composite wear have been proposed. One mode is based on direct contact of the restoration with an opposing cusp so that high stresses are developed in the small area of contact. The wear process in this region may be related to the higher stress levels induced by this cusp.

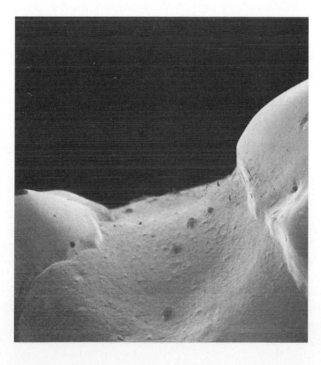

Figure 12–16. Nine-year-old small-particle–filled composite illustrating general wear. (Courtesy of R. L. Erickson.)

Loss of material in noncontact areas is most probably caused by contact with a food bolus as it is forced across the occlusal surface. This type of wear is probably controlled by a number of composite properties, such as porosity, stability of silane coupling, degree of monomer conversion, filler loading, and the size and type of filler particles. Variations among patients, such as differences in chewing habits, force levels, and oral environments also play a significant role in the wear process. A typical wear pattern for a composite is shown in Figure 12–16 for a 9-year-old chemically activated, small particle–filled composite restoration. Although the loss of material is more severe than for newer materials, it illustrates the wear phenomenon. (Notice the smoother anatomic contours and the exposed cavity walls where the composite has been worn away by abrasion.)

Clinically, the loss of material caused by contact area wear appears to be greater than that associated with abrasion by food. Composites in which the filler particles are small, high in concentration, and well bonded to the matrix are the most resistant to wear. Large restorations tend to wear more than do smaller ones, as do restorations that are subjected to higher forces such as those in molars compared with those in premolars.

With these thoughts in mind, a brief summary of the current state of the art in this somewhat controversial area is in order. The major indications for composites in Class II restorations place emphasis on the demand for aesthetics by the patient or by the dentist. A conservative preparation is preferred so that the tooth, rather than the composite, absorbs more of the stress. The dentist must also make the effort to become familiar with the rigorous placement procedures that are essential to success.

There are, however, obvious contraindications. A composite Class II restoration is doomed to failure in the mouth of a patient who bruxes because of the greater potential for wear. Use of posterior composites in a caries-active mouth is questionable, because the current materials have no capability to provide an anticariogenic effect or to resist leakage. Nonetheless, with the greater demands on aesthetics and the improved composite formulations, the use of these materials in stress-bearing situations continues to increase.

Indirect Posterior Composites. The problem of wear in posterior resin applications has been considerably reduced with newer formulations, but difficulties still exist in high-stress situations that are related to inherent problems with both mechanical and chemical degradation of composites. Probably more important, though, are polymerization shrinkage, technique sensitivity, and difficulty in obtaining a predictable, reliable bond to dentin or cementum margins. These deficiencies raise a major concern over the potential leakage of Class II restorations.

The introduction of composite inlay systems that are polymerized outside of the mouth and cemented to the tooth with a compatible resin material represents an attempt to overcome the limitations of traditional posterior composites. Several different approaches to resin inlay construction have been proposed. These include both direct and indirect fabrication; light, heat, pressure, or a combination of these curing systems; and the use of both hybrid and microfilled composites.

The *direct inlay systems* (those processed in the clinical practice) apply a separating medium (agar solution or glycerin) to the prepared tooth. The restorative resin restoration is formed, light cured, and removed from the preparation. The rough inlay is then subjected to additional light (6 minutes) or heat (about

100° C for 7 minutes), after which the preparation is etched. The inlay is then cemented to place with a dual-cure resin and is then polished.

These systems are also available as indirect products. The *indirect inlay* resins require an impression and a dental laboratory technician to fabricate the inlay. In addition to conventional light and heat curing, laboratory processing may employ heat (140° C) and pressure (0.6 MPa for 10 minutes). This polymerization under heat and pressure is used for a homogenous microfilled resin that is claimed to have a higher filler content, less porosity, and greater color stability than light-activated versions. The delivery system is essentially the same as that for the direct systems.

The potential advantage of these materials is that a slightly higher degree of polymerization is attained which improves physical properties and resistance to wear. The polymerization shrinkage does not occur in the tooth, so induced stresses and bond failures are reduced. Theoretically, this reduces the potential for leakage. Furthermore, these resins are repairable in the mouth and they are not as abrasive to opposing tooth structure as ceramic inlays.

Even though laboratory studies support some of these claims, long-term clinical studies are needed to verify the longevity of these restorations in the oral environment. In addition, the technique sensitivity of these systems remains high, and their appropriateness as a substitute for amalgam or cast restorations in all posterior applications needs additional research support, even though the aesthetics are appealing.

PROSTHODONTIC RESINS

The initial resin veneering materials were heat-polymerized poly(methyl methacrylate), which subsequently were improved by the addition of fillers and cross-linking agents. Microfilled materials, which use bis-GMA, urethane dimethacrylate, or 4,8-di(methacryloxy methylene)-tricyclo-decane as resin matrices, have created renewed interest in resin-veneered metal restorations. These resins are polymerized using light of wavelengths in the range of 320 to 520 nm, or by a combination of heat and pressure. Generally, the new microfilled resins have physical properties superior to those of the original unfilled resin.

Originally, the resins were mechanically bonded to metal substrates using wire loops or retention beads. Recent improvements in the bonding mechanisms have included micromechanical retention created by acid etching the base metal alloy and the use of chemical bonding systems such as 4-META, phosphorylated methacrylate, epoxy resin, or silicon dioxide that is flame sprayed to the metal surface followed by the application of a silane coupling agent (silicoating).

Prosthetic resin-veneering materials have several advantages and disadvantages compared with ceramics. The advantages include ease of fabrication, predictable intraoral reparability, and less wear of opposing teeth or restorations. The disadvantages include low proportional limit and pronounced plastic deformation that contribute to distortion on occlusal loading. Therefore, the resin should be protected with metal occlusal surfaces. Leakage of oral fluids and staining below the veneers, particularly those attached mechanically, are caused by the dimensional change during thermal cycling and water sorption. Surface staining and intrinsic discoloration of these resins have been observed.

Resins are also susceptible to wear during tooth brushing. Thus, it is necessary to instruct the patient in proper cleaning procedures using a soft toothbrush and mild abrasive toothpastes. Resin-veneered metal restorations are unsuitable for use as removable partial denture abutment retainers where the clasp arm engages an undercut on the veneered surface, because the resin is not as wear resistant as porcelain or cast metal alloys.

Prosthodontic resins have also been used as a conservative alternative to conventional prosthodontic restorations, such as for masking tooth discoloration or malformation. The resins are used as preformed laminate veneers where resin shells are adjusted by grinding, and the contoured facing is bonded to tooth structure using the acid-etching technique with either autopolymerizing or visible light-activated or dual-cure luting resins.

BIOCOMPATIBILITY OF COMPOSITES

Concerns about biocompatibility of restorative materials usually relate to the effects on the pulp from two aspects: the inherent chemical toxicity of the material and marginal leakage.

Chemical insult to the pulp from composites is possible if components leach out or diffuse from the material and subsequently reach the pulp. Properly polymerized composites are relatively biocompatible, because they exhibit minimal solubility, and unreacted species are leached in small quantities. From a toxicologic point of view, these amounts are too small to cause toxic reactions. However, from an immunologic point of view, under extremely rare conditions, some patients and dental personnel can develop an allergic response to these materials.

Uncured composite materials at the floor of a cavity can serve as a reservoir of diffusable components that can induce long-term pulp inflammation. This situation is of particular concern for the light-activated materials. If a clinician attempts to polymerize too thick a layer of resin or if the exposure time to the light is inadequate, the uncured or poorly cured material can release leachable constituents adjacent to the pulp.

The second biologic concern is associated with shrinkage of the composite during polymerization and the subsequent marginal leakage. The marginal leakage might cause bacterial ingrowth, and these micro-organisms may cause secondary caries, pulp reactions, or both. The restorative procedure must therefore be designed to minimize the polymerization shrinkage and marginal leakage, as discussed in the following section.

TECHNIQUES FOR INSERTION OF COMPOSITES

Some of the matters involved in the manipulation and placement of composites have been noted previously but are explored further in this section. However, the discussion is limited to the handling of the composite itself. Other essential components in the total placement technique, such as agents for enamel and dentin bonding, are also discussed.

Chemically Activated Composites. Composites that are chemically activated are supplied as two-paste systems either in jars or syringes. One paste contains the benzoyl peroxide initiator and the other contains the tertiary amine activator.

Equal amounts of paste are dispensed onto a mixing pad and combined by rapid spatulation for about 30 seconds. If the materials are furnished in jars, cross-contamination must be avoided, because partial polymerization of the paste may occur in the contaminated container. Visual proportioning of pastes is adequate, but care must be taken to avoid any large differences. The mixing should be thorough, because uniform polymerization depends on a homogenous mixture of the activator and the initiator.

When the mix is completed, the resin should be promptly inserted into the cavity to avoid poor adaptation to the cavity walls and loss of plasticity because of the onset of polymerization. Care should be taken to avoid incorporating air during mixing and insertion of the resin. Because the polymerized mass is oxygen inhibited, such air inclusions can result in soft spots in the restoration.

Voids can be minimized by wiping the material into one side of the cavity with a placement instrument, then filling the cavity from the bottom outward. To prevent the material from sticking to the instrument, the instrument should be wiped with a gauze moistened with alcohol. Excess alcohol must be removed from the instrument before it contacts the composite material. Avoid using small instruments with sharp edges during insertion, because such instruments often leave imprints that can result in voids when a new portion of composite is added. Use of a matrix strip to apply pressure yields better adaptation to the walls by forcing the material to flow during the plastic stage of polymerization.

The matrix strip is removed after setting and the restoration is finished. If no matrix strip is used, the surface of the restoration will be sticky as a result of air inhibition. This layer is only a few microns thick and can be easily wiped away to expose the polymerized surface.

Light-activated Composites. Light-activated materials afford a number of advantages over chemically activated resins. The light curable materials are single-component pastes that require no mixing, thus eliminating some important variables. The working time is that chosen by the clinician, and the materials harden rapidly once they are exposed to the curing light. As discussed earlier, the depth of cure is limited and is dependent on several variables such as material, color, location of light source, and quality of the light source. Thus, in deep cavities, the restoration must be built up in increments. Each increment must be cured before insertion of the next increment. Although this appears to be a limitation, it is actually an advantage. A significant portion of the polymerization shrinkage is compensated for as the cavity is being filled and cured.

The resin paste should not be dispensed until it is to be used. Exposure to operatory lights for any appreciable time can initiate polymerization of the material, because these lights emit radiation in the 400- to 500-nm range.

Insertion of the material into the cavity should be done in a manner so as to minimize void formation, just as was described for the chemically activated composites. Once each increment is inserted, it can be shaped to the desired form and then cured. Additional increments are then added, shaped, and cured. A convenient method is to insert the material with a syringe.

The influence of optimal polymerization on color stability, physical properties, and biologic properties, and hence the clinical performance has already been discussed. Also covered were those factors affecting polymerization that are associated with the resins and light units.

Although manufacturers provide information on curing times for different shades, these times are based on a given thickness of a specific resin polymerized by a particular light unit. These recommended times usually are the absolute minimum. To ensure maximum polymerization and clinical success, a high-intensity light unit should be used, and the light intensity should be evaluated periodically. The light tip should be positioned as closely as possible to the resin surface. Ideally, curing should be initiated at the tooth-resin interface so that the resin shrinks toward the cavity walls rather than away from these walls. This can be achieved by first curing through the tooth structure adjacent to the proximal margins. However, because light is absorbed when it passes through the tooth tissue, additional curing is needed when such an approach is taken. The exposure time should be no less than 40 seconds, and the resin thickness should be no greater than 2.0 to 2.5 mm. Dark shades require longer exposure times, as do resins that are polymerized through enamel and dentin.

The light emitted by curing units can cause retinal damage if one looks directly at the beam for an extended period. To avoid such damage, never look directly into the light tip, and minimize observation of the reflected light for longer periods. Protective eye glasses and various types of shields that filter the light are available for increased protection.

Finishing. The differences in surface smoothness of the various types of composites have been described. Because all composites wear over time, they assume a surface roughness that is characteristic of the material. For initial finishing, as well as for refinishing of older restorations, a textbook on operative dentistry should be reviewed for an in-depth discussion of the procedure.

REPAIR OF COMPOSITES

Composites may be repaired by placing new material over the old composite. This is a useful procedure for correcting defects or altering contours on existing restorations. The procedure for adding new material differs depending on whether the restoration is freshly polymerized or an older restoration.

When a restoration has just been placed and polymerized, it may still have an oxygen-inhibited layer of resin on the surface. Additions can be made directly to this layer, because this represents, in essence, an excellent bonding substrate. Even after the restoration has been polished, a defect such as a porosity can still be repaired by adding more material. A restoration that has just been cured and polished may still have more than 50% of unreacted methacrylate groups to copolymerize with the newly added material.

As the restoration ages, fewer and fewer unreacted methacrylate groups remain, and greater cross-linking reduces the ability of fresh monomer to penetrate into the matrix. The strength of the bond between the original material and the added resin decreases in direct proportion to the time that has elapsed between polymerization and addition of the new resin. In addition, polished surfaces expose filler surfaces that are free from silane coating. Thus, the filler surface

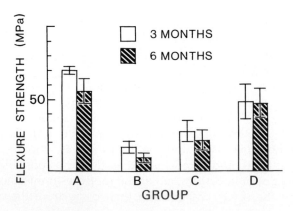

Figure 12–17. Histogram showing flexural strength of different composites after storage in distilled water at 37° C for 3 and 6 months. The four groups include unrepaired samples serving as a control *(A)*, repair without preceding acid etching *(B)*, repair after acid etching and the application of an unfilled resin *(C)*, and repair after toluene-silane treatment of the cut surface *(D)*. (From Söderholm K-J: Flexure strength of repaired dental composites. Scand J Dent Res 94:364, 1986.)

area does not chemically bond to the new composite layer. Under the most ideal condition, the strength of repaired composite is less than half the strength of the original material (Fig. 12–17).

SELECTED READING

Academy of Dental Materials: International Congress on Dental Materials Transactions. Houston, TX, Academy of Dental Materials, Baylor College of Dentistry, 1990.
A host of papers presented on many aspects of dental composite chemistry, systems usage, dentin bond agents, and microleakage.

Albers H: Tooth-colored Restoratives: A Syllabus for Selection, Placement, and Finishing, 7th ed. Cotati, CA, Alto Books, 1985.
Discusses the complete array of composite systems, with emphasis on clinical applications. The author combines the science of dental polymers with discussions of in vivo situations.

Baum L, Phillips RW, and Lund MR: Textbook of Operative Dentistry, 2nd ed. Philadelphia, WB Saunders, 1985.
The technical procedures in the placement of composite resins in various types of restorations are discussed and illustrated.

Bowen RL: Dental filling material comprising vinyl-silane–treated fused silica and a binder consisting of the reaction product of bisphenol and glycidyl methacrylate. US Patent 3,006,112, 1962.
This patent is a milestone in dentistry. It resulted in superior resin-based materials and came a few years after Buonocore's discovery that resins could be bonded to acid-etched enamel. With Bowen's and Buonocore's inventions, it became possible to restore class IV restorations in a conservative and predictable way, something that had been impossible previously.

Gallegos LL, and Nicholls JI: In vitro two-body wear of three veneering resins. J Prosthet Dent 60:172, 1988.
Three veneering resins were tested for wear. A significant difference in wear against porcelain was found among the three resins, but no difference was found against enamel.

Lambrechts P, Braem M, and Vanherle G: Evaluation of clinical performance for posterior composite resins and dentin adhesives. J Oper Dent 12:53, 1987.
These authors have been leaders in the clinical evaluation of resin systems. This paper is a superb treatment of the subject and emphasizes the limitations of current adhesives and composites.

Lutz F, and Phillips RW: A classification and evaluation of composite resin systems. J Prosthet Dent 50:480, 1983.
A classification scheme for composites, based on structure, is presented and has been almost universally accepted since that time. A knowledge of the structure makes it possible to make decisions as to the inherent properties and selection for specific situations.

Roulet JF: The problems associated with substituting composite resins for amalgam: A status report on posterior composites. J Dent 16:101, 1988.
A comprehensive review is presented of the factors to be considered in the use of posterior composites as an alternative to dental amalgam. It concludes that the indications for posterior composites are limited.

Swartz ML, Phillips RW, and Rhodes B: Visible light-activated resins: Depth of cure. J Am Dent Assoc 106:634, 1983.
Depth of cure, as determined by hardness measurements, is influenced by a number of parameters, such as color of the resin, type of system, and time of exposure to the light source.

Vanherle G, and Smith DS: Posterior Composite Resin Dental Restorative Materials. St. Paul, MN, 3M Dental Products Division, 1985.
Proceedings from an international symposium provide a basis for clinical decisions and for further research and development of resin-based composites.

Wendt SL Jr, and Leinfelder KF: The clinical evaluation of heat-treated composite resin inlays. J Am Dent Assoc 120:177, 1990.
One of a few papers available at this time that report the clinical performance of heat-polymerized composite inlays. Although marginal integrity was superior, no difference was detected in wear resistance as compared with light-cured inlays.

13 *Bonding*

- Acid-etch Technique
- Enamel Bonding Agents
- Dentin Bonding Agents
- Manipulation of Dentin Bonding Agents
- Treatment of Cervical Lesions
- Pit and Fissure Sealants

ACID-ETCH TECHNIQUE

Because of the polymerization shrinkage that occurs when methacrylate resins set, it should be apparent that the problem of interfacial leakage is more acute for existing restorative resins than it is with any other type of material. Most dental restorative materials provide some mechanism to counteract marginal leakage. For example, amalgam corrosion products along the tooth-restoration interface form a leakproof seal. Fluorides, known to inhibit secondary caries, are also present in some materials and thus provide some form of caries protection.

Current composite materials have no built-in capability to resist the effects of marginal penetration, and the leakage of oral fluids often occurs adjacent to these restorations. However, such materials can yield useful restorations, although they are extremely technique sensitive.

One of the most effective ways of improving mechanical bonding and the marginal seal is by use of the acid-etch technique. This procedure has markedly expanded the use of resin-based restorative materials because it provides a strong bond between resin and enamel, forming the basis for many innovative dental procedures, such as resin-bonded metal retainers, porcelain laminate veneers, and orthodontic brackets. It has also solved, to a large extent, the previous problems that plagued resin-based restorations, namely, marginal staining caused by interfacial leakage (Fig. 13–1).

The process of achieving a bond between enamel and resin-based restorative materials involves discrete etching of the enamel to provide selective dissolution with resultant microporosity. Figure 13–2 shows an etched surface of enamel in which the centers of the enamel rods have been preferentially dissolved. Other etch patterns show preferential dissolution of the rod peripheries. There can be combinations of the two dissolution patterns.

Etched enamel has a high surface energy, unlike the normal enamel surface, and allows a resin to readily wet the surface and penetrate into the microporosity. Once the resin penetrates into the microporosity, it can be polymerized to form

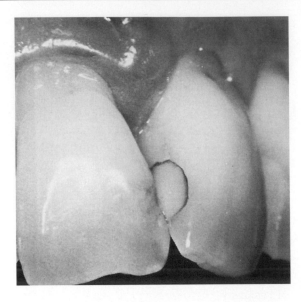

Figure 13–1. Clinical resin restoration with severe marginal discoloration, which resulted from poor adaptation and subsequent leakage. (Courtesy of J. Osborne.)

a mechanical bond to the enamel. These resin "tags" may penetrate 10 to 20 μm into the enamel porosity, as seen in Figure 13–3, but their lengths are dependent on the enamel etching time.

A number of acids have been used to produce the required microporosity, but the universally used acid is phosphoric acid at a concentration between 30% and 50%, with 37% being the concentration most commonly provided. Concentrations greater than 50% result in the formation of monocalcium phosphate monohydrate on the etched surface that inhibits further dissolution. Although aqueous solutions are available, generally the etchant is supplied in a gel form to allow control over the area of placement. These gels are often made by adding colloidal

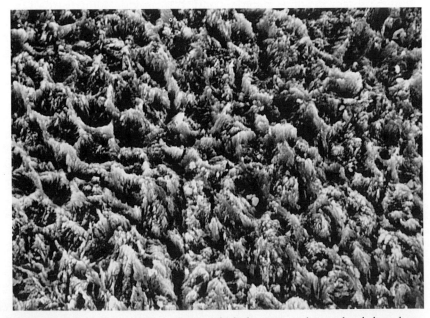

Figure 13–2. Surface of etched enamel in which the centers of enamel rods have been preferentially dissolved by the phosphoric acid.

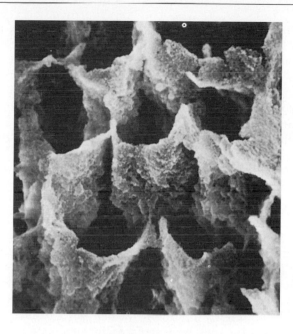

Figure 13–3. Scanning electron microscopy of tags formed by the penetration of resin into etched areas of enamel. The resin was applied to the etched enamel, and the enamel was then dissolved by acid to reveal the tags. ×5000.

silica (the same fine particles used in microfilled composites) or polymer beads to the acid. Brushes are used to place the gel material, or the acid is supplied in a syringe from which it can be dispensed onto the enamel. During placement, it is important to be aware of the risk of air bubbles that may be introduced at the interface. If these voids remain, these regions will not be etched.

The application time of the etchant may vary somewhat, depending on the particular history of the tooth. For example, a tooth with a high fluoride content derived from a fluoride water supply may require a somewhat longer etching time as does a primary tooth. In the latter instance, the increased etching time is needed to enhance the etching pattern on enamel that is more aprismatic than that of permanent enamel. Currently, the length of application of the etchant is often 15 seconds, a sufficient time to produce a bond equivalent to that produced by a 60-second etching time used routinely a few years ago. The advantage of a shorter etching time is that it yields an acceptable bond strength in most instances, and it also conserves enamel and saves time.

Once the tooth is etched, the acid should be rinsed off thoroughly with a stream of water for about 20 seconds, and the enamel dried completely. When the enamel is dry, it should have a white, frosted appearance, indicative of a successful etch. This surface must be kept clean and dry until the resin is placed to form a good bond. Because enamel etching raises the surface energy of the enamel, contamination can readily occur because of the tendency to reduce the energy level of the etched surface. Such a potential reduction in surface energy, in turn, makes it more difficult to wet the surface with a bonding resin that may have a higher surface energy than that of the contaminated surface. Thus, even momentary contact of saliva or blood can prevent effective resin tag formation and severely reduce the bond strength. Another contaminant could be oil that is released from the air compressor and transported along the air lines to the air-water syringe. If contamination occurs, the contaminant should be rinsed off, and the enamel should be dried and etched again for 10 seconds.

Bond strengths to etched enamel range from 15 to 25 MPa, depending on the resin and testing method that is used. A bis-GMA–triethylene glycol dimethacrylate (TEGDMA) resin tends to yield lower values, whereas some of the newer enamel and dentin bonding agents can yield larger values. These differences in bond strength are small, and because of large variations during testing, they are unlikely to be clinically significant. However, these *in vitro* differences may be associated with the better wetting capability of the etched enamel by the newer materials. It has also been shown that drying the enamel with warm air or using an ethanol rinse can increase the bond strength, suggesting that moisture may still be trapped in the micropores even when the surface appears dry.

In summary, the acid-etching technique has resulted in a simple, conservative, and effective use of resin in many dental procedures.

ENAMEL BONDING AGENTS

Because the resin-based composites are more viscous than unfilled acrylic resins, enamel bonding agents were developed to enhance the wettability to etched enamel. Generally, the viscosity of these materials is derived from that of the resin matrix, which is diluted by other monomers to lower the viscosity and to enhance wettability. These agents have no potential for adhesion but tend to improve mechanical bonding by optimum formation of resin tags within the enamel. These materials have now been replaced by agents designed to provide adhesion to dentin, as discussed in the following sections.

Chemistry. Traditionally, enamel bonding agents have been made by combining different dimethacrylates such as bis-GMA and TEGDMA to control viscosity. Because enamel can be kept fairly dry, these rather hydrophobic resins work well as long as they are restricted to enamel. During the last few years, these bonding agents have been replaced by the same systems as are used on dentin. This transition occurred because of the benefit of simultaneously bonding to both enamel and dentin rather than any substantial improvement in bond strength.

DENTIN BONDING AGENTS

As has been stated, acid etching of enamel has provided a superb mechanism for mechanical bonding. It has become an established procedure for the placement of restorative resins. Thus, leakage or loss of retention is no longer a hazard at the enamel-resin interface.

The challenge to adhesive researchers has been, and still remains, the development of agents that adhere to dentin and cementum. Although research in this area has been in progress since the 1950s, it has been a major priority during the last few years as practical applications of dentin adhesives have emerged.

Dentin poses greater obstacles to adhesive bonding than does enamel, because dentin is a living tissue. It is heterogeneous and consists of 50 vol% of inorganic material (hydroxyapatite), 30 vol% of organic material (mainly Type I collagen), and 20 vol% of fluid. Its high fluid content places stringent requirements on materials that can be effective coupling agents between dentin and a restorative material. The tubular nature of dentin provides a variable area through which dentinal fluid may flow to the surface to adversely affect adhesion. The tubules with their branching channels may also be used for enhanced mechanical retention. Further challenges to adhesion involve the presence of the smear layer on the cut dentin surface and the potential biologic side effects that different chemicals can cause within the pulp. It is for these reasons that the development of dentin bonding agents has been delayed compared with the development of the enamel bonding agents.

An important breakthrough in dentin bonding occurred in 1978, when Fusayama and associates started to use 37% phosphoric acid to etch both enamel and dentin. Their findings suggest that the procedure did not increase the frequency of pulp damage but in fact improved the restoration retention substantially. Later studies by Nakabayashi and colleagues revealed that acid etching left a layer of dentin-anchored collagen fibers on the surface of demineralized dentin and that hydrophilic resins infiltrated that layer to form a hybrid layer consisting of resin-infiltrated dentin. The dentin-etching procedure, though, was not generally accepted initially outside of Japan, because it was believed that such aggressive treatment would result in pulpal damage. It was not until the early 1990s that dentin etching gained acceptance throughout the world.

Ideally, dentin adhesives should be hydrophilic to displace the dentinal fluids and thereby wet the surface, permitting them to penetrate porosities within the dentin and eventually react with organic or inorganic components. Because most composite matrix resins are hydrophobic, the bonding agent should contain both hydrophilic and hydrophobic materials. The hydrophilic part should be designed to interact with the moist dentin surface, whereas the hydrophobic part should bond to the restorative resin.

Chemistry. Several years ago, the general belief was that dentin bonding could be achieved by forming chemical bonds between a resin system and either the inorganic or the organic component of dentin. The most commonly targeted components were either collagen or the calcium ions within hydroxyapatite. The molecules that were designed for these purposes can be represented by a M—R—X molecule, where M is a methacrylate group, R is a spacer such as a hydrocarbon chain, and X is a functional group that is targeted for adhesion to tooth tissue. Typical phosphate X groups were believed to bond to calcium during dentin priming. Then, during polymerization, the methacrylate group of the M—R—X molecule would react with the composite material and form a chemical bond between composite and dentin. Compounds that were believed to possess these properties were NPG-GMA (a condensation product of *N*-phenyl glycine and glycidyl methacrylate), polymerizable phosphates, and poly(alkenoic) acids (Fig. 13–4).

Another bonding agent used was glutaraldehyde, a compound that is known to bond to collagen. By attaching a molecule such as hydroxyethyl methacrylate (HEMA) to the collagen-bonded glutaraldehyde, and using the methacrylate group of the HEMA to bond to the composite during polymerization, the belief was that a chemical bond could be formed between the collagen and the composite (Fig. 13–5).

Although this concept might seem reasonable, clinical studies revealed that these systems did not work as well as originally believed. However, it was also found that as the conditioning procedures, such as acid etching or demineralization with ethylene–diaminetetra-acetic acid (EDTA), became more aggressive, the clinical results improved. The ability of resins to infiltrate the moist collagen mesh is probably more important than their ability to form chemical bonds to tooth structure. In other words, the key to adhesion is to find hydrophilic monomers that can easily infiltrate the collagen mesh produced by conditioning dentin with an acid often called a *conditioner*. Some of the systems that exhibit those properties include HEMA, polyacrylic acid, and NPG-GMA. To simplify the dentin bonding process, the current trend is to develop hydrophilic, multi-

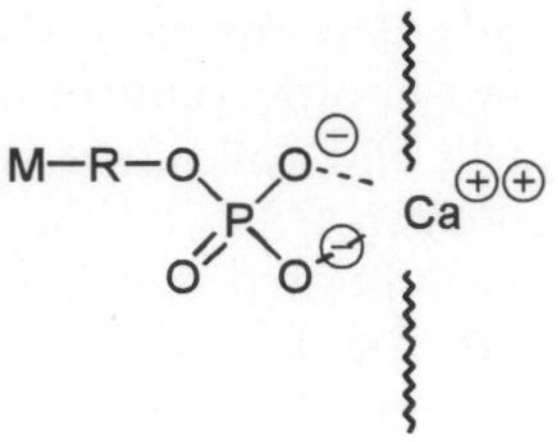

PHOSPHATE BASED BONDING AGENT

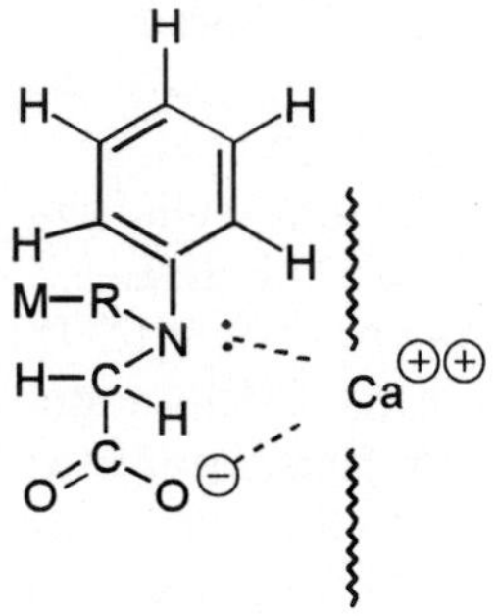

AMINO-CARBOXYLATE BASED BONDING AGENT
(NPG-GMA)

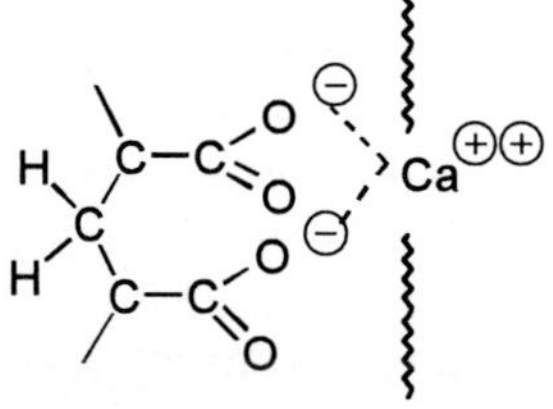

CARBOXYLATE BASED BONDING AGENT
(PAA)

Figure 13–4. Chemical bonding mechanisms to hard tooth tissues.

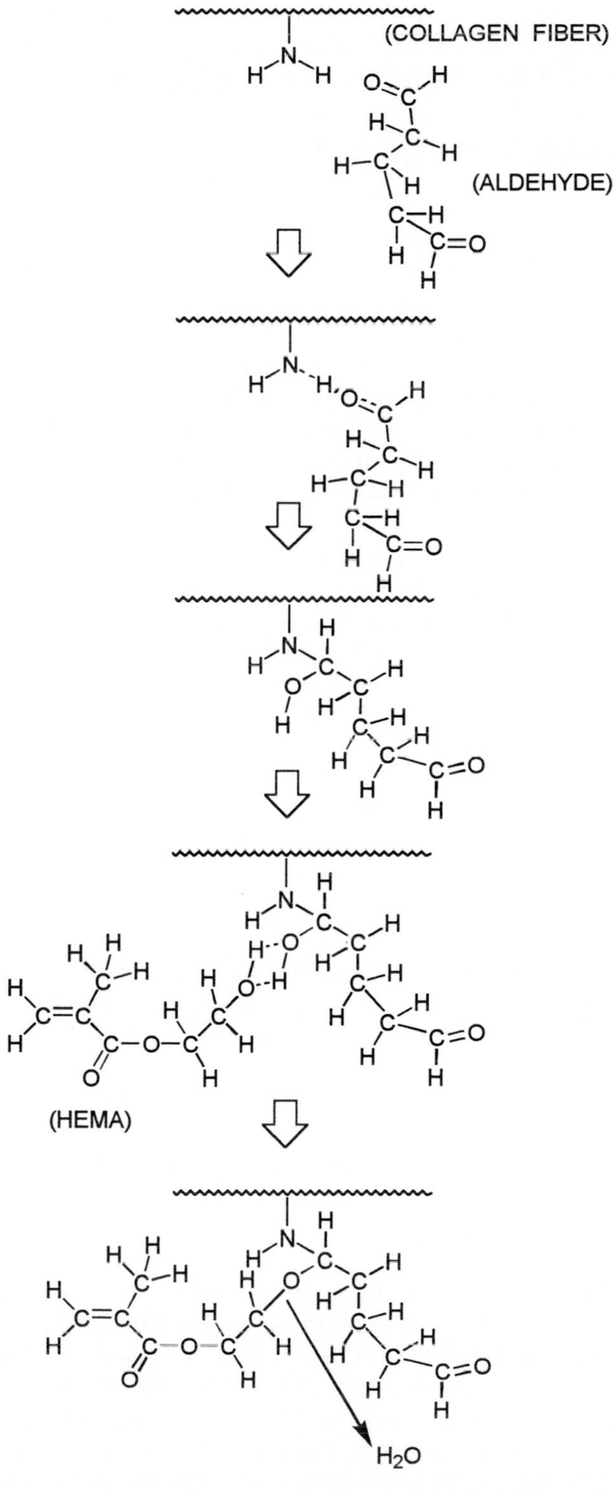

Figure 13–5. Theoretic bonding of collagen to a composite via attachment of hydroxyethyl methacrylate (HEMA) to collagen-bonded glutaraldehyde and use of the methacrylate group of the HEMA to bond to the composite. *A,* Aldehyde approaches an amino group present along the collagen molecule. *B,* A hydrogen bond forms between the hydrogen of the amino group and the oxygen of the carboxyl group of the aldehyde. *C,* The nitrogen of the amino group starts interacting with the carbon of the carbonyl group, and the hydrogen of the amino group leaves the nitrogen bonded to the oxygen of the carbonyl group of the aldehyde. At the same time, a covalent bond is formed between the nitrogen of the collagen and the carbon of the aldehyde. *D,* The OH group of the hydroxyethyl methacrylate (HEMA) approaches the OH group formed when the amino group and the aldehyde group reacted. *E,* A condensation reaction occurs between the aldehyde grafted collagen chain and the HEMA molecule resulting in the release of a water molecule. During this reaction, the remaining part of the HEMA molecule becomes covalently bonded to the collagen-aldehyde graft.

functional, and self-etching monomers such as penta-acrylate monophosphate (see Chapter 10, Fig. 10–16). In fact, with the bonding agents now available, it is possible under ideal conditions to achieve bond strengths that exceed the strength of the dentin. Whether these bond strength values are permanent, though, remains an open question, because little is known about degradation mechanisms that may occur at the dentin-collagen-resin interfaces.

MANIPULATION OF DENTIN BONDING AGENTS

Most dentin bonding systems are provided with a conditioner, often an acid, that can remove the smear layer and expose a collagen network. The dentin is conditioned most commonly for 15 seconds and the conditioner is subsequently rinsed away. Excess water is then removed from the etched and rinsed dentin surface, without desiccating the *collagen mesh*. If the mesh is desiccated, the collagen network collapses and forms a dense film that is difficult to infiltrate with the primer. The hydrophilic primer, in contrast with a hydrophobic primer, infiltrates the collagen network when placed on the somewhat moist dentin surface. To optimize bonding, the primer should cure as efficiently as possible. This curing process, though, is not easy to achieve because both dentinal fluids and oxygen, present either in the dentin or in the air jet used for drying, inhibit polymerization. To avoid this situation, the primer should contain a solvent that evaporates easily and removes water without the need for excessive air drying. In addition, the primer should also contain a resin that produces a cross-linked polymer network that is well retained within the collagen mesh.

A bonding resin is placed on the primed surface region of conditioned tooth surface. The resin should be thinned with a brush rather than with an air jet to avoid oxygen inhibition. The thickness of the bonding resin should be at least 50 μm to prevent diffusion of oxygen from the air through the coating to prevent oxygen inhibition of the primer and the adjacent bonding resin during polymerization. Because the light-activating compounds are contained commonly in the bonding resin, the primer and the bonding resin are cured simultaneously for the minimum time recommended by the manufacturer. Subsequently, layers of composites are placed and cured on the bonding agent layer.

Product chemistry and procedural variations make it imperative that the dentist understand not only the treatment sequence but also the function of each component of an adhesive system. For example, imagine that the treated tooth is contaminated with saliva after primer application and that the dentist decides to rinse it with water before the bonding agent is placed. Because most primers are hydrophilic monomers, a rinsing procedure would result in removal of the primer from the dentin surface. In this situation, no interpenetrating network formation within the collagen mesh would occur, and poor bonding would result.

Bond Strength and Leakage. Evaluation of the efficacy of dentin adhesives is generally based on measurement of bond strength determined by loading bond test specimens in shear or in tension until fracture occurs. Such tests are indicative of how the adhesive is likely to perform *in vivo*. Data published on bond strengths for a given material often vary widely, and the standard deviation of the mean value within a given series of tests is usually high. This wide variance in data may be attributed to the variables inherent at the dentin surface, such as water content, the presence or absence of the smear layer, dentin permeability, orientation of the tubules relative to the surface, and differences in the *in vitro* test methodology. Furthermore, although no universal agreement on the minimal bond strength necessary to provide successful bonding has been established, a value of 20 MPa or higher is a reasonable goal.

The degree of leakage at the restoration-tooth interface can be monitored by the penetration of tracers and staining agents. As is true for bond testing, there is also a large variation in leakage data from one laboratory to another, depending on the technique used and the manipulative variables adopted during placement of the bonding agents. Often, there is not a good correlation between bond strength values and microleakage. Nonetheless, the newer systems appear to be superior in inhibiting interfacial leakage between the conditioned tooth structure and adhesive resin.

TREATMENT OF CERVICAL LESIONS

Cervical lesions with exposed areas of cementum and dentin are becoming more common. People are living longer and the loss of teeth has been markedly reduced through preventive dentistry. When these two facts are considered, there is a greater likelihood that "eroded area" lesions may develop. They are a real concern to the patient, because they are often visible and unsightly, as can be seen in Figure 13-6A. Furthermore, the affected teeth may be sensitive to temperature changes, toothbrush abrasion, or both.

Four methods have been used to treat cervical lesions. The traditional method involves Class V cavity preparations and placement of a restorative material, such as resin, amalgam, and direct gold. Recently, several additional conservative procedures have become popular, all of which rely on bonding for retention of the restorative material. In each instance, no anesthesia and little or no instrumentation is required, as in the cases for Class V preparations.

One method takes advantage of the adhesive potential of glass ionomer cements. A modification of this procedure is the *sandwich technique*. In this instance, the glass ionomer cement is used to line the dentin for adhesion, and then a cosmetic resin is bonded to the ionomer cement and to etched enamel.

Another conservative approach involves the use of the acid-etching technique to bond a restorative resin to the enamel without the need for mechanical retention derived from cavity preparation. This concept is based on making use of the resin aesthetics and mechanical bonding of resin to etched enamel. When this technique was first introduced, several resins were designed specifically for such restorations. However, the resins need not be of a particular formulation, and light-cured microfilled composites are generally used. Originally, enamel bonding agents were also applied to the tooth surface to ensure good wetting and resin tag formation to the etched enamel. Now, dentin bonding agents are generally used in an attempt to attain adhesive bonding to dentin and cementum.

If enamel is present within the marginal area, one can anticipate a high success rate. When proper acid etching is accomplished, it will produce a satisfactory enamel bond to any resin system and ensure a certain longevity of the restoration. It is unfortunate that one seldom finds enamel surrounding the entire lesion. At the gingival margin, cementum or dentin is usually present.

From the previous discussion, the bond to cementum or dentin always represents the critical interface, because composition and morphology of these complex tissues are impossible to standardize. Therefore, bonding to dentin and cementum is not yet as predictable as is bonding to enamel. Thus, even though the restoration may remain in place for an extended period because of the

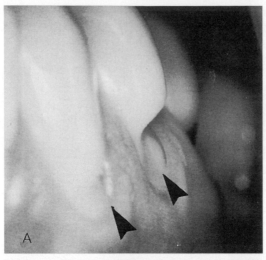

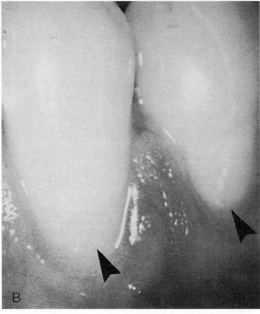

Figure 13–6. *A,* An example of the so-called eroded area *(arrowheads)* with exposed dentin, cementum, or both. *B,* The lesions are restored *(arrowheads)* by means of an acid-etch technique and a resin-based composite. (Courtesy of B. Matis.)

excellent mechanical bond to the etched enamel at the incisal or occlusal interface, leakage may be occurring at the gingival margin. One should not feel a false sense of security even though the restoration is still intact. In time, this leakage pattern can contribute to a degradation of the bond and loss of the restoration. Equally important, gross leakage is always a possible contributor to secondary caries, pulpal irritation, and postoperative sensitivity. Nonetheless, such a technique merits consideration because of the conservative nature of the procedure and the aesthetics of restorative resins as compared with metallic materials. Recognizing the problem of an inadequate bond to cementum or dentin, several suggestions can be offered if a resin-bonded restoration is to be used. Certainly, the patient should be advised that the restoration is not permanent, and repair or replacement may be required subsequently.

Relative to the tooth preparation technique for bonding, pumice is often used for the initial removal of plaque and debris from the area. A pumice paste should not be employed, because the glycerin type of vehicle used may leave a film on the tooth surface even if it is subsequently washed and cleaned with water. This oil film prevents proper etching of the cavity and wetting of the resin to the tooth. A pumice slurry, not a paste, should be used.

It is also advisable to use a small amount of instrumentation to the area. At the incisal, or occlusal, a bevel can be placed in the enamel (Fig. 13–7A) with a tapered fissure bur, for example. The removal of the surface exposes fresh enamel that is readily etched. Likewise, beveling provides the proper orientation of the enamel rods to the etching solution. The etch pattern on beveled enamel is markedly superior to that produced when the enamel rods are lying somewhat perpendicular to the action of the acid. Thus, the bevel enhances retention and reduces the likelihood of marginal stain caused from leakage.

Improving the retention at the gingival margin of a Class V restoration is even more important, if restoration retention is the key concern. This can be accomplished by placing a slight undercut in dentin by means of a small round bur, as illustrated in Figure 13–7B to D. However, although retention is enhanced, the potential for leakage remains, particularly if dentin etching and priming is not used.

It can be argued that the newer dentin bonding agents are sufficiently effective and gingival retention is not required. However, more information is needed on the long-term stability of these agents. Should such a mechanism prove to be effective over a long period, it would probably be possible to restore the eroded area without the necessity for any kind of mechanical retention. The end result of such a treatment is an aesthetic restoration, as shown in Figure 13–6B.

PIT AND FISSURE SEALANTS

Various materials and techniques have been advocated for preventing caries in the susceptible pit and fissure areas of posterior teeth, particularly in the child

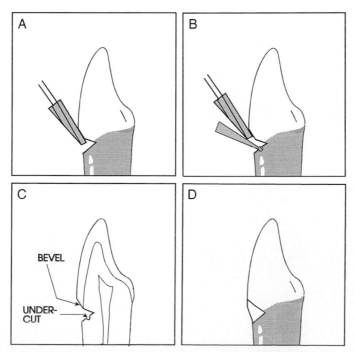

Figure 13–7. A, Placement of incisal bevel in the enamel of Class V preparation. B and C, Placement of a small retention groove in dentin using a small round bur. D, Finished composite restoration.

patient. The most popular sealant techniques make use of resin systems that can be applied to the occlusal surfaces of the teeth. The objective of sealant use is for the resin to penetrate into the pits and fissures and to polymerize and seal these areas against the oral bacteria and debris. A cross section of a tooth to which a pit and fissure sealant has been applied is shown in Figure 13–8.

Several types of resin, both filled and unfilled, have been employed as pit and fissure sealants. These resin systems include cyanoacrylates, polyurethanes, and bis-GMA. The commercially available products have been based on either the polyurethane resin or the bis-GMA resin. The bis-GMA material may be polymerized in the conventional manner by means of the amine-peroxide chemical activation-initiation system or by light activation. The unfilled resins are available as colorless or tinted transparent materials. The filled resins are opaque and available either as tooth-colored or white materials.

The success of the sealant technique is highly dependent on obtaining and maintaining an intimate adaptation of the sealant to the tooth surface. Therefore, the sealants must be of relatively low viscosity so that they will flow readily into the depths of the pits and fissures and wet the tooth. To enhance wetting and mechanical retention of the sealant, the tooth surface is first conditioned by etching with acid, as described earlier. The physical properties of the sealants are closer to those of unfilled direct resins than to those of resin-based composites.

The reduction in occlusal caries resulting from the careful use of pit and fissure sealants has been impressive. Consequently, the use of sealants has been endorsed as an effective therapy by the American Dental Association, the American Academy of Pediatric Dentistry, the American Society of Dentistry for Children, and the American Association of Public Health Dentistry.

Clinical studies have shown that the failure frequency of sealants is approximately 5% per year after one single application of the sealant. In one report, at the end of 10 years, 78% of first permanent molars were free of caries when a single application of sealant had been placed, as compared with only 31% of caries-free teeth in the unsealed matched pairs.

If doubt exists whether the pit or fissure is free from caries or not, it is still justified to place a sealant. Clinical trials in which sealants were intentionally placed in pits and fissures that were diagnosed as having caries have shown that as long as the sealant is well retained, no caries progression will occur.

If a dentist feels uncomfortable about sealing in a potential caries lesion and

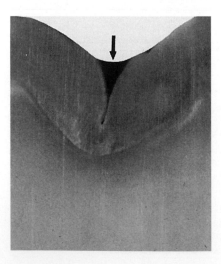

Figure 13–8. Cross section of a tooth showing penetration of a sealant into an occlusal fissure (*arrow*).

believes that a visual inspection of the potential lesion is required, another conservative approach can be taken. This option consists of a minimal cavity preparation and the placement of an enamel-dentin bonded composite restoration combined with a sealant application. With such an approach, most of the occlusal surface is sealed. This restoration is called a *preventive-resin restoration* (PRR). The PRR treatment has exhibited a success rate of 75% after 9 years, a remarkably high success rate even when compared with traditional amalgam treatment.

SELECTED READING

Asmussen E, and Munksgaard EC: Bonding of restorative resins to dentine: Status of dentine adhesives and impact on cavity design and filling techniques. Int Dent J 38.97, 1988.
The chemistry of dentin bond agents is covered and bond strength data are presented. In addition, factors involved in clinical usage that influence retention are cited.

Bowen RL, Eichmiller FC, Marjenhoff WA, and Rupp NW: Adhesive bonding of composites. J Am Coll Dent 56:10, 1989.
A discussion of several of the popular dentin and enamel bonding systems, noting differences in chemical components and instructions for use.

Buonocore MG: A simple method of increasing the adhesion of acrylic filling materials to enamel surfaces. J Dent Res 34:849, 1955.
This article, published 40 years ago, is worthy of citation. It was this research that suggested that etching of enamel would improve mechanical bonding of an unfilled resin (composites were nonexistent at that time). The technique is now an essential step in the use of all modern composites.

Buonocore MG: The Use of Adhesives in Dentistry. Springfield, IL, Charles C Thomas, 1975.
This book deserves citation, being authored by the late Dr. Buonocore, who initiated the acid-etch technique. The problems associated with the use of adhesives in dentistry are still germane to current systems such as dentin bond agents. These matters, and the clinical application, are well covered.

Douglas WH: Clinical status of dentine bonding agents. J Dent 17:209, 1989.
An excellent review and update of the evolution of dentin bonding agents, the problems associated with adhesion, and the clinical criteria involved in phenomena such as microleakage and tooth strengthening. Essential reading for the person interested in this highly controversial area.

Fusayama T, Nakamura M, Kurosaki M, and Iwaku M: Nonpressure adhesion of a new adhesive restorative resin. J Dent Res 58:1364, 1979.

Houpt M, Fuks A, and Eidelman E: The preventive resin (composite resin/sealant) restoration: Nine-year results. Quint Int 25:155, 1994.
Nine-year data presented to show the efficiency of using preventive resin restorations to treat cavities with caries lesions.

Mertz-Fairhurst EJ: Current status of sealant retention and caries prevention. J Dent Educ 48(2 Suppl):18, 1984.
Ten-year data presented to show a substantial reduction in caries after the placement of sealant as compared with untreated control surfaces.

Nakabayashi N, Kojima K, and Masuhara E: The promotion of adhesion by the infiltration of monomers into tooth substrates. J Biomed Mater Res 16:265, 1982.

Sealants Consensus Development Conference Statement on Dental Sealants and The Prevention of Tooth Decay. J Am Dent Assoc 108:233, 1984.
Recommendations from a consensus conference on the state-of-the-art of sealant therapy. The posture taken was decidedly positive.

Simonsen RJ: Retention and effectiveness of dental sealant after 15 years. J Am Dent Assoc 122:34, 1991.
This article represents a long-term evaluation of sealants after a single placement.

14 *Solidification and Microstructure of Metals*

- **Metals**
- **Metallic Bonds**
- **Alloys**
- **Solidification of Metals**

Chapters 14, 15, 20, 22, 23, and 27 provide an introduction to cast metals and alloys and physical metallurgy. Although the use of cast metals has decreased in recent years because of the increased consumer demand for aesthetics over durability, a knowledge of the structure and properties of cast metals and alloys is essential to properly handle these materials in a clinical practice and to diagnose clinical failures of cast restorations should they occur. Furthermore, cast metals are used as copings or substructures for metal-ceramic restorations, the most common crown and bridge prostheses, and the most durable of all aesthetic restorations, especially when used to restore posterior teeth.

METALS

In dentistry, metals represent one of the four major classes of materials used for the reconstruction of decayed, damaged or missing teeth. Although metals are easy to distinguish from ceramics, polymers, and composites, they are not easy to define. The *Metals Handbook* (1992) defines a metal as "an opaque lustrous chemical substance that is a good conductor of heat and electricity and, when polished, is a good reflector of light." We can also define metals in terms of their common characteristics. Gallium and mercury, elements that are commonly used as alloying elements in dental alloys, are liquid at body temperature. However, all metals and alloys used in dentistry are crystalline solids. With the exception of pure gold foil, commercially pure titanium, and endodontic silver points, most metals used for dental restorations, partial denture frameworks, and orthodontic wires are alloys.

A clean metallic surface exhibits a luster that is difficult to duplicate in other types of solid matter. Most metals emit a metallic ring when they are struck, although certain silica compounds can emit a similar sound. A unique characteristic of metals is that they are good thermal and electrical conductors. Compared with ceramics, polymers, and composites, metals have a high fracture toughness, which is the ability to absorb energy under increasing tensile stress before fracture occurs. For example, the fracture toughness of most metals varies between 25 and 60 MPa·m$^{1/2}$ compared with a range of 0.75 to 2.5 MPa·m$^{1/2}$ for dental ceramics. Generally, solid metals are stronger and more dense than other chemical elements. Most metals also are more ductile and malleable than nonmetals, most of which are brittle. A few metals (iron, nickel, and cobalt) can be magnetized, but they can also be produced in a nonmagnetic state.

Metals are generally resistant to chemical attack, but some metals require alloying elements to resist tarnish and corrosion in the oral environment. For example, chromium is required as an alloying element in alloys based on iron, nickel, or cobalt to provide passivation of the alloy through the formation of a thin layer of chromium oxide. Noble metals are highly resistant to chemical corrosion and oxidation and do not require alloying elements for this purpose. However, pure noble metals must be alloyed to provide sufficient resistance to deformation and fracture when they are used for cast restorations.

Of the 103 elements currently listed in the periodic table of the elements, approximately 81 can be classified as metals. It is of scientific interest that these metallic elements can be grouped according to density, ductility, melting point, and nobility. This indicates that the properties of metals are closely related to their valence electron configuration. The groupings of pure light and heavy metal elements are shown in Table 14–1.

To the chemist and physicist, all metallic elements have one common characteristic. The outermost electrons around the neutral atom are freely given up. For example, the chemist knows that sodium, zinc, and aluminum all tend to

TABLE 14–1. Periodic Chart of the Elements

Modified after Grosvenor AW (ed): Basic Metallurgy Principles, Vol. 1. Cleveland, American Society for Metals, 1954. The preferred symbol for element 41 is now Nb.

sacrifice their few valence electrons to become positive ions in solution. In addition, if two different metals are the electrodes of a galvanic cell, the negative electrode (the one supplying the electrons to an outer circuit) is the more metallic. This ease of giving up the valence electrons is indeed responsible for their malleability and their luster, or mirror-reflecting property.

Most metals, including silver, nickel, tin, aluminum, and zinc, are "white." However, there are slight differences in color among the white metals. Two important metal components of cast dental alloys—gold and copper—are non-white.

The properties of the pure elements do not change abruptly from metallic to a nonmetallic nature as one moves to the right side of the periodic chart (see Table 14–1). Rather, the boundary between metals and nonmetals is somewhat arbitrary, and the elements near the boundary exhibit characteristics of both metals and nonmetals. The elements carbon, boron, and silicon are often combined with metals to form important alloys. Silicon and germanium are termed *semiconductors* because their electrical conductivity is intermediate between that of a metal and that of an insulator. These two elements form the basis for many of the modern electronic devices.

METALLIC BONDS

In addition to covalent and ionic bonds, matter can be held together also by a primary atomic interaction known as the *metallic bond* that occurs between valence electrons. One of the chief characteristics of a metal is its ability to conduct heat and electricity. Such energy conduction is associated with the mobility of the free electrons present in metals. The outer shell valence electrons can be removed easily from the metallic atom, leaving the balance of the electrons tied to the nucleus, thus forming a positive ion.

The free valence electrons are able to move about in the metal space lattice to form an electron "cloud" or "gas." The electrostatic attraction between this electron cloud and the positive ions in the lattice provides the force that bonds the metal atoms together as a solid. These free electrons act as conductors of both thermal energy and electricity. They transfer energy by moving readily from areas of higher energy to those of lower energy, under the influence of either a thermal gradient or an electrical field (potential gradient).

ALLOYS

The use of pure metal elements is quite limited. Pure metals are apt to be soft and, like iron, many of these tend to corrode rapidly. The metals most useful to civilization along with some of their physical constants are listed in Table 14–2. It is fortunate that metallic elements maintain their metallic behavior even when they are not pure and that they can tolerate a considerable addition of other elements in the liquid or solid state.

Thus, to optimize properties, most of the metals commonly used are mixtures of two or more metallic elements or, in some instances, a metal and a nonmetal. Although such mixtures can be produced in a number of ways, they are generally produced by fusion of the elements above their melting points. A solid mixture of a metal with one or more other metals or with one or more nonmetals is called an *alloy*. For example, a small amount of carbon is added to iron to form steel. A certain amount of chromium is added to iron and carbon to form stainless steel, an alloy that is highly corrosion resistant. To impart corrosion

TABLE 14–2. Physical Constants of the Alloy-forming Elements

Element	Symbol	Atomic Weight	Melting Point (° C)	Boiling Point (° C)	Density (g/cm³)	Linear Coefficient of Thermal Expansion (10⁻⁴/° C)
Aluminum	Al	26.98	660.2	2450	2.70	0.236
Antimony	Sb	121.75	630.5	1380	6.62	0.108
Bismuth	Bi	208.98	271.3	1560	9.80	0.133
Cadmium	Cd	112.40	320.9	765	8.37	0.298
Carbon	C	12.01	3700.0	4830	2.22	0.06
Chromium	Cr	52.00	1875.0	2665	7.19	0.062
Cobalt	Co	58.93	1495.0	2900	8.85	0.138
Copper	Cu	63.54	1083.0	2595	8.96	0.165
Gold	Au	196.97	1063.0	2970	19.32	0.142
Indium	In	114.82	156.2	2000	7.31	0.33
Iridium	Ir	192.2	2454.0	5300	22.5	0.068
Iron	Fe	55.85	1527.0	3000	7.87	0.123
Lead	Pb	207.19	327.4	1725	11.34	0.293
Magnesium	Mg	24.31	650.0	1107	1.74	0.252
Mercury	Hg	200.59	−38.87	357	13.55	0.40
Molybdenum	Mo	95.94	2610.0	5560	10.22	0.049
Nickel	Ni	58.71	1453.0	2730	8.90	0.133
Palladium	Pd	106.4	1552.0	3980	12.02	0.118
Platinum	Pt	195.09	1769.0	4530	21.45	0.089
Rhodium	Rh	102.91	1966.0	4500	12.44	0.083
Silicon	Si	28.09	1410.0	2480	2.33	0.073
Silver	Ag	107.87	960.8	2216	10.49	0.197
Tantalum	Ta	180.95	2996.0	5425	16.6	0.065
Tin	Sn	118.69	231.9	2270	7.298	0.23
Titanium	Ti	47.90	1668.0	3260	4.51	0.085
Tungsten	W	183.85	3410.0	5930	19.3	0.046
Zinc	Zn	65.37	420.0	906	7.133	0.397

Data from Lyman T (ed): Metals Handbook, 8th ed., Vol. 1. Cleveland, American Society for Metals, 1964.

resistance to either nickel or cobalt, chromium is also added to form two of the predominantly base metal alloys used in dentistry. Although pure gold is also highly corrosion resistant, copper is added to it to enhance its strength and resistance to plastic deformation. Early alloys evolved by trial and error, but special-purpose alloys currently in use are the result of technologic advances.

The term *metal* is used all-inclusively to include alloys as well as pure metals. In this book, if the phenomenon discussed does not apply to both alloys and pure metals, a distinction will be made as to which is meant. In a later chapter, the physical and chemical properties of alloys are discussed in some detail. However, before proceeding to alloys, the fundamental principles that control how a solid is formed from the molten (liquid) state are first described.

SOLIDIFICATION OF METALS

Pure metals, in common with other chemical elements, can be identified by their melting points, boiling points, and similar basic physical and chemical properties. Some of these properties for metals of dental interest are tabulated in Table 14–2.

The solidification phenomena that occur during the freezing of a pure metal are considered first. The solidification of alloys is discussed in a subsequent chapter. If a metal is melted and then allowed to cool, and its temperature during cooling is plotted as a function of time, a graph similar to that in Figure 14–1 results. As can be noted, the temperature decreases steadily from A to B′.

An increase in temperature then occurs to point B, at which time the temperature becomes constant until the time indicated at point C. After time C has elapsed, the temperature decreases steadily to room temperature.

Temperature T_f, as indicated by the straight or "plateau" portion of the curve at BC, is the freezing point, or solidification temperature. This is also the melting point, or *fusion temperature*. During melting, the temperature remains constant. During freezing or solidification, heat is evolved as the metal changes from the liquid to the solid state. This heat is the latent heat of solidification and is equal to the heat of fusion studied in physics courses. It is defined as the number of calories of heat liberated from 1 g of a substance when it changes from the liquid to the solid state.

The interpretation of the curve in Figure 14–1 is that all temperatures above T_f, as indicated by the plateau BC, are associated with a molten metal, and all temperatures below this temperature are associated with a solid. The initial cooling to B′ is called *supercooling*. During this period of supercooling, crystallization begins. Once the crystals begin to form, the latent heat of fusion causes the temperature to rise to temperature T_f, where it remains until crystallization is completed.

The fusion temperature of metals and alloys is of considerable interest to the dentist. Many metallic dental structures are cast. A wax or plastic *pattern* is prepared that is an exact replica of the dental appliance or restoration to be cast. A mold is prepared from the pattern, into which a molten alloy can be flowed under pressure. When the alloy solidifies, the original pattern is thus reproduced in metal, and a *casting* is produced. Such metals are called *casting alloys*. The casting procedures and materials involved are discussed in subsequent chapters.

Nucleus Formation. Although the surface tension of liquid metals is approximately 10 times greater than that of water, molten or liquid metals are not much different in structure than any other liquids. Like other liquids, metal atoms can migrate through the molten liquid at a rapid rate determined by its diffusion coefficient of approximately 10^{-5} cm²/s. Liquid metals do not differ in structure

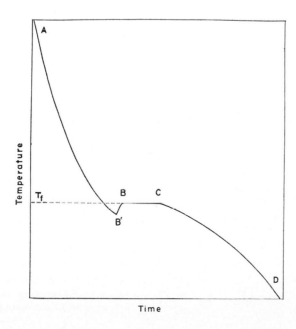

Figure 14–1. A time-temperature cooling curve for a pure metal that illustrates supercooling.

from one another as much as do solid metals. The liquids all exhibit a tendency toward a short-range order arrangement.

As the molten metal approaches its melting temperature or plateau (see Fig. 14–1), its energy relationships change. During supercooling below the freezing point (BC), the atoms begin to diffuse toward the regular space lattice arrangement and an interface tends to form between the liquid and the embryonic solid phase.

As previously explained, the surface energy of a solid is greater than its internal energy because the unequal attraction of the surface atoms tends to draw them closer together, which is a state of increased surface tension. It follows, therefore, that the solid space lattice arrangement cannot be permanent and a liquid-solid interface is created until a proper relationship is established between the surface energy and the internal energy of the system. The internal energy can be related to the *volume free energy,* which, at this state of the solidification, decreases because of the change from the liquid to the solid state. On the other hand, the *surface free energy* increases as the supercooling increases, that is, as the surrounding temperature decreases below the fusion temperature.

The liquid state can be visualized as one of a multitude of random atoms or molecules surrounding numerous unstable atomic aggregates or clusters that tend to form crystal nuclei. These temporary nuclei are usually called *embryos.*

The embryos at high temperatures are few in number and generally very small in size. Thus, they dissolve readily back into the matrix of the random atoms. On approaching the solidification temperature, these embryos increase in number and get larger, but they are still unstable and tend to dissolve into the matrix. However, once the supercooled region is reached, there is a tendency for some of these embryos to survive and thus form a solidification nucleus.

To understand this phenomenon in detail, one needs to make use of thermodynamics. It may be explained by a study of Figure 14–2. Imagine a spherical

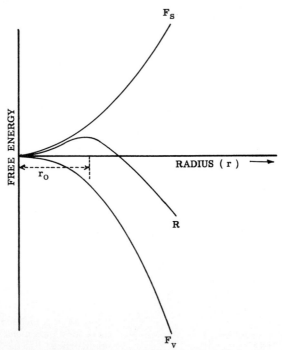

Figure 14–2. Free energy of formation of a nucleus as a function of its radius.

embryo of radius y, as scaled on the horizontal axis in the figure. Envision about 50 atoms making up such an embryo at the start. The vertical axis is the difference in the average useful energy per atom as compared with that which it possesses at precisely the melting temperature. The word *useful* is somewhat important, because this energy must be used for the nucleus to form. This free energy is positive in the upper half of the graph and negative in the lower half. At the horizontal line, it is zero; that is, there is true equilibrium between liquid and solid.

Three curves are shown, all three representing a specific amount of super-cooling. The volume free energy of the embryo is shown in curve F_v. The atoms in the interior of the embryo have a little negative free energy. Because the number of atoms in a sphere is proportional to the value of r^3, the negative contribution to this curve increases rapidly as the radius gets larger. Because it would take work to break up the embryo, it tends to become stable when the free energy is strongly negative. Meanwhile, the surface of the embryo is also increasing. Every surface atom has a little positive surface free energy, because it takes "work" to hold an atom on the surface of the embryo. An atom on the surface has fewer nearest neighbor atoms with which to bond. Curve F_s represents the increase in the surface free energy as a function of the increase in the radius of the embryo.

Now, because the embryo is ambiguously increasing and decreasing in its free energy while it is growing, one would like to know what the net result will be. As the surface energy increases proportionately to the square of the radius, the F_s curve increases mildly with the increase in radius. This means that eventually the steeply descending F_v curve becomes dominant and the embryo becomes stable.

Curve R is drawn to represent the resultant free energy existing at any instant. The *critical radius*, indicated as r_o in the figure, is the embryo radius obtained when the resultant free energy first begins to decrease with an increase in radius. It is also the minimal radius at which a nucleus of crystallization, or the first permanent solid space lattice, is formed.

The greater the supercooling, or the rate of temperature decrease, the smaller this critical radius, r_o, as is seen in Figure 14–3. Hence, an increasing number of embryos become stable as supercooling is increased. If the melt is cooled rapidly so that solidification must occur at a low temperature, there will be a tendency for many very small solidification centers to form. If one wants a single crystal, little supercooling is needed, and the melt must be cooled slowly. This method of nucleus formation is called *homogeneous nucleation*, because the formation of nuclei in the molten metal is a random process and has an equal probability of occurring at any point in the melt.

Another method for reducing the surface energy of the embryo is for the atoms to contact some surface particle or particles in the mold that it can wet; thus, the surface energy can be reduced and a nucleus formed. Such a process is known as *heterogeneous nucleation* because a foreign body "seeded" the nucleus, and the distribution of these foreign bodies is not random. For example, if the metal is gold, very fine particles of gold sifted into the molten metal can cause nucleation. Even the walls of the containing vessel or particles of dust and other impurities in the melt may produce heterogeneous nucleation.

Supercooling is not necessary for heterogeneous nucleation. In fact, this type may account for most of the nucleation when no supercooling occurs. The distribution uniformity of heterogeneously formed nuclei is difficult to control because the distribution of the "seeds" is not likely to be uniform.

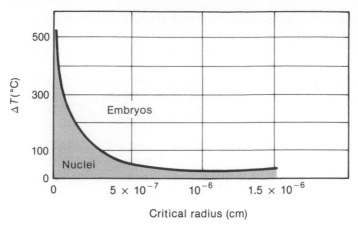

Figure 14–3. The critical radius of copper as a function of the degree of supercooling. T denotes the number of degrees of supercooling below $T_f = 584°$ C. The shaded area represents nuclei; the unshaded area represents embryos. (From INTRODUCTION TO MECHANICAL PROPERTIES OF MATERIALS by Eisenstadt, M., © 1971. Reprinted by permission of Prentice-Hall, Inc., Upper Saddle River, NJ.)

Mechanism of Crystallization. The crystallization is controlled by atomic diffusion from the melt to the nuclei. The crystals do not form regularly along one plane at a time but rather the atomic diffusion to lattice positions is pictured as being irregular, with lattice discontinuities and imperfections being constantly formed in a random manner.

Characteristically, a pure metal may crystallize in a tree-branch pattern from

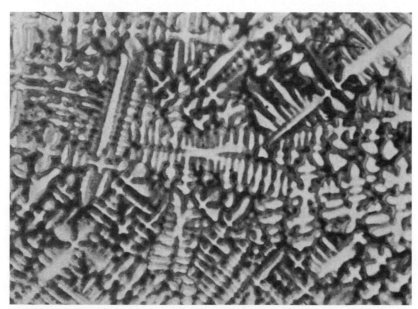

Figure 14–4. Microstructure of a brass alloy showing branchlike dendritic formations. (From INTRODUCTION TO MECHANICAL PROPERTIES OF MATERIALS by Eisenstadt, M., © 1971. Reprinted by permission of Prentice-Hall, Inc., Upper Saddle River, NJ.)

a nucleus. Such crystal formations are called *dendrites*. In three dimensions, they are not unlike the two-dimensional frost crystals that form on a window pane in the winter. Figure 14–4 shows the dendritic structure that can be observed in alloy microstructures.

A schematic representation of such a crystallization in two dimensions is shown in Figure 14–5. As can be observed, the growth starts from the nuclei of crystallization, and the crystals grow toward each other (Fig. 14–5*B* to *E*). When two or more crystals collide, their growth is stopped. Finally, the entire space is filled with crystals as diagrammed in Figure 14–5*F*. However, each crystal remains a unit in itself. It is oriented differently from its neighbors. The metal is, therefore, made of thousands of tiny crystals. Such a metal is said to be *polycrystalline*, and each crystal in the structure is known as a *grain*.

If any metal is highly polished, and if the polished surface is etched with an appropriate reagent, the grain structure can be made visible in a microscope. The photomicrograph of the grain structure of a gold casting prepared in this manner is shown in Figure 14–6. The resemblance between the grain structure in Figure 14–6 and that of the diagram in Figure 14–5*F* is evident. The lines in Figure 14–6, somewhat indistinct in certain areas, represent the periphery of the grains, or the boundaries at which the grains met during their original growth.

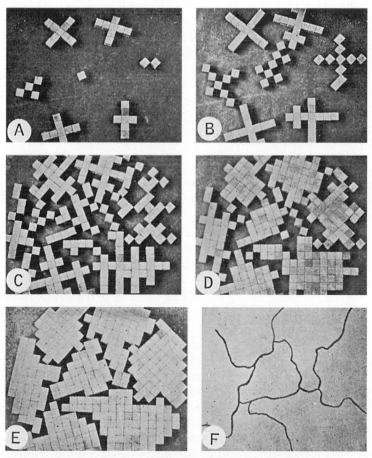

Figure 14–5. Stages in the formation of metallic grains during the solidification of a molten metal. (From Rosenhain W: Introduction to Physical Metallurgy, 3rd ed. London, Constable and Co, 1935.)

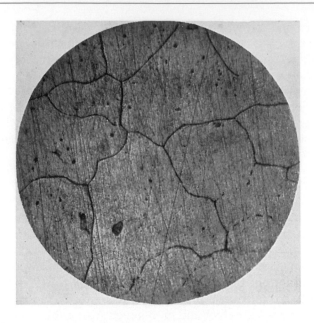

Figure 14–6. Microstructure of a gold casting. ×100. (Courtesy of S. D. Tylman.)

Grain Size. The size of metal grains depends on the number and location of the nuclei at the time of the solidification. If the nuclei are equally spaced with reference to each other, the grains will be approximately equal in size. The solidification can be pictured as proceeding from the nuclei in all directions at the same time in the form of a sphere that is constantly increasing in diameter. When these spheres meet, they are flattened along various surfaces. The tendency for each grain to remain spherical still exists, however, and the grain tends, therefore, to be the same diameter in all dimensions. Such a grain is said to be *equiaxed*. Dental castings generally tend to exhibit an equiaxed grain structure, and such a structure is of considerable dental importance.

Control of Grain Size. In general, the smaller the grain size of the metal, the better its physical properties. For example, the yield strength of many types of materials has been found to vary inversely with the square root of the grain size. Consequently, obtaining a small grain size during casting is an advantage.

Because the grains crystallize from nuclei of crystallization, it follows logically that the number of grains formed is directly related to the number of nuclei of crystallization present at the time of solidification. This factor can be controlled to a degree by the amount of supercooling and the rate of cooling. In other words, the more rapidly the liquid state can be changed to the solid state, the smaller or finer the grains will be.

Another factor of equal importance is the rate of crystallization. If the crystals form faster than do the nuclei of crystallization, the grains will be larger than if the reverse condition prevails. Conversely, if the nucleus formation occurs faster than the rate of crystallization, a small grain size can be obtained. Consequently, slow cooling results in large grains. For example, some metals can be held at their fusion temperatures and caused to crystallize in contact with a crystal or seed of the metal. If the crystal is withdrawn at a constant speed as the crystallization proceeds, a rod or bar made up of a single grain can be formed. Such a metal is known as a *single crystal* in contrast with the polycrystalline form that is usually present.

In a polycrystalline metal, the shape of the grains may be influenced by the shape of the mold in which the metal solidifies. The latent heat of solidification of the metal must be absorbed by the surroundings. This heat transfer requires the existence of temperature gradients, which in turn greatly influence the size and shape of the solidifying grains. For example, if a metal solidifies in a square mold that is at a temperature considerably below the melting temperature of the metal, the crystal growth proceeds from the edges to the center, as shown in Figure 14–7. The first grains to form are quite small and many in number as a result of a great amount of supercooling. This results in an equiaxed zone of crystal growth immediately adjacent to the mold walls.

The latent heat given up by this initial solidification raises the temperature in the vicinity of the solidification front, and the condition then becomes favorable for dendritic growth, resulting in grains called *columnar grains.* If the mold had been cylindrical, the grains would have grown perpendicular to the wall surface, thereby giving the radial grain structure appearance. Such grains are called *radial grains.*

Grain Boundaries. As previously noted, the orientation of the space lattice of the various grains is different, although each grain may possess the same space lattice as its neighbor. The probability is small for two neighboring grains to grow from different nuclei and to meet so that the planes of their space lattices join in exact continuity. Consequently, there must be a discontinuity of lattice structure at the *grain boundaries,* as this area is designated.

It follows logically that the structure of the grain boundaries is different from that in the grain proper. The grain boundary is assumed to be a region of transition between the differently oriented crystal lattices of the two neighboring grains. The structure is more nearly noncrystalline, particularly toward the central region of the grain boundary. This region, therefore, must be considered to be of higher energy than the interior of the grain. Its tendency toward amorphism indicates the possibility of a greater rate of diffusion. As a consequence, impurities in the metal may be found in greater concentration at the grain boundaries than in the grain proper. Also, the region is more readily attacked by chemicals, as indicated by grain boundaries that are revealed after chemical etching in Figure 14–6.

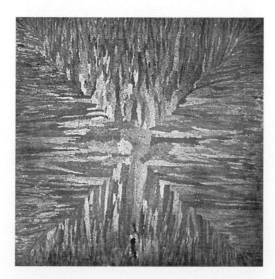

Figure 14–7. Metallic grains formed by the solidification of a metal in a square mold. (From Williams RS, and Homerberg VO: Principles of Metallography, 5th ed. New York, McGraw-Hill, 1948.)

SELECTED READING

Eisenstad MM: Introduction to Mechanical Properties of Materials. New York, Macmillan, 1971, pp 95–110.

A very readable discussion of solidification, including nucleation and growth. Also includes some examples of growth kinetics as influenced by temperature gradients that have dental applications.

Metals Handbook, Desk Edition. Metals Park, OH, American Society of Metals, 1992.

A comprehensive reference book on the structure, properties, and processing of metals. It also describes testing methods for metals and provides an excellent review of fractographic analysis procedures for fractured metals.

15 *Constitution of Alloys*

- Classification of Alloys
- Solid Solutions
- Constitution or Equilibrium Phase Diagrams
- Eutectic Alloys
- Physical Properties
- Peritectic Alloys
- Solid-state Reactions
- Other Binary Systems

An *alloy* is defined for dental purposes as a metal containing two or more elements, at least one of which is a metal, and all of which are mutually soluble in the molten state. Although there are some similarities between the characteristics of pure metals and alloys, the addition of other metals to a pure metal complicates the picture relative to certain fundamental aspects not yet considered. For example, most alloys solidify over a range in temperature rather than at a single temperature, as does a pure metal. Within this temperature range, two phases (solid and liquid) exist. The presence of more than one metal may also cause certain reactions in the solid state that cannot occur with a pure metal and that directly affect the properties of the alloy. These and other alloy phenomena are now discussed.

Before the technical discussion continues, several terms must be explained to ensure that a common ground of understanding is reached. An *alloy system* is an aggregate of two or more metals in all possible combinations. For example, the "gold-silver system" includes all possible concentrations of gold and silver, varying from 100% gold to 100% silver.

To specify a particular alloy, it is necessary to list the elements contained in the alloy and the amount of each element present. Two systems are commonly employed to define composition: the weight percentage (wt%) of each element may be given or, alternatively, the atomic fraction or percentage (at%) can be used. As an example, the $AuCu_3$ phase, which can form during slow cooling of a molten gold-copper alloy, contains 51 wt% gold but only 25 at% gold.

From a biocompatibility viewpoint, predominantly nickel-based metal alloys contain an apparently small amount (1.8 wt%) of beryllium, a relatively toxic element. However, on an atomic percentage basis, these nickel-chromium-molybdenum-beryllium alloys contain a much larger proportion of beryllium (approximately 10.7 at%). For alloys with elements that differ considerably in atomic weight, the weight percentage and atomic percentage obviously differ substantially. Usually, the properties of an alloy relate more directly to the atomic percentage rather than the weight percentage of each element present.

From a metallurgic standpoint, a *phase* is any physically distinct, homogeneous, and mechanically separable portion of a system. We are familiar with the existence of matter in three different physical states or phases: liquid, solid, and gas. However, in metallurgy, one finds that more than one phase is present in the solid state. For example, grains (crystals) of two or more different compositions may be present that are mechanically separable. The region between any two grains is called a *grain boundary*.

Alloys must be in *equilibrium* before a true phase can exist. Polycrystalline metals and alloys never reach true equilibrium conditions in the solid state because of slow solid-state diffusion rates and other factors. If an alloy has been cooled rapidly from a high temperature at which the rate of atomic diffusion is considerable, an unstable structure may be made permanent and apparently stable at room temperature. Nevertheless, equilibrium conditions are assumed in the subsequent discussions. The conditions to be described are approached as a limit only under conditions of slow cooling and prolonged times at temperatures high enough to allow ample opportunity for atomic diffusion.

CLASSIFICATION OF ALLOYS

Alloys can be classified according to (1) use (such as all-metal inlays, crowns and bridges, metal-ceramic restorations, removable partial dentures, and implants); (2) major element (gold, palladium, silver, nickel, cobalt, or titanium); (3) nobility (high noble, noble, and predominantly base metal); (4) principal three elements (gold-palladium-silver, palladium-silver-tin, nickel-chromium-beryllium, cobalt-chromium-molybdenum, titanium-aluminum-vanadium, or iron-nickel-chromium); and (5) the dominant phase system (isomorphous [single phase], eutectic, peritectic, or intermetallic).

If two elements are present, a *binary alloy* is formed; if three or four metals are present, *ternary and quaternary alloys,* respectively, are produced, and so forth. As the number of elements increases above two, the structure becomes increasingly complex. Consequently, only binary alloys are studied in detail in this section.

The simplest alloy is one in which the atoms of the two metals intermingle randomly in a common space lattice. Under the microscope, the grains of such alloys may resemble those of pure metals; the structure is homogeneous because only one phase is formed during solidification. The two metals are said to be mutually soluble in the solid state, and the alloys are called *solid solutions*. Most of the gold alloys used in dentistry are predominantly the solid-solution type, although they usually contain more than two metals.

Like the components of many liquid solutions, the metals that form solid solutions may not be completely soluble in each other in all proportions; they may be only partially soluble. In such a case, *intermediate phases* may also appear that are not mutually soluble in the solid state. Once the solubility limit has been exceeded, the solid state is composed of a mixture of two or more distinct solid phases. Some of the alloys that are not solid solutions are *eutectic alloys, peritectic alloys, intermetallic compounds*, and *combinations*. These types are discussed later.

SOLID SOLUTIONS

By far the greatest number of alloys used for dental restorations are solid solutions. Therefore, special attention should be given to this type of alloy. The term *solution* as applied to liquids is familiar from high school chemistry courses. For example, a solution of sugar and water connotes a homogeneous system in which molecules of sugar diffuse through and intermingle at random with those of water. The same is true of a molten solution of silver in palladium. However, if the sugar and water are frozen, each component solidifies separately, but a palladium-silver alloy solidifies in such a manner that the the silver atoms are distributed randomly through the space lattice of the solid palladium, replacing the palladium atoms in a manner analogous to the molecular arrangement of the solute in the liquid solution. Such an alloy is called a *solid solution.* Because the atoms of silver enter directly into the space lattice of palladium, the system is not mechanically separable and only one phase is formed. Furthermore, if the atoms of silver are segregated for any reason and are not scattered randomly throughout the palladium space lattice, they can be made to diffuse at high temperatures in a manner analogous to that of undissolved sugar in water until equilibrium is reached.

Solutes and Solvents. When sugar is dissolved in water, the water is referred to as the *solvent* and the sugar as the *solute.* When two metals are soluble in one another in the solid state, the solvent is that metal whose space lattice persists, and the solute is the other metal. In palladium-silver alloys, the two metals are completely soluble in all proportions, and the same type of space lattice persists throughout the system. In such a case, the solvent may be defined as the metal whose atoms occupy more than one half the total number of positions in the space lattice.

The configuration of the space lattice of solid solutions may be of several types: substitutional, interstitial, and ordered. In the *substitutional* type, the atoms of the solute occupy the space lattice positions that normally are occupied by the solvent atoms in the pure metal. In a palladium-silver alloy in which the palladium is the solvent, the silver atoms replace the palladium atoms randomly in lattice positions.

Another type of solid solution of considerable importance is the *interstitial solid solution.* In this case, the solute atoms are present in positions between the solvent atoms (the interstices between regular lattice positions). This type of solid solution ordinarily requires that the solute atoms be much smaller in diameter than the solvent atoms. These solid solutions usually are limited to relatively small concentrations of solute. The interstitial solid solution of carbon in iron is one of the most important, because it forms the basis for the family of alloys called *steels.*

In some substitutional solid solutions, the solvent and solute atoms have a slight affinity for each other. From an energy point of view, the random arrangement of atoms represents a higher energy than if the atoms are ordered in such a way as to have unlike nearest neighbors. For such an alloy, at a sufficiently low temperature, diffusion may cause an ordering of a random solid solution. Because the ordering process implies a definite proportion of solute and solvent atoms, such ordered structures usually exist over small compositional ranges. For example, the gold-copper alloys exhibit a random or substitutional solid solution structure of the face-centered type at high temperatures (Fig. 15–1A), but if an alloy of the composition 50.2 wt% gold and 49.8 wt% copper is allowed

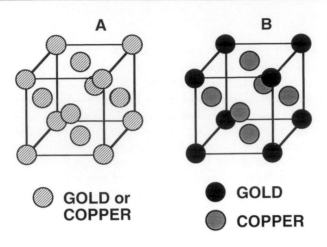

Figure 15–1. Structure of AuCu₃. In a unit cell of a face-centered cubic space lattice of a copper-gold substitutional type *(A)*, the positions of the gold atoms cannot be distinguished from the positions of the copper atoms. In the superlattice or ordered arrangement *(B)*, the gold atoms are situated at the corners, and the copper atoms are on the faces of the cube.

to cool slowly to below 400° C (752° F), the gold atoms are located at the corners of the cube of the unit lattice cell and the copper atoms are positioned on the faces (Fig. 15–1*B*).

When the unit cells are combined to form the space lattice, there are three times as many copper atoms as there are gold atoms, and as a result such a structure is represented as AuCu₃. The structure is called a *superlattice,* or an *ordered* structure.

Conditions for Solid Solubility. In any substitutional type of solid solution, the distance between the atoms changes according to the size of the solute atom. The entire lattice may be expanded or contracted sometimes nonuniformly, according to the size of the solute atom relative to the solvent atom. Generally, however, such changes in atomic distances are not great because one of the primary requisites for two or more metals to form solid solutions is that their atomic diameters be approximately the same.

There are at least four factors that determine the extent of solid solubility of two or more metals.

1. Atom size—if the sizes of two metallic atoms differ by less than approximately 15%, they possess a favorable size factor for solid solubility. If the size factor is greater than 15%, multiple phases appear during solidification. Probably none of the metals is completely lacking in solid solubility with other metals. Even if the solid solubility is only a fraction of a percent, such a limited solubility can be of importance in certain instances.

2. Valence—metals of the same valence and size are more likely to form extensive solid solutions than are metals of different valences. If the valences differ, the metal with the higher valence may be more soluble in a metal of lower valence.

3. Chemical affinity—when two metals exhibit a high degree of chemical affinity, they tend to form an intermetallic compound on solidification rather than a solid solution.

4. Lattice type—only metals with the same type of crystal lattice can form a complete series of solid solutions, particularly if the size factor is less than 8%. Most of the metals used for dental restorations are face-centered cubic (see Fig. 15–1*A*) and can form a continuous series of solid solutions.

Although the diameter of the copper atom differs as much as 12% from that of the other four metals under consideration, it is an important alloy component. As discussed later, it forms a limited series of solid solutions with silver. Solid solutions of copper in gold, platinum, and palladium are continuous at high temperatures, but on cooling, superlattice changes take place, as already discussed for the formation of the $AuCu_3$ superlattice.

According to Table 15–1, the difference between the silver and the tin atomic diameters is approximately 4%. However, the two metals are different in valence and have different crystal structures, and they are not closely associated in the electromotive series. Silver is a limited solvent for tin. As the tin content increases, an intermetallic compound (Ag_3Sn) forms, which is an important constituent of dental amalgams.

Physical Properties of Solid Solutions. It was previously noted that the lattice structure of a solvent metal is expanded or contracted by substitution of solute atoms. Such a statement is true only if the situation is considered as an average condition over the entire space lattice. Wherever a solute atom displaces or substitutes for a solvent atom, the difference in size of the solute atom results in a localized distortion or strained condition of the lattice, and slip becomes more difficult. As a consequence, the strength, proportional limit, and surface hardness are increased, whereas the ductility is usually decreased. In other words, the alloying of metals may be a means of strengthening the metal. The general theory of slip interference in alloys is the same as in strain hardening, except that a different type of lattice distortion is present initially to inhibit slip before the structure is plastically stressed or worked.

Gold itself cannot be used as a restorative material unless it is strain hardened, as in the compaction of gold foil. Pure gold in the cast condition is too weak and ductile. However, if as little as 5% by weight of copper is alloyed with the gold, the latter loses practically none of its ability to resist tarnish and corrosion, yet adequate strength and hardness are imparted to it so that it can be used for the casting of small inlays.

The hardness and strength of any metallic solvent are increased by the atoms of a solute. The closer the atoms are in size, the less is the effect of the solute atoms, but some increase in strength can be expected nevertheless.

Generally, the more of the solute metal is added to the solvent, the greater are the strength and hardness of the alloy. In two metals that form a continuous series of solid solutions with one another, the maximal hardness is reached at approximately 50 at% of each metal. As might be expected from the theory, the ductility usually decreases progressively as the strength and hardness increase.

TABLE 15–1. Atomic Diameters of Metals of Dental Interest

Metal	Atomic Diameter (Angstroms)	Crystal Structure
Gold	2.882	Face-centered cubic
Platinum	2.775	Face-centered cubic
Palladium	2.750	Face-centered cubic
Silver	2.888	Face-centered cubic
Copper	2.556	Face-centered cubic
Tin	3.016	Body-centered tetragonal
Zinc	2.665	Close-packed hexagonal
Silicon	2.351	Diamond cubic

From Lyman T (ed): Metals Handbook, 8th ed., Vol. I. Cleveland, American Society for Metals, 1964.

CONSTITUTION OR EQUILIBRIUM PHASE DIAGRAMS

The concept of a constitution or equilibrium phase diagram is introduced using the table salt–water system. The dissolution of ordinary table salt (NaCl) in water to form a chemical solution (brine) is the starting point for the discussion. It is observed that at a particular temperature, a limit exists on how much salt can be dissolved before salt crystals begin to settle out. The chemist would refer to a solubility or miscibility limit. Notice that a pure single-phase liquid—brine—becomes a two-phase solid-liquid mixture (brine and salt) as the solubility limit is exceeded. If the temperature of the system is increased, the amount of salt that can be dissolved increases. If the temperature is decreased sufficiently, eventually another solid phase appears, called *ice*. Although pure water solidifies to form ice at 0° C, it is common knowledge that the addition of salt to water depresses its freezing point.

All this information concerning the salt-water system can be assembled in an orderly fashion to form a "map" showing what phases are present at a particular temperature and composition (amount of salt). Such a diagram is presented in Figure 15–2.

This diagram assumes that equilibrium conditions have been established, a reasonable assumption for a system dependent on solid diffusion in a liquid. In this figure can be seen one single-phase region (brine); two liquid-solid two-phase regions (ice plus brine and salt plus brine); and one solid-solid two-phase region (ice plus salt). The region labeled "ice plus brine" is probably not as familiar as the others. As the temperature of a salt solution is lowered for salt concentrations below 23.3%, almost pure water settles out of solution as ice to form the ice-brine mixture. This can be used to desalinate sea water (a 1.7% salt solution) and is an economical alternative to distillation.

Now let us turn to the alloy system of pure metal A and pure metal B. As previously noted, such a system is composed of all possible combinations of A and B, ranging from 100% A to 100% B. Further assume that A and B are completely soluble at all compositions in both solid and liquid states.

Cooling curve experiments like the ones discussed previously are now performed on a series of alloys from the A-B system as follows: (1) 100% A; (2) 80% A-20% B; (3) 60% A-40% B; (4) 40% A-60% B; (5) 20% A-80% B; and (6) 100% B. These are shown in Figure 15–3A. Curves 1 and 6 for the pure metals A and B are familiar from Chapter 14. Curves 2 through 5 illustrate that solid-solution alloys do not have a solidification temperature but instead solidify over a

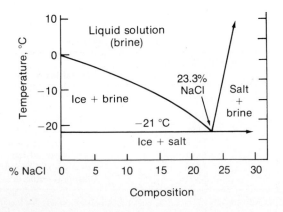

Figure 15–2. Solubility of table salt (NaCl) in brine (right upward-sloping line) and solubility of ice in brine (left curve). (Redrawn from Van Vlack LH: ELEMENTS OF MATERIALS SCIENCE AND ENGINEERING, 4th edition. © 1980 Addison-Wesley Publishing Company, Inc. Reprinted by permission of Addison-Wesley Publishing Company, Inc.)

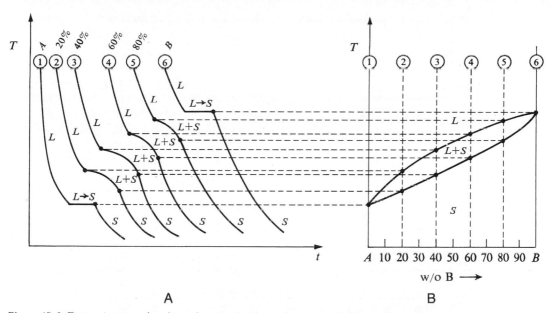

Figure 15–3. Determination of a phase diagram by thermal analysis. *A,* The cooling curves of six alloys of various compositions are determined experimentally. *B,* In addition, the temperature of fusion and the liquidus and solidus temperatures are plotted as a function of composition to form the phase diagram. (*A* and *B* from Richman M: An Introduction to the Science of Metals. Waltham, MA, Blaisdell, 1967, p 213.)

temperature range. The region labeled L+S is a two-phase region composed of liquid and solid analogous to the brine and salt region in the first example.

These cooling curves can now be used to determine the equilibrium phase diagram for the A-B alloy system, as shown in Figure 15–3B. The temperature at which the first solid begins to form (called the *liquidus temperature*) for each composition is determined from the cooling curves in Figure 15–3A and then plotted on the temperature-composition diagram (see Fig. 15–3B). Similarly, the temperature at which the last liquid solidifies (called the *solidus*) is determined and plotted. When these points are connected with a smooth curve, the *equilibrium phase diagram* (see Fig. 15–3B) results.

The upper solid line in Figure 15–3B is called the *liquidus line,* because the alloys are entirely liquid above this line. The lower line is called the *solidus,* because the alloys are entirely solid below this line. The region between is, of course, the two-phase liquid plus solid region. Consider now an alloy system that has considerable dental interest and resembles the theoretical system just described.

Figure 15–4 presents the silver-palladium phase diagram. Pure silver is represented at 0% palladium and pure palladium at 100%. These metals exhibit complete solubility in both liquid and solid states. Note that the liquid and liquid-solid region and the liquid-solid and solid regions are separated by liquidus and solidus lines, respectively.

Interpretation of the Constitution Diagram. As an illustration of how the constitution diagram can be used to advantage, consider an alloy of composition 65% palladium and 35% silver as indicated by the dotted line PO, erected perpendicularly from the base line through 65% palladium (see Fig. 15–4). If the point on the line PO corresponding to the temperature 1500° C (2732° F) is

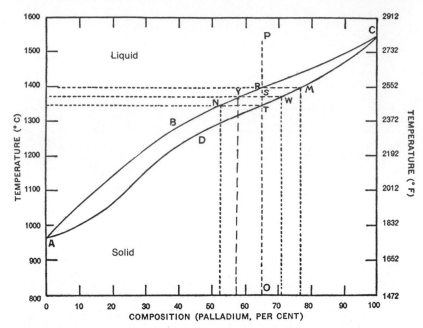

Figure 15–4. Equilibrium phase diagram for the silver-palladium system. Only the percentage composition for palladium is given; the percentage composition for silver is determined by subtracting the palladium composition from 100.

considered, only liquid is present with a composition of 65% palladium and 35% silver.

When the temperature decreases to approximately 1400° C (2552° F), the first solid forms at the point R that is situated on the liquidus. To determine the composition of the first alloy that solidifies, the line RM, called the *tie line,* is drawn through R, parallel to the base line. If the point of intersection (M) with the solidus is projected to the base line, the composition of the first solid can be determined as 77% palladium. Similarly, if the point R is similarly projected, the composition of the remaining liquid is found to be 65% palladium.

Now assume that the temperature decreases to approximately 1370° C (2498° F) as denoted by the point S. At this temperature, the material is partially solid and partially liquid. As before, the composition of the solid and liquid at this stage may be determined by drawing the tie line YW and locating its point of intersection with the liquidus and solidus, respectively, in terms of composition. Hence, the approximate composition of the liquid is 58% palladium, as given by the projection of the point Y on the base line, whereas that of the solid is about 71% palladium, determined by projecting the point W to the base line. At the temperature corresponding to the point T (approximately 1340° C, or 2444° F), the last portion of liquid solidifies. This liquid has the composition of 52% palladium and the solid phase is 65% palladium.

It should be reemphasized that this is an equilibrium phase diagram and that the system must be held at each of these temperatures for a time sufficient for diffusion to produce equilibrium conditions. After equilibrium has been achieved, the compositions of liquid and solid and the amounts of each phase present are stable.

When the temperature decreases below point T, the alloy is entirely solid with a composition of 65% palladium. Thus, the chemical composition of any phase

TABLE 15–2. Chemical Compositions and Phase Amounts of a 65% Palladium (Pd) and 35% Silver Alloy

Temperature		Chemical Composition	
°C	°F	Liquid-% Pd	Solid-% Pd
1500	2732	65	*
1400	2552	65	77
1370	2498	58	71
1340	2444	52	65
900	1652	*	65

*Phase not present at this temperature.

of the palladium-silver system at any temperature can be obtained in a similar manner. The percentage of each phase that is present at a given temperature with a given base composition can also be calculated.

Coring. It can be noted from Table 15–2 that the composition of a rapidly cooled dendrite or grain is not uniform. For example, the first embryo or nucleus that forms at the temperature R (or slightly below) in Figure 15–4 is rich in palladium, but as the temperature decreases, the palladium content decreases with an increase in the silver content as each succeeding "layer" solidifies. The palladium content of the liquid phase decreases, but its silver content increases as the solidification temperature is approached.

At the solidus temperature T (see Fig. 15–4) the composition of the outermost "layer" of the dendrite is 65% palladium and 35% silver. The last liquid to solidify is rich in silver and solidifies between the dendrites. Therefore, a cored structure results, with the core consisting of the dendrites composed of compositions with higher solidus temperatures and the matrix containing compositions with a lower solidus.

Excellent examples of cored structures can be observed in the photomicrograph in Figure 15–5 in the as-cast state (A) and after a homogenization heat treatment (B). The dark dendritic structure (A) represents the core composed of the high melting range compositions. The matrix that solidified between the dendrites is lighter in shade. Note that this cored structure is an equilibrium

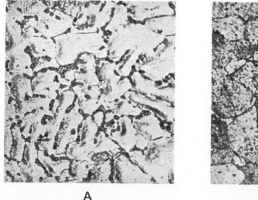
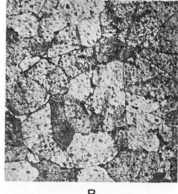

A   B

Figure 15–5. Copper-silver alloy (1%) as cast (A) and the same structure after homogenization (B). ×100. (A and B from Avner SH: An Introduction to Physical Metallurgy. New York, McGraw-Hill, 1964.)

structure. The cooling rates involved in normal casting procedures do not allow sufficient time for diffusion to achieve a state of equilibrium. Note also that the larger the temperature range between liquidus and solidus, the greater the tendency toward coring.

Homogenization. In the previous discussion, rapid cooling was assumed. The atoms tend to diffuse to reduce segregation. Under conditions of equilibrium, the alloy composition should be 65% palladium and 35% silver throughout, and atomic diffusion during cooling controls such a situation. However, the faster the alloy is cooled from its liquidus temperature, the more nearly the compositions in Table 15–2 are approached; on the other hand, during slow cooling, there is greater atomic diffusion and a greater probability of achieving equilibrium.

If the alloy is cooled rapidly from its liquidus temperature, the coring can be relieved by a heat-treating process similar to that described for wrought metal. The alloy is held at a temperature near its solidus temperature so that solid-state atomic diffusion can occur. Little or no grain growth occurs when a casting is heat treated, and higher temperatures are often employed than would be used with a wrought metal. The process of heating a cast alloy to eliminate composition differences caused by coring is called *homogenization*.

A second difference between annealing and homogenization is the time necessary for the homogenization. The rate of atomic diffusion in the cast structure is much slower than that in a cold-worked structure. The former may require hours, whereas, at the same temperature, the cold-worked structure may recrystallize in minutes. Consequently, if the cast structure can be cold worked, it can be homogenized much faster by recrystallization. However, casting alloys cannot always be cold worked, although they must be homogenized, a process that requires 6 hours at high temperature for the alloy shown in Figure 15–5B.

An inhomogeneous dental gold alloy is more subject to tarnish and corrosion than the same alloy after it has been homogenized. This consideration is also important for silver-palladium alloys, because silver-rich phases tend to tarnish readily in the mouth.

As might be expected, the heterogeneous grain structure offers more resistance to slip and less ductility than does the homogenized structure. After homogenization, the ductility of the alloy usually increases.

EUTECTIC ALLOYS

Many binary alloy systems are not as simple as the one just considered in that they do not exhibit complete solubility in both the solid and the liquid states. The eutectic alloy is an example in which the components exhibit complete liquid solubility but limited solid solubility.

The simplest illustration of a eutectic alloy is two metals, A and B, which are completely insoluble in each other in the solid state. In such a case, some of the grains are composed solely of metal A, whereas the remainder of the grains are composed of metal B. The situation is analogous to a frozen brine solution. Although in solution, the salt and the water molecules intermingle randomly. On freezing, the result is a mixture of salt crystals and ice crystals that form independently of each other.

However, all metals are probably soluble in one another to at least a limited extent. Therefore, a binary eutectic system in which the two metals are partially soluble in each other is used for purposes of illustration. Such a system of interest to dentistry is the silver-copper system.

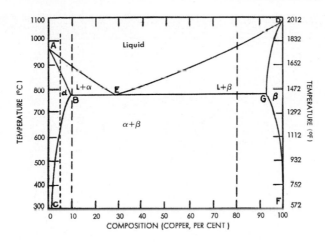

Figure 15–6. Equilibrium phase diagram for the silver-copper system.

Silver-Copper System. The constitution diagram for the silver-copper system is presented in Figure 15–6. The solidus can be identified as the boundary line ABEGD and the liquidus as AED. The limited solid solubility of Cu in Ag and Ag in Cu is evident in that the major portion of the diagram below 780° C is composed of a two-phase region labeled $\alpha + \beta$. This region is a mechanical mixture of α, the silver-rich alloy, and β, the copper-rich alloy.

The first difference to be noted in comparison with Figure 15–4 is that the liquidus and solidus meet at E. This composition (71.9% silver, 28.1% copper) is known as the *eutectic composition* or, simply, the *eutectic*. One should note the following characteristics of a eutectic alloy:

- The temperature (779.4° C [1434.9° F]) at which the eutectic occurs is lower than the fusion temperature of either silver or copper (eutectic literally means lowest melting) and is the lowest temperature at which any alloy composition of silver and copper is entirely liquid.
- There is no solidification range for composition E. In other words, it solidifies at a constant temperature, which is characteristic of a eutectic composition. In this respect only is the alloy similar to a pure metal. Eutectic alloys are often used when a lower fusion temperature is desired as, for example, in soldering. In other respects, they are generally inferior to solid solution alloys.

When a eutectic alloy solidifies, the atoms of the constituent metals must segregate to form regions of nearly pure parent metals. This results in a distinctive structure, as can be seen in Figure 15–7A. The layered structure forms because it requires the least amount of diffusion to produce the required segregation.

The eutectic reaction is sometimes written schematically as follows:

$$\text{Liquid} \rightarrow \alpha\text{-solid solution} + \beta\text{-solid solution}$$

It is referred to as an *invariant transformation*, because it occurs at a single temperature and composition.

Another feature of the diagram in Figure 15–6 is that the solidus at first gradually changes composition with a decrease in temperature until the eutectic temperature is attained. Its temperature then remains constant even though there is a phase change. For example, along the solidus from A to B, the silver becomes richer in copper as the temperature decreases. In fact, the copper content in-

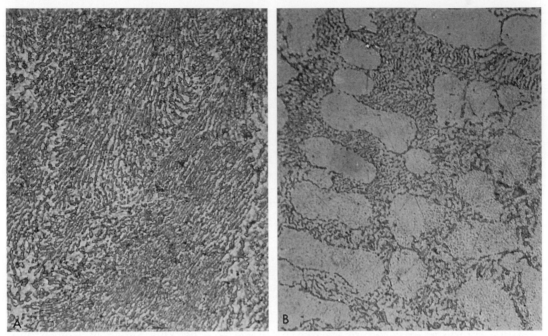

Figure 15–7. Microstructure of two lead-tin alloys. *A,* The alloy has the eutectic composition 62% Sn-38% Pb. The structure is composed of alternating layers (lamellae) of α-solid solution (dark) that is Pb rich and β-solid solution (light) that is Sn rich. ×1280. *B,* The alloy has a high tin content (75% Sn-25% Pb). The light islands are primary β phase that solidified first. They are surrounded by the eutectic that solidified when the eutectic temperature was reached ×560. (*A* and *B* courtesy of P. G. Winchell.)

creases from 0% to 8.8% at B with the reduction in temperature. At the copper end of the diagram, as the alloy cools from D to G, the number of silver atoms in the copper space lattice increases until 8% silver has alloyed with the copper. It is evident that the silver lattice contains the copper atoms in solution in the first instance and that the copper lattice contains the silver atoms in solution at the other end of the diagram. In other words, the copper is soluble in the silver to an extent of 8.8% provided the system is held at the eutectic temperature E or, similarly, the temperature indicated by the point B.

As with any solution in which the solute solubility in the solvent is limited, the solubility decreases with a decrease in temperature. The *solvus lines* and GF indicate the change in solid solubility of the copper in silver and silver in copper, respectively, as the temperature of the total solid phase decreases. The solid solution of copper in silver is called the α-*solid solution*, and that of silver in copper is called the β-solid solution.

The compositions of the various alloys and the amount of each phase present can be determined in the same manner as for solid solutions of silver and palladium. For example, if a silver-copper alloy of 10% copper is melted at a temperature above the liquidus and allowed to cool along the second dotted vertical line (see Fig. 15–6), the first solid crystallizes at approximately 900° C (1652° F). If a tie line is drawn from the liquidus at this point to the solidus, the first solid is the α-solid solution of the approximate composition of 4% copper and 96% silver.

If the temperature is allowed to fall to 850° C (1562° F), the points of intersection of the α tie line on the solidus and liquidus indicate an α-solid solution composition of 5% copper; the remaining liquid is 15% copper. When the temperature decreases to the eutectic temperature, the tie line becomes BE. As the eutectic temperature is reached, the last liquid to solidify has the eutectic composition and solidifies, forming α + β phases in the typical eutectic structure.

If the copper composition is greater than that of the eutectic, the composition change is similar except that the β-solid solution is the first solid solution to form instead of the α-solid solution, as in the previous case. Such an effect is evident if the compositions of the alloy, 80% copper, and 20% silver, are calculated during cooling as indicated by the dotted vertical composition line to the extreme right in Figure 15–6.

In summary, the first solids to form above the eutectic temperature are always of either the solid solution α or the solid solution β. The first grains so formed are large, at least compared with the mixture of small grains that form the eutectic. The larger grains are called *primary grains* because they form first. The α + β formed above the eutectic temperature is referred to as *primary α or β*.

To this point, the compositions below the eutectic temperature have not been considered. This is best illustrated by a cooling of the composition 5% copper, as indicated by the first vertical dotted line in Figure 15–6. It begins to solidify at a temperature slightly above 900° C (1652° F), and it freezes completely as an α-solid solution at approximately 860° C (1580° F). As the temperature falls, the solid solution phase remains intact until a temperature of 630° C (1166° F) is reached; then the copper-rich β phase appears in a mixture with the α-solid solution as a precipitated phase. The reason for this change is related to the solid solubility of copper in silver. Just as the line AB (liquidus) represents the solubility limit of the copper in the silver at the respective solidus temperatures, so does the line BC (solvus) represent the solubility limit of the two metals in the solid state. Again, this occurs only if very slow cooling has permitted equilibrium to be achieved. Rapid cooling of the 5% copper alloy results in almost pure α phase being retained at room temperature. As previously noted, if more than 8.8% copper is added to the melt, the eutectic appears on solidification. However, the solubility of the copper in the silver becomes less as the temperature decreases below the eutectic solidification temperature, as indicated by the line BC. Consequently, when this alloy is slowly cooled below 630° C, the solid solution becomes supersaturated with copper, and the excess copper is *precipitated*. The process is analogous to similar phenomena in supersaturated liquid solutions. At the other end of the diagram, it can be expected that silver precipitates from a supersaturated solution on cooling in the same manner.

The eutectic structure does not appear in alloys of less than 8.8% copper. Only the α-solid solution is present, with varying amounts of β according to the temperature.

PHYSICAL PROPERTIES

Unlike the silver-palladium system (see Fig. 15–4), the mechanical properties of the eutectic alloys do not vary linearly with the composition. For purposes of convenience, alloys with a composition less than that of the eutectic are called *hypoeutectic alloys*, and those with a composition greater than the eutectic are known as *hypereutectic alloys*. The primary crystals of the hypoeutectic alloys in the copper-silver systems are composed of α-solid solution, and those of the hypereutectic alloys are composed of β-solid solution; therefore, a linear relationship between composition and physical properties cannot be expected because two different phases exist on opposite sides of the eutectic composition.

The eutectic alloys are apt to be brittle because the presence of insoluble phases definitely inhibits slip. Consequently, the strength, and sometimes the hardness, of these alloys may surpass those of the constituent metals because of the composite structure of the alloy (an analogy may be made to resin-based composite structures). On the other hand, if the recrystallization temperature of one of the matrix metals is very low, creep may occur even at room temperature.

Except for the gold alloy solders (see Chapter 27), eutectic systems do not generally occur in high noble and noble dental alloys because of their poor tarnish and corrosion resistance. However, α-solid solution alloys of silver and copper have been used to some extent in pedodontics as casting alloys. The tarnish resistance of these alloys is superior to that of the alloys containing the eutectic (see Chapter 16). The silver-copper eutectic is found as the admixed component in some types of high-copper amalgam alloys (see Chapters 17 and 18).

It has been found that the grain size of a cast gold alloy can be reduced by the addition of a trace of another metal of very low solubility and high fusion temperature. It can be added to form a eutectic alloy with a eutectic composition very close to 100% gold. For example, iridium forms a eutectic alloy with gold at a eutectic composition of approximately 0.005% iridium. If approximately 0.005% iridium is added to pure gold, nucleation occurs with a resulting grain refinement. The iridium reduces the critical radius for nucleus formation. If greater amounts of iridium are added than in the eutectic composition with gold, the iridium tends to segregate, and a nonuniform grain size may result.

PERITECTIC ALLOYS

In addition to the eutectic system just described, limited solid solubility of two metals can result in a transformation referred to as *peritectic*. Peritectic systems are uncommon in dentistry, the exception being the silver-tin system, which is the basis for original dental amalgam alloys. However, the platinum-silver phase diagram exhibits a simple peritectic transformation; because these metals are found in many of the gold casting alloys, the system is quite appropriate for study.

Like the eutectic transformation, the peritectic reaction is an invariant reaction (i.e., it occurs at a particular composition and temperature). The reaction can be written as

$$\text{Liquid} + \beta \to \alpha$$

Figure 15–8 is the phase diagram for the silver-platinum alloy system. The α phase is a silver-rich phase, the β phase is platinum rich, and α + β is the two-phase region resulting from limited solid solubility. The peritectic transformation occurs at the point P at which the liquid plus the platinum-rich β phase transforms into the silver-rich α phase. The substantial composition change involved can lead to large amounts of coring if rapid cooling occurs.

If the alloy has a hypoperitectic composition (below line BD), as does alloy I in Figure 15–8, cooling of the alloy through the peritectic temperature results in the transformation

$$\text{Liquid} + \beta \to \text{liquid} + \alpha$$

Rapid cooling results in precipitation of α phase around the β grains before diffusion can occur. The solid α phase inhibits diffusion, and substantial coring

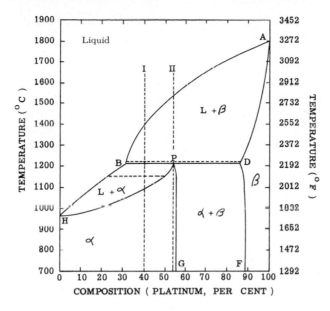

Figure 15–8. Equilibrium phase diagram of the silver-platinum system.

occurs. The cored structure is more brittle and has corrosion resistance inferior to that of the homogeneous α phase.

SOLID-STATE REACTIONS

Several methods for modifying the physical properties of metals have been discussed. The metal can be strengthened by strain hardening, and the strain-hardened metal can be rendered more ductile by an annealing heat treatment. In addition, the strength and toughness of a metal can be increased by reducing the grain size. It has been shown that the physical properties can also be controlled by alloying two or more metals. Each metal constituent contributes certain properties to the alloy.

A fourth and practical method is to cause atomic diffusion by heat treatment in the solid state. This method is now discussed in detail; it can be employed in either the cast or wrought condition.

At this point, two terms need to be clarified. *Heat treatment* is the thermal processing of an alloy for a length of time above room temperature but below the solidus temperature. The effects of such a treatment depend entirely on the temperature, the metal, and its previous history. Heat treating may, for example, harden a metal, soften a metal, or change its grain size or corrosion resistance.

The second term is *quenching*. This term means that a metal is rapidly cooled from an elevated temperature to room temperature or below. This is usually done for one of two reasons: (1) to preserve at room temperature a phase ordinarily stable only at elevated temperatures; and (2) to rapidly terminate a process that only occurs at elevated temperatures. The rapid cooling is often accomplished by immersing the hot metal in a liquid such as water, hence the term *quenching*.

The alloy systems discussed so far have involved either total solid solubility or limited solid solubility. However, another possibility exists in which the elements are completely soluble in the liquid state and at high temperatures in the solid state. At lower temperatures, the attraction of the solvent and solute atoms may be sufficient to convert the random solid solution into an ordered solid phase. The gold-copper alloy system exhibits this phenomenon at certain compositions.

Copper-Gold System. The phase diagram is shown in Figure 15–9. Note that the melting range is narrow for all compositions and that the liquidus and solidus touch at 80.1% gold. Also, addition of as little as 10% copper to the gold lowers the liquidus temperature substantially. Both of these facts are advantageous in the use of the alloy system for dental casting procedures. At temperatures below the solidus but above 410° C, gold and copper exhibit complete solid solubility.

Below 410° C, new solid phases appear. The phase α' is the ordered solid, $AuCu_3$ previously described and illustrated in Figure 15–1. Because of the large amount of copper in this phase, it is not found in dental applications. The α'' phase is another ordered structure and is shown in Figure 15–9. This phase is face-centered tetragonal and has the composition AuCu.

The composition of most of the harder casting gold alloys is compatible with the compositional limits for this phase to form. The transformation from the cubic lattice type at high temperatures to the tetragonal low-temperature phase produces localized strains that inhibit dislocation motion, effectively hardening the alloy. As usually happens when a gold-copper alloy is cooled rapidly (quenched) from the solidus temperature, the disordered solid solution is retained at room temperature, and the alloy is relatively soft. Slow cooling through the transition temperature, however, allows diffusion to occur. The alloy would partially transform to the ordered phase and would be harder than the quenched alloy.

Even after the gold alloy casting has been cooled to room temperature, the same principles can be used to alter its mechanical properties. If the casting is heated to a temperature slightly below the solidus temperature (e.g., 700° C) and held for a time, it will transform into a random solid solution. If it is then cooled rapidly to room temperature, this structure is retained, and the alloy will be

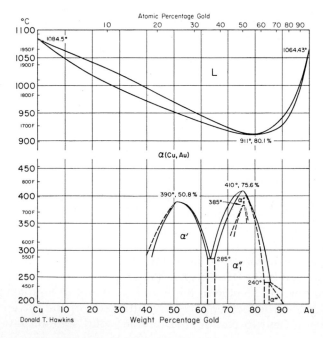

Figure 15–9. Equilibrium phase diagram for the copper-gold system. (From Metals Handbook, Vol 8, 8th ed. Metals Park, OH, American Society for Metals, 1973, p 267.)

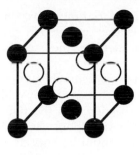

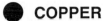 **COPPER**

 GOLD

Figure 15–10. Unit cell of the face-centered tetragonal superlattice of AuCu. The open circles represent the gold atoms.

relatively soft and ductile. This is called *solution heat treatment*. If the same casting is heated to a temperature slightly below that required to form the ordered structure and is held at temperature for a period, the ordered AuCu phase will form (Fig. 15–10) and the result will be a stronger, harder, but less ductile structure. This is referred to as an *age-hardening heat treatment*.

The formation of the AuCu tetragonal crystal lattice contributes to the age-hardening process in an interesting manner. The ordered phase per se is not particularly strong or hard. However, the tetragonal structure precipitates out in the age-hardening temperature range in thin alternate layers. The alternate layering is necessary because the short C axis of the tetragonal structure tends to produce elastic strain in the face-centered cubic parent structure. The strain is then relieved by a follow-up precipitated layer with the C axis perpendicular to the previous C axis. These alternations continue until the structure has precipitated the equilibrium quantity of the ordered structure.

These thin layers are seen as striations (fine parallel lines or markings) in the microstructure (Fig. 15–11), which represents the aged structure for a gold-

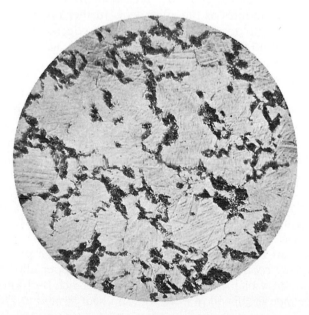

Figure 15–11. Photomicrograph of a dental gold alloy that was age hardened at 450° C for 100 hours. ×250. (Courtesy of E. M. Wise.)

copper-silver Type IV dental gold alloy. The dark-gray constituent is a silver-rich phase, and the white matrix phase is the copper-rich phase. The gray precipitate hardens by dispersed phase hardening; the striations harden by obstructing slip through the lattice alternations.

The time for heat treatment is also important. Presumably, the longer the time of the age-hardening treatment, the greater the change in physical properties.

The precipitated phase is not necessarily harder than the parent lattice. The slip interference can be attributed to the lattice distortions caused by the precipitated phase. Theoretically, if the parent lattice could be entirely transformed to the precipitated phase, it is conceivable that the strength would be less than that obtained during a proper age-hardening treatment but with an increase in ductility. That such a condition is not expected in an actual gold casting alloy is evidenced by the photomicrograph shown in Figure 15–11. Even though the alloy was age hardened for 100 hours, the amount of precipitated phase was minimal and apparently occurred near the grain boundaries.

Usually, the time for age hardening is limited according to the desired properties of the resulting structure. A low ductility in a dental alloy results in a brittleness that may prevent necessary adjustments of the dental appliance by the dentist. On the other hand, an increase in proportional limit is desirable to increase the modulus of resilience of the appliance. From a practical viewpoint, the time and temperature for age hardening should be specified for the particular alloy to provide a reasonable balance between the properties of strength and ductility.

In a solution heat treatment, the alloy should be held at the treatment temperature for sufficient time to allow diffusion of the copper atoms to a random substitutional arrangement. Usually, an arbitrarily selected time of 10 minutes at 700° C (1292° F) is employed, followed by quenching.

Silver-Copper System. The silver-copper alloys were possibly the first system investigated in which the changes in properties by precipitation hardening from a solid solution were demonstrated. For example, when the alloy of 5% copper in Figure 15–6 is allowed to cool slowly, copper is precipitated at 630° C (1166° F) at the point where the dotted line intersects the solvus line. Of course, additional copper precipitates as the alloy cools further but to a limited extent, because the diffusion rate decreases rapidly with the decrease in temperature.

Any localized concentration of copper atoms in the space lattice of the silver-copper solid solution is sufficient to inhibit slip.

If the alloy is again heated above the temperature indicated by the solvus line for a sufficient time to allow the copper atoms to diffuse to random positions in the silver space lattice, a single-phase solid solution structure again forms.

As in the case of the gold-copper alloy, the heat treatment of the alloy at the high temperature to produce the solid solution, followed by quenching, is known as *solution heat treatment*. After a solution heat treatment, heating to produce precipitation of a second phase is known as a precipitation *age-hardening heat treatment*.

One particularly useful silver-copper alloy, used in the past for inlay purposes in deciduous teeth, is known as *sterling silver.* It is used extensively in fine silverware and was the basis for silver coinage. It contains 7.5% copper and 92.5% silver. As can be concluded from the silver-copper phase diagram in Figure 15–6, on slow cooling from the melt the 7.5% copper alloy first solidifies as an α-solid solution, which precipitates out a copper-rich β-phase on continued cooling. If a specimen of this alloy were solution heat treated at 775° C (1427° F) for 30 minutes, then quenched to room temperature, and finally brought back up to 325° C (617° F) for 2 hours, it would produce an age-hardening effect, and the microstructure would exhibit a fine dispersed phase. Silversmiths use these processes to advantage, because the solution heat-treated alloy is soft and has high ductility, permitting it to be readily shaped by cold working. The finished utensil then can be subjected to age hardening, which hardens and strengthens the finished product, adding significantly to its durability.

OTHER BINARY SYSTEMS

Dental casting gold alloys may contain as many as six metals, including gold, platinum, silver, palladium, copper, and zinc. Many of these metals in binary combinations can form precipitation phases, leading to age hardening. A study of the binary phase diagrams for the various combinations provides information about phases that may be present in the multicomponent commercial gold alloys.

The platinum-gold system exhibits a considerable spread in temperature between the liquidus and solidus, and an undesirable cored structure results. Platinum and gold exhibit total solid solubility only at temperatures near the solidus. At lower temperatures, a large two-phase region develops in a manner similar to a eutectic structure. At 400° C (752° F), this heterogeneous structure may be spread over compositions that range from 4% to 90% gold.

The palladium-copper system is characterized by a relatively short melting range in comparison with that of the platinum-gold system. Although the liquidus temperature is never less than the melting temperatures of the constituents, the copper effectively reduces the liquidus and solidus temperatures over a considerable range of composition. In some respects, this system resembles that of the gold-copper system. Transformations that correspond to the superlattice compositions PdCu (62.6% palladium) and $PdCu_3$ (36% palladium) occur. The range of the ordered PdCu transformation is from 48% to 63% palladium, and it involves formation of an ordered body-centered cubic structure of essentially the same dimensions as the parent lattice.

The platinum-copper system resembles the palladium-copper system to some extent. The melting range is again fairly narrow. Alloys with less than 20% platinum have liquidus temperatures only slightly above the melting point of copper. At least two intermediate phases appear upon slow cooling: PtCu (75.5% platinum) and $PtCu_3$ (44% platinum). The precipitation of the PtCu phase results in age hardening. PdCu is not as effective in hardening unless silver is present, in which case a ternary superlattice forms.

A particularly effective age-hardening constituent in gold alloys is a platinum-iron intermetallic compound. It is useful in strengthening the gold alloys used in the metal-ceramic restoration when platinum is used to increase the melting range and lower the coefficient of thermal expansion of the alloy. Such alloys are discussed in Chapter 20.

The Ternary Gold-Silver-Copper System. Many dental gold alloys are ternary alloys of gold, silver, and copper, containing minor additions of such metals as platinum, palladium, and zinc. Most of these alloys can be hardened by heat treatment. They are usually homogeneous solid solutions when they are quenched immediately after solidification from the melt. This is the same as quenching for a solid solution heat treatment.

These alloys can be age hardened primarily because two phases precipitate out. One is a copper-rich phase, and the other is the typical AuCu ordered phase. In both precipitates, silver is also present, thus adding to the solid-solution hardening of each precipitated phase as well as to the residual random solid-solution phase.

A ternary phase diagram is available for the gold-silver-copper alloy system. It is more complex to visualize because it is three dimensional; there are two compositional variables plus temperature to specify. Pseudobinary diagrams that hold the concentration of one of the three components fixed are often used to study the influence of composition on phases present. Isothermal cross sections (fixed temperature) through the three-dimensional diagram also are available.

There are many other ternary combinations, quaternary combinations, and multicomponent systems used in dentistry. Such systems are complex, and the phase diagram information available is quite limited, with the exception of the silver-mercury-tin ternary system, which is discussed in detail in Chapters 17 and 18 on dental amalgam. Binary phase diagrams still are often useful in predicting the influence of individual components.

SELECTED READING

Flinn R, and Trojan P: Engineering Materials and Their Applications, 3rd ed. Boston, Houghton Mifflin, 1986, pp 116–169.
   A very readable discussion of equilibrium (phase diagram) and nonequilibrium conditions in systems as related to properties. Excellent photographs and examples.
Metals Handbook, Desk Edition. Metals Park, OH, American Society of Metals, 1992.
   A comprehensive reference book on the casting, structure, and properties of metals, including a section on metallography procedures.
Porter DA, and Easterling KE: Phase Transformations in Metals and Alloys, 2nd ed. London, Chapman & Hall, 1992.
   An undergraduate engineering course in phase transformations and the structure and properties of interfaces.
Van Vlack LH: Elements of Materials Science and Engineering, 5th ed. Reading, MA, Addison-Wesley, 1985.
   Chapter 10 includes phase diagrams on pages 374 to 426.
   Chapter 11 covers processes to develop and control microstructure on pages 417 to 464.

16 *Corrosion*

- Causes of Tarnish and Corrosion
- Classification of Corrosion
- Electrochemical Corrosion
- Protection Against Corrosion
- Corrosion of Dental Restorations
- Clinical Significance of Galvanic Currents

TERMINOLOGY

In most instances corrosion is undesirable. In dental practice, corrosion around the margins of dental amalgam restorations may be beneficial because the corrosion products tend to seal the marginal gap and inhibit the ingress of oral fluids and bacteria. Some metals and alloys are resistant to corrosion either because of inherent "nobility" or because of the formation of a protective surface layer.

The following definitions clarify some of the fundamental types and forms of metal degradation in the oral environment:

Concentration cell–an electrochemical corrosion cell, in which the potential difference is associated with the difference in the concentration of dissolved species, such as oxygen, in the solution at different parts of the metal surface.

Corrosion–a chemical or electrochemical process through which a metal is attacked by natural agents, such as air and water, resulting in partial or complete dissolution, deterioration, or weakening of any solid substance. Although glasses and other nonmetals are susceptible to environmental degradation, metals are generally more susceptible to such an attack because of electrochemical reactions.

Crevice corrosion–accelerated corrosion in narrow spaces, caused by localized electrochemical processes and chemistry changes, such as acidification and depletion in the oxygen content. Crevice corrosion commonly occurs when leakage takes place between a restoration and the tooth, under a pellicle, or under other surface deposits.

Galvanic corrosion–an accelerated attack occurring on a less noble metal when electrochemically dissimilar metals are in electrical contact in the presence of a liquid corrosive environment.

Galvanic shock–a pain sensation caused by electric current generated by a contact between two dissimilar metals, forming a battery in the oral environment.

Pitting corrosion–sharply localized corrosion occurring on base metals, such as iron, nickel, and chromium, which are protected by a naturally forming, thin film of an oxide. In the presence of chlorides in the environment the film locally breaks down, and rapid dissolution of the underlying metal occurs in the form of pits.

Stress corrosion–degradation by the combined effects of mechanical stress and a corrosive environment, usually in the form of cracking.

Tarnish–a process by which a metal surface is dulled in brightness or discolored through the formation of a chemical film, such as a sulfide and an oxide.

Wear, abrasion, and erosion–loss of material from a surface caused by a mechanical action alone or through a combination of chemical and mechanical action.

The most common example of corrosion is rusting of iron, a complex chemical reaction in which the iron combines with both the oxygen in air and water to form a hydrated oxide of iron, $Fe_2O_3 \cdot H_2O$. The oxide is a solid that is porous and is bulkier, weaker, and more brittle than the metal from which it is formed.

Four methods may be used to prevent the corrosion of iron: (1) covering it with an impermeable surface coating such as oil or paint so that air and water cannot reach it; (2) coating it with a material such as zinc that reacts with the corroding substances more readily than the iron and thus, while being consumed, protects the iron; (3) electroplating the surface with an element that resists corrosion; and (4) alloying the iron with chromium so that it becomes chemically resistant to corrosion. Alloying is the most satisfactory, but the most expensive, of these methods. Orthodontic wire can be made of stainless steel, an alloy containing iron, carbon, chromium, and sometimes nickel.

High noble alloys used in dentistry are so inactive chemically that they do not sustain corrosion in the oral environment; the major components of those alloys are one or more of the noble elements, gold, platinum, palladium, iridium, osmium, rhodium, and ruthenium. The first three of these elements are most commonly used in dental alloys. Silver is not considered noble by dental standards because it reacts with air, water, and sulfur to form silver sulfide, a dark discoloration product.

Metals undergo chemical or electrochemical reactions with the environment, resulting in dissolution or formation of chemical compounds. Commonly known as corrosion products, the chemical compounds may accelerate, retard, or have no influence on the subsequent deterioration of the metal surface. It is unfortunate that many of the commonly used metals derive little or no protection from the corrosion products that form under normal circumstances. The rusting of iron is a familiar example of the effects that may be produced by such a process.

One of the primary requisites of any metal that is to be used in the mouth is that it must not produce corrosion products that are harmful to the body. Some metallic elements that are completely safe in the elemental state can form hazardous or even toxic ions or compounds. If the corrosion process is not too severe, these products may not be recognized easily.

The oral environment is conducive to the formation of corrosion products. The mouth is moist and is continually subjected to fluctuations in temperature. The foods and liquids ingested have wide ranges of pH. Acids are liberated during the breakdown of foodstuffs. This food debris often adheres tenaciously to the metallic restoration, thus providing a localized condition that is extremely conducive to an accelerated reaction between the corrosion products and the metal or alloy. All these environmental factors contribute to the degrading process known as *corrosion*.

Gold resists chemical attack of this nature well; therefore, it was natural that this "noblest of the metals" was employed early for the construction of dental appliances.

CAUSES OF TARNISH AND CORROSION

A differentiation should be made between *tarnish* and *corrosion*. Even though there is a definite technical difference, it is difficult clinically to distinguish between the two phenomena, and the terms are often used interchangeably in the dental literature.

Tarnish is observable as a surface discoloration on a metal or even as a slight loss or alteration of the surface finish or luster. In the oral cavity, tarnish often occurs from the formation of hard and soft deposits on the surface of the restoration. Calculus is the principal hard deposit and its color varies from light yellow to brown. The soft deposits are plaques and films composed mainly of micro-organisms and mucin. Stain or discoloration arises from pigment-producing bacteria, drugs containing chemicals such as iron and mercury, and adsorbed food debris.

Although such deposits are the main cause of tarnish in the oral cavity, surface discoloration may also arise on a metal from the formation of thin films, such as oxides, sulfides, and chlorides. This phenomenon may then be only a simple deposition on the surface, and such a film may even be protective, as discussed subsequently. However, usually it is an early indication of corrosion.

Corrosion in the specific sense is not merely a surface deposit, but it is an actual deterioration of a metal by reaction with its environment. Frequently, especially with surfaces under stress or with intergranular impurities in the metal or with corrosion products that do not completely cover the substrate metal, the corrosion attack rate may actually increase with time. In due course it causes severe and catastrophic disintegration of the metal body. In addition, corrosion attack that is extremely localized may cause rapid mechanical failure of a structure even though the actual loss of material is quite small.

This disintegration of a metal may occur through the action of moisture, atmosphere, acid or alkaline solutions, and certain chemicals. Tarnish is often the forerunner of corrosion.

The film that is deposited and produces tarnish may in time form, or accumulate, elements or compounds that chemically attack the metallic surface. For example, eggs and certain other foods contain significant amounts of sulfur. Various sulfides, such as hydrogen and ammonium sulfide, corrode silver, copper, mercury, and similar metals present in dental alloys and amalgam.

In addition, water, oxygen, and chloride ions are present in saliva and contribute to corrosion attack. Various acids such as phosphoric, acetic, and lactic are present at times. At the proper concentration and pH these can lead to corrosion.

As discussed in the following chapters, specific ions may play a major role in the corrosion of certain alloys. For example, oxygen and chlorine are implicated in the corrosion of amalgam at the tooth interface and within the body of the alloy. Sulfur is probably most significant in surface tarnish developed on casting alloys that contain silver, although chloride has also been identified as a contributor.

CLASSIFICATION OF CORROSION

The exact phenomenon of corrosion is often complex and not completely understood. The less homogeneous the metal and the more complex the environment, the more complicated the corrosion process. The composition, physical state, and surface condition of the metal, as well as the chemical components of the surrounding medium determine the nature of the corrosion reactions. Other important variables affecting corrosion processes are the temperature, temperature fluctuation, movement or circulation of the medium in contact with the metal surface, and the nature and solubility of the corrosion products. In spite of all these complexities, if the general mechanism of corrosion is understood, it is usually possible to recognize the controlling variables in a given instance of corrosion.

There are two general types of corrosion reactions. One type is called *chemical corrosion*, in which there is a direct combination of metallic and nonmetallic elements. This type is exemplified by oxidation, halogenation, or sulfurization reactions. A good example is the discoloration of silver by sulfur. The formation of silver sulfide in this reaction is chemical corrosion. Silver sulfide appears to be the principal corrosion product of dental gold alloys that contain silver. Such corrosion is also referred to as *dry corrosion*, because it occurs in the absence of water or other fluid electrolytes.

Yet another example is the oxidation of alloy particles used in preparation of some dental amalgams. They contain a silver-copper eutectic phase, and their oxidation limits the reactivity with mercury, thereby affecting amalgamation. That is why it is prudent to store the alloy in a cool, dry location to ensure an adequate shelf life.

Chemical corrosion is seldom isolated and almost invariably is accompanied by a second type of corrosion known as *electrochemical corrosion*. This type is also referred to as *wet corrosion*, because it requires the presence of water or other fluid electrolytes. It also requires a pathway for the transport of electrons, an electrical current, if the process is to continue. Because the oral cavity is a wet environment, the remaining discussion is principally concerned with wet corrosion.

ELECTROCHEMICAL CORROSION

The starting point for the discussion of electrochemical corrosion is the electrochemical cell, illustrated in Figure 16–1. Such a cell is composed of four components: an anode, a cathode, an electrolyte, and an ammeter. In this figure, the anode simulates an amalgam restoration and the cathode represents a gold alloy restoration. Saliva represents the electrolyte fluid.

The anode represents the surface or sites on a surface where positive ions are formed, that is, the metal surface that is corroding. The reaction may be described as

$$\text{(1)} \qquad\qquad M^\circ \rightarrow M^+ + e^-$$

Notice that free electrons (e^-) are produced; hence, this is sometimes referred to as an *oxidation reaction.*

At the cathode or cathodic sites a reaction must occur that consumes the free electrons produced at the anode. Numerous possibilities exist and are dependent on the environment. For example, metal ions may be removed from the solution

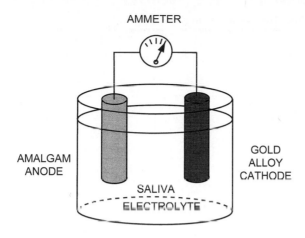

AMMETER

AMALGAM ANODE

GOLD ALLOY CATHODE

SALIVA ELECTROLYTE

Figure 16–1. Diagram of an electrochemical cell consisting of an amalgam anode, a gold alloy cathode, and saliva as the electrolyte.

to form metal atoms, hydrogen ions may be converted to hydrogen gas, or hydroxyl ions may be formed:

(2)
$$M^+ + e \rightarrow M^\circ$$

(3)
$$2H^+ + + 2e^- \rightarrow H_2 \uparrow$$

(4)
$$2H_2O + O_2 + 4e^- \rightarrow 4(OH)^-$$

These processes are referred to as *reduction reactions.* The electrolyte serves to supply the ions needed at the cathode and to carry away the corrosion products at the anode. The external circuit serves as a conduction path to carry electrons (the electric current) from the anode to the cathode. If a voltmeter is placed into this circuit instead of an ammeter, an electrical potential difference (a voltage [V]) can be measured. This voltage has considerable theoretical importance, as discussed in the following section. This simple electrochemical cell is, in principle, a battery because the flow of electrons in the external circuit is capable of lighting a light bulb in a flashlight or producing a physiologic sensation, such as pain.

For electrochemical corrosion to be an ongoing process, the production of electrons by the oxidation reactions at the anode must be exactly balanced by the consumption of electrons in the reduction reactions at the cathode. Often, the cathodic reactions can be considered to be the primary driving force in electrochemical corrosion. This is an important consideration in determining the rate of a corrosion process and can be used to advantage to reduce or eliminate corrosion.

The basis for any discussion of electrochemical corrosion is the *electromotive force* (EMF) series. This classification is an arrangement of the elements in the order of their dissolution tendencies in water. The potential values are calculated for the elements in equilibrium with solutions containing one atomic weight, in grams, of ions in 1000 mL of water at 25° C. These standard potentials may be considered as the voltage of electrochemical cells in which one pole is the hydrogen electrode (equation 3), designated arbitrarily as zero, and the other is the electrode of the element of interest. The sign of the electrode potential indicates the polarity in such a cell. The series for the elements that might be useful to the dentist is seen in Table 16–1. Metals with a more positive potential have a lower tendency to dissolve in aqueous environments.

If two metals are immersed in an electrolyte and are connected by an electrical

TABLE 16–1. Electromotive Series of the Metals

Metals	Ion	Electrode Potential (V)
Gold	Au^+	+1.50
Gold	Au^{3+}	+1.36
Platinum	Pt^{2+}	+0.86
Palladium	Pd^{2+}	+0.82
Mercury	Hg^{2+}	+0.80
Silver	Ag^+	+0.80
Copper	Cu^+	+0.47
Bismuth	Bi^{3+}	+0.23
Antimony	Sb^{3+}	+0.10
Hydrogen	H^+	0.00
Lead	Pb^{2+}	−0.12
Tin	Sn^{2+}	−0.14
Nickel	Ni^{2+}	−0.23
Cadmium	Cd^{2+}	−0.40
Iron	Fe^{2+}	−0.44
Chromium	Cr^{2+}	−0.56
Zinc	Zn^{2+}	−0.76
Aluminum	Al^{3+}	−1.70
Sodium	Na^+	−2.71
Calcium	Ca^{2+}	−2.87
Potassium	K^+	−2.92

conductor, an electric couple is formed. With the sign designation used in Table 16–1, the metal with the lowest electrode potential goes into solution. The strength and direction of the current thus depend primarily on the electrode potential of the individual metals. A familiar example of this phenomenon is the dissolution of the zinc electrode in a flashlight battery, in which the other electrode is graphite, and the electric contact is made through the filament of the light bulb. The disintegration of the surface of the zinc electrode is an example of the processes involved in corrosion.

The relative position of any of the elements in the electromotive series is dependent not only on the inherent solution tendencies but also on the effective concentration of ions of that element that are present in the environment. As the ionic concentration of the element increases in the environment, the tendency for that element to dissolve decreases. The EMF series provides information only about whether a given corrosion reaction can occur. In an actual situation, it predicts neither the occurrence nor the rate of corrosion.

The increase in metal content in the environment may eventually prevent further corrosion. Metals sometimes cease corroding merely because their immediate environments have become saturated with ions of the metals. Such a situation does not usually occur in dental restorations because the dissolving ions are removed by food, fluids, and toothbrushing. Thus, the corrosion continues.

Provided that an electrolyte is present, many types of electrochemical corrosion are possible and all may occur to some extent in the oral cavity because saliva, with the salts it contains, is a weak electrolyte. The electrochemical properties of saliva depend on its composition, the concentration of its components, pH, surface tension, and buffering capacity. All these factors may influence the strength of any electrolyte and thus the magnitude of the resulting corrosion process.

In a wet corrosion environment in which a metal is corroding, two types of reactions take place simultaneously on the surface of the metal. Metal ions pass into solution or form corrosion products because of the anodic reactions, and other ions are reduced in the cathodic reactions. These two reactions may occur at randomly distributed sites on the metal surface or, more frequently, there are areas at which mostly the metal dissolves (anodic) and those at which mostly other ions are discharged (cathodic). Several forms of electrochemical corrosion are based on the mechanisms that produce these inhomogeneous areas.

Galvanic Corrosion or Dissimilar Metals Corrosion. An important type of electrochemical corrosion occurs when *dissimilar metals* are in direct physical contact with each other. Here the dental reference is to two separate restorations in which the metal surfaces are chemically dissimilar. The metallic combinations that may produce *electrogalvanism* or "galvanic currents" may or may not be in intermittent contact.

The effect of "galvanic shock" is well known in dentistry. For example, assume that an amalgam restoration, as discussed in the following chapters, is placed on the occlusal surface of an upper tooth directly opposing a gold inlay in a lower tooth. Because both restorations are wet with saliva, an electrical couple exists, with a difference in potential between the dissimilar restorations. Such a situation is diagrammed in Figure 16–2. When the two fillings are brought into contact, the potential is suddenly short-circuited through the two alloys. The result may be a sharp pain. A similar effect may be observed by touching the tine of a silver fork to a gold foil or inlay restoration, and at the same time allowing some other portion of the fork to come in contact with the tongue. An undetected piece of aluminum foil in a baked potato can produce the same effect.

When the teeth are not in contact, the difference in electrical potential, or EMF, between the two fillings still exists. A circuit also exists. The saliva forms the electrolyte, and the hard and soft tissues can constitute the external circuit. The resistance of the external circuit is considerable in comparison with that which exists when the two fillings are brought into contact. The electric currents measured under these conditions between a gold crown and an amalgam restoration in the same mouth, but not in contact, appear to be approximately 0.5 to 1 μA with a corresponding EMF of approximately 500 mV. These currents are somewhat greater when dissimilar metals are present, but they also occur between restorations of similar metals, which are never exactly comparable in surface composition or structure.

A current is even present in a single isolated metallic restoration, although it

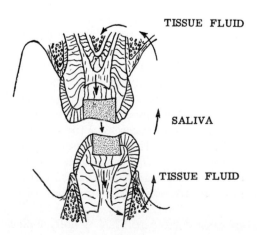

TISSUE FLUID

SALIVA

TISSUE FLUID

Figure 16–2. Possible path of a galvanic current in the mouth.

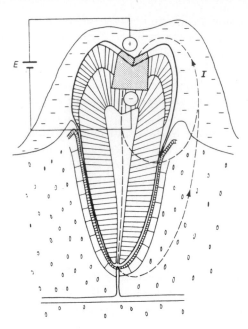

Figure 16–3. Schematic illustration of a single metallic restoration showing two possible current pathways between an external surface exposed to saliva and an interior surface exposed to dentinal fluid. Because the dentinal fluid contains a higher Cl⁻ concentration than does the saliva, it is assumed that the electrode potential of the interior surface exposed to dentinal fluid is more active; therefore, it is given a negative sign ($-$). The potential difference between the two surfaces is represented by *E*. (From Metals Handbook, 9th ed, Vol 13. Metals Park, OH, American Society for Metals, 1978, p 1342.)

is less intense. In such a situation, the cell is generated by the potential differences created by two electrolytes, saliva and tissue fluids. The term *tissue fluids* is used to denote the dentinal, fluid, soft tissue fluid, and blood that provide the means for completing external circuit. It contains a chloride ion concentration seven times higher than that of saliva. Thus, it is assumed that the interior surfaces of a dental restoration exposed to the dentinal fluid have a more active potential. The possible current pathways are diagrammed in Figure 16–3.

Although the magnitude of these currents usually diminishes somewhat as the restoration ages, it remains indefinitely at the approximate value cited. The clinical significance of these currents, other than their influence on corrosion, is discussed later in this chapter. Coating with varnish tends to eliminate galvanic shock.

Heterogeneous Composition. Another type of galvanic corrosion is that associated with *heterogeneous composition* of the metal surface. Examples of this type may be the eutectic and peritectic alloys. It was previously stated that the corrosion resistance of such alloys is generally less than that of solid solution. The reason should now be evident. When an alloy containing a eutectic is immersed in an electrolyte, the metallic grains with the lower electrode potential are attacked, and corrosion results. Likewise, in a solid solution, any cored structure is less resistant to corrosion than the homogenized structure because of differences in electrode potential caused by segregation and variation in composition between the individual dendrites. Even a homogenized solid solution is somewhat susceptible to corrosion because of the difference in structure between the grains and their boundaries. The grain boundaries may act as the anodes, and the interior of the grains as the cathodes. This results in the corrosion of the material in the anodic region at the grain boundaries. Solder joints may corrode because of the difference in composition of the alloy-solder combination.

Impurities in any alloy enhance corrosion. They usually collect in the grain boundary, which in itself is more easily attacked by virtue of being in an inherently higher energy condition. The impurities, such as mercury contamination of gold, have potentials different from those of the grains themselves. Pure metals corrode at much slower rates than alloys, because there is less chance of impurities or second phases, which act as miniature dissimilar electrode cells.

Stress Corrosion. On most dental appliances, the deleterious effects of stress and corrosion are most apt to occur because of fatigue of the metal when it is associated with a corrosive environment. Repeated removal and insertion of a partial denture, for example, may build up a severe stress pattern in certain types of alloys, especially at the grain boundaries. Combined with an oral condition that promotes corrosion, the stressed appliance develops *stress corrosion*. Slight surface irregularities at that point, such as a notch or pit, can accelerate the process so that ordinary fatigue starts below the normal limit and failure results.

Any cold working of an alloy by bending, burnishing, or malleting localizes stress in some parts of the structure. A couple composed of the stressed metal, saliva, and the unstressed metal is thus formed. The stressed area is then more readily dissolved by the electrolyte. This is one of the reasons that unnecessary burnishing of the margins of metallic restorations is contraindicated.

Concentration Cell Corrosion. The third form of electrochemical corrosion is called *concentration cell corrosion.* An important type of concentration cell corrosion is *crevice corrosion.* This situation exists whenever there are variations in the electrolytes or in the composition of the given electrolyte within the system. For example, there are often accumulations of food debris in the interproximal areas of the mouth, particularly if oral hygiene is poor. This debris then produces one type of electrolyte in that area, and the normal saliva provides another electrolyte at the occlusal surface. Therefore, electrochemical corrosion occurs, with preferential attack of the metal surface occurring underneath the layer of food debris.

A similar type of attack may be produced from differences in oxygen tension between parts of the same restoration. A cell is produced, with the greatest activity occurring around the areas containing the least oxygen. Irregularities, such as pits, contribute to this phenomenon. The areas at the bottom of the surface concavities do not have oxygen because they are covered with food debris and mucin. The material at the bottom of the pit then becomes the anode and the material at the periphery the cathode, as diagrammed in Figure 16–4. In this manner, metal atoms at the base of the pit ionize and go into solution, causing the pit to deepen. The rate of such corrosion may be rapid, and failure

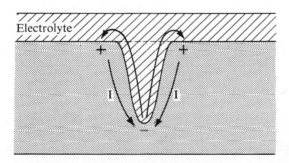

Figure 16–4. A pit as a corrosion cell. The pit bottom is an anode, and the surface around the rim of the pit is the cathode. The ionic current flows through the electrolyte and the electronic current through the metal. (From Richman MH: An Introduction to the Science of Metals. Waltham, MA, Blaisdell, 1967.)

may occur much before what would be anticipated if only a uniform surface attack were expected. For this reason, all metallic dental restorative materials should be polished.

Seldom is any one of these types of electrochemical corrosion found alone. Generally, two or more mechanisms act simultaneously and thus compound the problem. This situation can be illustrated by dissimilar metal corrosion between an inlay and an amalgam restoration.

If the two restorations are in contact, galvanic corrosion of the amalgam occurs because of the dissimilarity of the two materials and the more noble character of the inlay. At the same time, in the narrow gap between them, changes in the solution chemistry (such as depletion of dissolved oxygen) result in the formation of a concentration cell and crevice corrosion. In addition, the inhomogeneity of the structure of the amalgam and the possible presence of an incomplete or porous corrosion product generate local galvanic cells, which further accelerate the corrosion attack.

In the early stages of tarnish, apparently the principle of concentration cells, and thus localized galvanic action, operate. Careful microscopic examination of the progress of tarnish on dental gold alloys reveals that initially the deposited tarnish film is not actually continuous. Rather, it is a discrete or discontinuous deposit. The apparent continuity is an overlapping of these numerous microscopic, but discrete, tarnish regions. Such a situation exists even when the conditions remain constant. The oral environment is not stable because of pH fluctuations, oral hygiene habits, characteristics of the saliva, and continuous stress exerted on the restoration. All these variables, then, accelerate the multiple corrosion processes.

PROTECTION AGAINST CORROSION

It has been suggested that for dental castings, a coating of a noble metal may be applied to the surface of a second metal, for instance, a base metal. However, the noble metal is soft, and when its surface becomes scratched or pitted to such a depth that the base metal is exposed to the environment, the base metal will be corroded at a rapid rate. This occurs for three reasons: (1) a surface defect is created that could set up a concentration cell; (2) two dissimilar metals are in direct contact, thus producing a galvanic cell; and (3) there is an unfavorable anode:cathode surface area ratio. In general, a large anode surface coupled to a small cathode surface results in low corrosion rates. In this example, the reverse is true. The anode surface is small (the base metal at the bottom of the scratch) and the cathode surface is large (the noble metal coating covering the entire casting). Thus, rapid corrosion is expected where the coating has been scratched.

When paints or other types of inorganic or organic coatings are used for protection, any pit or scratch in the protective layer may lead to rapid corrosion of the base metal. In the case of dissimilar metal corrosion, a paint or other nonconductive film can be used to advantage if it is applied to the more noble of the two metals. The corrosion rate of the more active metal is reduced because the surface area available for the reduction reaction has been decreased. A scratch in this type of coating does not lead to a rapid attack on the active metal.

Metallic and nonmetallic coatings have been attempted on dental gold alloys. Generally, they were ineffective because they were too thin, were incomplete, did not adhere to the underlying metal, or were readily scratched or attacked by oral fluids.

Certain metals develop a thin, highly protective film by reaction with the environment; such a metal is said to be passive. Chromium is a good example of a passivating metal. This important metal forms a film of a corrosion product, which probably consists of closely packed chromic oxide. Iron, steel, and certain other metals that are subject to corrosion may be electroplated with nickel followed by chromium for protective and aesthetic reasons. The so-called stainless steels are alloys of iron and carbon with chromium in amounts sufficient to passivate the alloy.

Passivating metals are not without drawbacks, however. Tensile stresses and certain ions, such as chlorides, can disrupt the protective film, and rapid corrosion may ensue. Chromium passivated metals can be susceptible to stress corrosion and pitting corrosion. For this reason, it is imperative that patients be warned against using household bleaches for cleaning partial denture frameworks or removable orthodontic appliances that are alloyed with chromium. Aluminum and titanium are other passivating metals that have found application in dentistry.

Noble metals resist corrosion because their EMF is positive with regard to any of the common reduction reactions found in the oral environment. To corrode a noble metal under such conditions, an external current would have to be imposed.

CORROSION OF DENTAL RESTORATIONS

It is apparent from this discussion that the oral environment and dental structures present complex conditions that can promote corrosion and discoloration. The variables of diet, bacterial activity, drugs, smoking, and oral hygiene habits unquestionably account for a great portion of the differences in corrosion often noted in different patients in whom the same dental alloy, handled in the same manner, has been employed.

Corrosion resistance is an important consideration in the composition of the alloy itself. It is unfortunate that there is no laboratory test that duplicates oral conditions exactly and thus accurately predicts the susceptibility of the material to corrosion. Various accelerated tests using sulfide and chloride solutions have been advocated. With the use of these test methods, it has been shown that the noble metal content, particularly gold, influences the resistance to sulfide tarnishing. For this reason, it has been suggested that at least half the atoms in a dental alloy should be noble metals, such as gold, platinum and palladium, to ensure against corrosion. Palladium is effective in reducing the susceptibility to sulfide tarnishing of alloys containing silver. If noble metals are used to avoid corrosion, it is important that the more active constituents of the alloy be uniformly dispersed (i.e., a random solid solution). The formation of a second phase that is rich in active metal obviously produces a galvanic corrosion cell. Base metal alloys, such as stainless steels, nickel-chromium and cobalt-chromium alloys, and titanium, are virtually immune to sulfide tarnishing. They are susceptible to a localized attack in the presence of chlorides, such as pitting and crevice corrosion, however. Generally, titanium and its alloys are superior to the other alloys in their resistance to chloride attack.

CLINICAL SIGNIFICANCE OF GALVANIC CURRENTS

It has been proved that small galvanic currents associated with electrogalvanism are continually present in the oral cavity. Their influence on corrosion was discussed earlier. As long as metallic dental restorative materials are employed, there seems to be little possibility that these galvanic currents can be eliminated. The cement base itself, although it is a good thermal insulator, has little effect in minimizing the current that is carried into the tooth and through the pulp. Although many of these base materials are good electrical insulators when they are dry, they lose this property when they become wet through marginal seepage or from moisture in the dentin. For all practical purposes, the metallic restoration cannot be isolated electrically from the tooth.

Although the postoperative pain caused by galvanic shock is not a common occurrence in the dental office, it can be a real source of discomfort to an occasional patient. However, such postoperative pain usually occurs immediately after insertion of a new restoration, and generally it gradually subsides and disappears in a few days. It is likely that the physiologic condition of the tooth is the primary factor responsible for the pain resulting from this current flow. Once the tooth has recovered from the injury of preparing the cavity and has returned to a more normal physiologic condition, the current flow then produces no response.

Practically, the best method for reducing or eliminating galvanic shock seems to be to paint an external varnish on the surface of the restoration. As long as the varnish remains, the restoration is insulated from saliva and no cell is established. By the time the varnish has worn away, the pulp has usually healed sufficiently so that no pain remains.

It has been suggested that these currents, or the metallic ions that are liberated from the restoration because of the galvanic current, could account for many types of dyscrasias, such as lichenoid lesions, ulcers, leukoplakia, cancer, and kidney disorder. Other research, particularly a statistical analysis of 1000 patients, has failed to find any correlation between dissimilar metals and tissue irritation. One study (Phillips et al., 1968) is of particular interest. A high galvanic current flow of approximately 5 μA was induced through the tongue and lips of rats each time they drank water through a stainless steel tube. After a period of 1 year, there was no gross or microscopic evidence of tissue changes induced by a current of this magnitude.

The effects of these currents on pathologic changes in oral or other tissues have possibly been exaggerated. The problem will remain controversial as long as dissimilar metals are used in the mouth. It is the opinion of most research workers in pathology and dental materials that these currents exist but that they are probably deleterious only from the standpoint of patient discomfort on rare occasions.

It seems that the conservative procedure would be to avoid situations that might obviously produce an exaggerated condition. For example, the insertion of an amalgam restoration directly in contact with a gold crown seems to be contraindicated, although it is often done. Mercury released from the corroding amalgam (the anode) certainly interacts with the gold alloy (the cathode) and weakens it. A discoloration of both restorations will probably occur. Furthermore, whether it is harmful or not, a metallic taste is present subsequent to the dental operation, and it may persist indefinitely. For further reading on this topic, the papers by Marek (1983) and Mueller (1987) listed in the Selected Reading section are recommended.

SELECTED READING

Fontana MG: Corrosion Engineering, 3rd ed. New York, McGraw-Hill, 1986.
This text is the primary corrosion handbook used by engineers. Basic and advanced corrosion theory are presented in a readable format, and specific metal-environment interactions are included.

Marek M: The corrosion of dental materials. In: Scully JC (ed): Treatise on Materials Science and Technology. New York, Academic Press, 1983, pp 331–394.
A detailed treatment of corrosion phenomena associated with dental amalgam.

Mills RB: Study of incidence of irritation in mouths having teeth filled with dissimilar metals. Northwest Univ Bull 39:18, 1939.
Analysis of a large group of patients did not show a relationship between the presence of dissimilar metals and tissue irritation, casting doubt on the validity of this hypothesis.

Mueller HJ: Tarnish and corrosion of dental alloys. In: Metals Handbook, 9th ed, Vol 13. Metals Park, OH, 1987, pp 1336–1366.
An excellent overview of corrosion behavior of many dental alloy systems based on data from both in vitro and in vivo studies.

Phillips RW, Schnell RJ, and Shafer WG: Failure of galvanic current to produce leukoplakia in rats. J Dent Res 47:666, 1968.
A high galvanic current was generated in the mouths of rats. The model did not induce tissue changes, again suggesting that oral dyscrasia frequently associated with such currents is more probably due to other causes.

Reed GJ, and Willmann W: Galvanism in the oral cavity. J Am Dent Assoc 27:1471, 1940.
One of the first studies that demonstrated the presence of galvanic currents in the oral cavity and established approximate values for the magnitude of the currents.

Sarkar NK: The electrochemical behavior of dental amalgams and their component phases. PhD Thesis, Northwestern University, 1973. (Available through University Microfilms International.)
This classic work describes laboratory testing and corrosion behavior of dental amalgam. Its technical nature requires a fundamental understanding of corrosion theory.

17 *Dental Amalgam*

Structures and Properties

- **Alloy Composition**
- **Manufacture of Alloy Powder**
- **Amalgamation and Resulting Structure**
- **Dimensional Stability**
- **Strength**
- **Creep**
- **Clinical Performance of Amalgam Restorations**

An amalgam is a special type of alloy that contains mercury as one of its constituents. Because mercury is liquid at room temperature, it can be alloyed with other metals that are in the solid state. The modern process of amalgamation begins in a clinic when droplets of mercury are released from a sealed chamber within a capsule into another capsule chamber that contains a dental amalgam alloy powder; the components are then mixed together in a device called an *amalgamator*. The amalgamation process continues while segments of the plastic mass are condensed under firm pressure against the walls of prepared teeth and, if present, a matrix band. The reaction continues during the manipulation period in the mouth and decreases within a few minutes as the dental amalgam increases in strength and hardness. Although the reaction can continue for several days, the dental amalgam becomes sufficiently strong to support moderate biting forces within the first hour.

A detailed discussion of the structure, properties, and manipulation characteristics requires an understanding of a few terms that are commonly used by the dental profession.

TERMINOLOGY

Amalgam–an alloy of mercury.

Amalgamation–the process of mixing liquid mercury with one or more metals or alloys to form an amalgam.

Creep–the time-dependent strain or deformation that is produced by a stress. The creep process can cause an amalgam restoration to extend out of the

361

cavity preparation, thereby increasing its susceptibility to marginal break-down.

Delayed expansion–the gradual expansion of a zinc-containing amalgam over a period of weeks to months that is associated with hydrogen gas development caused by contamination of the plastic mass with moisture during its manipulation in a cavity preparation.

Dental amalgam–an alloy of mercury, silver, copper, and tin, which may also contain palladium, zinc, and other elements to improve handling characteristics and clinical performance. The general term *amalgam* is also used as a synonym by the dental profession.

Dental amalgam alloy–an alloy of silver, copper, tin, and other elements that is formulated and processed in the form of powder particles or as a compressed pellet.

Marginal breakdown–the gradual fracture of the perimeter or margin of a dental amalgam restoration that leads to the formation of gaps or ditching at the external interfacial region between the amalgam and the tooth.

Trituration–the process of grinding powder, especially within a liquid. In dentistry, the term is used to describe the process of mixing the amalgam alloy particles with mercury in an amalgamator.

ALLOY COMPOSITION

American Dental Association (ADA) Specification No. 1 requires that amalgam alloys be predominantly silver and tin. Unspecified amounts of other elements, such as copper, zinc, gold, and mercury, are allowed in concentrations less than the silver or tin content. Alloys containing zinc in excess of 0.01% are required to be designated *zinc containing*. Those alloys containing 0.01% or less of zinc are designated as *nonzinc*. There is no specification for a low-copper or high-copper alloy, per se.

It is less common to use the silver-tin (Ag-Sn) alloys (low-copper alloys) of G. V. Black in preparing amalgam restorations. Nevertheless, the Ag-Sn alloy is still an important alloy for amalgam, because a Ag-Sn alloy powder makes up the largest part of many high-copper alloy powders. Therefore, it is important to understand the characteristics of both low-copper and high-copper alloys.

Before these alloys combine with mercury, they are known as *dental amalgam alloys*. Historically, amalgam alloys contained at least 65 wt% silver, 29 wt% tin, and less than 6 wt% copper, a composition close to that recommended by G. V. Black in 1896. During the 1970s, many amalgam alloys containing between 6 wt% and 30 wt% copper were developed. Many of these high-copper alloys produce amalgams (high-copper amalgams) that are superior in many respects to the traditional low-copper amalgams.

To produce dental amalgam, mercury is mixed with a powder of the amalgam alloy. The powder may be produced by milling or lathe cutting a cast ingot of the amalgam alloy. The particles of this lathe-cut powder are irregularly shaped, as seen in Figure 17–1. Alternatively, the powder may be produced by atomizing the liquid alloy, producing essentially spherical particles. As can be seen in Figure 17–2, they may not be true spheres and can even have an oblong shape, depending on the atomizing and solidification technique that is employed. The alloy may also be supplied as a mixture of lathe-cut and spherical particles.

The powder may also be supplied in the form of pellets or pills. In this instance, the fine particles are subjected to pressure sufficient to cause them to form a "skin" over the outside of the pellet and to cohere slightly on the inside.

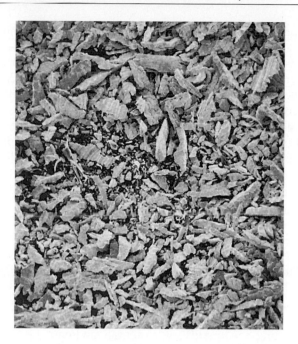

Figure 17–1. Particles of a conventional lathe cut amalgam alloy. ×100.

However, the cohesion is not so great that the particles cannot be readily separated when they are properly amalgamated.

Amalgam alloy is mixed with mercury by the dentist or the assistant. In dentistry, the mixing procedure is technically known as *trituration*. The product of trituration is a plastic mass similar to the one that occurs in the melt of alloys at temperatures between the liquidus and the solidus temperatures. Special instruments are used to force the plastic mass into the prepared cavity by a process known as *condensation*. The complete technique is discussed in detail in Chapter 18.

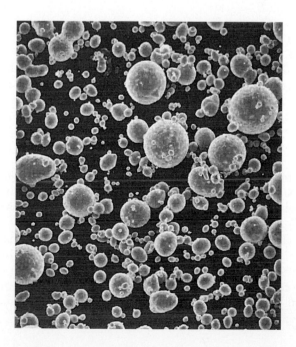

Figure 17–2. Particles of a spherical amalgam alloy. ×500.

During trituration of an alloy powder with mercury, the mercury dissolves the surface of alloy particles, and some new phases form. These new phases have melting points well above any temperature that might normally occur in the mouth. The transformation of the mercury-powder mixture to a composite plastic mass is followed by the setting and hardening of the amalgam as the liquid mercury is consumed in the formation of new solid phases.

The clinical success of the amalgam restoration is based on meticulous attention to detail. Each manipulative step from the time the cavity is prepared until the restoration has been polished can have an effect on the physical and chemical properties of the amalgam and the success or failure of the restoration. Violation of the fundamental principles of cavity preparation has contributed substantially to failure. These matters are treated in operative dentistry texts. The following discussion is concerned with failures associated with the alloy itself and its manipulation.

In a sense, the dentist and the assistant manufacture the amalgam. The two components, the alloy and the mercury, are purchased. In the process of combining the two and fashioning the restoration, the amalgam is formed. The manner in which this is accomplished controls the properties and performance of the amalgam.

The factors governing the quality of a dental amalgam restoration can be divided into two groups: (1) those that can be controlled by the dentist, and (2) those that are under the control of the manufacturer. The factors governed by the dentist are (1) the selection of an alloy; (2) the mercury:alloy ratio; (3) the trituration procedures; (4) the condensation technique; (5) the marginal integrity; (6) the anatomic characteristics; and (7) the final finish. Because many modern amalgam alloys are furnished by manufacturers in a capsule containing both alloy and mercury, selection of these pre-encapsulated alloys results in selection of mercury:alloy ratio as well.

The manufacturer controls (1) the composition of the alloy; (2) the heat treatment of the alloy; (3) the size, shape, and method of production of the alloy particles; (4) the surface treatment of the particles; and (5) the form in which the alloy is supplied.

Metallurgic Phases In Dental Amalgams. The setting reactions of alloys for dental amalgam with mercury are usually described by the metallurgic phases that are involved. These phases are named with Greek letters that correspond with the symbols found in the phase diagram for each alloy system. To facilitate the reading of subsequent sections, the Greek letters and stoichiometric information for these phases are given in Table 17–1.

The Silver-Tin System. Figure 17–3 is an equilibrium phase diagram of the Ag-Sn alloy system. Because silver and tin make up the major portion of amalgam alloys, the phase relations shown in this diagram are found in many amalgam alloys.

The low-copper alloys have a narrow range of compositions that fall within the $\beta + \gamma$ and the γ areas of the diagram shown in Figure 17–3. These areas are enclosed by the lines ABCDE. At point C is the intermetallic compound Ag_3Sn, the γ phase, which forms by peritectic reaction (see Chapter 15) from the liquid plus β area above it. The more silver-rich β phase is crystallographically similar to the γ phase.

TABLE 17–1. Symbols and Stoichiometry of Phases that Are Involved in the Setting of Dental Amalgams

Phases in Amalgam Alloys and Set Dental Amalgams*	Stoichiometric Formula
γ	Ag_3Sn
γ_1	Ag_2Hg_3
γ_2	$Sn_{7-8}Hg$
ϵ	Cu_3Sn
η	Cu_6Sn_5
Silver-copper eutectic	Ag-Cu

*The Greek letters are named as follows: γ (gamma); ϵ (epsilon); and η (eta).

The Influence of Ag-Sn Phases on Amalgam Properties. In the range of compositions around the γ phase, increases or decreases in silver influence the amounts of β and γ phases and the properties. Most commercial alloys fall within the limited composition range of B to C and are not exactly at the peritectic composition (point C). Because the effect of these phases is relatively pronounced, their control is essential if an alloy of uniform quality is to be produced.

If the tin concentration exceeds 26.8 wt%, a mixture of γ phase and a tin-rich phase is formed. The presence of the tin phase increases the amount of the tin-mercury phase formed when the alloy is amalgamated. The tin-mercury phase lacks corrosion resistance and is the weakest component of the dental amalgam. Amalgams of tin-rich alloys display less expansion than do silver-rich alloys.

Ag-Sn alloys are quite brittle and difficult to comminute uniformly unless a small amount of copper is substituted for silver. This atomic replacement is limited to about 4 wt% to 5 wt%, above which Cu_3Sn is formed. Within the limited range of copper solubility, increased copper content hardens and strengthens the Ag-Sn alloy.

The use of zinc in an amalgam alloy is a subject of controversy. Zinc is seldom present in an alloy to an extent greater than 1 wt%. Alloys without zinc are more brittle, and the amalgams produced tend to be less plastic during condensation and carving. The chief function of zinc in amalgam alloys is that of a deoxidizer. It acts as a scavenger during melting, uniting with oxygen to mini-

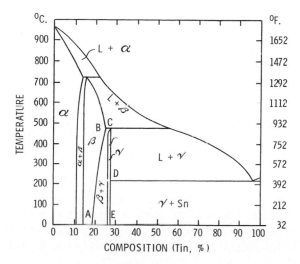

Figure 17–3. Equilibrium phase diagram of the silver-tin system.

mize the formation of other oxides. Zinc may have some beneficial effects related to early corrosion and marginal integrity, as shown in clinical trials. Zinc, even in small amounts, causes an abnormal expansion of the amalgam if the amalgam is condensed in the presence of moisture (discussed later).

The ADA specification for amalgam alloys allows mercury in the alloy powder. Some preamalgamated alloys are sold in Europe, but they have not been marketed extensively in the United States. Other elements may be included in the amalgam alloy if clinical and biologic data show that the alloy is safe to use in the mouth. Small amounts of indium or palladium have been included in some commercial systems.

MANUFACTURE OF ALLOY POWDER

Lathe-cut Powder. To make lathe-cut powder, an annealed ingot of alloy is placed in a milling machine or in a lathe and is fed into a cutting tool or bit. The chips removed are often needlelike, and some manufacturers reduce the chip size by ball-milling.

Homogenizing Anneal. Because of the rapid cooling conditions from the as-cast state, an ingot of an Ag-Sn alloy has a cored structure and contains nonhomogeneous grains of varying composition. A homogenizing heat treatment is performed to re-establish the equilibrium phase relationship (see Chapter 15). The ingot is placed in an oven and heated at a temperature below the solidus for sufficient time to allow diffusion of the atoms to occur and the phases to reach equilibrium. The time of heat treatment may vary, depending on the temperature used and the size of the ingot, but a thermal treatment time of 24 hours at the selected temperature is not unusual.

At the conclusion of the heating cycle, the ingot is brought to room temperature for the succeeding steps in manufacture. The proportion of phases present in the ingot after cooling is affected by the manner in which the ingot is cooled. If the ingot is withdrawn from the heat treatment oven rapidly and then quickly quenched, the phase distribution will remain essentially unchanged. On the other hand, if the ingot is permitted to cool very slowly, the proportions of phases will continue to adjust toward the room temperature equilibrium ratio. For example, in a Ag-Sn alloy, rapid quenching of the alloy ingot results in the maximum amount of β phase retained, whereas slow cooling results in the formation of the maximum amount of the γ phase.

Particle Treatments. Once the alloy ingot has been reduced to cuttings, many manufacturers perform some type of surface treatment of the particles. Although specific treatments are proprietary, treatment of the alloy particles with acid has been a manufacturing practice for many years. The exact function of this treatment is not entirely understood, but it is probably related to the preferential dissolution of specific components from the alloy. Amalgams made from acid-washed powders tend to be more reactive than those made from unwashed powders.

The stresses induced into the particle during cutting and ball-milling must be relieved or they slowly release over time, causing a change in the alloy, particularly in the amalgamation rate and the dimensional change occurring during hardening. The stress-relief process involves an annealing cycle at a moderate temperature, usually for several hours at approximately 100° C. The alloy generally then is stable in reactivity and properties when it is stored for an indefinite period.

Atomized Powder. Atomized powder is made by melting together the desired elements. The liquid metal is atomized into fine spherical droplets of metal. If the droplets solidify before hitting a surface, the spherical shape is preserved, and these atomized powders are called *spherical powders.* Like the lathe-cut powders, spherical powders are given a heat treatment that coarsens the grains and slows the reaction of these particles with mercury. As with the lathe-cut alloys, spherical powders are usually washed with acid.

Particle Size. Maximum particle size and the distribution of sizes within an alloy powder are controlled by the manufacturer. The average particle sizes of modern powders range between 15 and 35 μm. The most significant influence on amalgam properties is the distribution of sizes around the average. For example, very small particles (<3 μm) greatly increase the surface area per unit volume of the powder. A powder containing tiny particles requires a greater amount of mercury to form an acceptable amalgam.

In producing lathe-cut alloys, the cutting rate is precisely controlled to maintain the desired average particle size and size distribution. Similarly, parameters of the atomizing process are controlled to produce the desired particle sizes of spherical alloys. The particles may be graded according to size, and the graded particles are remixed to produce a powder with an optimal size distribution. The present trend in amalgam technique favors the use of a small-to-average particle size, which tends to produce a more rapid hardening of the amalgam with a greater early strength.

As discussed later, the bulk of the finished restoration is composed of particles of the original alloy surrounded by reaction products. The particle size distribution can affect the character of the finished surface. When the amalgam has partially hardened, the tooth anatomy is carved in the amalgam with a sharp instrument. During this carving, the larger particles may be pulled out of the matrix, producing a rough surface. Such a surface is probably more susceptible to corrosion than is a smooth surface.

Lathe-cut Compared with Atomized Alloys. Amalgams made from lathe-cut powders, or admixed powders of a blend of lathe-cut and spherical powders, tend to resist condensation better than amalgams made entirely from spherical powders. Because amalgams of spherical powders are extremely plastic, one cannot rely on the pressure of condensation to establish proximal contour. A contoured and wedged matrix band is essential to prevent flat proximal contours, improper contacts, and overhanging cervical margins. Good technique requires a matrix band, regardless of the amalgam's resistance to condensation.

Spherical alloys require less mercury than typical lathe-cut alloys because spherical alloys have a smaller surface area per volume than do the lathe-cut alloys. Amalgams with a low mercury content generally have better properties.

AMALGAMATION AND RESULTING STRUCTURE

Low-copper Alloys. Amalgamation occurs when mercury comes into contact with the surface of the Ag-Sn alloy particles. When a powder is triturated, the silver and tin in the outer portion of the particles dissolve into mercury. At the same time, mercury diffuses into the alloy particles. The mercury has a limited solubility for silver (0.035 wt%) and tin (0.6 wt%).

When that solubility is exceeded, crystals of two binary metallic compounds precipitate into the mercury. These are the body-centered cubic Ag_2Hg_3 compound (the γ phase) and the hexagonal close-packed $Sn_{7-8}Hg$ compound (the γ_2 phase). Because the solubility of silver in mercury is much lower than that of tin, the γ_1 phase precipitates first, and the γ_2 phase precipitates later.

Immediately after trituration, the alloy powder coexists with the liquid mercury, giving the mix a plastic consistency. As the remaining mercury dissolves the alloy particles, γ_1 and γ_2 crystals grow. As the mercury disappears, the amalgam hardens. As the particles become covered with newly formed crystals, mostly γ_1, the reaction rate decreases. The alloy is usually mixed with mercury in approximately a 1:1 ratio. This is insufficient mercury to completely consume original alloy particles; consequently, unconsumed particles are present in the set amalgam. Alloy particles (smaller now, because their surfaces have dissolved in mercury) are surrounded and bound together by solid γ_1 and γ_2 crystals.

Thus, a typical low-copper amalgam is a composite in which the unconsumed particles are embedded in γ_1 and γ_2 phases. The sequence of amalgamation of the Ag-Sn alloy is shown schematically in Figure 17–4.

The micrograph shown in Figure 17–5 illustrates the features found in a

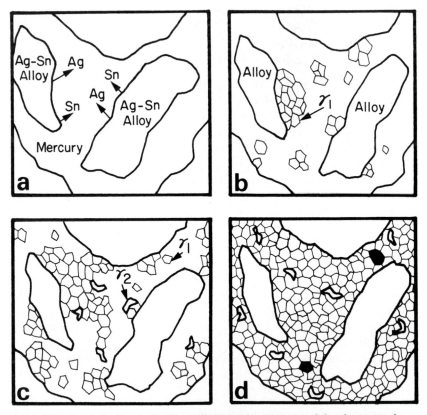

Figure 17–4. These schematic drawings illustrate the sequence of development of amalgam microstructure when lathe-cut low-copper alloy particles are mixed with mercury. In order, these show *(a)* dissolution of silver and tin into mercury; *(b)* precipitation of γ_1 crystals in the mercury; *(c)* consumption of the remaining mercury by growth of γ_1 and γ_2 grains; *(d)* and the final set amalgam. (*a* through *d* courtesy of T. Okabe, R. Mitchell, and C. W. Fairhurst.)

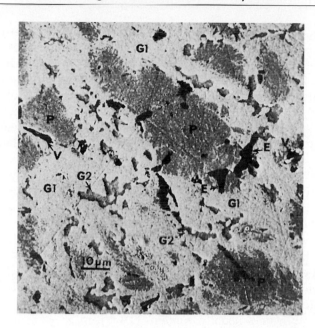

Figure 17–5. Scanning electron micrograph of a low-copper silver-tin amalgam. ×1000. (Courtesy of T. Okabe and M. B. Butts.)

typical amalgam made from a lathe-cut low-copper alloy. The features include the remaining alloy particles of β and γ Ag-Sn phases (larger dark-gray areas labeled P), ε (Cu_3Sn) particle (black area labeled E), γ_1 (Ag_2Hg_3) phase (labeled G1), γ_2 ($Sn_{7-8}Hg$) grains (labeled G2), and voids (left center and right center areas labeled V). These voids are always formed during γ_1 and γ_2 crystal growth when amalgam is condensed by the usual methods. The reaction can be conveniently expressed in terms of the phases that form during amalgamation:

Alloy particles (β + γ) + Hg → γ_1 + γ_2 + unconsumed alloy particles (β + γ)

The physical properties of the hardened amalgam depend on the relative percentages of each of the microstructural phases. The unconsumed Ag-Sn particles have a strong effect. The more of this phase that is retained in the final structure, the stronger is the amalgam. The weakest component is the γ_2 phase. The hardness of γ_2 is approximately 10% of the hardness of γ_1, whereas the γ phase hardness is somewhat higher than that of γ_1.

γ_2 phase is also the least stable in a corrosive environment and may experience corrosion attack, especially in "crevices" of the restorations. Generally, γ (Ag_3Sn) and pure γ_1 (Ag_2Hg_3) phases are stable in an oral environment. However, γ_1 in amalgam does contain small amounts of tin, which can be lost in a corrosive environment.

The interface between the γ phase and the matrix is important. The high proportion of the unconsumed γ phase does not strengthen the amalgam unless the particles are bound to the matrix.

High-copper Alloys. High-copper alloys have become the materials of choice because of their improved mechanical properties, corrosion characteristics, and better marginal integrity and performance in clinical trials, as compared with traditional low-copper alloys. Two different types of high-copper alloy powders are available. The first is an admixed alloy powder, and the second is a single-composition alloy powder. Both types contain more than 6 wt% copper.

Admixed Alloys. In 1963, Innes and Youdelis added spherical silver-copper (Ag-Cu) eutectic alloy (71.9 wt% silver and 28.1 wt% copper) particles to lathe-cut low-copper amalgam alloy particles. This was the first major change in the composition of alloy for dental amalgam since Black's work. These alloys are often termed *admixed alloys* because the final powder is a mixture of at least two kinds of particles. An admixed powder, showing lathe-cut low-copper alloy particles and spherical Ag-Cu alloy particles, is seen in Figure 17–6. Amalgam made from these powders is stronger than amalgam made from lathe-cut low-copper powder, because of the strength of the Ag-Cu particles rather than because of the dispersion strengthening mechanism originally suggested. Composite materials (materials that consist of a matrix and a filler) can be strengthened by the addition of strong fillers (see Chapter 12), and the Ag-Cu particles probably act as strong fillers, strengthening the amalgam matrix.

Several classic studies have shown that restorations made with this prototype admixed amalgam were clinically superior to low-copper amalgam restorations when they were evaluated for resistance to marginal breakdown. The suggested characteristics of the alloy that bring about this improved clinical performance are discussed later.

Admixed alloy powders usually contain 30 wt% to 55 wt% spherical high-copper powder. The total copper content in admixed alloys ranges from approximately 9 wt% to 20 wt%. The phases present in the copper-containing particles depend on their composition. The Ag-Cu alloy consists of mixtures of two phases—silver rich and copper rich—with the crystal structures of pure silver and pure copper, respectively. Each phase contains a small amount of the other element. In the atomized powder (which is fast cooled), the eutectic two-phase mixture forms very fine lamellae. Compositions on either side of the eutectic form relatively large grains of copper-rich phase or silver-rich phase amid the eutectic mixture (see Chapter 15).

When mercury reacts with an admixed powder, silver dissolves into the mercury from the Ag-Cu alloy particles, and both silver and tin dissolve into the mercury from the Ag-Sn alloy particles. The tin in solution diffuses to the

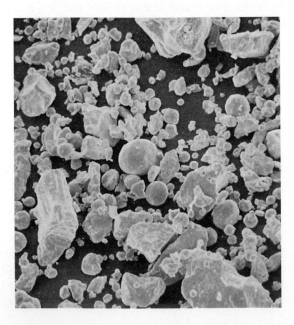

Figure 17–6. Typical admix high-copper alloy powder showing the lathe-cut silver-tin particles and the silver-copper spheres. ×500.

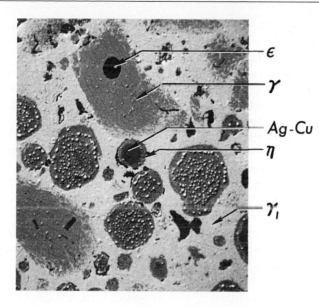

Figure 17–7. Scanning electron micrograph of an admixed (lathe-cut and spherical powder particles) high-copper amalgam. The various phases and reaction layer are labeled. The small, very light, drop-shaped areas are high in mercury owing to the freshly polished specimen. ×1000.

surfaces of the Ag-Cu alloy particles and reacts with the copper phase to form the η phase (Cu_6Sn_5). A layer of η crystals forms around unconsumed Ag-Cu alloy particles. The η layer on Ag-Cu alloy particles also contains some γ_1 crystals. The γ_1 phase forms simultaneously with the η phase and surrounds both the η-covered Ag-Cu alloy particles and the Ag-Sn alloy particles. As in the low-copper amalgams, γ_1 is the matrix phase, that is, the phase that binds the unconsumed alloy particles together.

Figure 17–7 illustrates the microstructure of an admixed amalgam. Included in the structures are the γ phase, Ag-Cu particles, ϵ particles, γ_1 matrix areas, and η reaction layers. In some admixed amalgams, a small number of η crystals are also found amid the γ_1 matrix.

Thus, the reaction of the admixed alloy powder with mercury can be summarized as follows:

$$\text{Alloy particles } (\beta + \gamma) + \text{Ag-Cu eutectic} + \text{Hg} \rightarrow \gamma_1 + \eta$$
$$+ \text{ unconsumed alloy of both types of particles}$$

Note that γ_2 has been eliminated in this reaction. γ_2 does form at the same time as η but is later replaced by it. There is not a precise definition for an amalgam alloy to qualify as a "high-copper" system, but it is generally accepted that it is a formulation whereby the γ_2 is virtually eliminated during the hardening reactions. To accomplish this, it is probably necessary to have a net copper concentration of at least 12% in the alloy powder.

Some set admixed amalgams do contain γ_2, although the percentage is smaller than that in low-copper amalgams. The effectiveness of the copper-containing particles in preventing γ_2 formation depends on their percentage in the mix.

Single-composition Alloys. Success of the admixed amalgams has led to the development of another type of high-copper alloy. Unlike admixed alloy powders, each particle of these alloy powders has the same chemical composition. Therefore, they are called *single-composition alloys*. The major components of the particles are usually silver, copper, and tin. The first alloy of this type contained 60 wt% silver, 27 wt% tin, and 13 wt% copper. The copper content in various single-composition alloys ranges from 13 wt% to 30 wt%. In addition, small amounts of indium or palladium are also found in some of the currently marketed single-composition alloys, as noted earlier.

A number of phases are found in each single-composition alloy particle, including β (Ag-Sn), γ (Ag$_3$Sn), and ε (Cu$_3$Sn). Some of the alloys may also contain some η phase (Cu$_6$Sn$_5$). Atomized particles have dendritic microstructures, consisting of fine lamellae.

When triturated with mercury, silver and tin from the Ag-Sn phases dissolve in mercury; little copper dissolves in mercury. The γ$_1$ crystals grow, forming a matrix that binds together the partially dissolved alloy particles. The η crystals are found as meshes of rod crystals at the surfaces of alloy particles, as well as dispersed in the matrix. These are much larger than the η crystals found in the reaction layers surrounding Ag-Cu particles in admixed amalgams.

Figure 17–8 shows the microstructure of a typical single-composition amalgam. The structure includes unconsumed alloy particles labeled P, γ$_1$ grains (G1), and η crystals (H).

Figure 17–9A shows a scanning electron micrograph of a high-copper single-composition amalgam fractured a few minutes after condensation when the amalgamation reaction was still taking place. Two kinds of crystals are seen on the surface: (1) polyhedral crystals *(arrow A)* between the unconsumed alloy particles, and (2) meshes of η rod crystals *(arrow B)* that cover the unconsumed alloy particles.

Figure 17–9B shows details of the marked areas in Figure 17–9A. In addition to a mesh of η crystals *(arrow B)* that formed on an unconsumed particle, η rods *(arrow C)* are seen embedded in a γ$_1$ crystal *(arrow A)*. Meshed η crystals on unconsumed alloy particles may strengthen bonding between the alloy particles and γ$_1$ grains, and η crystals dispersed between γ$_1$ grains may interlock γ$_1$ grains. This interlocking is believed to improve the amalgam's resistance to deformation.

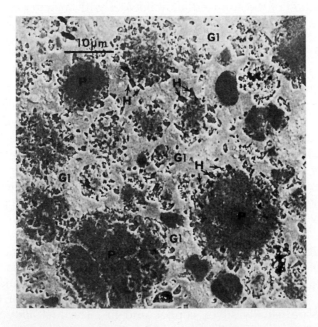

Figure 17–8. Scanning electron micrograph of a high-copper single-composition amalgam. A relief-polish technique was used to reveal the structure. ×560. (Courtesy of M. B. Butts, T. Okabe, and C. W. Fairhurst.)

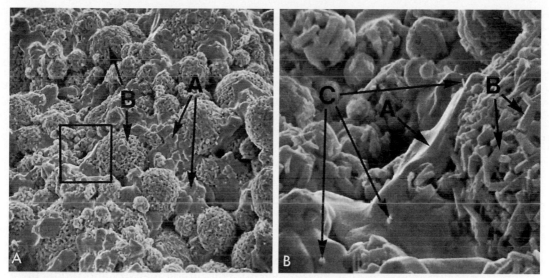

Figure 17–9. A, Scanning electron micrograph of a high-copper single-composition amalgam fractured shortly after condensation, showing reaction products being formed—γ (A), and η (B). ×1000. *B,* Higher magnification of marked area. η rods are embedded in γ ; crystals can be identified (C). ×5000. (*A* and *B* courtesy of T. Okabe, R. Mitchell, M. B. Butts, and C. W. Fairhurst.)

To summarize, the reaction of the single-composition alloy powder with mercury is as follows:

$$\text{Ag-Sn-Cu alloy particles} + \text{Hg} \rightarrow \gamma_1 + \eta$$
$$+ \text{ unconsumed alloy particles}$$

The undesirable γ_2 phase can also form in single-composition amalgams. This is particularly true if the atomized powder has not been heat treated or if the powder has been treated for too long at too high a temperature. Nevertheless, in most single-composition amalgams, little or none of this phase forms.

DIMENSIONAL STABILITY

Ideally, an amalgam should set with no change in dimensions and then remain stable for the life of the restoration. However, a variety of factors influence both the initial dimensions on setting and the long-term dimensional stability, as discussed in the following sections.

Dimensional Change. Amalgam can expand or contract, depending on its manipulation. Ideally, the dimensional change should be small. Severe contraction can lead to microleakage and to secondary caries. Excessive expansion can produce pressure on the pulp and postoperative sensitivity. Protrusion of a restoration can also result from excessive expansion.

The dimensional change of amalgam depends on how much the amalgam is constrained during setting and on when the measurement is initiated. ADA Specification No. 1 requires that amalgam neither contract nor expand more than 20 μm/cm, measured at 37° C, between 5 minutes and 24 hours after the beginning of trituration, with a device that is accurate to at least 0.5 μm. The specimen size is essentially equivalent to the bulk used in large amalgam restorations.

Theory of Dimensional Change. Most modern amalgams exhibit a net contraction when triturated with a mechanical amalgamator and evaluated by the ADA procedure. The classic picture of dimensional change is one in which the specimen undergoes an initial contraction for about 20 minutes after the beginning of trituration and then begins to expand. However, as Figure 17–10 illustrates, modern amalgams do not exhibit such simple behavior.

When the alloy and mercury are mixed, contraction results as the particles dissolve (and hence become smaller) and the γ_1 phase grows. Calculations show that the final volume of γ_1 is less than the sum of the initial volumes of dissolved silver and liquid mercury that are used to produce γ_1. Therefore, contraction continues as long as growth of γ_1 continues. As γ_1 crystals grow, they will impinge against one another. If conditions are right, this impingement of γ_1 can produce an outward pressure tending to oppose the contraction.

If there is sufficient liquid mercury present to provide a plastic matrix, expansion will occur when γ_1 crystals impinge. After a rigid γ_1 matrix has formed, growth of γ_1 crystals cannot force the matrix to expand. Instead, γ_1 crystals grow into interstices that contain mercury, consuming mercury and producing a continued reaction.

According to the aforementioned model, if sufficient mercury is present in the mix when the measurement of dimensional change begins, expansion will be observed. Otherwise, contraction is seen. Therefore, manipulation, such as lower mercury:alloy ratios and higher condensation pressures, that results in less mercury in the mix favors contraction. Higher condensation pressures squeeze mercury out of the amalgam, producing a lower mercury:alloy ratio and favoring contraction. In addition, manipulative procedures that accelerate setting and consumption of mercury also favor contraction, including longer trituration times and use of smaller particle size alloys. Smaller particle size accelerates the consumption of mercury because small particles have a larger surface area per

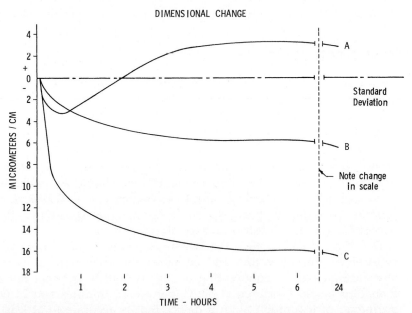

Figure 17–10. Dimensional change curves for three amalgam alloys. Curve A is for a high-copper admixed amalgam. Curve B is for a high-copper single-composition amalgam. Curve C is for a lathe-cut low-copper amalgam.

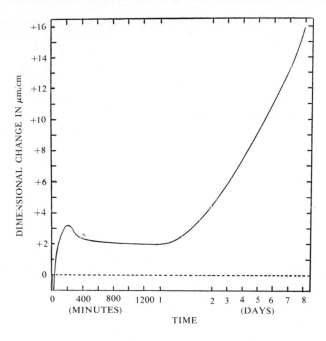

Figure 17–11. Delayed expansion of an amalgam.

unit mass than that of larger particles. Because a larger surface area is dissolving, silver enters the solution faster, γ_1 grows from the solution faster, and the consumption of mercury is accelerated.

Measurements of the dimensional change of many modern amalgams reveal a net contraction, whereas in the past measurements invariably indicated that an expansion occurred. Two reasons for the difference are that older amalgams contained larger alloy particles, and they were mixed at higher mercury:alloy ratios than present-day amalgams. Likewise, hand trituration was used in preparing the specimens. Currently, high-speed mechanical amalgamators are employed. The change to the modern method is equivalent to a large increase in trituration time, resulting in contraction of the specimens prepared by these techniques.

Effect of Moisture Contamination. All the observations presented thus far have been concerned with the dimensional change during the first 24 hours only. Some admixed amalgams continue to expand for at least 2 years. This expansion may be related to the disappearance of some or all of the γ_2 in these high-copper amalgams or other solid-state transformations that continue to occur for long periods. Nevertheless, if they are manipulated properly, most amalgams exhibit little further dimensional change after 24 hours.

If, however, a zinc-containing low-copper or high-copper amalgam is contaminated by moisture during trituration or condensation, a large expansion, such as that shown in Figure 17–11, can take place. This expansion usually starts after 3 to 5 days and may continue for months, reaching values greater than 400 μm (4%). This type of expansion is known as *delayed* or *secondary expansion*.

Delayed expansion is associated with the zinc in the amalgam. The effect is caused by the reaction of zinc with water and is absent in nonzinc amalgams. It has been clearly demonstrated that the contaminating substance is water. Hydrogen is produced by electrolytic action involving zinc and water. This hydrogen does not combine with the amalgam but rather collects within the restoration, increasing the internal pressure to levels high enough to cause the amalgam to creep, thus producing the observed expansion. The contamination of the amalgam can occur at almost any time during its manipulation and insertion into the cavity. If the zinc-containing amalgam is touched with the hands during trituration or condensation, skin secretions are likely to be introduced. If the operative area is not kept dry, the amalgam may become contaminated with saliva during condensation. In short, any contamination of zinc-containing amalgam with moisture, whatever the source, before it has been inserted into the prepared cavity causes a delayed expansion. The contamination must occur during trituration or condensation; after the amalgam is condensed, the external surface may come in contact with saliva without the occurrence of delayed expansion.

STRENGTH

A prime requisite for any restorative material is a strength sufficient to resist fracture. Fracturing of even a small area, especially at the margins, hastens corrosion, secondary caries, and subsequent clinical failure. A lack of adequate strength to resist masticatory forces has been recognized as one of the inherent weaknesses of the amalgam restoration.

An example of bulk fracture of an amalgam restoration is shown in Figure 17–12. In properly designed restorations, such failures are relatively rare. Defects at the margins of amalgams are more common. There is a difference of opinion on this subject as to whether the gaps produced at the interfacial region between the tooth and the amalgam is caused by fracture of the enamel or of the amalgam (marginal breakdown). Marginal defects are the most frequently occurring defects in amalgams. However, there are no general correlations between secondary caries and increasing gap size. In fact, one study revealed that more lesions were found beneath amalgams with smaller marginal gaps and at locations far removed from the larger gaps. The incidence of secondary caries may be quite low in patients with severely deteriorated margins, if oral hygiene is good. However, the influence of the patient may be an important parameter in the

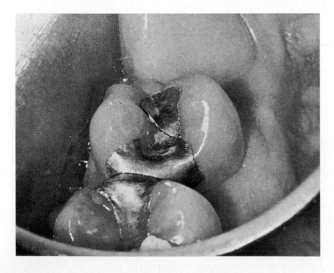

Figure 17–12. Fractured amalgam restoration. Such failures may occur from improper manipulation of the material. (Courtesy of J. T. Andrews.)

TABLE 17–2. Comparison of Compressive Strength and Creep of a Low-Copper Silver-Tin Amalgam and High-Copper Amalgams

Amalgam	Compressive Strength (MPa)		Creep (%)	Tensile Strength—24 h (MPa)
	1 h	7 Day		
Low copper*	145	343	2.0	60
Admix†	137	431	0.4	48
Single composition‡	262	510	0.13	64

*Fine Cut, L. D. Caulk Company, Milford, DE.
†Dispersalloy, Johnson & Johnson Dental Products, East Windsor, NJ.
‡Tytin, S. S. White Dental Manufacturing Company, Philadelphia, PA.

development of secondary caries. Thus, a more conservative approach to replacement of amalgams with defective margins, in the absence of other evidence of pathology, has gained acceptance.

Measurement of Strength. It is difficult to identify the principal property, or properties, responsible for the fractured amalgam restoration shown in Figure 17–12. Traditionally, the strength of dental amalgam has been measured under compressive stress using specimens of dimensions comparable with the volume of typical amalgam restorations. When strength is measured in this manner, the compressive strength of a satisfactory amalgam probably should be at least 310 MPa. When they are manipulated properly, most amalgams exhibit a compressive strength in excess of this value.

In Table 17–2, typical compressive strengths at 1 hour and 7 days after preparation are given for a low-copper amalgam and two high-copper amalgams. After 7 days, the compressive strengths of high-copper amalgams are generally higher than those of low-copper amalgams. In addition, note that the 1-hour compressive strength of the single-composition amalgam is almost double that of the other two amalgams. This trend is generally true for other single-composition amalgams.

The significance of the 7-day compressive strength to clinical performance has been questioned. The strength of amalgam is more than adequate to withstand potential compressive loads. It is unfortunate that amalgam is much weaker in tension than in compression. Both low-copper and high-copper amalgams have tensile strengths that range between 48 and 70 MPa (see Table 17–2).

Tensile stresses can easily occur in amalgam restorations. For example, a compressive stress on the adjacent restored cusp introduces complex stresses that result in tensile stresses in the isthmus area. Because dentin has a relatively low elastic modulus, as much tooth structure as possible should be preserved to prevent the dentin from bending away from the restoration, or fracturing under masticatory forces. It is important to re-emphasize that amalgam cannot withstand high tensile or bending stresses. The design of the restoration should include supporting structures whenever there is danger that it will be bent or pulled in tension. Use of a high-copper amalgam does not help. The tensile strengths of high-copper amalgams are not significantly different from those of the low-copper amalgams (see Table 17–2).

Effect of Trituration. The effect of trituration on strength depends on the type of amalgam alloy, the trituration time, and the speed of the amalgamator. Either undertrituration or overtrituration decreases the strength for both traditional and high-copper amalgams.

Effect of Mercury Content. An important factor in the control of strength is the mercury content of the restoration. Sufficient mercury should be mixed with the alloy to coat the alloy particles and to allow a thorough amalgamation. Each particle of the alloy must be wetted by the mercury; otherwise a dry, granular mix results. Such a mix results in a rough, pitted surface that may lead to corrosion. Any excess of mercury left in the restoration can produce a marked reduction in strength.

The effect of the mercury content on the compressive strength of amalgam is shown in Figure 17–13. For either low-copper or high-copper admixed amalgam, if the mercury content increases above approximately 54% to 55%, the strength is markedly reduced. Similar decreases in strength with increased final mercury content are observed for spherical high-copper amalgams, except that the critical mercury content is less. This subject is discussed further in Chapter 18.

The strength of an amalgam is a function of the volume fractions of unconsumed alloy particles and mercury-containing phases. Low-mercury-content amalgams contain more of the stronger alloy particles and less of the weaker matrix phases. Increasing the final mercury content increases the volume fraction of the matrix phases at the expense of the alloy particles. As a result, amalgams containing higher amounts of final mercury are weaker.

High-copper amalgams are particularly weakened by the presence of a small amount of γ_2 phase, because it is the weakest phase within the dental amalgam. This problem can be minimized by using low mercury:alloy ratios, because excess mercury promotes formation of the γ_2 phase in a high-copper amalgam.

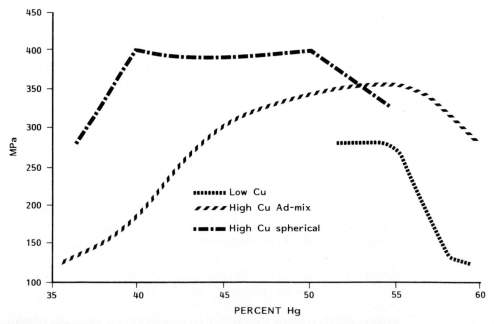

Figure 17–13. Effect of mercury:alloy ratio on the compressive strength of amalgam prepared with representative low-copper, high-copper admix and high-copper single-composition spherical alloys.

Effect of Condensation. Condensation pressure, technique, and alloy particle shape affect amalgam properties. When typical condensation techniques and lathe-cut alloys are employed, the greater the condensation pressure, the higher the compressive strength, particularly the early strength (e.g., at 1 hour). Good condensation techniques express mercury and result in a smaller volume fraction of matrix phases. Higher condensation pressures are required to minimize porosity and to express mercury from lathe-cut amalgams. On the other hand, spherical amalgams condensed with lighter pressures produce adequate strength.

Effect of Porosity. Voids and porosity are possible factors influencing the compressive strength of hardened amalgam. Voids are seen in micrographs of a low-copper amalgam (see Fig. 17–5), an admixed amalgam (see Fig. 17–7), and a single-composition amalgam (see Fig. 17–8).

Porosity is related to a number of factors, including the plasticity of the mix. Plasticity of amalgam mixes decreases over time from the end of trituration and condensation (delayed condensation). It also decreases with undertrituration. It could be anticipated that porosities would thereby be greater, and strength lower, under such conditions. Increasing condensation pressure steadily improves adaptation at the margins and decreases the number of voids.

The previous comments are related to lathe-cut or admix amalgams, which offer resistance to condensation. For spherical alloys, the condenser simply punches through the amalgam if heavy pressures are employed. It is fortunate that voids are not such a problem with these amalgams. Thus, lighter but firm pressure can be used without danger of sacrificing properties.

Effect of Amalgam Hardening Rate. The amalgam hardening rate is of considerable interest to the dentist. Because a patient may be dismissed from the dental chair within 20 minutes after trituration of the amalgam, a vital question is whether the amalgam has gained sufficient strength for its function. It is probable that a high percentage of amalgam restorations that fracture (see Fig. 17–12) do so shortly after insertion. The clinical manifestation may not be evident for months, but an initial crack within the restoration may occur within the first few hours.

Amalgams do not gain strength as rapidly as might be desired. For example, at the end of 20 minutes, compressive strength may be only 6% of the 1-week strength. The ADA specification stipulates a minimum comprehensive strength of 80 MPa at 1 hour. The 1-hour compressive strength of high-copper single-composition amalgams is exceptionally high (see Table 17–2). This strength may have some advantages clinically. For example, fracture is less probable if the patient accidentally bites on the restoration soon after leaving the dental office. Also, these amalgams may be strong enough shortly after placement to permit amalgam build-ups to be prepared for crowns and to permit taking impressions for crowns.

Even if a fast-hardening amalgam is used, its strength is likely to be low initially. Patients should be cautioned not to subject the restoration to high biting stresses for at least 8 hours after placement. By that time, a typical amalgam has reached at least 70% of its strength.

Even at the end of a 6-month period, some amalgams may still be increasing in strength. Such observations suggest that the reactions between the matrix phases and the alloy particles may continue indefinitely. It is doubtful that equilibrium conditions between them are ever attained.

CREEP

Significance of Creep on Amalgam Performance. During the 1970s, it was shown that the resistance of hardened dental amalgams to slow strain rate deformation seemed to correlate with long-term clinical performance. One such test measures the static creep of amalgam. Creep rate has been found to correlate with marginal breakdown of traditional low-copper amalgams, that is, the higher the creep, the greater the degree of marginal deterioration. This is illustrated in Figure 17–14, which shows marginal breakdown in amalgam restorations made of high and low creep-rate amalgams. The margins of the high creep amalgam are severely ditched.

However, for high-copper amalgams, creep is not necessarily a good predictor of marginal fracture. Many of these amalgams have creep rates of 0.4% (see Table 17–1) or lower. It is prudent to select a commercial alloy that has a creep rate below the level of 3% in ADA Specification No. 1. As tested by this specification, creep values of low-copper amalgams range between 0.8% and 8%. High-copper amalgams have much lower creep values, some even less than 0.1%. No data are available that suggest that reducing the creep value below approximately 1% influences marginal breakdown.

Influence of Microstructure on Creep. The γ_1 phase has been found to exert a primary influence on low-copper amalgam creep rates. Creep rates increase with larger γ_1 volume fractions and decrease with larger γ_1 grain sizes. The presence of γ_2 is associated with higher creep rates. In addition to the absence of γ_2, the very low creep rates in single-composition high-copper amalgams may be associated with η rods, which act as barriers to deformation of the γ_1 phase.

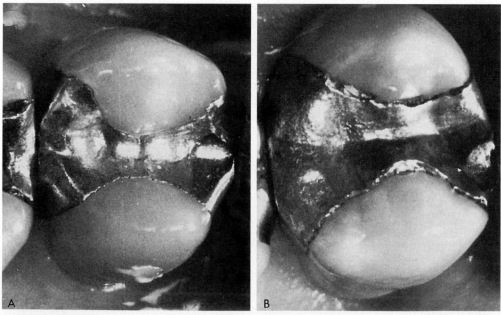

Figure 17–14. Four-year-old amalgam restorations. *A,* Amalgam placed with an alloy having minimal dynamic creep. *B,* Amalgam restoration of an alloy having a high creep value. (*A* and *B* courtesy of D. B. Mahler.)

Effect of Manipulative Variables on Creep. Those manipulative factors discussed previously that maximized strength also minimize creep rate for any given type of amalgam. Thus, mercury:alloy ratios should be minimized, condensation pressure should be maximized for lathe-cut or admixed alloys, and careful attention should be paid to timing of trituration and condensation, as discussed in Chapter 18.

CLINICAL PERFORMANCE OF AMALGAM RESTORATIONS

The exceptionally fine clinical performance of dental amalgam may be linked to its tendency to minimize marginal leakage. One of the greatest hazards associated with restoring teeth is the microleakage that may occur between the tooth walls and the restoration. With the exception of glass ionomer cement, no restorative material truly adheres to tooth structure; consequently, penetration of fluids and debris around the margins may be the greatest cause for secondary caries. At best, amalgam affords only a reasonably close adaptation to the walls of the prepared cavity. For this reason, cavity varnishes (see Chapter 24) are used to reduce the gross leakage that occurs around a new restoration. The use of dentin bonding agents with amalgam is another relatively new method to reduce microleakage. Although this technique shows promise, long-term results with this method are not yet available.

The small amount of leakage under amalgam restorations is unique. If the restoration is properly inserted, leakage decreases as the restoration ages in the mouth. This may be caused by corrosion products that form in the interface between the tooth and the restoration, sealing the interface and thereby preventing leakage. The presence of calcium and phosphorus and the demineralization of tooth structures adjacent to the amalgam restoration also strongly suggest a possible biologic interaction in this corrosion process.

The ability to seal against microleakage is shared by both the older low-copper amalgams and the newer high-copper amalgams. However, the accumulation of corrosion products is slower for the high-copper alloys.

Many amalgam restorations must be replaced because of problems, including secondary caries, gross fracture, "ditched" or fractured margins, and excessive tarnish and corrosion. The characteristics of an amalgam depend on its properties, which in turn depend on the alloy selected and how it is manipulated, as described in the previous sections. After placement, amalgams continue to undergo changes as a result of moisture contamination, corrosion, slow solid-state phase changes, and mechanical forces. The ultimate lifetime of an amalgam restoration is determined by a number of factors: (1) the material, (2) the dentist and the assistant, and (3) the patient environment. The dominant factors that control the performance during the early life of the restoration are the first two. As time proceeds, differences in the dynamics of the oral environment among patients contribute significantly to the variability of deterioration, particularly marginal ditching. Changes in the amalgam structure during clinical use and survival of amalgam restorations of various types are discussed later.

Tarnish and Corrosion. Amalgam restorations often tarnish and corrode in the oral environment. The degree of tarnish and the resulting discoloration appear to be dependent on the individual's oral environment and, to a certain extent, on the particular alloy employed. Electrochemical studies indicate that some passivation offering partial protection against further corrosion occurs as a result of the tarnish process. A tendency toward tarnish, although perhaps unaesthetic because of black silver sulfide, does not necessarily imply that active corrosion and early failure of a restoration will occur.

Active corrosion of a newly placed restoration occurs within the interface between the tooth and the restoration. The space between the alloy and the tooth permits the microleakage of electrolyte, and a classic concentration cell (crevice corrosion) process results. The build-up of corrosion products gradually seals this space, making dental amalgam a self-sealing restoration.

The precise role of corrosion in the process of marginal breakdown has not been established; however, several theories have been developed relating the two. There is indirect evidence that the γ_2 phase is implicated in both marginal failure and active corrosion in traditional alloys, but such a correlation is not possible for high-copper alloys.

The most common corrosion products found with traditional amalgam alloys are oxides and chlorides of tin. These are found at the tooth-amalgam interface and penetrating the bulk of old amalgam restorations, as shown in Figure 17–15. In the case of high-copper amalgams, many of the same products are found (Fig. 17–16).

Corrosion products containing copper can also be found in high-copper amalgams. However, the corrosion process is more limited, because the η phase is less susceptible to corrosion than is the γ_2 phase of traditional amalgams. Every effort should be made to produce a smooth, homogeneous surface on a restoration to minimize tarnish and corrosion, regardless of the alloy system used.

Whenever a gold restoration is placed in contact with an amalgam, corrosion of the amalgam can be expected as a result of the large differences in electromotive force of the two materials. The corrosion process can liberate free mercury, which can contaminate and weaken the gold restoration. Biologic effects such as galvanism can also result. Such a practice should be avoided.

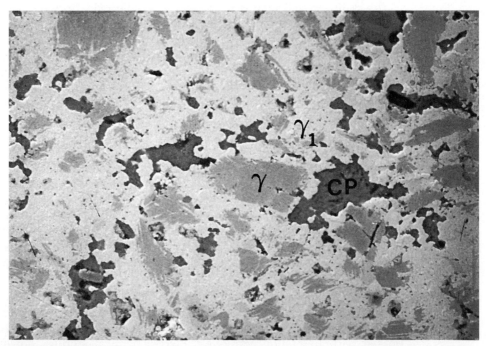

Figure 17–15. Microstructure of a 7-year-old traditional amalgam alloy restoration. The various phases are marked. Note that the γ_2 area has been replaced by tin-chloride corrosion products (CP).

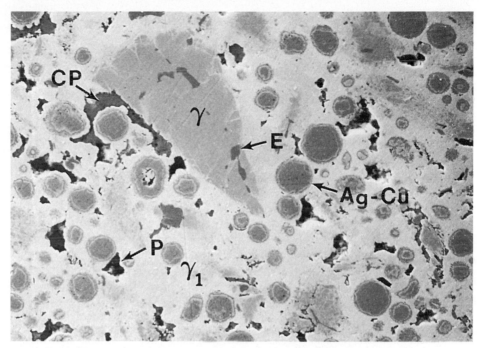

Figure 17–16. Microstructure of an 8-year-old high-copper alloy restoration. The phases are labeled. Although some porosity (P) is seen, it is less than that of the traditional alloy restoration seen in Figure 17–15, with fewer corrosion products (CP).

A high-copper amalgam is cathodic with respect to a conventional amalgam. Thus, concern has been expressed that if high-copper amalgam restorations were placed in the mouth of the same patient with existing restorations of traditional amalgam, corrosion and failure would be accelerated in the latter. Clinical observations do not indicate accelerated corrosion in such situations. Laboratory models established to monitor corrosion in adjacent restorations suggest that the current flow paths are such that electrochemical interaction between restorations is minimal.

Because the γ_2 phase is the most anodic of those present in set amalgam alloys, the high-copper amalgams, which virtually eliminate this phase, show improved laboratory corrosion behavior compared with traditional amalgams. However, as already noted, high mercury:alloy ratios can lead to the formation of γ_2 phase even in amalgams produced from high-copper alloys, thus promoting corrosion.

Compositional Effects on the Survival of Amalgam Restorations. Although many factors may contribute to the deterioration of dental amalgams as noted in the prior sections, the ultimate test is the long-term survival of the well-placed dental amalgam restoration. A number of clinical trials have attempted to determine differences in performance of dental amalgams based on amalgam type. Results of such long-term studies are illustrated in Figure 17–17. In this figure the survival of amalgam restorations are grouped into categories based on their content of copper and zinc. Modern high-copper amalgams with zinc (HCZ) have the best overall survival of nearly 90% after 12 years. High-copper amalgams without zinc (HC) performed the next best with survival rates of approximately 80%. The survival curves for these two groups of amalgams could

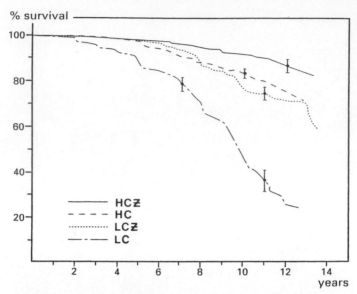

Figure 17–17. Survival curves for amalgam restorations classified according to copper and zinc content. Both copper and zinc appear to provide protection to restorations. Thus, many more high-copper restorations containing zinc survived than did low-copper restorations without zinc in these clinical trials. (Courtesy of H. Letzel, G. Marshall, S. Marshall, and M. Van't Hof.)

be distinguished only after approximately 8 years, when the better survival of the high-copper systems that contain a small quantity of zinc became apparent. The next group are traditional low-copper amalgams with zinc (LCZ). The worst performance was exhibited by low-copper amalgams that were zinc free. These systems exhibited failures in 50% of the restorations after only 10 years. The reasons for the differences seen in the survival are not completely clear. However, the combined and perhaps synergistic effects of the additional copper and zinc contents probably offer increased corrosion protection to the restorations.

SELECTED READING

Duperon DF, Nevile MD, and Kasloff Z: Clinical evaluation of corrosion resistance of conventional alloy, spherical-particle alloy, and dispersion-phase alloy. J Prosthet Dent 25:650, 1971; and Mahler DB, Terkla LG, Van Eysden J, and Reisbick MH: Marginal fracture versus mechanical properties of amalgam. J Dent Res 49:1452, 1970.
These two independent studies showed clinical superiority for the admix alloy developed by Innes and Youdelis (see later in list). These publications are classic, as they led to the introduction of the high-copper alloy.
Fairhurst CW, and Ryge G: X-ray diffraction investigation of the Sn-Hg phase in dental amalgam. In: Mueller WM (ed): Advances in X-ray Analysis, Vol. 5. New York, Plenum Press, 1962; Mahler DB, Adey JD, and Van Eysden J: Quantitative microprobe analysis of amalgam. J Dent Res 54:218, 1975; and Okabe T, Mitchell RJ, Butts MB, and Fairhurst CW: A study of high-copper amalgams. III. SEM observations of amalgamation of high-copper powders. J Dent Res 57:975, 1978.
Three publications representative of the literature that have defined the phases occurring in the setting reaction of the alloy and mercury and as influenced by parameters such as composition and particle configuration.
Ferracane JL, Mafiana P, Cooper C, and Okabe T: Time-dependent dissolution of amalgams into saline solution. J Dent Res 66:1331, 1987.
The rate of dissolution of ions from amalgams into saline is low once the amalgam has set, probably inhibited by formation of a surface film.
Greener EH: Amalgam—yesterday, today, and tomorrow. Oper Dent 4:24, 1979.

An excellent review of the history of amalgam, the evolution of newer formulations, and citation of what the future may hold. Incidentally, some of these predictions have been prophetic.

Innes DBK, and Youdelis WV: Dispersion-strengthened amalgams. Can Dent Assoc J 29:587, 1963.
Admix alloys were introduced via this research.

Letzel H, van't Hof MA, Vrijhoef MMA, Marshall GW Jr, and Marshall SJ. A controlled clinical study of amalgam restorations: Survival, failures, and causes of failure. Dent Mater 5:115, 1989.
A retrospective evaluation of a long-term clinical study highlighting failure frequencies and modes.

Lloyd CH, and Adamson M: The fracture toughness of amalgam. J Oral Rehabil 12:59, 1985.
Admix high-copper products have higher fracture toughness than those of a single-component powder, attributed to differences in microstructures.

Mahler DB, and Adey JD: Microprobe analysis of three high-copper amalgams. J Dent Res 63:921, 1984.
The composition and structure of three high-copper amalgams before and after their reaction were studied.

Mahler DB, Adey JD, and Marek M: Creep and corrosion of amalgam. J Dent Res 61:33, 1982.
Corrosion was directly related to the amount of γ_2 phase present, whereas creep was either high or low, depending on the absence or presence of γ_2.

Mahler DB: Research on dental amalgam, 1982–1986. Adv Dent Res 2:71, 1988.
One of the premier authorities on amalgam traces the pertinent trends and literature over a 5-year period. Excellent source reading that offers pertinent suggestions as to future avenues of meaningful research.

Marshall GW Jr, Marshall SJ, Letzel H, and Vrijhoef MMA: Microstructures of Cu-rich amalgam restorations with moderate clinical deterioration. Dent Mater 3:135, 1987.
The large variations in porosity and corrosion products in clinically retrieved restorations are described. The article also demonstrates a zinc-rich layer and other tin layers that form at the tooth-amalgam interface.

Marshall SJ, and Marshall GW: Dental amalgam: The materials. Adv Dent Res 6:94–99, 1992.
A recent review of setting reactions, microstructures, and properties of various amalgam types as related to clinical performance.

Sarkar NK, and Park JR: Mechanism of improved corrosion resistance of Zn-containing dental amalgams. J Dent Res 67:1312, 1988.
An in vitro study that may explain the mechanism of improved corrosion resistance of zinc-containing amalgams as compared with that of zinc-free alloys.

Schoonover IC, and Souder W: Corrosion of dental alloys. J Am Dent Assoc 28:1278, 1941.
The first suggestion of the potential for high-copper alloys, even though the subject then lay dormant for several decades.

Sutow EJ, Jones DW, and Hall GC: Correlation of dental amalgam crevice corrosion with clinical ratings. J Dent Res 68:82, 1989.
Marginal breakdown and the corrosion behavior of γ_2 and γ_2-free amalgams was studied in vitro. The methodology is of particular interest.

Swartz ML, and Phillips RW: In vitro studies on the marginal leakage of restorative materials. J Am Dent Assoc 62:141, 1961.
One of numerous studies demonstrating the reduction in microleakage as the amalgam restoration ages unique to restorative materials.

18 *Dental Amalgam*
Technical Considerations

- Factors Affecting the Quality of Amalgam Restorations
- Mercury:Alloy Ratio
- Mechanical Trituration
- Condensation
- Carving and Finishing
- Clinical Significance of Dimensional Change
- Side Effects of Mercury
- Marginal Deterioration
- Repaired Amalgam Restorations

FACTORS AFFECTING THE QUALITY OF AMALGAM RESTORATIONS

A good modern dental amalgam alloy can be manipulated so that the restoration lasts an average of 12 to 15 years. A defective restoration is most frequently associated with the dentist, auxiliary, or patient and not with the material, although amalgam is brittle and must be manipulated with this deficiency in mind. The cavity preparation must be designed correctly, and the amalgam must be manipulated properly so that no part of the amalgam restoration is placed under excessive tensile stress. The manipulative aspects of amalgam are discussed in detail relative to the influence of technique on the physical properties and clinical success of these restorations.

The criteria involved in the selection of an alloy vary with the individual practitioner. Certainly, the first criterion is to make sure that the alloy meets the requirements of the American Dental Association (ADA) Specification No. 1 or a similar specification.

The manipulative characteristics are extremely important and a matter of personal preference. The smoothness of the mix, ease of condensation, ease of finishing the working time and the setting time influence the final selection of the practitioner. For example, amalgams made from an admix blend of lathe-cut and spherical particles have an entirely different feel during condensation than do spherical particle amalgams. It is essential that the alloy selected be one with which the dentist and the assistant feel comfortable. The operator variable is a major factor influencing the clinical life span of the restoration. Use of alloys and techniques that encourage standardization in the manipulation and placement of the amalgam enhances the quality of the service rendered. Coincident with these manipulation considerations is the delivery system provided by the manufacturer—its convenience, expediency, and capability to minimize the technique sensitivity associated with human variables. The alloy may be purchased in powder or pellet form or as preproportioned alloy with mercury in disposable capsules. For the first form the mercury must be obtained from a mercury dispenser, a device that is somewhat technique sensitive. There are advantages and disadvantages to the use of preproportioned capsules, as discussed later. Nonetheless, the delivery system is an important consideration.

Obviously, the selection of one type of amalgam over others should be based on clinical performance and, lacking such information, on the physical properties. However, the initial analysis of properties should be compared with clinical performance as such data become available. This is especially necessary for alloy formulations that depart from traditional compositions and for which a consistent correlation between properties and performance has not as yet been established.

Alloys of traditional composition are still available, and acceptable amalgam restorations can be obtained from many of these products. However, it is obvious that the higher-copper alloy systems are now the materials of choice. Improved physical properties, the elimination of the γ_2 phase, and the better corrosion resistance associated with these alloys generally lead to superior clinical performance.

There is only one requisite for dental mercury: its purity. Common contaminating elements, such as arsenic, can lead to pulpal damage. Furthermore, a lack of purity may adversely affect the physical properties of the amalgam. It is unfortunate that terms such as *pure*, *redistilled*, and *triple distilled* do not indicate the chemical quality of the mercury.

The designation *USP* (United States Pharmacopeia) ensures mercury of satisfactory purity with no surface contamination and less than 0.02% nonvolatile residue. The requirements for dental mercury are encompassed in ADA Specification No. 6 and ISO 1560 for dental mercury.

MERCURY:ALLOY RATIO

Up until the early 1960s it was necessary to use an amount of mercury considerably in excess of that desirable in the final restorations to achieve smooth, plastic amalgam mixes. Because of the deleterious effects of an excessive mercury content on the physical and mechanical properties of amalgam, manipulative procedures were employed subsequently to reduce the amount of mercury left in the restoration to an acceptable level.

For conventional mercury-added systems, two techniques were used for achieving mercury reduction in the final restoration. Initially, the removal of excess mercury was accomplished by the operator's squeezing or wringing the mixed amalgam in a squeeze cloth before inserting the increments into the prepared cavity. Also, additional mercury-rich amalgam was worked to the top during condensation of each increment, and this excess was removed as the amalgam mix was built up to form a restoration. Although excellent restorations may be produced in this manner, the amount of mercury removed by the squeeze cloth and during condensation varied. Thus, there was a considerable chance for error.

The most obvious method for reducing the mercury content of the restoration is to reduce the original mercury:alloy ratio. The alloys currently available are designed for manipulation with reduced mercury:alloy ratios. This method is known as the *minimal mercury technique* (1959), or the *Eames technique* (1959), in recognition of the dentist who developed the concept. Sufficient mercury must be present in the original mix to provide a coherent and plastic mass after trituration, but it must be low enough that the mercury content of the restoration is at an acceptable level without the need to remove an appreciable amount during condensation. The mercury content of the finished restoration should be comparable with that of the original mercury:alloy ratio, usually approximately 50 wt%, with lesser amounts (approximately 42 wt%) being used with spherical alloys.

The obvious choice for placement of amalgam restorations with today's alloys is the minimal mercury technique, but manipulative procedures are still critical. The excellence of clinical restorations placed by this technique depends on proper manipulation, including proportioning of the mercury and alloy. Because the recommended amount of mercury is always the minimum amount required to produce a usable mix, proportioning of the two components must be exact. Trituration and condensation of the amalgam must be done with equal care and attention to detail.

Proportioning. The amount of alloy and mercury to be used can be described as the *mercury:alloy ratio*, which signifies the parts by weight of mercury and of alloy to be used for the particular technique employed. For example, a mercury:alloy ratio of 4:5 indicates that four parts of mercury are to be used with five parts of alloy by weight. Sometimes, instead of a mercury:alloy ratio, manufacturers' instructions specify the percentage of mercury by weight to be employed in the mix. A mix of amalgam prepared with a mercury:alloy ratio of 4:5 would contain 44.4% mercury.

The recommended ratio varies for different alloy compositions, particle sizes, particle shapes, and heat treatments. The particular manipulative and condensation technique favored by the dentist can also be a factor in selecting the desired ratio. The recommended mercury:alloy ratios for most modern lathe-cut alloys is 1:1 or 50% mercury, as noted earlier, although some may vary by a few percentages. With spherical alloys, the recommended amount of mercury is closer to 42%.

Regardless of the ratio, proportioning is critical for the minimum mercury alloys. If the mercury content is slightly low, the mix may be dry and grainy with insufficient matrix present to cohesively bond the mass. As discussed in Chapter 17, the use of too little mercury impairs the strength of high-copper amalgams as much as an excessive quantity of mercury. Corrosion resistance is also reduced.

A wide variety of mercury and alloy dispensers, or proportioning devices, are available. The most common type is the dispenser based on volumetric proportioning. Preweighed pellets or tablets are a more convenient method for correctly dispensing the alloy. The individual pellets are quite uniform in weight, provided that normal care is exercised in handling to avoid chipping of the pellet. With preweighed pellets, all that is required is an accurate mercury dispenser.

As a liquid, mercury can be measured by volume without appreciable loss of accuracy. Standard deviations in weights of mercury dispensed as low as ±0.5% may be attained with a number of commercial mercury dispensers. However, precautions must still be exercised in their use. The dispenser should be held vertically to ensure consistent spills of mercury. Tilting the bottle to a 45-degree angle results in unreliable mercury:alloy ratios. The dispenser should be at least half full when it is used. If it is not, the weight of mercury dispensed may be erratic. Probably the most common cause of inaccurate delivery of the mercury is use of contaminated mercury, which leads to entrapment of the contaminants in the reservoir and orifice of the device.

If such variables are not controlled, variation in individual spills of mercury may amount to 3% or 4%. With the use of low mercury:alloy ratios, variations of this magnitude result in an unusable mix.

Disposable capsules containing preproportioned aliquots of mercury and alloy are widely used. They contain alloy either in pellet form or as a preweighed portion of powder in conjunction with the appropriate quantity of mercury. To prevent any amalgamation from occurring during storage, the mercury and alloy are physically separated from each other. The older types of preproportioned capsules require activation before trituration to allow the mercury to enter the compartment with the alloy. Some alloys are now available in *self-activating capsules*, which bring the alloy and mercury together automatically during the first few oscillations of the amalgamator. Although the preproportioned material is more expensive, it is convenient, it eliminates the chance of mercury spills and exposure to mercury vapor during proportioning, and it should result in a reliable mercury:alloy ratio. At the same time, there is no opportunity to make minor adjustments in the mercury:alloy ratio to accommodate personal preference.

Regardless of the method used, the proper amount of mercury and alloy always must be proportioned before the start of trituration. The addition of mercury after trituration is contraindicated.

MECHANICAL TRITURATION

Originally, the alloy and mercury were mixed, or *triturated*, by hand with a mortar and pestle. Today, however, mechanical amalgamation saves time and standardizes the procedure. In fact, it is probably impossible to employ hand trituration for mixing modern amalgams prepared with low mercury:alloy ratios.

The object of trituration is to provide proper amalgamation of the mercury and alloy. The alloy particles are coated with a film of oxide that is difficult for the mercury to penetrate. This film must be rubbed off in some manner so that a clean surface of alloy can come in contact with the mercury. The oxide layer is removed by abrasion when the alloy particles and mercury are triturated.

A large number of commercial brands of amalgamator are available. Two representative ones are shown in Figure 18–1. The basic principle of operation is comparable for most of them. A capsule serves as a *mortar*. A cylindrical metal or plastic piston of smaller diameter than the capsule is inserted into the capsule, and this serves as the *pestle*. Capsules for disposable systems also usually contain an appropriate pestle.

The alloy and mercury are dispensed into the capsule, or if a disposable-capsule system is being used, the capsule may require activation. When the capsule has been secured in the machine and the machine has been turned on, the arms holding the capsule oscillate at high speed; thus, trituration is accomplished. There is an automatic timer for controlling the length of the mixing time, and most modern amalgamators have two or more operating speeds. Multiple-speed amalgamators provide greater versatility, often permitting the amalgamator to be used for mixing other preproportioned materials,

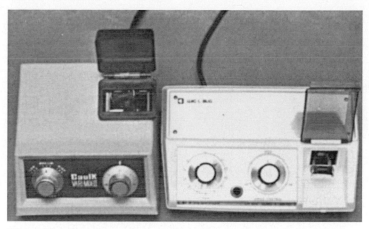

Figure 18–1. Two representative commercial mechanical amalgamators.

such as cements and composites. Some amalgam alloys and certain types of preproportioned capsule systems have specific recommendations for trituration speeds.

New amalgamators must have hoods that cover the reciprocating arms holding the capsule, as shown in Figure 18–1. The purpose of the hood is to confine mercury that might be sprayed into the room or a capsule that might be thrown from the amalgamator during trituration.

Reusable capsules are available with friction fit and screw-cap lids. With either type, it is important that the lid on the capsule fit tightly. If it does not, a fine mist of mercury will be sprayed out of the capsule during trituration. Loss of mercury can alter the mercury:alloy ratio to the extent that the mix is unusable. Much more important, an aerosol of mercury droplets is created, producing a risk of mercury inhalation. Capsule lids should be carefully checked before use, and any that appear to be loose should be discarded. Also, with long use, the fit may deteriorate. Disposable capsules should never be reused, because leakage or fracture of the capsule is likely to occur.

A wide variety of capsule-pestle combinations are available. One type of capsule is of a one-piece construction such that no mercury is released during trituration. After trituration, the capsule is broken open by bending across a notched area. Pestles may be either plastic or metal and come in a variety of sizes, shapes, and weights. In selecting a capsule-pestle combination, the size of the pestle is an important consideration. The diameter and length of the pestle should be considerably less than the comparable dimensions of the capsule. For example, the capsule-pestle combination shown in Figure 18–2A is acceptable from this standpoint. If the pestle is too large (Fig. 18–2B), the resultant mix may not be homogeneous. When the pellet form of alloy is used, the pellet or a piece of it may become wedged between the wall of the capsule and the pestle and may not be completely broken up during mixing.

The pellets produced by different manufacturers differ to some extent in the ease with which they are reduced to powder. In instances when pellets are difficult to break, one should consider employing a small metal pestle rather than a plastic one of a lighter weight. Trituration of alloy in a capsule without a pestle should be limited to those alloys for which that mode of mixing is specifically recommended.

An amalgamator should be used at the speed recommended by the alloy

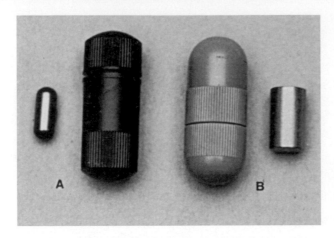

Figure 18–2. Capsule-and-pestle combinations, demonstrating a satisfactory size relationship between the capsule and pestle (A) and an unsatisfactory pestle size (B).

manufacturer. Some older amalgamators do not operate at a sufficient rate of speed to properly amalgamate newer high-copper alloys mixed with minimal mercury. Self-activating capsules are usually quite sensitive to trituration speed. Regardless of the alloy or amalgamator used, no more than two pellets of alloy should be mixed in a capsule at one time.

A reusable capsule should be clean and free of previously mixed, hardened alloy. Scraping out hardened alloy usually produces scratches that compound the sticking problem in the future. In the long run, it is well to discard the capsule. This sticking problem can often be minimized by the following procedure: at the end of amalgamation, quickly remove the pestle from the capsule, replace the lid, reinsert the capsule in the amalgamator, turn it on for a second or two, and then remove it. This *mulling process* generally causes the mix to cohere so that it can be readily removed from the capsule.

No exact recommendations for mixing time can be given because of such factors as the wide variety of amalgamators, differences in speed and oscillating patterns, and different capsule designs. The amount of work required for amalgamation of various alloys differs from one to another. Spherical alloys, for example, usually require less amalgamation time than do lathe-cut alloys. Also, a larger mix requires slightly longer mixing time than a smaller one. Manufacturers' directions contain a time schedule for mixing the alloy. However, because of the speed variations in amalgamators, even of the same brand, this schedule should serve only as a rough guide.

An important factor to be decided by the dentist and assistant is the optimum amalgamation time required to attain a mix of correct consistency. A general rule is that for a given alloy and mercury:alloy ratio, increased trituration time or speed, or both, shortens the working and setting times. Alloys differ in the sensitivity to trituration time, as can be seen in Figure 18–3.

Consistency of the Mix. It is evident that the proper combination of the alloy and mercury is a prime manipulative consideration. At this stage, the composition of the final amalgam is largely determined, and the composition is a major determinant of the physical properties.

Provided that the same weights of alloy and mercury are used each time and are triturated by the same amalgamator, attainment of a proper mix can be controlled by timing the trituration. The proper time can be determined by observing the consistency of the mix. For example, the somewhat grainy mix

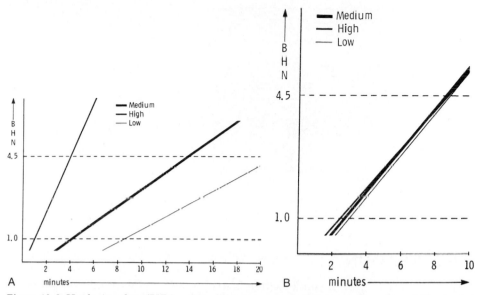

Figure 18–3. Hardening data (BHN = Brinell hardness number) for two alloys (*A* and *B*) mixed at low, medium, and high settings. Broken lines at 1.0 and 4.5 represent working and carving consistency, respectively. (From Brackett WW, Swartz ML, Moore BK, and Clark HE: The influence of mixing speed on the setting rate of high-copper amalgam. J Am Dent Assoc 115:289, 1987.)

shown in Figure 18–4 is undertriturated. Not only will the amalgam restoration made from this mix be weak, but also the rough surface left after carving of the granular amalgam will increase the susceptibility to tarnish.

If the trituration has produced an amalgam of the general appearance shown in Figure 18–5, the strength will approach the maximum value and the smooth carved surface will retain its luster longer after polishing. Such an amalgam mix may be warm (not hot) when it is removed from the capsule. This result has no effect on the physical properties of the amalgam other than to shorten the working time somewhat. With experience, the proper consistency can be recognized, and the timing of the mix can be adjusted to ensure this optimum level of plasticity.

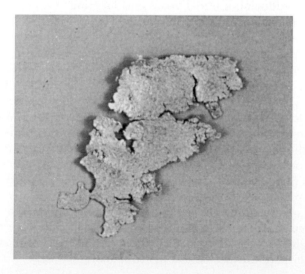

Figure 18–4. Undertriturated mix of amalgam. Such a mix has low strength and poor resistance to corrosion.

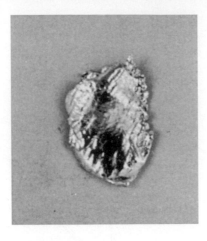

Figure 18–5. Properly triturated amalgam having maximum properties.

CONDENSATION

The goal of condensation is to compact the alloy into the prepared cavity so that the greatest possible density is attained, with sufficient mercury present to ensure complete continuity of the matrix phase between the remaining alloy particles. If this goal is achieved, the strength of the amalgam is thereby increased, and creep is decreased. Also, mercury-rich amalgam must be brought to the top of each increment as it is being condensed, so that successive increments bond to each other. A major objective is to remove any excess mercury from each increment as it is worked to the top by the condensing procedure. With the minimum mercury technique, removal of the soft, mushy material during condensation of the alloy is, of course, less critical. Under proper conditions of trituration and condensation, there is little danger of removing too much mercury during condensation.

After the mix is made, condensation of the amalgam should be promptly initiated. As can be seen in Figure 18–6, the longer the time lapse between mixing and condensation, the weaker is the amalgam. In addition, the mercury content and creep of the amalgam are increased. Condensation of partially set material probably fractures and breaks up the matrix that has already formed. Also, when the alloy has lost a certain amount of plasticity, it is difficult to condense without producing internal voids and layering.

The loss in strength incurred depends on the hardening rate of amalgam. A fast-setting amalgam, such as that obtained for alloy A in Figure 18–6, is affected to a greater extent than the slower setting alloy B. Most modern alloys mixed with minimal amounts of mercury harden with considerable rapidity. The working time is short, and the effects would be analogous to those observed with alloy A. Therefore, condensation should be as rapid as possible, and a fresh mix of amalgam should be made if condensation takes longer than 3 or 4 minutes.

The field of operation must be kept absolutely dry during condensation. The incorporation of the slightest moisture in a zinc-containing amalgam at this state can result in a delayed expansion, as discussed previously, and associated problems such as corrosion and loss of strength. The ultimate result of moisture contamination is premature failure of the restoration.

Because of the nature of the operation, condensation must always be accomplished within four walls and a floor; one or more walls may be a thin sheet of stainless steel, called a *matrix band* or *matrix strip*. Condensation can be accomplished with either hand or mechanical instruments.

Hand Condensation. The amalgam mixture should never be touched with bare hands. The freshly mixed alloy contains free mercury, and skin contact should be avoided because there is moisture on the surface of the skin that is a source of contamination of the amalgam. The increments of alloy should be carried to, and inserted in, the prepared cavity by means of instruments such as small forceps and an amalgam carrier designed for that purpose. The condensing instrument generally has a working point that is usually larger than that used in a direct-filling gold condenser.

Once the increment of amalgam is inserted into the cavity preparation, it should immediately be condensed with sufficient pressure to remove voids and to adapt the material to the walls. The condenser point, or face, is forced into the amalgam mass under hand pressure. Condensation is usually started at the center, and then the condenser point is stepped little by little toward the cavity walls. The force requirements depend on the shape of the alloy particle.

After condensation of an increment, the surface should be shiny in appearance. This indicates that there is sufficient mercury present at the surface to diffuse into the next increment so that each increment, as it is added, bonds to the preceding one. If this is not done and the increments do not bond, the restoration will be laminated. Such a restoration might be likened to a stack of bricks with no mortar cementing them together. It may subsequently fracture, probably when the matrix is removed. At best it would lack homogeneity, and it will subsequently sustain severe corrosion damage.

Even with the minimal mercury techniques now in general use, it is probably desirable to remove some of the soft or mushy material that is brought to the surface of each increment. This step is far less critical than it was when the percentage of mercury recommended for the mix was far above the acceptable level for the final restoration.

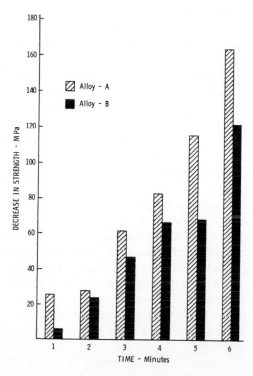

Figure 18–6. Effect of the elapsed time between trituration and condensation on the reduction in strength of the hardened amalgam. The greater the elapsed time, the lower the strength.

The procedure of adding an increment, condensing it, adding another increment, and so forth is continued until the cavity is overfilled. Any mercury-rich material at the surface of the last increment, constituting the overfill, is removed when the restoration is carved.

If the cavity is a large one or, for some reason, undue time is taken to complete condensation, another mix should be made just before original one is depleted or loses its plasticity. This can easily be accomplished, because mechanical mixing requires only a few seconds.

A well-condensed amalgam restoration can be achieved only if the mix has a proper consistency. A dry, grainy mix (see Fig. 18–4) has insufficient mercury and plasticity, as described previously, and a mix that is hard and hot to the touch has probably been mixed too long. In either case, condensation of mix should not be attempted. Rather, a new mix should be prepared.

One of the most important factors in condensation is the size of amalgam increments carried into the cavity. The larger the piece, the more difficult it is to reduce the voids and to adapt the alloy to the cavity walls. However, when a large restoration is being produced, a compromise is for speed, and a large increment may be added to increase the time available for condensation. In general, however, relatively small increments of amalgam should be used throughout the condensation procedure to reduce void formation and to obtain maximum adaptation to the cavity. Likewise, sufficient condensation pressure must be used to force the alloy particles together, reduce voids, and work mercury to the surface to achieve bonding between the increments.

Condensation Pressure. The area of the condenser point, or face, and the force exerted on it by the operator govern the condensation pressure. When a given force is applied, the smaller the condenser, the greater the pressure exerted on the amalgam. For example, a thrust of 44 N (10 lb) exerted on a circular condenser point 2 mm in diameter results in a condensation pressure of 13.8 MPa (2000 psi). The same thrust applied to a condenser 3.5 mm in diameter produces a condensation pressure of only 4.6 MPa (670 psi). If the condenser point is too large, the operator cannot generate sufficient condensation pressure to condense the amalgam adequately and force it into retentive areas.

Although forces as great as 66.7 N (15 lb) are recommended for condensation, it is doubtful that forces of that magnitude are generally used. A study of the condensation forces applied by 30 practitioners showed that forces in the range of 13.3 to 17.8 N (3 to 4 lb) represent the average force employed. To ensure maximum density and adaptation to the cavity walls, the condensation force should be as great as the alloy will allow, consistent with patient comfort. It is doubtful that condenser points larger than 2 mm in diameter provide adequate condensation of lathe-cut alloys.

One of the advantages of spherical amalgam alloys is that the strength properties tend to be less sensitive to condensation pressure. In fact, many of the spherical alloys immediately after trituration are "mushy" and have little "body." Thus, they offer only mild resistance to the condensation force. In many instances, condensation becomes a matter of attaining good adaptation. When these alloys are being condensed, a large condenser can often be used. The potential disadvantages of a spherical alloy compared with an admixed alloy (lathe-cut and spherical articles) is the tendency for overhangs in proximal areas and weak proximal contacts (i.e., unwaxed floss can pass through the contact area with little or no resistance).

The shape of the condenser points should conform to the area under condensation. For example, a round condenser point is ineffective adjacent to a corner or angle of a prepared cavity; a triangular or square point is indicated in such an area. Points of various shapes are available to provide effective condensation.

Mechanical Condensation. The procedures and principles of mechanical condensation are the same as those for hand condensation, including the need to use small increments of amalgam. The only difference is that the condensation of the amalgam is essentially done by an automatic device. Various mechanisms are employed for those instruments. Some provide an impact type of force, whereas others use rapid vibration.

Whether the device is of the impact or vibratory type, less energy is needed than for hand condensation, and the operation may be less fatiguing to the dentist. Similar clinical results can be achieved using either hand or mechanical condensation. The method selected is based usually on the preference of the dentist.

CARVING AND FINISHING

After the amalgam has been condensed into the prepared cavity, the restoration is carved to reproduce the proper tooth anatomy. The objective of carving is to simulate the anatomy rather than to reproduce extremely fine detail. If the carving is too deep, the bulk of amalgam, particularly at the marginal areas, is reduced. If this area is too thin, it may fracture under masticatory stress.

If the proper technique is followed, the amalgam should be ready for carving soon after completion of condensation. Carving should proceed in a direction parallel to or slightly toward the margin of the prepared tooth whenever possible. This is best accomplished with a bladed instrument such as a Hollenbeck carver. It is also beneficial to maintain contact with the tooth surface to minimize the risk for ditching or "hypomargination."

After carving is completed, the surface of the restoration should be smoothed. This process may be accomplished by judiciously burnishing the surface and margins of the restoration. If the alloy is a reasonably fast-setting one, it should have achieved sufficient strength by this time to support firm but not heavy rubbing pressure.

Burnishing of the occlusal anatomy can be accomplished with a ball burnisher. A rigid flat-bladed instrument is best used on smooth surfaces. Final smoothing can be concluded by rubbing the surface with a moist cotton pellet or by lightly going over it with a rubber polishing cup and polishing paste. Burnishing has been a somewhat controversial subject, and its effect on marginal adaptation and hardness is not well understood. There is ample evidence that amalgam surfaces that have been burnished, or burnished and lightly polished, are much smoother than carved surfaces. Clinical data on performance of restorations support the desirability of burnishing the fast-setting, high-copper systems. Burnishing slow-setting alloys can damage the margins of the restoration. Undue pressure should not be exerted in burnishing, and heat generation should be avoided. Temperatures higher than 60° C (140° F) cause a significant release of mercury. The mercury-rich condition thus created at the margins results in accelerated corrosion, fracture, or both.

Regardless of the alloy, the trituration method, and the condensation technique, the carved surface of the restoration is rough, as demonstrated by the dull surface of the restorations shown in Figure 18–7A. The surfaces are covered with scratches, pits, and irregularities. Even though the restoration surfaces have

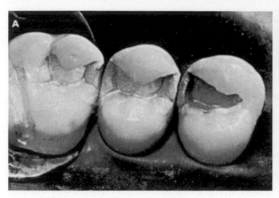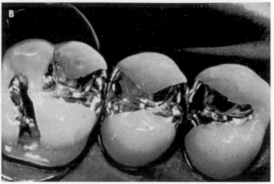

Figure 18–7. *A*, Amalgam restorations as they appear after carving. *B*, The same restorations after final finishing. (*A* and *B* courtesy of L. V. Hickey.)

been carefully finished by burnishing and smoothing, they are rough at the microscopic level. If these defects are not removed by further finishing after the amalgam is completely set, they can result in concentration cell-type corrosion. The smooth surface on the restorations shown in Figure 18–7*B*, produced by the final finishing procedure, is caused by the reduction in surface defects.

As previously stated, the final finishing of the restoration should not be done until the amalgam is fully set. It should be delayed for at least 24 hours after condensation, and preferably longer. The need for extremely high luster is questionable, but the metal surface should be smooth and uniform. The use of dry polishing powders and disks can easily raise the surface temperature above the 60° C (140° F) danger point. Thus, a wet abrasive powder in a paste form is used.

Polishing technique is a matter of personal preference, and textbooks on operative dentistry should be consulted. Essentially, one should use diminishing grades of abrasives and avoid heat production. The importance of finishing cannot be overemphasized. The restoration is not completed until its margins have been fully adjusted and its surfaces have been finely polished.

CLINICAL SIGNIFICANCE OF DIMENSIONAL CHANGE

After the amalgam is placed, a variety of changes occur at both the microstructural and the visual levels. Amalgams do deteriorate, and many are considered eventual failures. The leading causes for failures include (1) secondary caries; (2) marginal fracture; (3) bulk fracture; and (4) tooth fracture. At the microstructural level, changes occur as a result of (1) corrosion and tarnish; (2) γ_1 to β_1 transformation; and (3) stresses associated with mastication forces. All of these factors are probably interrelated, and the exact contribution of each to a specific case of failure is difficult to define. Thus, the dentist can expect to observe such deterioration over extended periods, but the rate of failures should generally decrease as a result of improvement in alloys. Modern amalgams should have survival rates of at least 90% after 5 years. Some amalgams are probably replaced prematurely for minor defects and because of uncertainty in diagnosis of early secondary caries. However, there are several types of dimensional instability that are under the direct control of the dentist.

CRITICAL QUESTION   *A patient reports pain on chewing one day after an amalgam restoration has been placed. What are most likely causes of this condition, and what are the best solutions?*

Expansion. In an early survey of the causes for failures of amalgam restorations, 16.6% of a large group of defective restorations failed because of excessive expansion. There are several causes for excessive expansion of amalgam. One is insufficient trituration and condensation, and another is the delayed expansion brought about by the contamination of the zinc containing amalgam with moisture during trituration or condensation. The latter is unquestionably the principal cause for such failures.

Delayed expansion is probably caused by the internal pressure exerted by hydrogen gas that is one of the corrosion products between the zinc in the amalgam and the incorporated moisture. This matter was discussed to a certain extent in Chapter 17. The large expansion begins 4 or 5 days after condensation (see Fig. 17–11 in Chapter 17). Thus, a patient who complains of pain 1 day after a restoration is placed cannot be experiencing the effects of delayed expansion caused by incorporation of moisture into the setting amalgam. One should examine the surface of the restoration for shiny abrasion marks that indicate the possibility of hyperocclusion. If this condition exists, the pain will disappear soon after the occlusion is properly adjusted. Another possibility is the development of cracks in the tooth that may have developed by removing too much remaining tooth structure and weakening the cusps. This situation may require replacement of the amalgam and *hooding* of the weakened cusp or cusps such as is done with a cast-onlay restoration. It is also possible that the cracks are minor and do not threaten the integrity of the cusps or the vitality of the tooth. In this case, etching of the crack walls and bonding of the fissure may provide a sufficient interim solution. The last resort is to restore the tooth with an onlay or full crown to minimize the risk of fracture.

Delayed expansion of amalgam often causes intense pain. It is presumed that when an expansion of this magnitude occurs, the restoration may become wedged so tightly against the cavity walls that a pressure toward the pulp chamber results. Such pain may be experienced 10 to 12 days after the insertion of the restoration. If it is not removed, a contaminated amalgam restoration continues to expand, and the final result may be similar to the protruding restoration shown in Figure 18–8. Undoubtedly, moisture was incorporated into the amalgam mix because the dry field was not maintained. Excessive expansion and corrosion of the restoration have ensued, and the restoration has extruded from the prepared cavity. Because the brittle amalgam margins are unsupported,

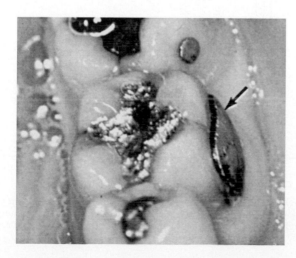

Figure 18–8. A Class V amalgam restoration *(arrow)* that has failed because of excessive expansion. (Courtesy of J. Osborne.)

they are susceptible to fracture, and marginal defects result. Leakage of the restoration can produce marginal discoloration, with further corrosion and pitting caused by the concentration cells formed.

Pitting and corrosion, regardless of the cause, definitely reduce the strength of the amalgam restoration. If this process proceeds far enough, the amalgam may become so pitted that it crumbles under stress.

Delayed expansion, occurring with moisture contamination of zinc-containing amalgams of either high or low copper content, is illustrated in Figure 18–9. At 20 weeks, amalgam specimens prepared from both types of alloys (alloy A is low copper and alloy B is high copper), when they were contaminated by moisture, expanded far in excess of the same uncontaminated amalgams. The expansion of the alloys at 20 weeks was also accompanied by a substantial reduction in strength (Fig. 18–10).

Contraction. Undertrituration results in reduced strength and possibly undue expansion during hardening. In addition, a slight contraction occurs with many modern amalgam alloys when they are properly triturated.

For many years it was believed that a slight expansion of the amalgam during setting would result in a restoration that seals the cavity against ingress of oral fluids. Laboratory tests indicate no difference in the sealing properties of expanding and contracting alloys. Clinical studies of restorations placed with amalgams that contract 2 to 40 μm/cm failed to reveal a marginal contraction gap after several years.

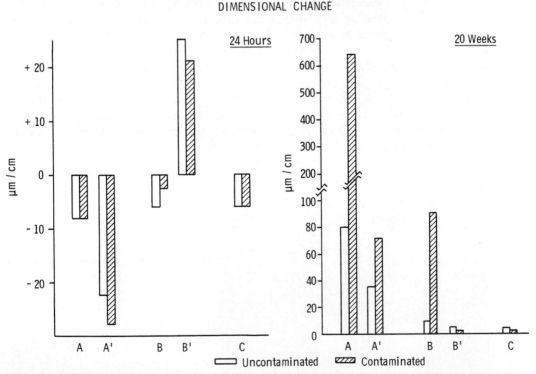

Figure 18–9. Effect of moisture contamination on the dimensional change of various types of amalgam alloys. A, Zinc-containing low-copper lathe-cut alloy; A', zinc-free low-copper lathe-cut alloy; B, zinc-containing high-copper lathe-cut alloy; B', zinc-free high-copper lathe-cut alloy; and C, zinc-free high-copper spherical alloy.

COMPRESSIVE STRENGTH

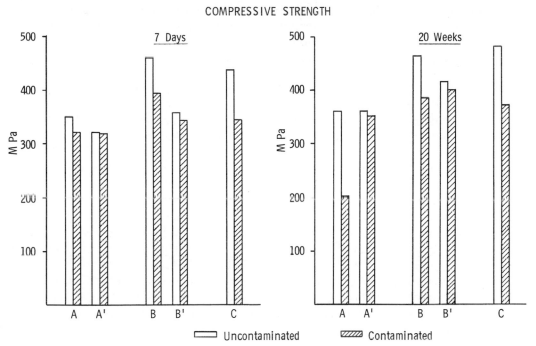

Figure 18–10. Effect of moisture contamination on the compressive strength of various types of amalgam alloys. A, Zinc-containing low-copper lathe-cut alloy; A′, zinc-free low-copper lathe-cut alloy; B, zinc-containing high-copper lathe-cut alloy; B′, zinc-free high-copper lathe-cut alloy; and C, zinc-free high-copper spherical alloy.

It is difficult to estimate whether an amalgam restoration in the mouth has contracted or expanded within the required 20-μm limits of such dimensional change. When it is recognized that the average human hair is 40 μm in diameter, it is virtually impossible to detect margins that may be open a few micrometers, either with the eye or with a dental instrument such as an explorer. It is for these reasons that through the years ADA Specification No. 1 has been broadened in terms of the permissible dimensional change on hardening, as measured on an unrestricted specimen.

These observations should not be construed as a recommendation for a contracting amalgam. They merely emphasize that small contractions during hardening do not appear to be clinically significant.

Zinc-free Alloys. As might be expected, the deleterious effects of moisture spurred interest in zinc-free alloys. Their use is certainly justified in those areas where it is virtually impossible to keep the operating region dry, such as the posterior teeth in the mouth of a child patient. In such instances, if a zinc-containing alloy is used, the dentist must sacrifice normal condensation procedures for the sake of speed. The restoration must be placed before any moisture contamination occurs; for example, the condensation should be accomplished by filling the prepared cavity with a few large increments rather than with small increments, as previously recommended.

The use of zinc-free alloys provides some measure of safety in this regard, as seen in Figures 18–9 and 18–10. When they are contaminated by moisture, the expansion at 20 weeks of specimens of zinc-free alloys (A′, B′, and C) was not appreciably different from that of specimens prepared from the uncontaminated alloys. Also, at 20 weeks, contaminated zinc-free alloys A' and B' showed virtually no reduction in strength. However, the spherical single composition high-copper alloy C, even though it contained no zinc, experienced a loss in strength both at 24 hours and 20 weeks when it was contaminated by moisture. Although the mechanism by which moisture reduces strength of alloys of this type has not been defined, it can be assumed that moisture present in the mix may interfere with the binding of the matrix. The present trend is toward reduction of the zinc content of alloys. Many of the spherical, single-composition, high-copper alloys are zinc free, and although contaminated nonzinc alloys do not exhibit high expansion, the strength of some is impaired (see Fig. 18–10).

Zinc was added primarily to aid in alloy manufacture, as discussed previously. There are no great differences in the mechanical properties of the two types of alloys. It is clear that zinc can have undesirable effects associated with delayed expansion. However, there is also evidence that in controlled clinical trials zinc-containing alloys have better marginal integrity and longer survival times than similar zinc-free alloys. This may be the result of preferential zinc corrosion leading to an early or good amalgam-tooth seal, which offers some advantage. Thus, the influence of the zinc on clinical performance still needs further clarification. Regardless of composition, moisture is to be avoided in the manipulation and placement of amalgam restorations or of any other restorative material.

CRITICAL QUESTION *Can the mercury vapor that is inhaled from amalgam restorations cause systemic diseases with symptoms that mimic multiple sclerosis and epilepsy? Isn't it possible that such symptoms can be experienced by a small percentage of patients who are "hypersensitive" to mercury?*

SIDE EFFECTS OF MERCURY

The amalgam restoration is possible only because of the unique characteristics of mercury. This metal provides the plastic mass that can be inserted and finished in the teeth, hardening to a structure that resists the rigors of the oral environment surprisingly well. However, it is also the element that so markedly influences the basic properties necessary to clinical services. The use of mercury in the oral environment has raised concerns over safety for more than 160 years. Currently, several countries are phasing out the use of dental amalgam because of environmental concerns as well as alleged side effects that may be sustained by the patients who receive amalgam restorations. Although this topic cannot be discussed thoroughly in this section, some aspects of the current controversy are mentioned to place the issue in perspective relative to the safety of amalgam and other materials that may be considered as alternatives to amalgam. Additional information on biocompatibility or bioacceptance is given in Chapter 5. To understand the possible side effects of dental amalgam, the differences between allergy and toxicity must be defined.

Allergy. Typically, allergic responses represent an antigen-antibody reaction marked by itching, rashes, sneezing, difficulty in breathing, swelling, or other symptoms. Contact dermatitis or Coombs' Type IV *hypersensitivity reactions* represent the most likely physiologic side effect to dental amalgam, but these reactions are experienced by less than 1% of the treated population. When allegations of certain signs and symptoms of amalgam toxicity have been made in recent years, some health care professionals have mistakenly concluded that patients with symptoms that mimicked those of various diseases and symptoms, including multiple sclerosis, epilepsy, and arthritis, were "hypersensitive" to mercury and this misconception prompted a few dentists to test for this hypersensitivity with a cutaneous patch test kit. Because the classic signs and symptoms of type IV hypersensitivity are hyperemia, edema, vesicle formation, and itching, the term *hypersensitivity* was incorrectly applied in these cases. Inappropriate use of patch test kits with instructions for additional analyses of blood pressure, pulse rate, indigestion, blurred vision, headaches, irritability, fatigue, depression, and redness of the eyes has led to an erroneously high estimate of 25% positive responses in one report. To confirm suspicions of true hypersensitivity, especially when a reaction has been sustained for 2 weeks or longer, the patient should be evaluated by an allergist. A small percentage of the public is allergic to mercury, as they are to many other elements. When such a reaction has been documented by a dermatologist or an allergist, an alternative material, such as a composite, cast metal alloy, cast titanium, or a ceramic must be used. However, none of these materials has yet been proven to be as economical and as technique insensitive as dental amalgam.

Toxicity. From its earliest use, mercury's possible side effects have been questioned. It is still sometimes conjectured that mercury toxicity from dental restorations is the cause for certain undiagnosed illnesses and that a real hazard may exist for the dentist or dental assistant when mercury vapor is inhaled during mixing, placement, and removal. In fact, only about 100 documented reports of mercury toxicity and allergy attributable to dental amalgam have been published over the past 60 years in the scientific literature. Of these cases, most of the affected persons were dentists or assistants (nurses) in a dental clinic. Few such cases have been reported during the past several decades, presumably because of improvements in encapsulation technology, capsule design, and scrap storage methods and the elimination of carpets and other mercury retention sites. The matter has again come to the fore with recent concern over mercury pollution of the environment. In some countries, amalgam particle collectors with efficiencies greater than 99% are required in dental clinics.

Undoubtedly, mercury penetrates from the restoration into tooth structure. An analysis of dentin underlying amalgam restorations reveals the presence of mercury, which in part may account for a subsequent discoloration of the tooth. Use of radioactive mercury in silver amalgam has also revealed that some mercury might even reach the pulp.

Small amounts of mercury are released during mastication. However, the possibility of toxic reactions occurring in patients from these traces of mercury penetrating the tooth or sensitization from mercury salts dissolving from the surface of the amalgam is extremely rare. The danger has been evaluated in numerous studies.

The most significant contribution to mercury assimilation from dental amalgam is via the vapor phase. The patient's encounter with mercury vapor during insertion of the restoration is brief, and the total amount of mercury vapor released during function is far below the "no effect" level. The most reliable estimates suggest that mercury from dental amalgam does not contribute a significant amount to the total exposure of patients. The results of one study in which patients with amalgam restorations were monitored with mercury vapor detectors over a 24-hour period showed that the amount of vapor inhaled was 1.7 μg/day. Three other studies have confirmed that the magnitude of vapor exposure for a patient with 8 to 10 amalgam restorations is in the range of 1.1 to 4.4 μg/day. The threshold value for workers in the mercury industry is 350 to 500 μg/day, depending on activity level, and is based on an exposure of 40 hours per week.

Dentists and their auxiliaries are exposed daily to the risk of mercury intoxication. Although metallic mercury can be absorbed through the skin or by ingestion, the primary risk to dental personnel is from inhalation. The maximum level of occupational exposure considered safe is 50 μg of mercury per cubic meter of air. This is actually an average value of instantaneous exposures over a standard work day. Mercury is volatile at room temperature and has a vapor pressure of 20 mg per cubic meter of air, about 400 times the maximum level that is considered acceptable. Mercury vapor has no color, odor, or taste and cannot be readily detected by simple means at levels near the maximum safe exposure. Because liquid mercury is almost 14 times more dense than water in terms of volume, a small spill can be significant. An eyedropper-sized drop of mercury contains enough mercury to saturate the air in an average operatory. The ADA has estimated that 1 in 10 dental office exceeds the maximum safe exposure level for mercury. However, only few cases of serious mercury intoxication caused by dental exposure have ever been reported.

Mercury blood levels that were measured in one study indicated that the average level in patients with amalgam was 0.7 ng/mL compared with a value of 0.3 ng/mL for subjects with no amalgam. This difference was found to be statistically significant ($P \leq 0.01$). However, one should be aware of a study in Sweden that demonstrated that one saltwater seafood meal per week raised average blood levels of mercury from 2.3 to 5.1 ng/mL, a sevenfold increase (2.8 ng/mL) compared with that (0.4 ng/mL) associated with amalgam restorations. The normal daily intake of mercury is 15 μg from food, 1 μg from air, and 0.4 μg from water.

The potential hazards of mercury can be greatly reduced by attention to a few precautionary measures. First, the operatory should be well ventilated. All excess mercury, including waste, disposable capsules, and amalgam removed during condensation, should be collected and stored in well-sealed containers. Proper disposal through reputable dental vendors is mandatory to prevent environmental pollution. Increasing legal attention is being focused on correct disposal of potentially hazardous waste materials, including dental amalgams and mercury. Amalgam scrap and materials contaminated with mercury or amalgam should not be incinerated or subjected to heat sterilization. If mercury is spilled, it must be cleaned up as soon as possible. It is extremely difficult to remove mercury from carpeting. Ordinary vacuum cleaners merely disperse the mercury further through the exhaust. Mercury suppressant powders are helpful but should be considered as temporary measures. If mercury comes in contact with the skin, the skin should be washed with soap and water.

As noted earlier, the reusable capsule used with a mechanical amalgamator should have a tightly fitting cap to avoid mercury leakage. When grinding amalgam, a water spray and suction should be used. Eye protection, a disposable mask, and gloves are standard requirements for dental practices.

The use of an ultrasonic amalgam condenser is not recommended because a spray of small mercury droplets has been observed surrounding the condenser tip during condensation. More detailed recommendations can be obtained by consulting the most recent reports of the ADA Council on Scientific Affairs.

An important part of a program for handling toxic materials is periodic monitoring of actual exposure levels. Current recommendations suggest that this procedure be conducted annually. Several techniques are available. Instruments can be brought in that yield a time-weighted average for mercury exposure to sample the air in the operatory. Film badges are also available that can be worn by office personnel in a manner similar to radiation exposure badges. Biologic determinations can be performed on office staff members to measure mercury levels in their blood or urine. The risk from mercury exposure to dental personnel cannot be ignored, but close adherence to simple hygiene procedures helps ensure a safe working environment.

Influence of Mercury Content on the Quality of the Restoration. Mercury is extremely important to the physical behavior of the amalgam restoration. Analysis of clinical restorations indicates a wide variation in their mercury content. Characteristically, the mercury concentration is higher in the marginal areas. This is true regardless of the condensation method or the "dryness" of the increments used to build the restoration. Mercury analysis of a large number of restorations reveals that the mercury content of the marginal areas averaged between 2% and 3% higher than the bulk of the restoration. The higher mercury content at the margins is important because these areas are critical in terms of corrosion, fracture, and secondary caries.

Restorations that have an unduly high mercury content have been judged clinically unsatisfactory by visual examination. Such a relationship is to be expected in that a marked decrease in the strength of traditional silver-tin amalgams occurred at a mercury content of approximately 55% by weight, as noted. When clinical restorations were placed with a low-copper alloy containing various quantities of mercury, the restorations containing mercury in excess of 55% showed an appreciably higher incidence of marginal fracture and surface deterioration than did restorations that contained mercury in the 50% range. The higher the mercury content, the greater the incidence and severity of failure that occurred as the restorations aged.

Because high mercury content has the same effect on strength and creep of high-copper alloys as on the older low-copper amalgams, it would be expected that high-copper amalgam restorations with an excessively high mercury content would also exhibit a greater incidence of marginal degradation and other effects. Certainly, if the mercury content is too high, the weaker and corrosion-susceptible γ_2 phase will be formed. Analysis of high-copper amalgam restorations, prepared with proper mercury:alloy ratios, has shown that after 7 years there is little or no change in overall mercury content of the restorations.

MARGINAL DETERIORATION

As has been repeatedly mentioned, one of the most common types of amalgam deterioration is the so-called "ditched" restoration shown in Figure 18–11. Although the ditching may not have progressed to the point at which secondary caries has developed, the restoration is unsightly, and further deterioration may be anticipated. Examination of clinical restorations has associated secondary caries with marginal discrepancies that exceeded 50 μm. Many such restorations are replaced as a preventive measure. However, the need to replace such restorations may be highly dependent on the oral hygiene status of the patient. Recent studies have shown that in a population with good oral hygiene, the incidence of secondary caries may be quite low even in the presence of severe marginal deterioration. Thus, a more conservative approach to amalgam restoration replacement has been suggested.

Marginal gaps are often attributed to a contraction of amalgam, but, as

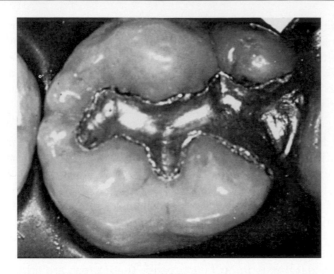

Figure 18–11. Typical "ditched" amalgam restoration. (Courtesy of H. W. Gilmore.)

explained earlier, this is not probable. Instead, marginal breakdown of amalgam restorations may be caused by, or related to, several factors.

Improper Cavity Preparation or Finishing. If unsupported enamel is left at the marginal areas of the cavity preparation, the tooth structure itself may in time fracture. Thus, the ditched amalgam may involve fracture of adjacent enamel as well as the amalgam.

Improper carving and finishing of the restoration may leave a thin ledge of amalgam extending over the enamel (Fig. 18–12). Such thin ledges are often

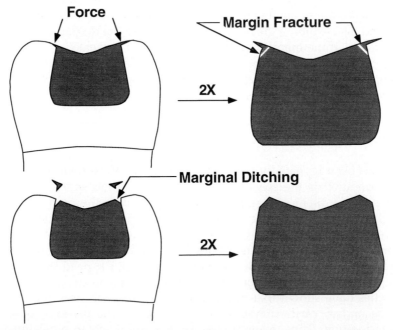

Figure 18–12. A common cause of marginal failure: If a feather edge of the amalgam is left overlapping the enamel at the margin, it will fracture under masticatory stress.

difficult to detect and remove. One method mentioned is to finish the margins after carving with a soft, unribbed, prophylactic polishing cup and a fine, slightly moist prophylactic paste. However, the cup should be tipped such that the edge rotates from amalgam to tooth, as shown in Figure 18–13. Light pressure should be used.

Excess Mercury. The effect of a high final mercury content on marginal deterioration has been discussed. Control of the mercury:alloy ratio, use of thorough trituration, and proper condensation reduce the possibility of such failures.

Creep. If the creep of the alloy is unduly high or if the manipulation is such that it tends to increase the creep, the potential for marginal breakdown is greatly enhanced. Certainly there is ample evidence that when other factors are controlled, the alloy used for the restoration is a highly significant factor in the incidence and severity of marginal failure of clinical restorations.

There appears to be little correlation between creep and marginal breakdown with alloys having creep values lower than 1%. However, when creep values are higher than this level, restorations of higher-creep alloys generally experience greater marginal breakdown than do restorations of lower-creep alloys.

The absence of the corrosion-susceptible γ_2 phase in the microstructure of high-copper amalgams is assumed to be the principal factor responsible for the superior resistance of these alloys to marginal breakdown. If this assumption is correct, the property of creep is not an important one for the prediction of marginal breakdown in high-copper amalgams. Theoretically, expansion of the amalgam from moisture contamination of a zinc-containing alloy can also cause this type of failure.

Thus, several mechanisms, separately or working synergistically, may be responsible for marginal breakdown. At this time, the exact mechanism of marginal breakdown and these specific properties are still under study. However, it is advisable to select alloys that inherently have low creep and possess maximum resistance to corrosion.

REPAIRED AMALGAM RESTORATIONS

Occasionally, when an amalgam restoration fails, as from marginal fracture, it is repaired. A new mix of amalgam is condensed against the remaining part of the existing restoration. Thus, the strength of the bond between the new and the old amalgam is important.

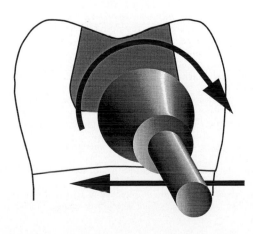

Figure 18–13. Final finishing of an amalgam margin with a soft, unribbed prophylaxis cup and fine prophylactic paste. The cup should be used with light pressure to avoid flattening of anatomic contours. Only the trailing edge (to the right) is in contact with the amalgam to ensure closure of the marginal space. (Artwork by Joel Anusavice.)

The flexure strength of repaired amalgam is less than 50% of that of unrepaired amalgam. The bond is a source of weakness. Factors such as corrosion and saliva contamination at the interface present formidable barriers that interfere with bonding of the old and new amalgam.

Repair of amalgam restorations probably falls into the category of a hazardous procedure. Repair should be attempted only if the area involved is small, one that is not subjected to high stresses, capable of adequately supporting and retaining two restoration parts.

In conclusion, let us place the amalgam restoration in proper perspective. In Chapter 12, we saw that resin-based composites are now being used frequently in posterior Class II sites. Likewise, ceramic inlays and onlays are becoming popular in such situations (see Chapter 26). The principal advantage for the use of such materials compared with amalgam is their tooth-colored appearance.

However, there are several major advantages of amalgam. It is far less technique sensitive, more durable, and less costly than the current Class II composites. The time involved for placement is less, and that is reflected in a lower fee charged to the patient. Wear resistance is excellent, and, via corrosion, the material tends to seal itself against leakage and bacterial invasion. Furthermore, bacteria do not tend to be as adherent to amalgam as to composite surfaces. Thus, for situations in which aesthetics is not a prime consideration and for restorations that have large contact-bearing surfaces, dental amalgam is still considered the most reliable direct-filling material. In fact, amalgam still represents the material of choice for more than 50% of all Class II restorations in many countries as we approach the twenty-first century.

SELECTED READING

Anusavice KJ: Quality Evaluation of Dental Restorations: Criteria for Placement and Replacement. Chicago, Quintessence, 1989.
Six chapters of the book are written by various experts who deal with clinical studies, methods of evaluation, and differences in diagnosis related to dental amalgam restorations. Evidence supporting a more conservative approach to replacement of the "ditched" amalgam restoration is presented.

Barbakow F, Gaberthuel T, Lutz F, and Schuepbach P: Maintenance of amalgam restorations. Quint Int 19:861, 1988.
A step-by-step procedure for recontouring, finishing, and polishing existing amalgam restorations. Proper selection of instruments is illustrated.

Bauer JG: A study of procedures for burnishing amalgam restorations. J Prosthet Dent 57:669, 1987.
This report describes the combined factors of time from the end of trituration and burnishing force for a high-copper admixed amalgam. Burnishing with few strokes and moderately high forces (1 to 3 lb) within 4 to 6 minutes after trituration gave the best marginal adaptation.

Berglund A: Estimation of a 24-hour study of the daily dose of intra-oral mercury vapor inhaled after release from dental amalgam. J Dent Res 69:1646, 1990.
A pioneering study conducted by measuring the intraoral vapor levels over a 24-hour period in patients with at least nine amalgam restorations. The average daily dose of inhaled mercury vapor was 1.7 μg (range from 0.4 to 4.4 μg), which is approximately 1% of the threshold limit value of 300 to 500 μg/day established by the World Health Organization, based on a maximum allowable environmental level of 50 μg/day in the workplace.

Duke ES, Cochran MA, Moore BK, and Clark HE: Laboratory profiles of 30 high-copper amalgam alloys. J Am Dent Assoc 105:636, 1982.
Laboratory profiles identify the alloy systems and reflect the performance of the alloy. A classification for various types is presented.

Eames WB: Preparation and condensation of amalgam with a low mercury:alloy ratio. J Am Dent Assoc 58:78, 1959.
This technique revolutionized the procedure in constructing an amalgam restoration by use of minimal amounts of mercury in the original mix.

Fédération Dentaire Internationale: Technical Report 33: Safety of dental amalgam. Int Dent 39:217, 1989.
This authoritative organization reviewed the literature on mercury toxicity and concluded that there is no documented scientific evidence to show adverse effects from mercury in amalgam restorations except in rare cases of mercury hypersensitivity.

Gale EN, Osborne JW, and Winchell PG: Fracture at the margins of amalgam as predicted creep, zinc content, and γ_2 content. J Dent Res 61:678, 1982.
Suggested that equations based on in vitro data to predict marginal breakdown for alloys might not be predictive for non-γ_2 alloys.

Klauoncr LH, Green TC, and Charbeneau GT: Placement and replacement of amalgam restorations: A challenge for the profession. J Oper Dent 12:105, 1987.
A national survey assessed factors underlying the placement and replacement of amalgam restorations. The reactions to questions such as expected length of service and reasons for failure are interesting, and a challenge to the profession is identified.

Leinfelder KF: Clinical evaluation of high-copper amalgam. Gen Dent March-April:105, 1983.
This review emphasizes that criteria in selecting an alloy include documented clinical studies, manipulative characteristics, physical properties, and quality control.

Letzel H, and Vrijhoef MMA: The influence of polishing on the marginal integrity of amalgam restorations. J Oral Rehabil 11:89, 1984.
The effect of polishing on the marginal integrity of amalgam restorations continues to be a matter of some controversy, particularly with high-copper alloys. This study questions the necessity for polishing, at least with respect to marginal dyscrasia.

Letzel H, van't Hof MA, Vrijhoef MMA, et al: A controlled clinical study of amalgam restorations: Survival, failures, and causes of failure. Dent Mater 5:115, 1989.
Bulk fracture or fracture at the marginal ridge was reported as the leading mode of failure. It was suggested that further improvements in mechanical properties and corrosion resistance are needed.

Mackert JR Jr: Factors affecting estimation of dental amalgam mercury exposure from measurements of mercury vapor levels in intra-oral and expired air. J Dent Res 66:1775, 1987.
This analytical study demonstrates that a previous paper on vapor release based on animal models was flawed and that the investigators in this previous study overestimated the daily dose by a factor of 16 or more.

Mahler DB, and Van Eysden J: Dynamic creep of dental amalgam. J Dent Res 48:501, 1969.
The first suggestion that creep may be a major factor in marginal breakdown of amalgam restorations. Although modern alloys have low creep values, the test is a useful screening tool in selecting commercial alloys.

Marshall GW, Marshall SJ, and Letzel H: Mercury content of amalgam restorations. Gen Dent November-December:473, 1989.
Amalgam restorations removed after prolonged clinical use contained nearly all the original mercury present, suggesting that mercury loss contributes only a minor amount to total daily dosage.

May KN, Wilder AD, and Leinfelder KF: Burnished amalgam restorations: A two-year clinical evaluation. J Prosthet Dent 49:193, 1983.
A study of the clinical behavior of amalgam restorations found that precarved burnishing improved the marginal integrity of lathe-cut alloys. Coupled with postcarved burnishing, it was suggested as a viable substitute for conventional polishing.

Mjör IA: The safe and effective use of dental amalgam. Int Dent J 37:147, 1987.
Many pertinent matters related to the amalgam restoration are discussed in this review, including mercury toxicity, longevity of the restoration, common causes for failure, and certain properties that relate to performance.

Powell LV, Johnson GH, and Bales DJ: Effect of admixed indium on mercury vapor release from dental amalgam. J Dent Res 68:1231, 1989.
Addition of indium decreased the release of mercury by reducing the amount of mercury required to wet the alloy particle.

Rogers KD: Status of scrap (recyclable) dental amalgams as environmental health hazards or toxic substances. J Am Dent Assoc 119:159, 1989.
A review presenting available evidence to show amalgam scrap is not a toxic substance or environmental health hazard. It also covers portions of the literature indicating that intraoral amalgams do not present an adverse health hazard.

Vrihjoef MMA, Vermeersch AG, and Spanauf AJ: Dental Amalgam. Chicago, Quintessence, 1980.
A comprehensive treatment of the various factors involved in the design of amalgam alloys, their properties, and the parameters that influence clinical behavior. The lifetime of an amalgam is determined by the material, the dentist and assistant, and the patient.

19 *Direct Filling Gold and Its Manipulation*

- Properties of Pure Gold
- Forms of Direct Filling Gold
- Gold Foil
- Electrolytic Precipitate
- Powdered Gold
- Removal of Surface Impurities
- Compaction of Direct Filling Gold
- Physical Properties of Compacted Gold
- The Direct Gold Restoration

PROPERTIES OF PURE GOLD

Few metals are used in the pure state for dental restorative purposes. Gold and titanium are the prominent exceptions. The purity of the gold products currently in use (99.99%) is higher than that used when it was first introduced as a restorative material. For direct filling restorations, gold has fallen in popularity considerably over the past four decades, but it has experienced a slight resurgence as a direct filling material in North America, Sweden, and Germany, in part because of environmental concerns about amalgam and the limitations of composites, glass ionomers, and ceramics. However, because of its technique sensitivity, metallic appearance, cost, and reduced emphasis in dental schools, it is likely that it will be used only with limited indications in the future.

Pure gold is the noblest of all dental metals, rarely tarnishing or corroding in the oral cavity. It is inactive chemically, and it is not affected by air, heat, moisture, and most solvents. It is the most ductile of all metals, as demonstrated by its ability for a 29-g (1-oz) cylinder to be drawn into a wire 100 km (62 miles) in length. It is the most malleable of metals, as shown by its ability to be hammered to a thickness of 0.00013 mm (0.13 μm), about one third of the thinnest gold foil used in dentistry.

Pure gold is extremely soft, but after cold working, its hardness (52 to 75 Vickers hardness number [VHN]) is equivalent to and may exceed that of conventional Type I (soft) gold alloy (50 VHN) in its softened state, and after work hardening, its hardness approaches that of Type II gold alloy (90 VHN).

411

Although its percent elongation (ductility) decreases during cold working, it has a reasonably high value (12.8%) during condensation to allow sufficient lateral displacement to occur to produce the wedging that is required to enhance retention. Because of these properties and certain other respects, pure gold is an almost ideal dental restorative material for permanently preserving tooth structure in nonaesthetic, low-stress areas. Its chief disadvantages are its color, high thermal conductivity, and technical difficulties in forming a dense restoration. It has one of the highest densities of all elements (19.3 g/cm^3). That represents a drawback from an economic viewpoint because a greater mass of gold is required to restore a given volume of a prepared tooth compared with metals of lower densities.

The low hardness of pure gold would seem to contraindicate its use as a restorative material. However, its malleability and lack of surface oxide after "degassing" permit the condensation of a restoration directly in the cavity. During the condensation process, the strength of the gold is increased by *cold working* or *work hardening*. The lack of a surface oxide for gold and a few other metals allows *cold welding* to occur; that is, welding of increments together under pressure at mouth temperature rather than by melting, such as occurs during the welding of most metals.

Pieces of gold are placed in the prepared cavity and are welded together by the pressure of a suitable *condensing instrument*. This process is referred to as *compaction* or *condensation*, and the gold restoration is built up into a coherent mass by this cold-welding technique. The cohesion results from *metallic bonding* between overlapping increments of gold under the pressure of compaction. This process requires the gold atoms to be forced into intimate contact with atoms in an adjacent segment and clearly indicates that impurity surface atoms, gaseous films, oily residues, or other intermediate contaminants must be avoided or eliminated before use.

FORMS OF DIRECT FILLING GOLD

Although the dental profession sometimes refers to direct filling golds (DFGs) or direct golds as *foils*, the products that are currently available may be divided into three categories: (1) foil (also known as fibrous gold); (2) electrolytic precipitate (also known as crystalline gold); and (3) powdered gold. The first two types have several subcategories or forms, as shown in the following classification:

I. Foil
   A. Sheet
      1. Cohesive
      2. Noncohesive
   B. Ropes
   C. Cylinders
   D. Laminated foil
   E. Platinized foil
II. Electrolytic precipitate
   A. Mat gold
   B. Mat foil (mat gold plus gold foil)
   C. Gold-calcium alloy
III. Powdered gold (encapsulated gold powder)

All three types have certain characteristics in common. All can be cold welded. Furthermore, the efficacy of restorations made from these materials is strongly affected by mishandling, contamination, deviations from ideal cavity design principles, placement methods, and finishing techniques. Finally, as shown in the following classification, their chemical purity is 99.99% or higher, with the exception of platinized foil and alloyed electrolytic precipitate.

GOLD FOIL

Historically, gold foil is the oldest of all the products described; it has been used for thousands of years. Although gold jewelry was found in Sumerian, Babylonian, and Assyrian tombs built between 3000 and 2000 B.C. and in Egyptian tombs built between 1570 and 1293 B.C., the first evidence of gold foil used for jewelry may be traced to the Greek and Roman cultures that began about 2500 B.C. Because gold is so malleable, it can be reduced in thickness almost to transparency. It is reduced by rolling to 25 μm (0.001 inch) or less. In its manufacture for dental use, 25 μm is the starting thickness for a beating operation that reduces it to a submicron thickness.

Standard No. 4 gold foil is supplied in 4 × 4-inch (100 × 100-mm) sheets that weigh 4 grains (0.259 g) and are about 0.51 μm thick. The numbering system refers to the weight of a standard sheet, so it reflects the thickness as well. Thus, No. 3 foil weighs 3 grains (0.194 g) and is about 0.38 μm thick. Other 100 × 100-mm gold foil sheets are available including No. 20 (20 grains), No. 40 (40 grains), No. 60 (60 grains), and No. 90 (90 grains). The No. 3 foil is used in the electrolytic and powder products that are described later. The surface of gold foil is shown in Figure 19–1.

Cohesive and Noncohesive Gold. Although the forms of DFG can be supplied in both the cohesive and the noncohesive conditions, only the sheet foil is typically furnished in either of these two conditions. As previously noted, the ability of two gold surfaces to cohere by welding at oral temperature is dependent on an *atomically clean surface*. Gold, like most metals, attracts gases to its surface, and any adsorbed gas film prevents the intimate atomic contact required for cold welding. For this reason, the manufacturer can supply the foil to the dentist essentially free of surface contaminants and, therefore, inherently cohe-

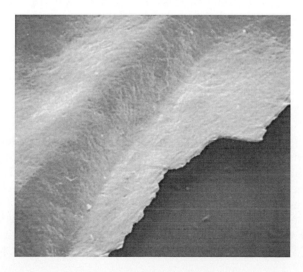

Figure 19–1. Scanning electron micrograph of the surface of gold foil × 750. (Courtesy of C. E. Ingersoll.)

sive. Although some adsorption of gases may occur during storage, this type is referred to as *cohesive foil*.

However, most gold sheets are provided with an adsorbed protective gas film, such as ammonia. This substance minimizes adsorption of other less volatile substances and prevents premature cohesion of sheets or segments of sheets that may come into contact. The ammonia-treated foil is called *noncohesive foil*. The volatile film is readily removed by heating to restore the cohesive character of the foil. Truly noncohesive foils, which have a permanent film, are not currently available.

Gold Foil Cylinders. This form is produced by rolling cut segments of No. 4 foils into a desired width, usually 3.2 mm, 4.8 mm, and 6.4 mm, using a modified No. 22 tapestry needle. An alternative method is to use No. 60 or 90 gold foil.

Preformed Gold Foils. Although in the past some dentists made their own ropes, cylinders, and laminates, cylinders and ropes are now available in preformed shapes. Both are made from No. 4 foil that has been "carbonized" or "corrugated." This form of gold foil is of historical interest because it was an outcome of the great Chicago fire of 1871. A dental dealer had some books of gold foil in a safe. After the fire, it was found that the paper between the sheets of foil had charred. However, the gold foil was unharmed, except that it had become "corrugated" because of the shriveling of the paper during carbonizing in the air-tight safe.

The ropes and cylinders are rolled in various diameters and then cut to various lengths to provide many sizes of increments for filling the preparation. The laminates are not available as preforms, but they can be made in a dental office by placing a number of sheets on top of each other and then cutting the laminate into pieces of a desired size.

Platinized Gold Foil. This form of gold foil is a laminated structure that can be produced in one of two ways: (1) two sheets of No. 4 pure gold foil and a layer of pure platinum foil sandwiched between them can be hammered until the thickness of a No. 4 sheet is obtained; and (2) layers of platinum and gold can be bonded together by a cladding process during the rolling operation and thus the "sandwich" is already welded together before the beating procedure begins. This product is available only in No. 4 sheet form. The object of adding platinum to the gold foil is to increase the hardness and wear resistance of restorations that are made from this material.

ELECTROLYTIC PRECIPITATE

Another form of gold for direct filling is crystalline gold powder formed by electrolytic precipitation. It cannot be described as a foil because it is not formed by a thickness reduction process such as hammering and rolling. The powder is formed into shapes by sintering at an elevated temperature well below the melting point of gold. Sintering causes self-diffusion between particles where they are in contact, so that the particles actually grow together (coalesce). This self-diffusion and the original dendritic structure of the mat gold powder are evident in Figure 19–2.

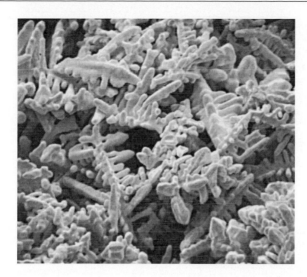

Figure 19–2. Scanning electron micrograph of mat gold. × 750. (Courtesy of C. E. Ingersoll.)

Mat Gold. Mat gold is a crystalline, electrolytically precipitated gold form that is formed into strips. These strips are cut by the dentist into the desired size. This form is often preferred for its ease in building up the internal bulk of the restoration because it can be more easily compacted within, and adapted to, the retentive portions of the prepared cavity. Because it is loosely packed, it is friable and contains numerous void spaces between particles. Therefore, foil is generally recommended for the external surface of the restoration. Using this two-material technique, the mat is covered with a veneer of foil. The loosely packed crystalline form of the mat powder with its large surface area does not permit easy welding into a solid mass as does gold foil. Therefore, there is a greater tendency for voids that may be seen as pits to form if mat gold is used on the surface of the restoration.

Mat Foil. Mat foil is a sandwich of electrolytic precipitated gold powder between sheets of No. 3 gold foil. The sandwich is sintered and cut into strips of differing widths. The dentist can cut these to the desired lengths. The purpose of sandwiching mat gold between foil sheets was to try to eliminate the need to veneer the restoration with a layer of foil. This type is no longer marketed.

Alloyed Electrolytic Precipitate. The newest form of electrolytic precipitate, Electralloy RV, is alloyed with calcium. The calcium content of the finished product is about 0.1%. Its purpose is to produce stronger restorations by dispersion strengthening.

POWDERED GOLD

Since the middle of the nineteenth century, chemically precipitated gold powders have been available in agglomerated form. These agglomerates usually disintegrated when compaction was attempted. The first successful use of powdered gold started in the early 1960s, when the gold powder was enclosed in No. 3 gold foil. Figure 19–3 illustrates the mix of atomized and chemically precipitated gold powders in a pellet from which the foil has been removed. The maximum particle size is about 74 μm (atomized), and the average is about 15 μm. The atomized and chemically precipitated powders are first mixed with a soft wax

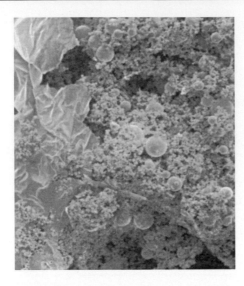

Figure 19–3. With the wax burned away, the spherical atomized particles can be seen. The finer and rougher surface particles are the chemically precipitated portion. ×100. (Courtesy of C. E. Ingersoll.)

to form pellets. These wax-gold pellets are wrapped with foil. The resulting pellets are cylindrical in shape and are available in several diameters and lengths.

REMOVAL OF SURFACE IMPURITIES

With the exception of noncohesive golds, the DFGs are received by the dentist in a cohesive condition. During manufacture and packaging, these products are never handled manually, and there are various heating stages that remove gaseous surface contamination. However, during storage and packaging, they are exposed to the atmosphere. Because gas can adsorb on the surface of the gold, it is necessary for the dentist or dental assistant to heat the foil or pellet immediately before it is carried into the prepared cavity. This step is commonly called *annealing, heat treatment,* or *degassing.* Although it is possible that a certain amount of recrystallization or stress relief may occur, these are unintentional because the primary purpose is to produce an atomically clean surface.

Rather, the gold is heated as a precautionary measure to remove any surface gases and to ensure a totally clean surface. Consequently, the term *annealing* is a misnomer. A more appropriate term would be *desorption,* because the object is to remove the adsorbed impurities.

Desorption is essential to the achievement of a cohesive mass. In the storage container, air (oxygen and nitrogen) is present. When the gold is not in the container, either in storage at the manufacturer's plant or in the dental office, other gases such as water vapor, sulfur dioxide, and ammonia are present as possible contaminants. If the dentist or assistant manipulates foil by hand, chamois finger tips should be worn to protect the gold from contamination. A totally dry cavity is mandatory throughout the compaction process to ensure complete cohesion.

From the foregoing discussion, it is obvious that decontamination of the gold surface is essential to ensure cohesion and to maximize the physical properties in the restoration. Proper desorption is a matter of heating long enough at a temperature that removes gases and, in the case of powdered gold, burns away the wax.

Underheating should be avoided because it does not adequately remove the impurities. The result is incomplete cohesion because of the remaining impurities or carbon deposited by the flame. Overheating should be avoided because it leads to excessive sintering and, possibly, contamination from tray, instruments, or flame. The result may be incomplete cohesion, embrittlement of the portion being heated, and poor compaction characteristics. Overheating can result from too long a time, even at a proper temperature, or from too high a temperature. However, heating times vary depending on the size and configuration of the gold segment. For example, powdered gold pellets may take 15 to 20 seconds, whereas gold foil pellets and electrolytic gold pellets may require only 1 or 2 seconds.

To determine the optimum temperature for removal of surface impurities, specimens were uniformly compacted from gold foil that had been heated for 5 minutes at various temperatures. The Brinell hardness numbers obtained are shown in Figure 19–4. The data indicate that temperatures below 315° C (600° F) are inadequate to attain optimum hardness of the compacted gold. The values were not significantly different in the temperature range between 315° C (600° F) and 760° C (1400° F).

It is not known whether these data are typical of other properties or for other forms of DFGs. The amount and form of DFG and the amount and type of surface contamination can influence the time-temperature combination needed to completely clean the surface. Aside from the purification of the gold surface, the total result of the heating process is not entirely known. Neither is it known what effect the structure or properties of the DFG have on the final properties of the restoration.

As previously noted, the primary purpose of desorption (degassing) is to remove surface impurities. In practice, all but the powdered gold may be desorbed on a tray heated electrically. An alternative method is to pass each pellet through a well-adjusted alcohol flame. Powdered gold must be heated in a flame to ensure the complete burning away of the wax. When heating in bulk on a tray, an excessive amount of gold should be avoided, because the difficulties of prolonged heating, referred to earlier, can arise from repeated heating as well. Care should be taken to handle pieces with stainless steel wire points or similar instruments that will not contaminate the gold.

Problems that may cause incomplete tray desorption include adhesion of

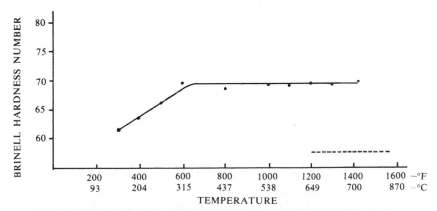

Figure 19–4. Brinell hardness number of specimens prepared from gold foil that was heated to various temperatures for surface decontamination. The dotted line indicates the general temperature range produced by an open alcohol flame. (Adapted from Hollenback GM, and Collard EW: J So Cal State Dent Assoc 29:280, 1961.)

pellets, air currents that affect heating uniformity, use of an excessive amount of gold to heat, oversintering, and greater exposure to contamination. The method of flame desorption consists of picking up each piece individually, heating it directly in the open flame, and placing it in the prepared cavity. Regardless of the type of direct gold type that is used, flame desorption has occurred when the gold segment has exhibited a dull-red glow. Overheating causes the material to become stiffer, less ductile, and more difficult to condense. Underheating may lead to partial cohesiveness and subsequent peeling away of adjacent segments or layers.

The fuel for the flame may be alcohol or gas, but alcohol is preferred because there is less danger of contamination. The alcohol should be pure methanol or ethanol without colorants or other additives. Denatured alcohol can be used if the only other denaturant available is methanol. Some denaturants may be solid inorganic compounds or higher alcohol-containing residues that release smoke when they are burned. Advantages of flame desorption include the ability to select a piece of appropriate size, desorption of only those pieces used, and less exposure to contamination.

COMPACTION OF DIRECT FILLING GOLD

Two of the main processes that control the quality of the final direct gold restoration are welding and wedging. *Welding* refers to the process of forming atomic bonds between pellets, segments, or layers as a result of condensation. *Wedging* refers to the pressurized adaptation of the gold form within the space between tooth structure walls or corners that have been slightly deformed elastically. Although a detailed account of the technique for insertion of DFG is not within the scope of this text, a brief description of foil compaction is given for illustration. Starting points are cut in the prepared cavity, and the first pieces of foil are wedged into these areas. Originally, compaction was accomplished by placing a condenser in contact with the foil and striking the other end of the condenser with a mallet. Subsequently, additional foil is welded to these pieces in the same manner. The compaction is continued, and the prepared cavity is gradually filled. This is one of several methods used for compaction.

Condensers. The original foil condensers had a single pyramid-shaped face, but current instruments have a series of small pyramids or serrations on the face. These act as swaging tools that exert lateral force on their inclines, in addition to providing direct compressive forces as the load is applied to the condenser. They also tend to cut through the outer layers to allow air trapped below the surface to escape.

Each increment of gold must be carefully "stepped" by placing the condenser point in successive adjacent positions as the compacting force is applied. This permits each piece to be compacted over its entire surface so that voids are not bridged. The surface texture of condensed foil, seen in Figure 19–5, illustrates the variation in condensation effectiveness from one region to another. The most dense structure occurs directly under the face of the condenser. To ensure dense masses in corners and at the junction between two walls, the line of force must be directed to bisect line angles and to trisect point angles. Loose or moderately compacted layers lie adjacent to, or below, the areas of greatest density. Thus, the condenser should traverse the entire surface of each increment as nearly as possible.

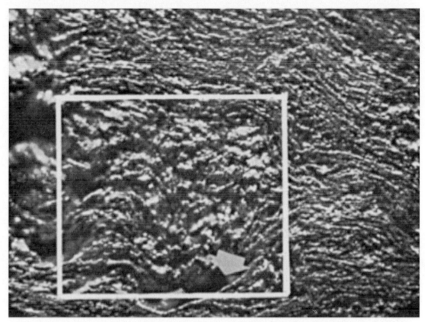

Figure 19–5. A cross section of compacted gold foil. A portion of loosely compacted foil is outlined by the rectangle, and the arrow indicates a void. The dense layers above the rectangle show good compaction directly under the face of the condenser. (Hodson JT: Dent Progr 2:55, 1961.)

Size of the Condenser Tip. The size of the condenser tip is an important factor in determining the effectiveness of compaction. The force distribution to the gold depends on the area of the point. For example, a given amount of force is distributed over four times as much area for a 2-mm tip as compared with a 1-mm tip. In other words, the concentration of the energy, and consequently, the compaction area welded, are four times as great with a 1-mm condenser as with a 2-mm condenser. Conversely, it takes four times as much force to compact fully the area under a 2-mm point as it does for a 1-mm point.

It follows that small condenser tips are indicated to achieve the desired compaction without using forces that might damage oral structures. The diameter of circular tips should be 0.5 to 1 mm. The lower limit is based on possible penetration by tips of smaller size.

Pressure Application. In recent years, there has been a tendency to apply condensation pressure by hand, although this is often supplemented by a mallet. Using this method, gold foil and electrolytic gold are subjected to a direct thrust from the hand followed by use of a mallet. For powdered gold, in addition to direct thrusts, heavy hand pressure using a rocking motion is also employed. Mechanical condensers are also available that have provided a consistent force.

PHYSICAL PROPERTIES OF COMPACTED GOLD

The physical properties of the various forms of DFG and the influence of various methods of compacting have been reported extensively. It is difficult to compare data between studies because each investigation involves somewhat different conditions. However, some representative property values can be established, as summarized in Table 19–1.

TABLE 19–1. Representative Physical Properties of Direct Filling Golds

Material and Technique	Transverse Strength		KHN	Apparent Density* (g/cm³)
	MPa	psi		
Mat gold				
Hand	161	23,000	52	14.3
Mechanical	169	24,100	62	14.7
Combined	169	24,100	53	14.5
Powdered gold				
Hand	165	23,600	55	14.4
Mechanical	155	22,200	64	14.5
Combined	190	27,100	58	14.9
Gold foil				
Hand	296	42,300	69	15.9
Mechanical	265	37,900	69	15.8
Combined	273	39,000	69	15.8
Mat gold and gold foil				
Hand	196	28,000	70	15.0
Mechanical	206	29,400	71	15.1
Combined	227	32,400	75	15.0

*Density measured by dividing the weight of the specimen by its volume.
KHN, Knoop hardness number.
From Richter WA, and Cantwell KR: J Prosthet Dent 15:722, 1965.

Transverse (bending) strength is chosen as being most representative of clinical applications. It is a reflection of three types of stress: compressive, tensile, and shear (see Chapter 4). Any failure can propagate from an area of weakness. In DFGs, the failure occurs usually from tensile stress, because of incomplete cohesion. Bending strength represents an indicator of cohesive strength.

Hardness may not be a valid measure of the effectiveness of a particular restorative material for its intended purpose of preserving the tooth. It may, however, indicate the overall quality of compacted gold; low hardness probably indicates the presence of porosity.

The density values shown in Table 19–1 should more properly be called "apparent density" because they were determined by linear measurement. No allowance is made for voids. Without such voids, the density should be 19.3 g/cm³. It is evident from the table that true density is not achieved. The direct gold restoration may be characterized by nonuniform density (see Fig. 19–5). It is evident from this figure that deformation is limited to short distances that are confined to areas immediately below the condenser point. Porosities are caused by lack of sufficient pressure to force the layers or crystals of gold into close enough contact to cause them to weld together. The greatest strength of compacted gold is in the most dense (solid) area. The weakest part is the porous area, where layers or crystals are not closely compacted. Thus, the maximum restoration strength is attained by minimizing the formation of internal voids.

Voids on the restoration surface (pits) increase the susceptibility to corrosion and deposition of plaque. Furthermore, voids at the restoration-tooth interface may be present to the extent that gross leakage and secondary caries may occur. However, one of the merits of properly compacted gold restorations is the small amount of leakage that takes place.

Apparently, voids are inevitable but they should be kept to a minimum, a factor that depends on the skill of the dentist. The size and shape of the condenser face, the dimensions of the prepared cavity, and the dynamics of the compacting system all influence the density of the compacted gold restoration.

The amount of voids can be estimated by the apparent density of the restoration. The apparent density is the measured density, decreased from true density by the amount of voids. The true density of pure gold is 19 g/cm³. A survey of the apparent density of restorations placed by different operators using different forms of direct gold with varying techniques revealed values ranging from 16 to 19 g/cm³. These results suggest that the theoretical density of a completely solid restoration is never achieved, regardless of the form of gold or the technique used.

The restorations made with the DFGs do not exhibit the high strength and hardness as those made with dental casting alloys to be discussed in the next chapter. Consequently, they cannot be used for large stress-bearing areas, such as a cast crown, nor can they withstand mastication stresses if they are used to restore a single cusp. Therefore, the use of DFGs is generally limited to areas where they simply "fill" a space rather than serve as a high stress-bearing member of a restored tooth. In addition, present means of compacting DFGs provide little opportunity for producing large variations in the form or shape that can be constructed. Thus, they are used principally for pits and small Class I restorations, for repair of casting margins, and for Classes III and V restorations.

The transverse strength, hardness, and apparent density are evidently somewhat greater when gold foil is used alone or in combination with mat gold, as compared with the other forms. Such data would imply a somewhat better compaction of foil (and better cohesion). It is more probable that the dentist or dentists were more familiar with the use of foil than with the other forms.

There is no evidence that the differences in physical properties (shown in Table 19–1) among the various forms of gold, including the gold-calcium alloy, and the method of compaction, are clinically significant. The physical properties of the compacted gold (restoration) are probably more greatly influenced by the competence of the dentist in manipulating and placing the gold, as has been suggested.

THE DIRECT GOLD RESTORATION

Compared with other materials, properly inserted direct gold restorations provide a reasonably long clinical service. With the variety of forms that are now available and the modern equipment for manipulating and compacting the gold, the time involved in placing the restoration has been reduced. The concern for a possible damaging effect on the pulp has been disputed. Apparently, direct gold that is compacted properly into sound tooth structure produces only a minimal pulpal response.

However, the technical skill of the dentist is of paramount importance to success. A direct gold restoration of poor quality can prove to be one of the most inferior of all clinical restorations. The proper insertion of a direct gold restoration challenges the technical proficiency of the dentist as does no other type of restoration.

SELECTED READING

Bauer JG: Microleakage of direct filling materials in class V restorations using thermal cycling. Quint Int 16:765, 1985; and Welsh EL, Nuckles DB, and Hembree JH Jr: Microleakage of direct gold restorations: An in vivo study. J Prosthet Dent 51:33, 1984.
Two recent studies showing that although microleakage does occur with direct gold restorations, the incidence is comparable to that of other restorative materials when the restorations are well placed. Thus, technique sensitivity of the material plays a major role in the quality of these restorations.

Baum L, Phillips RW, and Lund MR: Textbook of Operative Dentistry, 2nd ed. Philadelphia, WB Saunders, 1985.

A step-by-step coverage of the technical aspects of preparing and placing direct gold and finishing the restoration.

Craig RG: Biocompatibility testing of dental materials. In: Restorative Dental Materials, 9th ed. St. Louis, CV Mosby, 1993.

This review of the biocompatibility of restorative materials suggests that the placement of condensed gold restorations causes a moderate-to-severe pulpal inflammation 10 to 20 days postoperatively, but after 35 days, only a mild response remains and reparative dentin may form under the restorations. Thus, the use of direct gold is considered to be "biologically sound."

Hodson JT: Structure and properties of gold foil and mat gold. J Dent Res 42:575, 1963.

The data indicate that in clinical usage the theoretic density of direct gold is never attained.

Medina JE, Bridgeman RG, and Frazier KB: Compacted gold restorations. In: Clark's Clinical Dentistry, Vol 1, 2nd ed. Philadelphia, JB Lippincott, 1991.

An excellent review of the materials, tooth preparation requirements, placement techniques, and finishing techniques for Classes I, II, V, and VI restorations and for the repair of cast gold alloy restorations.

Richter WA, and Cantwell KR: A study of cohesive gold. J Prosthet Dent 15:722, 1965.

One of the most comprehensive surveys of the physical properties of various types of direct gold and compaction techniques.

Thomas JJ, Stanley HR, and Gilmore HW: Effect of gold foil condensation on human dental pulp. J Am Dent Assoc 78:788, 1969.

The compaction of direct gold does not produce a significant pulp response, as documented by this study.

20 Dental Casting Alloys

- Historical Perspective on Dental Casting Alloys
- Desirable Properties of Casting Alloys
- Alternatives to Cast Metal Technology
- Classification of Dental Casting Alloys
- Alloys for All-metal and Resin Veneer Restorations
- High Noble Alloys for Metal-ceramic Restorations
- Noble Alloys for Metal-ceramic Restorations
- Base Metal Alloys for Cast Metal and Metal-ceramic Restorations
- Laboratory Fees for Metal-ceramic Restorations
- Metals for Partial Denture Alloys

HISTORICAL PERSPECTIVE ON DENTAL CASTING ALLOYS

A brief description of the evolution of the present alloys is appropriate to understand the rationale for development of the current alloy formulations. The history of dental casting alloys has been influenced by three major factors: (1) the technologic changes of dental prostheses; (2) metallurgic advancements; and (3) price changes of the noble metals since 1968.

Taggart's presentation to the New York Odontological Group in 1907 on the fabrication of cast inlay restorations often has been acknowledged as the first reported application of the *lost wax technique* in dentistry. The inlay technique described by Taggart was an instant success. It soon led to the casting of complex inlays such as onlays, crowns, fixed partial dentures, and removable partial denture frameworks. Because pure gold did not have the physical properties required of these dental restorations, existing jewelry alloys were quickly adopted. These gold alloys were further strengthened with copper, silver, or platinum.

In 1932, the dental materials group at the National Bureau of Standards surveyed the alloys being used and roughly classified them as Type I (soft: Vickers hardness number [VHN] between 50 and 90), Type II (medium: VHN between 90 and 120), Type III (hard: VHN between 120 and 150), and Type IV (extra hard: VHN ≥ 150). At that time, some tarnish tests indicated that alloys with a gold content lower than 65% to 75% tarnished too readily for dental use.

In the following years, several patents were issued for alloys containing palladium as a substitute for platinum. By 1948, the composition of dental noble metal alloys for cast metal restorations had become rather diverse. With these formulations, the tarnishing tendency of the original alloys apparently had disappeared. It is now known that in gold alloys, palladium is added to counteract the tarnish potential of silver.

In the late 1950s, a breakthrough occurred in dental technology that was to influence significantly the fabrication of dental restorations. This was the successful veneering of a metal substructure with dental porcelain. Until that time, dental porcelain had a markedly lower coefficient of thermal expansion than did gold alloys, making it impossible to attain a bond between the two structural components. It was found that adding both platinum and palladium to gold would lower the alloy's coefficient of thermal contraction sufficiently to ensure physical compatibility between the porcelain veneer and the metal substructure. By serendipity, the melting range of the alloy was also raised sufficiently to permit firing of the porcelain onto the gold-based alloy at 1040° C (1900° F) without deforming the metal substructure. The metal-ceramic restoration that evolved from this development is discussed in Chapter 26.

The base metal removable partial denture alloys were introduced in the 1930s. Since that time, both nickel-chromium and cobalt-chromium formulations have become increasingly popular compared with conventional Type IV gold alloys, which previously were the predominant metals used for such prostheses. The obvious advantages of the base metal alloys are their lighter weight, increased mechanical properties (although exceptions to this statement may be found), and reduced costs. For these reasons, such nickel- and cobalt-based alloys have largely replaced the noble metal alloys for removable partial dentures.

The success of the base metal alloys for constructing a removable partial denture framework led to some early interest in applying these same alloys to fabricate other types of restorations. However, intensive research into the characteristics of alloys for that purpose did not start until the 1970s, when stimulated by the rapidly escalating price of noble metals. Naturally, the track record of the nickel-chromium and cobalt-chromium partial denture alloys made them a logical choice for evaluation as probable alternatives for other dental applications. Likewise, by 1978 the price of gold was climbing so rapidly that attention focused on the noble metal alloys—to reduce the precious metal content yet retain the advantages of the noble metals for dental use. The result was new alloys, as discussed subsequently.

Because of the multitude of casting alloys of widely diverse compositions and varied applications, it has been extremely difficult to devise a classification system with sufficient flexibility to accommodate newer formulations or alterations to the existing systems as they emerge without a constant revision of the classification.

DESIRABLE PROPERTIES OF CASTING ALLOYS

Cast metals are used in dental laboratories to produce inlays, onlays, crowns, conventional all-metal bridges, metal-ceramic bridges, resin-bonded bridges, endodontic posts, and removable partial denture frameworks. The metals must exhibit biocompatibility, ease of melting, casting, brazing (or soldering) and polishing, little solidification shrinkage, minimal reactivity with the mold material, good wear resistance, high strength and sag resistance (metal-ceramic alloys), and excellent tarnish and corrosion resistance. Generally, conventional type 2 and 3 gold alloys represent the standards against which the performance of other casting alloys are judged.

ALTERNATIVES TO CAST METAL TECHNOLOGY

All-metal restorations can be made intraorally by direct compaction of gold and direct condensation of amalgam. A mercury-free condensable intermetallic compound has been developed recently at the National Institute of Standards and Technology for direct placement of restorations as an alternative to dental amalgam, but the feasibility of this technique in general practices has not been established in controlled clinical studies.

Metal inlays, crowns, copings, endodontic posts, and bridges have been produced predominantly by a metal casting process for many years. Cast gold alloy restorations have demonstrated superior durability and fracture resistance compared with other types of restorative materials. Metal-ceramic restorations that are fabricated with cast alloy copings have demonstrated nearly the same clinical survivability, and because they are more aesthetic, they are used for most crown and bridge restorations.

For the production of metal copings as the substructure for metal-ceramic crowns, metal foil technology has been used as an alternative to the metal casting process. These layered metallic foils are swaged on dies and heat treated over a gas flame to strengthen the copings before the application of porcelain. Although the process avoids the need for preparation of a wax pattern, fabrication of a refractory mold, melting and casting of metal into the mold, a significant amount of time is required to swage the metal and to trim the margins accurately. Furthermore, metal folds on the surface to which porcelain is bonded represent stress concentration areas that may severely reduce the fracture resistance of the resulting metal-ceramic crown. However, for low stress applications, this technique allows the fabrication of metal-ceramic crowns with coping thickness of 100 µm or less, thereby permitting either a conservation of tooth structure or an improvement in aesthetics through the use of a greater porcelain thickness.

A *CAD-CAM process* can be used to prepare metal and ceramic inlays and crowns without the need for either an impression of the prepared teeth or a casting procedure. CAD-CAM technology has been introduced for imaging of prepared teeth, for computer-aided designing (CAD) of restoration size and shape, and computer-aided machining (CAM) of inlays and crowns made from ceramic blocks or metals that are difficult to cast, such as pure titanium and titanium alloys. Titanium is considered one of the most biocompatible metals for dental applications. The dentist can record a video image of a prepared tooth using an intraoral imaging device. After the boundaries of the restoration are selected on a video monitor, a command to cut the desired restoration is transmitted by computer to a milling machine. The inlay or crown is milled using a diamond-coated disk. Depending on the CAD-CAM system used, occlusal and proximal contours may need to be finished by hand using rotary instruments.

Another method of preparing all-metal crowns or copings for metal-ceramic crowns without using casting techniques consists of copy milling to produce the outer surface morphology and electrical discharge machining based on tracings of a master die to replicate the internal surface. The copy milling process starts with a master die of a prepared tooth whose three-dimensional coordinates are recorded in a computer from surface profiling of the prepared surface or a replica die prior to milling. These coordinates can be transformed in the computer yield to an enlarged copy of the original die and thus provide space for the luting material. Similarly, the outer crown surface can be milled from a block of metal based on surface profiles of the original tooth or of a tooth model. An additional graphite die is also prepared during the copy milling process. The internal surface of the crown form can then be created by placing the metal in an electrically conductive liquid and placing the graphite die in proximity to the metal block. A voltage is applied to the circuit and electrical discharge removal of metal occurs such that the surface eventually is transformed to the shape of the graphite die surface.

However, melting and casting of alloys still represent the most widely used procedures for extraoral fabrication of metallic restorations. For conventional metal casting procedures, a pattern of the lost tooth structure or the desired dental prosthesis is first constructed in wax on a die made from an intraoral impression. The wax is enveloped by a mold material called an *investment*, which is a mixture of water, silica, and a binder (such as calcium sulfate hemihydrate, magnesium ammonium phosphate, and ethyl silicate). After the investment slurry has set, the wax is burned out of the mold, and molten metal is cast under pressure or by centrifugal force into the mold cavity that was formed by the wax pattern. The resulting metal structure is an accurate duplication of the pattern if proper techniques are employed. A complete description of the casting procedure is presented in following chapters.

Many of the technical considerations of the procedure are dependent on a knowledge of the casting alloy. Therefore, it is necessary to discuss this subject before the details of the casting process are presented. Like so many other areas in dentistry, there have been major advances in the development of dental casting alloys during the past 20 years. Because of the large number and types of casting metals available for use, one of the most complex challenges of dentists is the proper selection of casting alloys for resin-bonded bridges, metal-ceramic restorations, and all-metal cast restorations. In many instances, the laboratory technician is required to make alloy selections because most dentists are not fully aware of the benefits and drawbacks of these many alloy systems. However, the technicians also have only limited experience with a few of these metals and they may not always make an optimum choice for a given clinical requirement. Thus, it is essential that the dentist-technician team become more communicative on the advantages and disadvantages of casting alloys to make more informed decisions on alloy selection. To accomplish this goal, this chapter summarizes the properties, relative technique considerations, and potential clinical performance of casting alloys.

CLASSIFICATION OF DENTAL CASTING ALLOYS

Several hundred brands of crowns and bridge alloys are currently available on the world market. Slightly more than half of these alloys are designed for all-metal crowns, bridges, onlays, and inlays that are described according to American Dental Association (ADA) Specification No. 5 as Types I through IV. In the past, this specification referred to gold-based alloys. Since 1989, ADA-approved casting alloys can have any composition as long as they pass the tests for toxicity, tarnish, yield strength, and percentage of (percent) elongation. As shown in Table 20–1, the minimum values for yield strength and percent elongation determine whether an alloy is classified as Type I (soft: for restorations subject to very slight stress such as inlays), Type II (medium: for restorations subject to moderate stress such as onlays), Type III (hard: for high-stress situations, including onlays, crowns, thick veneer crowns, and short-span fixed partial dentures),

TABLE 20–1. Mechanical Property Requirements of American Dental Association Specification No. 5

Alloy Type	Yield Strength (MPa) (0.1% offset)		Minimum Elongation (%)	
	Annealed	*Hardened*	*Annealed*	*Hardened*
I (soft)	140 maximum	None	18	None
II (medium)	140–200	None	18	None
III (hard)	200–340	None	12	None
IV (extra hard)	≥340	500	10	2

and Type IV (extra hard: for extremely high-stress states, such as endodontic posts and cores, thin veneer crowns, long-span fixed partial dentures, and removable partial dentures). The remainder are alloys designed for metal-ceramic restorations and removable partial denture frameworks.

Over the past decade or so, base metal alloys have captured a significant share of the market. Introduced originally during the upward spiral of gold prices in the late 1970s and early 1980s, base metal alloys have been developed to the point where they are superior to high noble and noble alloys in several respects. Most removable partial denture frameworks have been made from base metal alloys for some time, and about 40% of PFMs are currently made from base metal alloys in the United States.

This chapter presents a comparative evaluation of the positive and negative features of existing noble metal alloys and base metal alloys. The noble metals include gold, platinum, palladium, rhodium, ruthenium, iridium, and osmium. Virtually all noble alloys are based on gold or palladium as the principal noble metal species. Numerous classification systems have been proposed to categorize the wide variety of commercial gold-based and palladium-based alloys. In 1984 the ADA proposed a simple classification for dental casting alloys. Three categories are described: *high noble* (HN), *noble* (N), and *predominantly base metal* (PB). This classification is presented in Table 20–2. Many manufacturers have adopted this classification to simplify communication between dentists and dental laboratory technologists. Some insurance companies use it as well to determine the cost of crown and bridge treatment. This system lacks the potential to discriminate among alloys within a given category (HN or N) that may have quite different properties.

The dental casting alloy classification is useful for estimating the relative cost of alloys because the cost is dependent on the noble metal content as well as on the alloy density. It is also useful for identification of the billing code that is used for insurance reimbursement. Because insurance companies may pay more for high noble than for noble alloys or predominantly base metal alloys, it is important for dentists to correctly identify the noble metal category of the alloy they are using.

TABLE 20–2. Alloy Classification of the American Dental Association (1984)

Alloy Type	Total Noble Metal Content
High noble metal	Contains ≥40 wt% Au and ≥60 wt% of the noble metal elements (Au + Ir + Os + Pt + Rh + Ru)
Noble metal	Contains ≥25 wt% of the noble metal elements
Predominantly base metal	Contains <25 wt% of the noble metal elements

The principal cast metals and alloys used for all-metal restorations, metal-ceramic restorations, and removable partial dentures are listed in Table 20–3. Note that the alloys that are listed for metal-ceramic restorations can be used for all-metal (or resin-veneered) restorations, whereas the alloys for all-metal restorations should not be used for metal-ceramic restorations. The principal reasons that alloys for all-metal restorations cannot be used for metal-ceramic restorations are that the alloys may not form thin, stable oxide layers to promote bonding to porcelain; their melting range may be too low to resist sag deformation or melting at porcelain firing temperatures; and their thermal contraction coefficients may not be close enough to those of commercial porcelains.

The descriptors *precious* and *semiprecious* should be avoided because they are imprecise terms. Rather the terms *high noble*, *noble*, and *predominantly base metal* should be used. As used by laboratory technologists, the term *semiprecious* usually refers to alloys that are based either on palladium or on silver. Alloys that contain at least 50 wt% of palladium include palladium-silver (Pd-Ag), palladium-copper (Pd-Cu), palladium-cobalt (Pd-Co), palladium-gallium-silver (Pd-Ga-Ag), palldium-gold (Pd-Au), and palladium-gold-silver (Pd-Au-Ag). Most of these alloys are classified as *noble*. The term *noble* can also apply to silver-palladium alloys if they contain at least 25% by weight of palladium and other noble metals. High noble and noble dental alloys are usually packaged and priced in 1, 2, and 20 pennyweight (dwt) lots.*

Noble Metals. The periodic table of the elements (see Table 14–1) shows eight noble metals: gold, the platinum group metals (platinum, palladium, rhodium, ruthenium, iridium, osmium), and silver. However, in the oral cavity, silver is more reactive and therefore is not considered a noble metal. Noble metals have traditionally been used for the inlay, crown and bridge, and metal-ceramic alloys, by virtue of their tarnish and corrosion resistance. The term *noble metal* is relative. As discussed in Chapter 16, the lower the position of an element in the standard

---

*1 troy ounce = 20 pennyweights (dwt).

TABLE 20–3. Classification of Alloys for All-Metal Restorations, Metal-Ceramic Restorations, and Frameworks for Removable Partial Dentures

Alloy Type	All-Metal	Metal-Ceramic	Removable Partial Dentures
High Noble	Au-Ag-Cu-Pd Metal-ceramic alloys	Au-Pt-Pd Au-Pd-Ag (5–12 wt% Ag) Au-Pd-Ag (> 12 wt% Ag) Au-Pd (no Ag)	Au-Ag-Cu-Pd
Noble	Ag-Pd-Au-Cu Ag-Pd Metal-ceramic alloys	Pd-Au (no Ag) Pd-Au-Ag Pd-Ag Pd-Cu Pd-Co Pd-Ga-Ag	Ag-Pd-Au-Cu Ag-Pd
Base Metal	Pure Ti Ti-Al-V Ni-Cr-Mo-Be Ni-Cr-Mo Co-Cr-Mo Co-Cr-W Al bronze	Pure Ti Ti-Al-V Ni-Cr-Mo-Be Ni-Cr-Mo Co-Cr-Mo Co-Cr-W	Pure Ti Ti-Al-V Ni-Cr-Mo-Be Ni-Cr-Mo Co-Cr-Mo Co-Cr-W

electromotive force series, the more active it is. Conversely, the, higher a metal is in the series, the more inert it is, and thus the greater is its nobility. Of the seven noble metals that are considered noble by dental standards, only gold, palladium, and platinum are currently of major importance in dental casting alloys.

Predominantly Base Metal Alloys. These alloys are based on 75 wt% or more of base metal elements or less than 25 wt% of noble metals. *Base metals* are invaluable components of dental casting alloys because of their low cost and their influence on weight, strength, stiffness, and oxide formation (which is required for bonding to porcelain). Compared with noble metals, base metals are more reactive with their environment. Certain base metals, as noted in Chapter 16, can be used to protect an alloy from corrosion by passivation. Although these metals are still frequently referred to as *nonprecious* or *nonnoble,* the preferred designation is *predominantly base metal*. One reason for this designation is that some base metal alloys in the past have contained a minor amount of palladium, but because the properties of these alloys were controlled primarily by the base metals present, these alloys should not be classified as noble alloys. In this text, the terms *base metal* and *predominantly base metal* are used interchangeably because noble metals are not currently included in most of the base metal alloys in use.

Karat and Fineness. Traditionally, the gold content of a dental alloy has been specified on the basis of karat or fineness. *Karat* refers to the parts of pure gold in 24 parts of an alloy. For example, 24-karat gold is pure gold, whereas 22-karat gold is an alloy containing 22 parts pure gold and 2 parts of other metals.

Fineness describes gold alloys by the number of parts per 1000 of gold. For example, pure gold has a fineness of 1000, and 650 fine alloy has a gold content of 65%. Thus, the fineness rating is 10 times the gold percentage in an alloy. An alloy that is three-fourths (75%) pure gold is 750 fine. Fineness is considered a more practical term than karat. The terms *karat* and *fineness* are rarely used to describe the gold content of current alloys. However, fineness is often used to identify gold alloy solders described in Chapter 27.

Identification of Alloys by Principal Elements. Because so many alternative alloy systems have emerged, it is necessary to discuss them in relation to their numerous applications. At the same time, an understanding of their composition is vital, in view of differences in formulations and the resulting properties. Thus, the crown and bridge, metal-ceramic, and removable partial denture alloys are classified according to not only *function* but also according to their composition (principal element or elements). When an alloy is identified according to the elements it contains, the components are listed in declining order of composition, with the largest constituent first followed by the second largest constituent. This is the basis for the general alloy classification given in Table 20–3 for all-metal restorations, metal-ceramic restorations, and removable partial denture frameworks. An exception to this rule is the identification of certain alloys by elements that significantly affect physical properties or that represent potential biocompatibility concerns, or both. For example, nickel-chromium-molybdenum-beryllium alloys are often designated as *nickel-chromium-beryllium alloys* because of beryllium's contributions to the control of castability and surface oxidation at high temperatures, and because of its relative toxicity potential compared with other metals. Molybdenum (Mo) or tungsten (W) often exist in greater concentrations than beryllium to decrease the thermal coefficient of expansion. However, the concern for the biocompatibility of beryllium is a more important factor, and some research reports list these alloys as Ni-Cr-Be rather than Ni-Cr-Mo or Ni-Cr-Mo-Be. The general classification adopted in Table 20–3 is based on the latter designation.

ALLOYS FOR ALL-METAL AND RESIN VENEER RESTORATIONS

In 1927, the Bureau of Standards (now the National Institute of Standards and Technology) established gold casting alloy Types I through IV according to dental function, with hardness increasing from Type I to Type IV. Typical compositions of these alloys are given in Table 20–4. Properties of eight alloys used for all-metal (and resin veneer) restorations and four alloys used for metal-ceramic restorations are given in Table 20–5. Based on the 1989 revision of Specification No. 5 by the ADA, the following four alloy types are classified by their properties and not by their compositions:

Type I (soft)—small inlays, easily burnished and subject to very slight stress
Type II (medium)—inlays subject to moderate stress, including thick three-quarter crowns, abutments, pontics, and full crowns
Type III (hard)—inlays subject to high stress, including thin three-quarter crowns, thin cast backings, abutments, pontics, full crowns and denture bases, and short-span fixed partial dentures. Some Type III gold alloys usually can be age hardened, especially those containing at least 8 wt% of copper
Type IV (extra hard)—inlays subject to very high stresses, including denture base bars and clasps, partial denture frameworks, and long-span fixed partial dentures. (Full crowns are often made of this type.) The compositions of these alloys are usually based on a majority of either gold or silver; gold alloys can be age hardened by an appropriate heat treatment

Types I and II alloys are often referred to as *inlay alloys.* The development of modern direct and indirect tooth-colored filling materials has virtually eliminated the use of Types I and II gold alloys. Traditional Types III and IV alloys

TABLE 20–4. Composition Range (weight percent) of Traditional Types I to IV Alloys and Four Metal-Ceramic Alloys

Alloy Type	Main Elements	Au	Cu	Ag	Pd	Sn, In, Fe, Zn, Ga
I	High noble (Au base)	83	6	10	0.5	Balance
II	High noble (Au base)	77	7	14	1	Balance
III	High noble (Au base)	75	9	11	3.5	Balance
III	Noble (Au base)	46	8	39	6	Balance
III	Noble (Ag base)			70	25	Balance
IV	High noble (Au base)	56	14	25	4	Balance
IV	Noble (Ag base)	15	14	45	25	Balance
Metal-ceramic	High noble (Au base)	52			38	Balance
Metal-ceramic	Noble (Pd base)			30	60	Balance
Metal-ceramic	High noble (Au base)	88		1	7 (+4 Pt)	Balance
Metal-ceramic	Noble (Pd base)	0–6	0–15	0–6	88	Balance

TABLE 20–5. Physical Properties of Some Modern Noble Metal Dental Alloys

Alloy Type	Main Elements	Melting Range	Density (g/cm³)	Yield Strength‡ (MPa)	Yield Strength‡ (psi)	Hardness (VHN)	Percent Elongation
I	High noble	943–960° C (1730–1760° F)	16.6	103	(15,000)	80	36
II	High noble	924–960° C (1695–1760° F)	15.9	186	(27,000)	101	38
III	High noble	924–960° C (1710–1760° F)	15.5	207 H275	(30,000) (H40,000)	121 H182	39 H19
	Noble	843–916° C (1550–1680° F)	12.8	241 H586	(35,000) (H85,000)	138 H231	30 H13
	Ag-Pd noble	1021–1099° C (1870–2010° F)	10.6	262 H323	(38,000) (H47,000)	143 H154	10 H8
IV	High noble	921–943° C (1690–1720° F)	15.2	275 H493	(40,000) (H71,500)	149 H264	35 H7
	High noble	871–932° C (1600–1710° F)	13.6	372 H720	(54,000) (H104,500)	186 H254	38 H2
	Noble	930–1021° C (1705–1870° F)	11.3	434 H586	(63,000) (H85,000)	180 H270	10 H6
Metal-ceramic	*High noble	1271–1304° C (2320–2380° F)	13.5	572	(83,000)	220	20
	Noble	1232–1304° C (2250–2380° F)	10.7	462	(67,000)	189	20
	†High noble	1149–1177° C (2100–2150° F)	18.3	450	(65,300)	182	5
	Noble	1155–1302° C (2111–2375° F)	10.6–11.5	476–685	(68,000–95,000)	235–270	10–34

*White colored.
†Yellow colored.
‡H, Age hardened condition. Other values are for the quenched (softened) condition.
VHN, Vickers hardness number.

are generally called *crown and bridge alloys,* although Type IV alloys also are used occasionally for high-stress applications such as removable partial denture frameworks. Typical compositions of these four types of alloys are given in Table 20–4.

Heat Treatment of High Noble and Noble Metal Alloys. As previously discussed in Chapter 15, gold alloys can be significantly hardened if the alloy contains a sufficient amount of copper. Types I and II alloys usually do not harden, or they harden to a lesser degree than do the Types III and IV alloys. The actual mechanism of hardening is probably the result of several different solid-state transformations. Although the precise mechanism may be in doubt, the criteria for successful hardening are time and temperature.

Alloys that can be hardened can, of course, also be softened. In metallurgic terminology the softening heat treatment is referred to as solution heat treatment. The hardening heat treatment is termed age hardening, as discussed in Chapter 15.

Softening Heat Treatment. The casting is placed in an electric furnace for 10 minutes at a temperature of 700° C (1292° F), and then it is quenched in water. During this period, all intermediate phases are presumably changed to a disordered solid solution, and the rapid quenching prevents ordering from occurring during cooling. The tensile strength, proportional limit, and hardness are reduced by such a treatment, but the ductility is increased.

The softening heat treatment is indicated for structures that are to be ground, shaped, or otherwise cold worked, either in or out of the mouth. Although 700° C is an adequate average softening temperature, each alloy has its optimum temperature, and the manufacturer should specify the most favorable temperature and time.

Hardening Heat Treatment. The age hardening or hardening heat treatment of dental alloys can be accomplished in several ways. One of the most practical hardening treatments is by "soaking" or aging the casting at a specific temperature for a definite time, usually 15 to 30 minutes, before it is water quenched. The aging temperature depends on the alloy composition but is generally between 200° C (400° F) and 450° C (840° F). The proper time and temperature are specified by the manufacturer.

Ideally, before the alloy is given an age-hardening treatment, it should be subjected to a softening heat treatment to relieve all strain hardening, if it is present, and to start the hardening treatment with the alloy as a disordered solid solution. Otherwise, there would not be a proper control of the hardening process, because the increase in strength, proportional limit, and hardness and the reduction in ductility are controlled by the amount of solid-state transformations allowed. The transformations, in turn, are controlled by the temperature and time of the age-hardening treatment.

Because the proportional limit is increased during age hardening, a considerable increase in the modulus of resilience can be expected. The hardening heat treatment is indicated for metallic partial dentures, saddles, bridges, and other similar structures. For small structures, such as inlays, a hardening treatment is not usually employed.

The *yield strength*, the proportional limit, and the elastic limit are all measures of essentially the same property, as discussed in Chapter 3. This property reflects the capacity of an alloy (and hence the cast prosthesis) to withstand mechanical stresses without permanent deformation. In general, the yield strengths increase when progressing from Type I to Type IV alloys. Age hardening substantially increases the yield strength (in one case by nearly 100%).

The *hardness* values for noble metal alloys correlate quite well with the yield strengths. Traditionally, hardness has been used for indicating the suitability of an alloy for a given type of clinical application.

The *elongation* is a measure of ductility or the degree of plastic deformation an alloy can undergo before fracture. A reasonable amount of elongation is essential if the clinical application requires deformation of the as-cast structure, such as is needed for clasp and margin adjustment and burnishing. Age hardening reduces the elongation, in some cases very significantly. Alloys with low elongation are brittle materials and fracture readily if deformed.

Casting Shrinkage. As noted in a previous chapter, most metals and alloys, including gold and the noble metal alloys, shrink when they change from the liquid to the solid state. As will be seen, such a consideration is important in the dental casting procedure. For example, if a mold for an inlay is an accurate reproduction of the missing tooth structure, the cast gold inlay will be too small by the amount of its casting shrinkage.

The shrinkage occurs in three stages: (1) the thermal contraction of the liquid metal between the temperature to which it is heated and the liquidus temperature; (2) the contraction of the metal inherent in its change from the liquid to the solid state; and (3) the thermal contraction of the solid metal that occurs down to room temperature.

The first-mentioned contraction is probably of no consequence, because as the liquid metal contracts in the mold, more molten metal can flow into the mold to compensate for such a shrinkage. The casting technique, to be described in subsequent chapters, allows for such a flow of molten metal. The relative solidification shrinkage of various alloys cast as smooth cylinders is listed in Table 20–6.

The values for the casting shrinkage differ for the various alloys presumably because of differences in their composition. It has been shown, for example, that platinum, palladium, and copper all are effective in reducing the casting shrinkage of an alloy. It is of interest that the value for the casting shrinkage of pure gold closely approaches that of its maximal linear thermal contraction.

In general, it is apparent that the values obtained for the casting shrinkage are less than the linear thermal shrinkage values given in Table 20–6, even though the casting shrinkage as obtained included both the solidification shrinkage and the thermal shrinkage. This seemingly anomalous condition can be accounted for by two logical assumptions: (1) When the mold becomes filled with molten metal, the metal starts to solidify at the walls of the mold because the temperature of the mold is less than that of the molten metal; and (2) during initial cooling, the first layer of metal to solidify against the walls of the mold is weak, and it tends to adhere to the mold until it gains sufficient strength as it cools to pull away. When it is sufficiently strong to contract independently of the mold, it shrinks thermally until it reaches room temperature.

The important consideration is that the thermal shrinkage of the first weak solidified layer is initially prevented by its mechanical adhesion to the walls of the mold. During this period, it is actually stretched because of its interlocking with the investment material. Thus, any contraction occurring during solidification can be eliminated. Also, part of the total thermal contraction can be eliminated, with the result that the observed casting shrinkage is less than might be expected on the basis of the possible stages of the shrinkage.

Because the thermal contraction as the alloy cools to room temperature dominates the casting shrinkage, the higher melting alloys tend to exhibit greater shrinkage. This must be compensated for in the casting technique if good fit is to be obtained.

Silver-Palladium Alloys. These alloys are white and predominantly silver in composition but have substantial amounts of palladium (at least 25%) that provide nobility and promote the silver tarnish resistance. They may or may not contain copper and a small amount of gold. Casting temperatures are in the range of the yellow gold alloys. The copper-free Ag-Pd alloys may contain 70% to 72% silver and 25% palladium and may have physical properties of a Type III gold alloy. Other silver-based alloys might contain roughly 60% silver, 25% palladium, and as much as 15% or more of copper and may have properties

TABLE 20–6. Linear Solidification Shrinkage of Casting Alloys

Alloy	Casting Shrinkage (%)
Type I, gold base	1.56
Type II, gold base	1.37
Type III, gold base	1.42
Ni-Cr-Mo-Be	2.3
Co-Cr-Mo	2.3

more like a Type IV gold alloy. Despite early reports of poor castability, the Ag-Pd alloys can produce acceptable castings. The major limitation of Ag-Pd alloys, in general, and the Ag-Pd-Cu, in particular, is their greater potential for tarnish and corrosion. They should not be confused with Pd-Ag alloys that are designed for metal-ceramic restorations.

Because of the increasing interest in aesthetics by dental patients, a decreased use of all-metal restorations has occurred during the past decade. The use of metal-ceramic restorations in posterior sites has increased relative to the use of all-metal crowns and onlays. Because most crown and bridge restorations in posterior teeth are based on metal-ceramic systems, the alloys for these restorations are discussed more completely.

As mentioned previously, a comparison of typical physical properties of high noble and noble alloys (including the Ag-Pd alloys) for all-metal restorations (Type I to Type IV) and metal-ceramic restorations is given in Table 20–5.

Nickel-Chromium and Cobalt-Chromium Alloys. These alloys are described in more detail in the sections on metal-ceramic and partial dentures. They are rarely used for all-metal restorations.

Titanium and Titanium Alloys. These metals can be used for all-metal and metal-ceramic restorations as well as for removable partial denture frameworks. Because they have not been used often for the first two applications, their properties are described at the end of the section on partial dentures.

Aluminum Bronze Alloy. At least one alloy based on copper as the major element has been approved by the ADA. Although bronze is traditionally defined as a copper-rich copper-tin (Cu-Sn) alloy with or without other elements such as zinc and phosphorus, there exist essentially two-component (binary), three-component (ternary), and four-component (quaternary) bronze alloys that contain no tin such as aluminum bronze (copper-aluminum [Cu-Al]), silicon bronze (copper-silicon [Cu-Si]), and beryllium bronze (copper-beryllium [Cu-Be]). The aluminum bronze family of alloys including the one approved by the ADA may contain between 81 and 88 wt% copper, 7 to 11 wt% aluminum, 2 to 4 wt% nickel, and 1 to 4 wt% iron. Little clinical data are available on this aluminum bronze dental alloy. There is a potential for copper alloys to react with sulfur to form copper sulfide, which may tarnish the surface of this alloy in the same manner that silver sulfide darkens the surface of gold-base or silver-base alloys that contain a significant silver content.

HIGH NOBLE ALLOYS FOR METAL-CERAMIC RESTORATIONS

The chief objection to the use of dental porcelain as a restorative material is its low tensile and shear strength. Although porcelain can resist compressive stresses with reasonable success, substructure design does not permit shapes in which compressive stress is the principal force.

A method by which this disadvantage can be minimized is to bond the porcelain directly to a cast alloy substructure made to fit the prepared tooth. If a strong bond is attained between the porcelain veneer and the metal, the porcelain veneer is reinforced. Thus, the risk of brittle fracture can be avoided or, at least, minimized.

To fabricate this restoration, a metal substructure is waxed, cast, finished, and heat treated (oxidized). A thin layer of opaque porcelain is fused to the metal substructure to initiate the porcelain-metal bond and mask the color of the substructure. Then dentin and enamel porcelains, sometimes referred to as *body and incisal porcelains,* are fused onto the casting, shaped, stained to improve the aesthetic appearance, and glazed.

The original metal-ceramic alloys contained 88% gold and were much too soft for stress-bearing restorations such as fixed partial dentures. Because there was no evidence of a chemical bond between these alloys and dental porcelain, mechanical retention and undercuts were used to prevent detachment of the ceramic veneer. A stress bond test was developed in which the stress was concentrated at the porcelain-metal interface. Using this test, it was found that the bond strength of the porcelain to this type of alloy was less than the cohesive strength of the porcelain itself. This meant that if a failure occurred in the metal-ceramic restoration, it would most probably arise at the porcelain-metal interface. By adding less than 1% of oxide-forming elements such as iron, indium, and tin to this high-gold-content alloy, the porcelain metal bond strength was improved by a factor of three. Iron also increases the proportional limit and strength of the alloy.

This 1% addition of base metals to the gold, palladium, and platinum alloy was all that was necessary to produce a slight oxide film on the surface of the substructure to achieve a porcelain-metal bond strength level that surpassed the cohesive strength of the porcelain itself. This new type of alloy, with small amounts of base metals added, became the standard for the metal-ceramic restoration. In response to economic pressures, other gold- and palladium-based metal-ceramic alloys emerged. In time, base metals were also developed for this same purpose.

Despite the large number of alloys possessing the technical capability to bond to dental porcelain, they all can be arranged in a classification based on alloy composition. As shown in Table 20–3, metal-ceramic alloys fall into one of the three general categories—high noble, noble, or base metal—and are arranged according to composition. Using this approach, alloys with similar compositions, physical properties, and handling characteristics can be grouped together. Groups of high noble and noble alloys are listed in Table 20–7.

In spite of vastly different chemical compositions, all the alloys in the following categories share at least three common features: (1) they have the potential to bond to dental porcelain; (2) they possess coefficients of thermal contraction compatible with those of dental porcelains; and (3) their solidus temperature is sufficiently high to permit the application of low-fusing porcelains. The integrity and longevity of that bond are dependent on a multitude of factors, as presented in Chapter 26.

The coefficient of thermal expansion (CTE) tends to have a reciprocal relationship with the melting point of alloys and the melting range of alloys; that is, the higher the melting temperature of a metal, the lower its CTE. This fact is important in formulating metal-ceramic alloys for different dental porcelains. Metal-ceramic alloys are also often referred to as *porcelain-fused-to-metal* or *ceramometal* alloys. The preferred descriptive term is *metal-ceramic.* Likewise, the preferred acronym is PFM rather than other acronyms such as PBM (porcelain bonded to metal) and PTM (porcelain to metal). The classification system used for the high noble, noble, and predominantly base metal alloys is shown in Table 20–2.

TABLE 20–7. Typical High Noble and Noble Alloys for Metal-Ceramic Restorations

Alloy Class	Name (Supplier)	Principal Elements (WT%)*						
		Au	Pt	Pd	Ag	Cu	Co	Ga
High Noble Alloys								
Au-Pt-Pd or	SMG-3 (Ney)	81	6	11				
Au-Pd-Pt	Jelenko "O" (Jelenko)	87	5	6	1			
(0–4.99% Ag)	Degudent H (Degussa)	85	8	5				
Au-Pd-Ag	Micro-Bond #6 (Howmedica)	77	3	10	9			
(5–11.99% Ag)	Rx Sp. CG (Jeneric/Pentron)	75		13	9			
Au-Pd-Ag	Rx WCG (Jeneric/Pentron)	49		32	15			
(≥12% Ag)	Cameo (Jelenko)	53		27	16			
	Special White (Degussa)	45		40	16			
Au-Pd	Olympia (Jelenko)	52		39				2
(no Ag)	Lodestar (Williams)	52		37				
	Orion (Ney)	51		39				
	Deva 4 (Degussa)	51		39				
Noble Alloys								
Pd-Au	Olympia II (Jelenko)	35		57				5
(no Ag)	30 NS (Nobilium)	30		60				
Pd-Au-Ag	Rx SWCG (Jeneric)	32	3	42	13			
	Regent (Sterngold)	19		48	26			
	Shasta (Wilkinson)	16		62	6			
Pd-Au-Ag-Ga	Integrity (Jensen)	6		75	6.5			6
	Protocol (Williams)	6		75	6			6
	300SL (Leach & Dillon)	6		75	6.5			6
Pd-Ag	Jelstar (Jelenko)			60	28			
	Will-Ceram W-1 (Williams)			54	38			
	Pors On (Degussa)			58	30			
Pd-Cu-Ga	Naturelle (Jeneric)	2		79		10		9
	Spirit (Jensen)	2		80		9		9
	Athenium (Williams)			74		15		9
Pd-Co	Bond-On (Aderer)			78			10	
	APF (Jeneric)			79			8	1.5
	PTM-88 (Jelenko)			88			4	8

*Bond-forming elements such as tin and indium are not shown.

Gold-based Metal-Ceramic Alloys. PFM alloys containing more than 40 wt% gold at least 60 wt% of noble metals (gold plus platinum and palladium and/or the other noble metals) are generally classified as high noble to satisfy the compositional rule given in Table 20–2.

Gold-Platinum-Palladium Alloys. These alloys have a gold content ranging up to 88% with varying amounts of palladium, platinum, and small amounts of base metals. Some of these alloys are yellow in color. Alloys of this type are susceptible to sag deformation, and fixed partial dentures should be restricted to three-unit spans, anterior cantilevers, or crowns.

Gold-Palladium-Silver Alloys. These gold-based alloys contain between 39% and 77% gold, up to 35% palladium, and silver levels as high as 22%. The silver increases the thermal contraction coefficient, but it also has a tendency to discolor some porcelains.

Gold-Palladium Alloys. A gold content ranging from 44% to 55% and a palladium level of 35% to 45% is present in these metal-ceramic alloys, which have remained popular despite their relatively high cost. The lack of silver results in a decreased thermal contraction coefficient and the freedom from silver discoloration of porcelain. Alloys of this type must be used with porcelains that have low coefficients of thermal contraction to avoid the development of axial and circumferential (hoop) tensile stresses in porcelain during the cooling part of the porcelain firing cycle.

NOBLE ALLOYS FOR METAL-CERAMIC RESTORATIONS

Palladium-Based Alloys. According to the ADA classification of 1984, noble alloys must contain at least 25 wt% of the noble metals but do not necessarily contain any gold. The noble classification generally refers to all palladium-based alloys that contain between 54 and 88 wt% palladium, but it also describes the Ag-Pd alloys for all-metal or resin-veneer restorations that contain only 25 wt% palladium. Noble palladium-based alloys offer a compromise between the high-noble gold alloys and the predominantly base metal alloys. The price per ounce of a palladium alloy is generally one half to one third that of a gold alloy. The density of a palladium-based alloy is midway between that of base metal and of high noble alloys. Palladium-based alloys offer moderate price compared with gold alloys, workability similar to gold, and scrap value.

Palladium-Silver Alloys. Pd-Ag alloys were introduced widely in the late 1970s as an attempt by manufacturers to take advantage of the disenchantment of some dentists and laboratory technicians with the castability, porcelain bonding, and workability problems with the early base metal alloys. Pd-Ag alloys enjoyed widespread popularity for a few years after they were introduced, but their popularity has declined somewhat in recent years because of their tendency to discolor porcelain during firing. One theory that has been proposed for this greenish-yellow discoloration, popularly termed "greening," is that the silver vapor escapes from the surface of these alloys during firing of the porcelain, diffuses as ionic silver into the porcelain, and is reduced to form colloidal metallic silver in the surface layer of porcelain. Not all porcelains are susceptible to silver discoloration, because some apparently do not contain the necessary elements to reduce the ionic silver.

Other palladium alloys contain 75% to 90% palladium and no silver and were developed to eliminate the greening problem. Some of the high-palladium alloys develop a layer of dark oxide on their surface during cooling from the degassing cycle, and this oxide layer has proven difficult to mask by the opaque porcelain. Other high-palladium alloys such as the Pd-Ga-Ag-Au type seem not to be plagued by this problem. Because palladium is more expensive than silver, the elimination of silver and its replacement by palladium in these alloys naturally results in their being more expensive than Pd-Ag alloys.

This alloy type was introduced to the U.S. market in 1974 as the first gold-free noble metal available for metal-ceramic restorations. These alloys, like all palladium-based products, have been occasionally called *semiprecious*. As stated previously, this term should not be used because it cannot be precisely defined and because it tends to encourage the association of many dissimilar alloys in the same group.

The compositions of Pd-Ag alloys fall within a narrow range: 53% to 61% palladium and 28% to 40% silver. Tin or indium or both are usually added to increase alloy hardness and to promote oxide formation for adequate bonding of porcelain. In some of these alloys, the formation of an internal oxide rather than an external oxide has been reported. As shown in Figure 20–1, nodules are

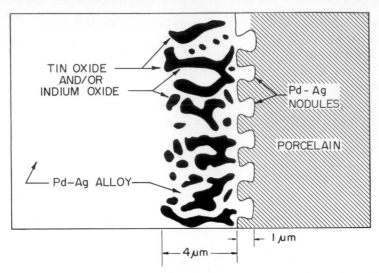

Figure 20–1. Internal oxide formation and creep-induced nodule formation in a Pd-Ag-In-Sn alloy for metal-ceramic restorations.

formed on the external surface as a result of the internal oxidation process. This phenomenon apparently produces a clinically acceptable result, although it is not an ideal situation. A proper balance is needed to maintain a reasonably low casting temperature and a compatible coefficient of thermal contraction. The replacement of gold by palladium raises the melting range but lowers the contraction coefficient of an alloy. Increasing the silver content tends to lower the melting range and raises the contraction coefficient.

Because of their high silver contents compared with the gold-based alloys, the silver discoloration effect is most severe for these alloys. Gold metal conditioners or ceramic coating agents may minimize this effect. The use of porcelains that are advertised as "nongreening" is another option that a dental technician might choose to help overcome this problem. One should proceed with caution when these alloys are to be used for anterior restorations or in cases where light shades are desired. Except for posterior restorations, experience should be gained with isolated single-unit restorations before proceeding with the fabrication of fixed partial dentures.

The low specific gravity of these alloys (10.7 to 11.1) combined with their low intrinsic cost makes these alloys attractive as economical alternatives to the gold-based alloys. Some of the alloys in this class with lower silver contents (approximately 28%) appear to be easily burnishable compared with other noble metal alloys. One would expect an alloy with a hardness of 170 to 180 DPH, a yield strength of about 462 MPa (67,000 psi), and an elongation value of 25% to be readily burnishable. In addition, the alloy would be easy to grind and polish.

Adherence of porcelain is considered to be acceptable for most of the Pd-Ag alloys. However, one study indicates that some of these alloys may form internal rather than external oxides. Instead of the formation of the desired external oxide, Pd-Ag nodules may develop on the surface that effect retention of porcelain by mechanical rather than chemical bonding. However, this condition has not apparently produced a significant number of clinical failures to warrant concern.

The thermal compatibility of these alloys is generally good except with certain European porcelains. As is true for all alloys, one should consult with the alloy manufacturer to determine which porcelains may be incompatible with a given alloy. In addition, the alloys should be approved through the ADA Acceptance Program.

Palladium-Copper Alloys. This alloy type is comparable in cost to the Pd-Ag alloys. Because alloys of this type are recent introductions to the dental market, little clinical information is available on their long-term clinical success. Thus, one should gain initial experience with single units rather than fixed partial dentures.

Because of their low melting range of approximately 1170° C to 1190° C (2140° F to 2170° F), these alloys are expected to be susceptible to creep deformation (sag) at elevated firing temperatures. Thus, one should exercise caution in using these alloys for long-span fixed partial dentures with relatively small connectors. Shown in Figure 20–2 is the microstructure of a Pd-Cu-Ga alloy in the as-cast state (A) and after porcelain firing cycles (B). Obviously, a structural change has occurred. Whether a volumetric change and potential distortion of the coping

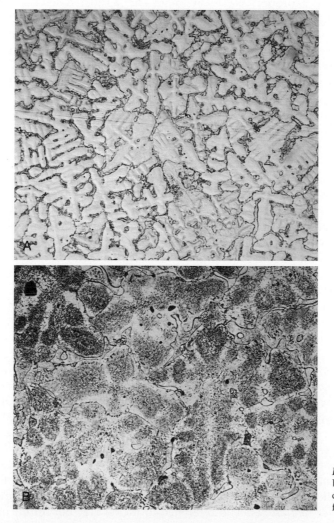

Figure 20–2. Microstructures of a Pd-Cu-Ga alloy in the as-cast condition (A) and after porcelain firing cycles (B).

occurred is not known, although these types of alloys have been associated with such problems.

As is true for some Pd-Ag alloys, several of these products contain 2% gold. This small amount of gold serves no useful purpose except possibly to allow these alloys to be considered gold-containing alloys for certain dental insurance policies. These alloys contain between 74% and 80% palladium and 9% to 15% copper. Porcelain discoloration due to copper is possible but does not appear to be a major problem. There has been some concern recently over the potential cytotoxic effect of copper released intraorally from certain Pd-Cu alloys. However, although research studies of this effect are inconclusive, there appears to be little reason for concern about their use.

One should be aware of the potential effect on aesthetics of the dark brown or black oxide formed during oxidation and subsequent porcelain firing cycles. Care should be taken by the technician to mask this oxide completely with opaque porcelain and to eliminate the unaesthetic dark band that develops at metal-porcelain junctions. It is also important that the technician ensure that a brown rather than a black oxide is formed on the metal surface during the oxidation treatment. Otherwise, poor adherence to porcelain may result.

Some of these alloys are somewhat technique sensitive with respect to casting, presoldering, and proper oxidation treatment (as just discussed). In some instances, the molten alloy should have a thin oxide film appearing on its surface at the casting temperature. Some instructions specify that heating be maintained for an additional 7 seconds beyond the point at which a rolling motion of the alloy is observed. Because of the lack of a specifically defined melt appearance, there may be a tendency to overheat the alloy to eliminate this film. This error could cause significant changes in the properties of the alloy and a decrease in metal-porcelain bond strength. Underheating of the molten alloy is also possible because of the difficulty in judging the proper melt appearance. This could result in incomplete castings or rounded margins.

The Pd-Cu alloys have yield strengths of up to 1145 MPa (166,000 psi), elongation values of 5% to 11%, and hardness values as high as some base metal alloys. Thus, these alloys would appear to have a poor potential for burnishing, except when the marginal areas are relatively thin. However, laboratory technicians report that most of these alloys are easier to handle than base metal alloys. Although thermal incompatibility is not considered to be a major concern, distortion of ultrathin metal copings (0.1 mm) has been occasionally reported. The principal cause of this effect is not known. Metal-porcelain incompatibility stresses may be responsible for this distortion, especially because Pd-Cu alloys have relatively high creep rates at temperatures near the glass transition temperature of porcelain. Other factors that may also cause distortion include the relaxation of elastic stresses due to solidification, grinding, and sandblasting, which occurs during subsequent heating procedures.

The solutions to problems involving distortion of single-unit or multiple-unit castings include using thicker copings or connectors, changing the brand of porcelain conversion to a more technique-insensitive alloy, or adopting a different metal-ceramic system that has demonstrated acceptable overall properties. Using another dental laboratory should also be considered if atypical laboratory procedures are suspected to be the cause of this problem.

Palladium-Cobalt Alloys. This alloy group is comparable in cost to the Pd-Ag and Pd-Cu alloys. They are often advertised as gold-free, nickel-free, beryllium-free, and silver-free alloys. The reference to nickel and beryllium indicates that these alloys, as is true with the other noble metals, are generally considered biocompatible. Like many noble metals, these alloys have a fine grain size to minimize hot tearing during the solidification process. This Pd-Co group is the most sag resistant of all noble metal alloys.

The noble metal content (based on palladium) ranges from 78% to 88%. The cobalt content ranges between 4 and 10 wt%. One commercial alloy contains 8% gallium. An example of typical properties of a Pd-Co alloy is as follows: hardness, 250 DPH; yield strength, 586 MPa (85,000 psi); elongation, 20%; and modulus of elasticity, 85.2 GPa (12.35×10^6 psi). These alloys should have good handling characteristics.

Although these alloys are silver free, discoloration of porcelain can still result because of the presence of cobalt. This is not considered a significant problem. Failure of the technician to completely mask out the dark metal oxide color with opaque porcelain is a more common cause of unacceptable aesthetic results. No metal coating agents are required to mask the oxide color or to promote adherence to porcelain. Like the Pd-Ag and Pd-Cu alloys the Pd-Co alloys generally tend to have a relatively high thermal contraction coefficient and would be expected to be more compatible with higher-expansion porcelains.

Palladium-Gallium-Silver and Palladium-Gallium-Silver-Gold Alloys. These alloys are the most recent of the noble metals. This group of alloys was introduced because they tend to have a slightly lighter-colored oxide than the Pd-Cu or Pd-Co alloys and they are thermally compatible with lower expansion porcelains. The oxide that is required for bonding to porcelain is relatively dark, but it is somewhat lighter than those of the Pd-Cu and Pd-Co alloys. The silver content is relatively low (5 to 8 wt%) and is usually inadequate to cause porcelain greening. Caution should be exercised in their initial use until clinical data are available. Little information is available on metal-ceramic bond strength or thermal compatibility. These Pd-Ga-Ag alloys generally tend to have a relatively low thermal contraction coefficient and would be expected to be more compatible with lower expansion porcelains such as Vita porcelain. Remember, to protect yourself from unnecessary clinical failures, it is recommended that any alloy you select should be certified as "acceptable" by the ADA. Furthermore, you should also ask the alloy manufacturer (not the sales representative or the laboratory technician) to provide a list (in writing, if possible) of the porcelain products with which the selected alloy will be compatible.

Physical Properties of High Noble and Noble Alloys. Important physical properties of alloys for all-metal and metal-ceramic restorations are provided in Table 20–5. Similar listings of properties are generally available for the alloys of any particular manufacturer. The melting range sets the basis for the casting temperature. The upper limit of the range is the liquidus. To this should be added 75° C to 150° C (150° F to 300° F) to obtain the proper casting temperature. The lower limit of the melting range can similarly be used to estimate maximum soldering temperatures.

The metal-ceramic alloys must have a high melting range so that the metal is solid well above the porcelain sintering temperature to minimize distortion (sag) of the casting during porcelain application. On the other hand, the Type I to Type IV alloys must have considerably lower fusion temperatures if they are to be cast with conventional equipment and if gypsum investments are used. The width of the melting range is also of interest since the wider the melting range, the greater is the tendency for coring during solidification.

The specific volume (cm³/g), which is the reciprocal of density (g/cm³), is an indication of the number of average dental units that can be cast from a unit weight of the metal. The ratio of the extreme densities in the table (e.g., from 10.7 to 18.3 for the metal-ceramic alloys) indicates that more equivalent castings can be cast from the lower-density alloy than from the one with higher density (in this example, 70% more).

BASE METAL ALLOYS FOR CAST METAL AND METAL-CERAMIC RESTORATIONS

A survey of 1000 dental laboratory owners in 1978 revealed that only 29% of these laboratories were using Ni-Cr or Co-Cr alloys for cast metal or metal-ceramic restorations. In 1980 and 1981, the percentage of laboratories using these base metal alloys increased to 66% and 70%, respectively, because of the unstable price of noble metals during this period. The percentage of base metal use in dentistry has decreased between 1981 and 1995. Most of these dental laboratories indicated a preference for Ni-Cr alloys over Co-Cr alloys. Although the increased acceptance of these alloys during this period was greatly influenced by the rapidly fluctuating international cost of gold and other noble metals, the subsequent decline in the cost of noble metals has had a small effect on reversing this trend. Ni-Cr-Be alloys have retained their popularity despite the potential toxicity of beryllium and the allergenic potential of nickel. In some regional areas, an increase in the use of palladium alloys has been observed. This chapter has been prepared to provide a critical assessment of the risks and benefits of base metal alloys when compared with gold-based or palladium-based alloys.

Since the development of cobalt-chromium alloys for cast dental appliances in 1928 and the subsequent introduction of Ni-Cr and Ni-Co-Cr alloys in later years, base metal alloys have demonstrated widespread acceptance in the United States as the predominant choice for the fabrication of removable partial denture frameworks. Compared with ADA-certified Type IV gold alloys, cobalt-based alloys, nickel-based alloys, and pure titanium feature lower cost, lower density, greater stiffness, (modulus of elasticity) higher hardness, and comparable clinical resistance to tarnish and corrosion.

Most Ni-Cr alloys for crowns and fixed partial denture prostheses contain 61 to 81 wt% nickel, 11 to 27 wt% chromium, and 2 to 5 wt% molybdenum. Typical compositions of several commercial alloys used in the past (some of which are currently used) for metal-ceramic restorations are given in Table 20–8. Chromium is essential to provide passivation and corrosion resistance. Other alloy formulations include Cr-Co and Fe-Cr. These alloys may also contain one or more of the following elements: aluminum, beryllium, boron, carbon, cobalt, copper, cerium,

TABLE 20–8. Typical Base Metal Alloys for Metal-Ceramic Restorations

Alloy Name (Supplier)	Composition (Weight Percent)						
	Ni	*Co*	*Cr*	*Be*	*Mo*	*W*	*Ru*
Rexillium III (Jeneric/Pentron)	76	0.3	14	1.8	5		
Litecast B (Williams Dental Co.)	78		13	1.7	4		
Neptune (Jeneric/Pentron)	62		22		9		
Forte (Unitek/3M)	62		22		9		
Genesis II (J. F. Jelenko & Co.)		53	27				3
Ultra 100 (Unitek/3M)		52	28				
Novarex (Jeneric/Pentron)		55	25			10	5

gallium, iron, manganese, niobium, silicon, tin, titanium, and zirconium. The Co-Cr alloys typically contain 53 to 67 wt% cobalt, 25 to 32 wt% chromium, and 2 to 6 wt% molybdenum. As is the case with base metal partial denture alloys, base metal alloys melt at elevated temperatures. In general, the use of phosphate- or silica-bonded investments is indicated. In addition, the use of high-temperature heat sources is required for casting. More important is the compensation for casting shrinkage required at these elevated temperatures if a clinically acceptable fit is to be obtained. Recently, chemically pure titanium and Ti-Al-V alloys have been introduced for metal-ceramic restorations.

Handling Hazards and Precautions. Laboratory technicians may be exposed occasionally or routinely to excessively high concentrations of beryllium and nickel dust and beryllium vapor. Although the beryllium concentration in dental alloys rarely exceeds 2 wt%, the amount of beryllium vapor released into the breathing space during the melting of Ni-Cr-Be alloys may be significant over an extended period. Actually, the potential hazards of beryllium should be based on its atomic concentration rather than its weight concentration in an alloy. One can readily demonstrate that an alloy which contains 80% nickel, 11.4% chromium, 5% molybdenum, 1.8% iron, and 1.8% beryllium on a weight basis contains 73.3% nickel, 11.8% chromium, 2.6% molybdenum, 1.6% iron, and 10.7% beryllium on an atomic basis. Thus, toxicity evaluations for beryllium should be based on a concentration level of approximately 11 atomic percent. The vapor pressure of pure beryllium is approximately 0.1 Torr (mm Hg) at an assumed casting temperature of 1370° C. Comparable vapor pressures for chromium, nickel, and molybdenum are 5×10^{-3} Torr, 8×10^{-4} Torr, and 3×10^{-11} Torr, respectively. If one assumes that the vapor pressure of beryllium in an alloy is proportional to its atomic concentration, beryllium would have a vapor pressure approximately 18 times greater than that of either chromium or nickel.

The risk of beryllium vapor exposure is greatest for dental technicians during alloy melting, especially in the absence of an adequate exhaust and filtration system. The Occupational Health and Safety Administration (OSHA) specifies that exposure to beryllium dust in air should be limited to a particulate beryllium concentration of 2 $\mu g/m^3$ of air (both respirable and nonrespirable particles) determined from an 8-hour time-weighted coverage. The allowable ceiling concentration is 5 $\mu g/m^3$ (not to be exceeded for a 15-minute period). For a minimum duration of 30 minutes, a maximum ceiling concentration of 25 $\mu g/m^3$ is allowed. The National Institute for Occupational Safety and Health (NIOSH) currently recommends a limit of 0.5 $\mu g/m^3$ based on a 130-minute sample. High levels of beryllium have been measured during finishing and polishing when a local exhaust system was not used. When an exhaust system was used, the concentration of beryllium in the breathing zone was reduced to levels considered safe by the authors.

Exposure to beryllium may result in acute and chronic forms of beryllium disease. Workers exposed to moderately high concentrations of beryllium dust over a short period, or prolonged exposure to low concentrations, may experience signs and symptoms representing acute disease states. Physiologic responses vary from contact dermatitis to severe chemical pneumonitis, which can be fatal. The chronic disease state is characterized by symptoms persisting for longer than 1 year with the onset of symptoms separated by a period of years from the time of exposure. Symptoms range from coughing, chest pain, and general weakness to pulmonary dysfunction.

Research has shown that airborne levels of beryllium can be controlled with a local exhaust system. One should not conclude, however, that melting and grinding of Ni-Cr alloys without beryllium and grinding of other dental materials pose no major risk to the health of laboratory technicians. The profession should be aware of a 1976 report that indicated that white male dental laboratory technicians, 20 to 64 years of age, exhibited an incidence of lung cancer 4.05 times higher than the incidence for all of the occupations identified. Compared with a standard mortality ratio (SMR) of 100 for all occupations and an SMR value lower than 70 for dentists, the SMR value for dental technicians was 405. Dental laboratory technicians were ranked fourth on a list of 24 occupations with SMR values above 125. This report was based on a review of 2161 death certificates and 1777 incident cases of lung cancer in the Los Angeles area between 1968 and 1973. A higher frequency of cigarette smoking among dental technicians cannot yet be ruled out as a possible cause. This high incidence of lung cancer may be due to inhalation of numerous other hazardous airborne particles released from materials such as asbestos, polycyclic aromatic hydrocarbon compounds, investment powder, gypsum products, dental porcelain, and grindings from other base metal elements such as nickel and chromium. Thus, good ventilation and exhaust facilities should be employed whenever any material is ground. The dental profession should investigate methods to minimize such risks.

Potential Patient Hazards. Of greater concern to dental patients is the intraoral exposure to nickel, especially for patients with a known allergy to this element. Dermatitis resulting from contact with nickel solutions was described as early as 1889. Inhalation, ingestion, and dermal contact of nickel or nickel-containing alloys are common because nickel is found in environmental sources such as air, soil, and food as well as in synthetic objects such as coins, kitchen utensils, and jewelry. The air concentration of nickel is relatively low except where environmental pollution conditions exist owing to nickel-processing operations or burning of fossil fuels.

A comprehensive study of 3287 Swedish patients with eczema was reported in 1953 (Skog and Thyresson, 1953). Nickel allergy was determined by patch testing using 5% nickel sulfate. Positive reactions were exhibited by 9.4% of the women and 7.9% of the men. When classified by occupation, a significantly increased sensitivity to nickel compared with other allergens was found for men employed in the building trades ($P \leq .01$) and shops and warehouses ($P \leq .02$), and by women employed in offices ($P \leq .001$). The overall higher nickel sensitivity by women was attributed to increased contact with nickel-plated objects at work and at home. The higher incidence of nickel sensitivity among men in the building trade, shops, and warehouses was explained by the increased handling of nickel-plated tools.

Based on a study of 621 persons in Denmark who developed nickel dermatitis between 1936 and 1955, it was concluded that the risk of sensitization was greater for people involved with the private use of nickel items than from people who have industrial exposure to nickel. Confirmation of these cases was established on the basis of patch test reactions to 5% nickel sulfate.

Eleven dermatologists in six European countries jointly investigated 4000 patients with contact dermatitis. These patients were exposed to 20 potential allergens, including 5% nickel sulfate. Of the 769 persons considered to have occupational dermatitis, positive reactions to nickel sulfate were shown in 59 (7%) of these cases. For the nonoccupational subjects, positive reactions to nickel sulfate were also observed in 59 (7%) of these cases. It was concluded that no difference in nickel dermatitis was found between the two groups. Despite the widespread use of nickel-based alloys for dental applications, research data are insufficient to determine the long term risks of nickel-containing prostheses to patients who demonstrate an extraoral allergic response to nickel-based alloys or a positive response to nickel patch tests.

A recent study was performed to determine the intraoral response to a nickel-based alloy by patients known to be allergic to nickel. Two groups of 10 patients each were subjected to patch tests using 0.5% potassium dichromate, 2.5% nickel sulfate, a Ni-Cr dental alloy, and a gold alloy. The control group of 10 patients had no known allergy to nickel. The nickel and gold dental alloys were also inserted in a removable acrylic appliance such that the alloys were exposed to palatal mucosa. This phase of testing was performed 3 weeks after the skin tests. None of the control patients responded to any of the dermal test materials. All 10 of the sensitized patients reacted positively to nickel sulfate, whereas 8 exhibited positive extraoral responses to the nickel alloy. After the intraoral exposure, none of control patients and only one of the sensitized patients developed any positive signs or symptoms of nickel allergy. The sensitized patient reported a burning and tingling sensation during the first 24 hours and exhibited a slight erythematous reaction on the palatal mucosa. Three patients indicated itching at the site of the nickel sulfate patch test while the intraoral appliances were in use. Such reactions at remote sites may result in underestimations of the incidence of allergic response triggered by intraoral appliances.

A recent study revealed that there is a tendency for patients who demonstrated a positive nickel patch test response to exhibit an allergic reaction within the buccal mucosa that was exposed to pure nickel foil bonded to premolar teeth. Such an effect was not found for patients with known allergy to palladium who were exposed in a similar manner to pure palladium foil. However, this response to pure nickel may not occur when nickel alloys are employed.

For patients between 24 and 44 years of age who possessed a nickel alloy fixed prosthesis, 9.7% of the women and 0.8% of the men experienced a positive reaction to 2.5% nickel sulfate in one study. The nickel allergy incidence for all age groups was 4.5% for women and 1.5% for men. Of the positive reactions to nickel, women with pierced ears accounted for 90% of the total. None of the males with pierced ears exhibited positive reactions. No correlation was found between the incidence of nickel hypersensitivity and the presence intraorally of nickel alloy restorations.

For a woman who reports that she is allergic to certain metals, the following three options can be pursued:

1. If, after a thorough medical history that includes questions on dermatologic reactions to coins, jewelry, or dental metals, you can conclusively identify the allergen as the component of a base metal alloy, a gold-based or palladium-based alloy can be selected on a trial basis.

2. If the patient states that she is allergic to gold alloy, this situation is highly unlikely (although not impossible) because the incidence of such an allergy is far less than 1% compared with an allergy potential of 10% for women to nickel under extraoral conditions. Further questioning should be conducted to determine whether some of the "gold jewelry" was actually a nickel-containing alloy which had been gold plated. If the examination does not resolve this issue, a palladium-based alloy (free of gold) should be selected on a trial basis.

3. If a patient insists that she is allergic to all metals and your examination

fails to identify the most probable allergen, the patient should be referred to a dermatologist or allergist for a medical diagnosis.

Numerous cases of respiratory organ cancer have been documented in studies of workers involved in the plating, stripping, refining, sintering, grinding, chipping, and polishing of nickel and nickel alloys. The effects of nickel exposure to humans have included dermatitis, cancer of the lungs, cancer of the nasal sinus and larynx, irritation and perforation of the nasal septum, loss of smell, asthmalike lung disease, pulmonary irritation, pneumoconiosis, a decrease in lung function, and death.

Because of the concerns over the carcinogenic potential of nickel, NIOSH has recommended that OSHA adopt a standard to limit employee exposure to inorganic nickel in the laboratory or office to 15 $\mu g/m^3$ (air) determined as a time-weighted average (TWA) concentration for up to a 10-hour work shift (40-hour work week). The existing OSHA standard specifies an 8-hour TWA concentration limit of 1000 $\mu g/m^3$. This limit is of the same magnitude as the established in Japan but is far higher than the 10 $\mu g/m^3$ limit specified in Sweden. In Sweden, the National Board of Health issued a warning against the use of dental casting alloys containing more than 1 wt% nickel.

It appears that the potential carcinogenic risks of nickel are far less likely to be incurred by dental patients and dentists as compared with dental technicians. Because of a far greater time-weighted exposure to nickel and beryllium dust and vapor, dental technicians should be provided with adequate protection facilities so that such risks are minimized.

To minimize exposure of metallic dust to patients and dentists during metal grinding operations, a high-speed evacuation system should be employed when such procedures are performed intraorally. Patients should be informed of the potential allergic effects of nickel exposure, and a thorough medical history should be taken to determine if the patient is at risk of exhibiting an allergic reaction to nickel. As a conservative approach, one should adopt the policy that evidence of a previous allergic response to any alloy should be sufficient grounds to contraindicate the use of nickel-based alloys.

Summary of Biocompatibility Considerations. Despite the widespread use of nickel-based alloys, claims for the safety of these alloys have not yet been universally accepted. The allergenic effects of nickel on dental patients and the potential toxic effects of nickel and beryllium on laboratory technicians continue to cause concern within the dental profession. The systemic response to metallic nickel and nickel compounds due to intraoral corrosion and dissolution of nickel-based restorations over extended periods have not been studied adequately. The dental profession may be overgeneralizing the relative safety of nickel alloys owing to the lack of allergy-induced intraoral lesions observed in private practices. Additional animal studies are needed to characterize the acute and chronic toxicity of nickel compounds. One should not overlook the potential for dermatologic and systemic effects that may result from patient and personnel exposure to cobalt alloys. Although allergic reactions may be of some concern, the toxicity potential of Co-Cr alloys appears to be insignificant.

Little research has been performed to determine the carcinogenic potential of nickel on dental laboratory technicians. In addition, animal and human studies are needed to determine the effect of nickel and beryllium exposure on the reproductive system. In the interim period, specific equipment and facilities that minimize dust and vapor exposure to dental technicians should be identified to reduce airborne concentrations of nickel and beryllium in commercial dental laboratories and dental offices so as to minimize the exposure of personnel to airborne debris from noble metal alloys, amalgams, porcelains, and other dental materials.

A recent workshop sponsored by the National Institute of Dental Research was devoted to the assessment of biocompatibility of metals in dentistry. As a result of this workshop the following recommendations were made for clinical implementation. Manufacturers, laboratories, and dentists should be encouraged to identify alloys used in the fabrication of prosthetic devices in terms of elements (such as nickel, chromium, and cobalt) that may affect a patient's health. Dentists and administrators of dental laboratories should be encouraged to inform employees who work as technicians regarding the need to avoid inhalation exposure to dusts from alloys. Practitioners are encouraged to document in patient records the content (or specific brand name) of alloys used in restorative materials. Health histories should include documentation of patients sensitive to metals. Patch testing for sensitivity to metals should not be performed by dentists but by professionals trained in the administration and interpretation of these tests. Practitioners are encouraged to report case histories of adverse reactions to metals and other biomaterials to the ADA.

Properties of Ni-Cr, Ni-Cr-Be, and Co-Cr Alloys. Several questions should be addressed whenever one considers the use of a nickel-based alloy as an alternative or replacement for a time-tested gold-based alloy. Is there any evidence to show that the alloy is technique sensitive with respect to castability, adherence to porcelain, thermal compatibility with porcelain, porcelain discoloration potential, or solderability? Do the advantageous properties and cost benefits outweigh the potential biological hazards? How many years of proven success has the laboratory technician had with this alloy? How long has the alloy been available to the dental profession? Which physical properties of the alloy are relevant to clinical practice? Has the alloy been classified as acceptable according to the acceptance program established by the Council on Scientific Affairs for alloys used to fabricate dental restorative and prosthetic devices?

Before attempting to answer these questions, one should recognize that no alloy is ideal in all respects. Compared with other alloys for metal-ceramic restorations, base metal alloys generally have higher hardness and elastic modulus (stiffness) values and are more sag resistant at elevated temperatures, but they may be more difficult to cast and presolder than Au-Pd or Pd-Ag alloys. Some claims have been made that base metal alloys are, in general, more technique sensitive than well-established noble metal alloys. It is well known that presoldering of Ni-Cr alloys with a high degree of reliability requires considerable experience. A recent survey by the National Association of Dental Laboratories indicated that only 46% of the laboratory owners surveyed were satisfied with the soldering performance of these alloys. The ability to obtain acceptable-fitting base metal castings represents a challenge to technicians and may require special procedures to adequately compensate for their higher solidification shrinkage. Another potential disadvantage of nickel-based or cobalt-based alloys is their potential for porcelain delamination due to separation of a poorly adherent oxide layer from the metal substrate. In addition, relatively small differences in composition may produce wide variations in metal-ceramic bond strength.

In general, nickel alloys without beryllium demonstrate poorer castability than those alloys that contain up to 1.8 wt% beryllium. The subject of castability is controversial because some researchers claim that all alloys theoretically produce complete castings under optimum burnout, melting, and casting conditions. The point to be made here, however, is that generalized statements on the superiority of beryllium or nonberyllium alloys should not be made without appropriate supporting research data and statistical analyses.

The creep resistance of nickel-based alloys at porcelain firing temperatures is considered to be far superior to the resistance of gold-based and platinum-based alloys under the same conditions. Higher creep values for high noble and noble alloys indicate that greater distortion of long-span frameworks is more likely to result at elevated temperatures unless special precautions are taken by the dental technician.

The tarnish and corrosion resistance of base metal alloys containing nickel is of principal concern because of the allergic potential of nickel and nickel compounds. Little information is available on the corrosion products that form under *in vivo* conditions. However, *in vitro* studies can provide some reasonable predictions of clinical performance. In one study it was reported that there was comparable resistance to pitting and tarnish among six Ni-Cr alloys, a Co-Cr alloy, an Fe-Cr-Ni alloy and a gold alloy containing 46% gold, 40% silver, 8% copper, and 6% palladium. These alloys were studied during immersion in a solution with a chloride concentration equivalent to that of saliva.

With the use of data from other studies, some predictions may be made about the potential for galvanic corrosion induced by the contact of base metal alloys with other metallic restorations. Amalgams are expected to sustain less galvanic attack when they are placed in contact with Ni-Cr or Co-Cr alloys than with gold alloys. Amalgams should be more susceptible to galvanic corrosion relative to base metal alloys. Therefore, the amalgams should corrode while the cast base metal alloys they contact are protected from corrosion. When in contact with type 3 gold alloys, however, the base metal alloys are more susceptible to corrosive degradation.

As shown by the property chart in Table 20–9 of Ni-Cr alloys whose compositions are given in Table 20–10, the bond strength values of Ni-Cr and Co-Cr

TABLE 20–9. Physical and Mechanical Properties of Base Metal Alloys and a Gold Alloy

Properties	A	B	C	D	E	F	Gold Alloy
Tensile strength							
MPa	1,142	1,139	1,355	661	540	703	490
(psi)	(165,600)	(165,200)	(196,500)	(95,900)	(73,300)	(101,900)	(71,000)
Yield strength							
Mpa	591	782	838	360	260	543	400
(psi)	(85,700)	(113,400)	(121,500)	(52,200)	(37,700)	(78,700)	(58,000)
Modulus of elasticity							
MPa ($\times 10^3$)	207	190	210	193	154	208	88
(psi) ($\times 10^6$)	30.0	27.6	30.4	28.0	22.3	30.2	12.8
Percent elongation (%)	23.9	11.6	18.0	27.9	27.3	2.3	9.1
Vicker's hardness (DPH)	293	348	357	211	175	316	161
Density (g/cm^3)	8.1	8.0	7.9	8.0	8.7	8.3	18.3
Porcelain bond							
MPa	97.9	51.0	87.6	70.3	80.7	106.2	111.0
(psi)	(14,200)	(7,400)	(12,700)	(10,200)	(11,700)	(15,400)	(16,100)

Adapted from Physical and Mechanical Properties of Gold and Base Metal Alloys, J. P. Moffa, Alternatives to Gold Alloys in Dentistry, DHEW Publication No. (NIH) 77-1227, 1977.

TABLE 20–10. Composition of Base Metal Alloys for Metal Ceramic Restorations

Element	A	B	C	D	E	F
Nickel	80.75	79.67	78.51	68.96	80.86	68.75
Chromium	12.58	13.24	19.47	16.54	11.93	19.57
Iron	0.34	0.11	0.43	0.37	0.20	0.38
Aluminum	3.42	3.87	0.21	4.15	2.95	—
Molybdenum	1.53	1.52	—	5.10	1.87	4.22
Silicon	0.29	0.30	1.10	0.83	0.18	2.72
Beryllium	0.57	0.65	—	—	1.55	—
Copper	0.15	—	—	—	0.13	1.54
Manganese	0.13	0.12	—	3.05	0.14	1.24
Cobalt	—	—	—	0.42	—	—
Tin	—	—	—	—	—	1.25

Adapted from Physical and Mechanical Properties of Gold and Base Metal Alloys, J. P. Moffa, Alternatives to Gold Alloys in Dentistry, DHEW Publication No. (NIH) 77 1227, 1977.

alloys to porcelain as determined from *in vitro* studies have not generally been shown to be superior or inferior to those for noble metal alloys. Furthermore, clinical studies have not demonstrated a difference in the failure incidence between metal-ceramic restorations made from base metal alloys and those fabricated from noble metal alloys. However, some research indicates that certain characteristics of the oxide layer that forms on these alloys during preoxidation and porcelain firing cycles may adversely affect the bond strength of metal-ceramic restorations. An oxide layer that is nonadherent to the alloy substrate may be more susceptible to delamination under relatively low stresses. Contrary to previous theories, the thickness of this oxide layer or wettability of the oxide layer by porcelain may not be as important in the control of metal-ceramic adherence as the bond strength between the alloy and its oxide layer.

For the laboratory technician to produce the optimum metal oxide characteristics, the manufacturer's instructions must be followed precisely. However, some instructions are relatively imprecise. For example, some alloys require a "light" sand-blasting procedure after the initial oxide is formed during the preoxidation cycle. Although a 50-μm aluminum oxide abrasive is generally recommended, the purity level is not usually specified. The use of more economical, lower-purity aluminum oxide abrasives by dental technicians could contaminate the metal surface and subsequently affect the integrity of the metal-ceramic adherence zone. The ability of a laboratory technician to discriminate light from moderate grit-blasting to remove these surface oxides is one example of the technique sensitivity of base metal alloys. Other procedures that may be more technique sensitive than those for noble metal alloys include the determination of the proper casting temperature and the judgment of the proper flow point of solder during the presoldering process.

The thermal contraction differential between base metal alloys and dental porcelains may, under certain conditions, contribute to high levels of stress that could induce checking of porcelain or delayed failure. Although the thermal expansion and contraction values of base metal alloys generally fall within the range of noble metal alloys, porcelain checking occasionally results when the thermal expansion and contraction differences between metal and porcelain are excessive. Additional research is needed to predict these results and to determine methods to minimize these failures.

Perhaps the greatest disadvantage of nickel-based alloys is the variability in quality and strength of brazed (presoldered) connectors. Flexure tests of presoldered specimens reveal relatively brittle fracture patterns that typically propagate within the solder. Tensile tests have demonstrated both intrasolder and interfacial types of failure. The principal defects within the solder alloy are voids, localized shrinkage porosity, and flux inclusions. Beryllium-containing alloys are generally more difficult to braze (solder), and these specimens contain relatively high concentrations of voids within the solder joint.

To circumvent the uncertainties and variations associated with presoldering procedures, some dental technicians prefer to avoid the soldering process by a cast-joining procedure. A pontic is cut diagonally in half, and each half is prepared with large undercut channels. After each half of the bridge is stabilized on an occlusal index, the undercut areas are waxed to full contour, sprued, invested, burned out, and cast with new metal. This process is known as *cast-joining*. Little research has been performed to identify the adequacy of this approach. However, the two components are retained by mechanical interlocking effects, and the excessive displacement of these regions will likely cause porcelain fracture.

The elastic modulus of base metal alloys is as much as two times greater than the values for some of the more popular noble metal alloys. To take advantage of this property, some clinicians have proposed that the coping thickness in veneered areas can be reduced from 0.3 mm, recommended for noble metal alloys, to a uniform thickness of 0.1 mm. It has also been claimed that the cross section area of cast interproximal connectors can be reduced from 4 to 8 mm^2 to 1 to 2 mm^2 when base metal alloys are used. This approach has been criticized on the basis that the deflection of a base metal alloy beam will be greater than that of a gold alloy beam if the former is reduced in thickness by 50%, even though its modulus of elasticity is higher. The deflection of a cantilever beam is inversely proportional to t^{3}E, where t is the beam thickness and E is the elastic modulus. Thus, the connector thickness can be reduced by only 16% when the elastic modulus is doubled. Furthermore, a reduction of the coping thickness from 0.3 mm to 0.1 mm may increase the risk of porcelain fracture owing to the increased flexibility of the coping. However, a recent study based on finite element stress analysis of stresses induced in anterior PFM crowns under intraoral forces indicates that a reduction of base metal coping thickness (in veneered areas) from 0.3 mm to 0.1 mm has only a slight effect on porcelain stresses.

The mechanical properties of nickel base alloys are known to vary considerably. For example, the 0.2% offset yield strength of 14 nickel-based alloys ranged from 310 MPa (45,000 psi) to 828 MPa (120,000 psi) in the as-cast condition. After a heat treatment process, the yield strength decreased to between 241 MPa (35,000 psi) and 724 MPa (105,000 psi). The hardness value of these 14 alloys were comparable.

In general, the high hardness and high strength of base metal alloys contribute to certain difficulties in clinical practice. Grinding and polishing of fixed restorations to achieve proper occlusion occasionally require more chair-side time. Removal of defective restorations may also require more time. Crowns with fractured porcelain veneers, which may be simply performed on noble metal substrates using pin-retained facings or metal-ceramic onlays, are more difficult to accomplish when the failed restoration has a framework cast with nickel-based or cobalt-based alloys. Such difficulties may partially offset the economic advantage of these alloys.

Before selecting a base metal alloy for your practice, there are three basic questions you should ask your technician to ensure that you are approaching the selection from a conservative point of view. These questions are as follows:

1. What is the brand name of the alloy, the alloy type, and the porcelain you are using?

The response to this question allows you to classify the alloy (Co-Cr, Ni-Cr, or Ni-Cr-Be) to determine if the product is an ADA-approved product. The porcelain brand name can be used to determine if a compatible system is being used. A telephone call to the company should answer this question.

2. How long have you been using the alloy, and what are the main problems you have experienced?

If the alloy-porcelain system has been used for less than 3 years, find another laboratory. If he or she mentions porcelain debonding or crack formation as the major problems, find another laboratory or a more reliable product.

3. Have you had any difficulty in brazing (soldering) this alloy?

Generally, this is the main problem with all base metal alloys, particularly when presoldering operations are performed. If he or she states that their laboratory does not solder base metal alloys but casts everything as a single unit, this approach is acceptable. However, if cast joining is the technique used to mechanically attach pontics to crowns, then I would select another laboratory or a noble metal alloy that the laboratory had used successfully for 3 years or more and that is routinely soldered when multiple units or bridges do not fit during try-in.

Mechanical Properties. The clinical success of a metal-ceramic restoration is dependent in large measure on the ability of the underlying alloy substructure to resist the potentially destructive masticatory stresses. Although the aesthetic fused porcelain veneer has relatively high resistance to compressive stresses, its low tensile strength and characteristic lack of ductility make this brittle material extremely susceptible to the destructive types of stresses that accompany flexure of the metal substructure. Therefore, it is imperative that the metal-ceramic restorations be formulated and designed in such a way as to maximize the rigidity of the prosthesis. The obvious approach would be to increase the thickness of the metal substructure, because doubling the thickness increases the rigidity in bending by a factor of eight. However, the maximum thickness of the overall restoration is limited externally by occlusion and proper anatomic contour and internally by the desire to retain as much tooth structure as possible. Aesthetics requires at least a minimal thickness of about 1.0 mm for the overlying porcelain, which results in severe limits as to the maximum thickness of the metal.

An examination of the mechanical properties (see Table 20–9) of base metal alloys whose compositions were given in Table 20–10 and a gold alloy shows that in general the base metal alloys have a modulus of elasticity approximately twice that of previously used gold alloys. Because elastic modulus is a measure of the stiffness or rigidity of materials, this property would enhance the application of base metal alloys for long-span bridges where flexure is a major cause of failure. Given an equal thickness of precious metal alloy and base metal alloy, the base metal alloy bridge would flex only half as much as the precious alloy material under the same occlusal forces. In a similar manner, the higher modulus of elasticity may be used to permit thinner castings.

The Vickers hardness of base metal alloys may range from approximately 175 to 360 diamond pyramid hardness (DPH). Although certain of the base metal alloys may approach the hardness of noble metal alloy (approximately 160 DPH), most of these alloys are considerably harder. Because of this relatively high hardness, cutting of sprues and grinding and polishing of the prosthesis require the use of high-speed equipment. Clinically, it is improbable that significant occlusal wear of these alloys will occur. Therefore, particular attention must be directed toward perfecting occlusal equilibration. The removal of defective clinical units is also more difficult than with noble metal alloys, because the high hardness results in rapid wear of carbide burs and diamond points.

The ductility (percent elongation) of base metal alloys ranges between approximately 10% and 28%. Noble metal alloys have an elongation of approximately 5% to 10%. Although the base metal alloys would appear to be more burnishable, one must consider the yield strength of the alloys as well before this advantage can be proven.

The density of base metal alloys is approximately 8.0 g/cm³ as compared with 18.4 g/cm³ for comparable high noble metal metal-ceramic alloys (see Table 20–5). Because casting alloys are purchased on a weight basis, a lower density is indirectly reflected to the purchaser, who receives more than twice the volume of material for each unit weight acquired. Also, the intrinsic value of the component elements in base metal alloys is significantly less than that of comparable noble metal alloys. Thus, on the basis of their lower density and the low intrinsic value of the component metals, the cost differential between base metal and noble metal alloys can be substantial.

In addition to the obvious economic considerations, the lower density of base metal alloys may also be a factor in producing adequate dental castings. Because most dental castings are fabricated by centrifugal casting machines, the lower density may play a role in the difficulty reported by some investigators in attaining precision castings with certain of these alloys.

When porcelain is first fired to a metal substructure, the alloy is subjected to considerable temperature variations and stresses induced by the shrinkage of the overlying porcelain. Sag resistance is the property that has been used to describe the ability of an alloy to resist the permanent deformation or creep induced by thermal stresses. It is particularly important in long-span bridges where the porcelain firing temperature may cause the unsupported structure to deform permanently. Under controlled conditions, it has been found that a base metal alloy deforms less than 25 μm, whereas a noble metal alloy deforms 225 μm. It is likely that the higher fusion temperature common to base metal alloys is a factor that contributes to the superior sag resistance properties of these alloys.

The question of metal-ceramic compatibility is basic to the selection of an alloy system for this type of restoration. Two requirements are implicit: the metal must not interact with the ceramic in such a way as to visibly discolor the porcelain at the interface or marginal regions, and the metal-ceramic system must form a stable bond at the interface that can withstand normal stresses which occur in the mouth.

Evaluation of the metal-ceramic bond is complicated by the lack of an accepted laboratory test with proven clinical significance. Different bond strength tests have resulted in widely varying results with regard to the strength of base metal-ceramic bonds. Some tests indicate that the strength of such bonds equals or exceeds that of the high noble metal alloys, whereas other tests indicate the reverse. However, these tests do make clear that different base metal alloys vary widely in their abilities to bond to porcelain. These differences are related to the minor constituents of the alloy. It is also clear that certain base metal-ceramic combinations are incompatible. The ADA acceptance program for metal-ceramic alloys suggests certain screening tests for such compatibility. It is also apparent that the base metal alloys are much more technique sensitive than their high noble metal alloy counterparts. It is fortunate that from a practical point of view, these considerations are primarily a concern for the dental laboratory and the technicians who fabricate prosthetic devices from these alloys.

Clinical Performance. On the basis of recent surveys, the use of base metal alloys has increased rapidly, largely at the expense of the traditional high noble metal-ceramic alloys. Laboratories report a high degree of satisfaction with most of these alloys in terms of the casting, finishing, and application of porcelain veneers.

Comparison of the long-term (10- to 15-year) clinical performance of these alloys has been difficult, because data based on well-controlled scientific clinical studies have not been available. One 5-year study compared several nickel based alloys with a gold alloy. In addition, a 10-year study that includes several other base metal (Ni-Cr) alloy systems is in progress, and the 5-year preliminary results have been reported. Although 5-year data provide important information, the time period is relatively short for detecting clinically significant differences as to long-term behavior. However, both studies indicate that during a period of 5 years the performance of the base metal alloys was acceptable and was comparable to a gold-containing alloy.

As has been stressed throughout this text, the performance of any restoration is related to multiple factors, for example, the design of the appliance, the skill and accuracy with which it has been fabricated, and the properties of the materials used. The successful use of the base metal alloys requires some modification of the laboratory procedures, but it appears to provide clinically acceptable and durable restorations. In the 10-year study noted, all restorations are deteriorating slightly; however, at 5 years, only 4% of all study restorations failed and had to be removed. This included those fabricated using the control alloy. Of these failures, slightly less than half could be associated with the materials themselves, and the rest were the result of patient-related reasons or technical errors in the making of the restorations.

LABORATORY FEES FOR METAL-CERAMIC RESTORATIONS

Density and Cost. Density may be thought of as how much a given volume of material weighs and it is usually expressed in grams per cubic centimeter. Another way of expressing the same idea is specific gravity, which is the ratio of the density of a given material to the density of water. Because the density of water in the metric system is 1 g/cm³, the specific gravity of a material is equal to its density in grams per cubic centimeter. Some manufacturers seem to prefer specific gravity, whereas others seem to prefer density, but as long as the values of density are expressed in grams per cubic centimeter, they can be compared with specific gravity.

The cost of a framework is primarily determined by two factors: the price per ounce of the alloy and the density of the alloy. Gold alloys are of course much more expensive per ounce than base metal alloys. In addition, they have densities that are about twice as great as those of base metal alloys. As a result, a given weight of gold alloy has only half of the volume of the same weight of base metal alloy. Hence, it takes about twice as much gold alloy by weight to make the same casting as base metal alloy.

Premium gold alloys are often priced 30 or more times higher per ounce than base metal alloys. As with the partial denture alloys, the price differential is further aggravated by the large difference in density. PFM gold alloys are even more dense than the type 4 gold removable partial denture alloys. As shown below, when both the price per ounce and the density are considered, the difference in metal cost between a premium gold alloy PFM coping and a base metal alloy coping can be as high as a factor of 80. There are other considerations however, that affect the actual fabrication cost to the laboratory. The gold alloys have scrap value, but the base metal alloys do not. Also, the base metal alloys are generally more difficult and time consuming to finish, and this factor results in higher labor costs.

$$\text{Alloy cost} = \left(\frac{\text{mass}}{\text{volume}}\right)\left(\frac{\text{cost}}{\text{mass}}\right) = \frac{\text{cost}}{\text{volume}}$$

$$\text{Cost of high noble alloy} = (18.2 \text{ g/cm}^3)\left(\frac{\$600}{\text{oz}}\right)\left(\frac{1 \text{ oz}}{31.1 \text{ g}}\right) = \$350/\text{cm}^3$$

$$\text{Cost of base metal alloy} = (8.0 \text{ g/cm}^3)\left(\frac{\$20}{\text{oz}}\right)\left(\frac{1 \text{ oz}}{31.1 \text{ g}}\right) = \$5.20/\text{cm}^3$$

Thus, the cost ratio in this case is 67 to 1 for a cubic centimeter of metal.

Shown in Table 20–11 are some typical laboratory prices on crown and bridge units. Note that the cost difference between crowns or bridges made of Ni-Cr and Pd-Ag alloys is negligible. Based on a 1994 national survey of laboratory owners (Laboratory Management Today, June/July, 1994), this fee schedule was obtained for a variety of crown and bridge procedures. Note that there is a considerable variation in fees for a specific procedure. For example, the national average fee for a three-unit PFM bridge is $252, but this fee ranges from $40 to $492. Likewise, the cost of preparing a porcelain butt-joint margin on a single PFM crown costs an additional $25 on the average, but ranges from $5 to $159. The insurance codes used in the United States for the three ADA classes of alloys are shown in Table 20–12.

TABLE 20–11. U.S. Laboratory Fees for Crown and Bridge Prosthetics and Services—1994

Type of Crown and Bridge Unit	Southeast United States Average Fee ($)	Lowest Price in United States ($)	Highest Price in United States ($)	National Average Fee ($)
3-unit PFM FPD (high noble alloy, excluding alloy cost)	263	37	510	249
3-unit PFM FPD (Pd-Ag or Ni-Cr alloy, including alloy cost)	252	40	492	252
PFM crown (high noble alloy, excluding alloy cost)	90	50	398	89
PFM crown (Pd-Ag or Ni-Cr alloy, including alloy cost)	92	50	252	90
Gold crown (excluding alloy cost)	64	25	135	61
Post and core (base metal)	33	13	109	34

PFM, porcelain fused to metal; FPD, fixed partial denture.

TABLE 20–12. Insurance Codes for American Dental Association's Classes of Alloys

Alloy Type	Insurance Code and Name
High Noble	2750 Single crown—porcelain
	6240 Bridge pontic—porcelain
	6750 Bridge retainer—porcelain
Noble	2752 Single crown—porcelain
	6242 Bridge pontic—porcelain
	6752 Bridge retainer—porcelain
Predominantly Base Metal	2751 Single crown—porcelain
	6241 Bridge pontic—porcelain
	6751 Bridge retainer—porcelain

METALS FOR PARTIAL DENTURE ALLOYS

In this section, base metal (Ni-Cr, Co-Cr, and Ni-Co-Cr) alloys are compared with Type IV gold alloys, which are now used only rarely for partial dentures. The general properties of removable partial denture alloys are listed in Table 20–13.

Base Metal Alloys. According to the ADA classification of 1984, any alloy that contains less than 25 wt% of the noble metals gold, platinum, and palladium is considered a predominantly base metal alloy. Alloys within this category include Co-Cr, Ni-Cr, Ni-Cr-Be, Ni-Co-Cr, and Ti-Al-V. Pure titanium is a base metal element, but it is not a base metal alloy.

Tarnish, Corrosion, and Passivation. High gold alloys contain a high percentage of noble metal elements and thus have an inherent resistance to corrosion because of their low reactivity to oxygen in the atmosphere. Elements in some base metal alloys have a high affinity for oxygen, but the oxide film formed can serve as a protective layer against further oxidation and corrosion. This formation of a protective film by a reactive substance is called *passivation*. Three metals are well known for their passivation potential: aluminum, chromium, and titanium. The most corrosion resistant of these is titanium, which is used for surgical implants, partial denture frameworks, and, most recently, for crowns

TABLE 20–13. Mechanical Properties of Removable Partial Denture Alloys

Alloy	Yield Strength MPa (psi × 10³)	Tensile Strength MPa (psi × 10³)	Percent Elongation	Hardness (VHN)	Modulue of Elasticity MPa × 10³ (psi × 10⁶)
A (Co-Cr)*	710 (103)	870 (120)	1.6	432	223.5 (32.4)
B (Ni-Cr)*	690 (100)	800 (116)	3.8	300	182 (26.4)
C (Co-Cr-Ni)*	470 (68)	685 (99)	8	264	198 (28.7)
D (Fe-Cr)*	703 (102)	841 (122)	9	309	202 (29.3)
Type IV Gold Alloy†	493 (71.5)	776 (112.5)	7	264	90 (13)

*Bench cooled in the investment after casting.
†Age hardened.
VHN, Vickers hardness number.
A, B, C, and D data from Morris HF, Asgar K, Rowe AP, et al: J Prosthet Dent 41:388, 1979.

and bridges. Alloys of Ni-Cr, Ni-Cr-Be, Ni-Co-Cr, and Co-Cr form a coherent, uniform, and nonporous layer of chromium oxide (Cr_2O_3) on their surfaces after exposure to atmospheric oxygen because the oxide is in a lower energy state. This film is self-limiting because it acts as a barrier to the flow of oxygen and metal ions necessary for further oxidation. It also protects the surface from corrosive liquids. For alloys to be protected from corrosion, they must contain a minimum of 12% chromium. Thus, base metal alloys are resistant to tarnish and corrosion not because of their low reactivity (as is the case with high noble and noble alloys) but because of their passivity when protected by a chromium oxide layer.

Castability. When the base metal alloys were first widely introduced in the early 1970s, they were inferior to the gold alloys in castability. Shown in Figure 20–3 is a schematic illustration of rounded or incomplete casting margins that can result from poor alloy castability. Improvements in both alloy composition and operator technique have brought base metal alloys to the point where they are able to cast sharper margins and more intricate patterns than the gold alloys. In particular, the presence of beryllium in Ni-Cr alloys greatly improves the castability of fine details. In PFM alloys it also improves the quality of the oxide layer, an essential aspect of bond formation to porcelain.

Modulus of Elasticity. The modulus of elasticity of a material is a measure of its stiffness or rigidity. This property is important in partial denture alloys, because it determines how thick the various portions of the framework must be to resist deflection. Base metal alloys in general have moduli of elasticity that are more than twice those of Type IV gold alloys. For example, one Co-Cr alloy has an elastic modulus of 218 GPa, whereas a Type IV gold alloy has an elastic modulus of 81 GPa. The result of this large difference in moduli is that base metal alloys can be designed with the same resistance to deflection but in thinner sections than lower modulus alloys. This result holds true even after the Type IV alloys are subjected to a hardening heat treatment (base metal alloys cannot be hardened by heat treatment), because modulus of elasticity is unaffected or only slightly affected by heat treatment. It is a structure-insensitive property, as discussed in Chapter 4. The density of the alloy is also insensitive to heat treatment. Heat treatment of base metal alloys has little effect on their properties.

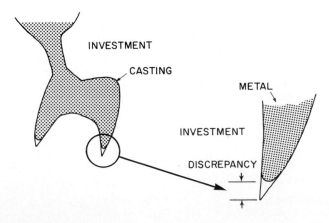

Figure 20–3. Incomplete or rounded casting margin caused by poor alloy castability.

Strength, Hardness, and Ductility. The base metal removable partial denture alloys are generally both harder and stronger than the Type IV gold alloys. The high hardness of some base metal alloys (which varies considerably among brands) is a detriment to finishing and polishing. After a Type IV gold alloy is subjected to a hardening heat treatment, its strength is comparable to that of a typical base metal alloy. For example the yield strength (0.1% offset) for a typical Type IV alloy increases from 320 MPa to 445 MPa after a hardening heat treatment. This value is slightly lower than the yield strength values for base metal alloys. For example, yield strength values (0.1% offset) are 644 MPa for Vitallium (a Co-Cr alloy); 651 MPa for Dentillium P-D (an Fe-Cr alloy); 359 MPa for Howmedica II (an Ni-Cr alloy); and 710 for Ticonium 100 (a Ni-Cr-Be alloy). The gold alloy's hardness, of course, is also increased by the treatment (150 to 185 VHN), but it remains somewhat below the hardness of the base metal alloy (330 VHN for Howmedica III [a Ni-Cr alloy]).

The ductility of Type IV gold alloys is usually much higher (7% elongation) than that of base metal alloys (1.1% elongation for Howmedica III, 1.5% for Vitallium, and 2.4% for Ticonium 100). This property represents a measure of the amount of plastic deformation that a denture framework can withstand before it fractures. The most likely fracture area is the junction between a cast clasp and the metal framework or any point on the clasp arm in which a major nick or other flaw exists, such as porosity.

Commercially Pure Titanium. The element titanium is a lightweight metal with a density of 4.51 g/cm^3 compared with a density of 7.6 g/cm^3 for Ni-Cr and Co-Cr alloys. It has a low elastic modulus of 110 GPa, which is about half that of Ni-Cr and Co-Cr alloys. It has a relatively high melting point of 1668° C and a low thermal expansion coefficient of $8.4 \times 10^{-6}/°$ C. This coefficient is far below the values (12.7 to $14.2 \times 10^{-6}/°$ C) for the porcelains that are typically used for metal-ceramic restorations. Thus, a special low-fusing porcelain is required to minimize the development of thermal tensile stresses in the porcelain veneers. Although its corrosion resistance is excellent at body temperature, it has a relatively poor oxidation resistance above 650° C (1200° F). The room-temperature pure titanium exists as the lower strength, but ductile (17% elongation) α phase. When one heats commercially pure titanium above 883° C, a stronger, more brittle β phase forms.

For general dental applications titanium has the ability to passivate, that is, to change its surface from a chemically active state to much less reactive state by the formation of an extremely thin oxide layer. Even when the surface is scratched or abraded it can reform this protective oxide layer instantaneously. This passivation potential provides a high degree of resistance to attack by most mineral acids and chlorides. Its most prominent attribute is that it is nontoxic and biocompatible with soft and hard tissues. Because of its excellent corrosion resistance, titanium is used for artificial heart pumps, pacemaker cases, heart valve components, and load-bearing hip joints, bone splints, and dental implants. Recently, commercially pure titanium has been used for crowns and removable partial dentures. For treatment of patients with a known hypersensitivity to nickel, pure titanium represents an excellent alternative to base metal alloys that contain nickel.

Titanium Alloys. The most common alloy for dental and medical purposes is the Ti-6Al-4V composition. The main benefits of alloying are significant strengthening and stabilization of the alloy against the formation of either the α phase (through aluminum additions) or the β phase (through additions of copper, palladium, or vanadium). The α-phase alloys are more resistant to high-temperature creep, a most important property for metal-ceramic applications. Because these alloys are insensitive to heat treatment, they are more amenable to brazing or soldering. β-phase alloys are less resistant to creep deformation at elevated temperatures, but they can be hardened and strengthened significantly.

SELECTED READING

Association Report: Classification System for Cast Alloys. J Am Dent Assoc 109:838, 1984.
  A brief description of the revised classification system for all dental casting alloys and a description of the guidelines for each of the three categories.

Council on Dental Materials, Instruments, and Equipment: Report on base metal alloys for crown and bridge applications: Benefits and risks. J Am Dent Assoc 111:479, 1985.
  This report updates the status of base-metal crown and bridge alloys and includes recommendations for handling them, and it includes a discussion of their potential hazards, carcinogenic potential, mechanical properties, and porcelain-metal bond strength.

Covington JS, McBride MA, Slagle WF, and Disney AL: Quantization of nickel and beryllium leakage from base metal casting alloys. J Prosthet Dent 54:127, 1985.
  The results of this in vitro study indicate that Ni-Cr-Be alloys possess a beryllium-rich surface, and both nickel and beryllium may be leached from dental restorations made from such alloys.

Lewis AJ: A metallographic evaluation of porosity occurring in removable partial denture castings. Aust Dent J 24:408, 1979; Lewis AJ: Porosity in base metal partial denture alloys, related industrial alloys, and pure metals. Aust Dent J 22:208, 1977; Lewis AJ: The effect of variations in mould temperature, metal temperature, and mould size on the development of internal porosity in cast structures. Aust Dent J 22:243, 1977; and Lewis AJ: The influence of the refractory investment on the development of porosity in cast structures. Aust Dent J 22:455, 1977.
  A collection of articles evaluating the causes and appearance of porosity in base metal alloy castings.

Lofstrom LH: A comparison of some alternative dental casting alloys. J Mich Dent Assoc 62:443, 1980; and Nitkin DA, and Asgar K: Evaluation of alternative alloys to type 3 gold for use in fixed prosthodontics. J Am Dent Assoc 93:622, 1976.
  These studies compared the castability and handling characteristics of alternative alloys to type 3 gold. In contrast with the earlier work of Nitkin and Asgar, Lofstrom found the silver-palladium alloys to be comparable to type 3 gold alloys in terms of castability and handling characteristics.

Moffa JP, Jenkins WA, Ellison JA, and Hamilton JC: A clinical evaluation of two base metal alloys and a gold alloy for use in fixed prosthodontics: A five-year study. J Prosthet Dent 52:491, 1984.
  This article compares the performance of several base metal alloys in a 5-year well-controlled clinical study. The performances of the various alloys were found to be acceptable.

Morris HF: Veterans Administration Cooperative Studies Project No. 147. IV. Biocompatibility of base metal alloys. J Dent 58:1, 1987.
  This part of a Veterans Affairs study provides an overview and update on the sensitivity levels and carcinogenesis of key base metals such as nickel, chromium, and beryllium.

Morris HF: Veterans Administration Cooperative Studies Project No. 147. I. A multidisciplinary, multicenter experimental design for the evaluation of alternative metal-ceramic alloys. J Prosthet Dent 56:402, 1986.
  This article summarizes the experimental design of one of the more comprehensive long-term (10-year) clinical evaluations of the nickel-based (Ni-Cr) and palladium-based alloys for metal-ceramic restorations. Their performances for 11 criteria are compared with a gold-containing control alloy along with their overall performances. Although some slight differences were noted during the first 5 years of the study, they were not clinically significant.

Morris HF: Veterans Administration Cooperative Studies Project No. 147. VI. Comparison of costs associated with restorations cast from several alternative metal-ceramic alloys. J Prosthet Dent 60:164, 1988.
  This article compares the time required for each of the fabrication procedures involved in making metal-ceramic restorations using each of the study alloys. Although each alloy took slightly longer for different procedures, the total time involved, which included remakes, was essentially the same for each of the alloys. The difference in restoration cost was in the initial cost of the alloy used.

Morris HF: Veterans Administration Cooperative Studies Project No. 147. VII. Comparison of the mechanical properties of different metal-ceramic alloys in the as-cast condition and after simulated porcelain firing cycles. J Prosthet Dent 61:160, 1989.
  This article compares the mechanical properties of several alloys and the changes that result after the porcelain veneer is applied. The nickel-based alloys became weaker, but their elongation increased considerably. Although of interest, these changes were not considered to be large enough to influence the clinical performance of the alloys.

Naylor WP: Introduction to Metal-Ceramic Technology. Chicago, Quintessence, 1992.
  This nine-chapter book covers many aspects of metal-ceramic restorations, including terminology, compari-

sons of alloy properties, alloy classification, and technical aspects of producing and finishing these restora
tions. Although no classification system has been universally accepted, this proposed system is a logical but
more complex alternative to the American Dental Association classification of 1984.*

Naylor WP, and Young JM: Nongold base dental casting alloys, Vol 1: Alternatives to Type 3 Gold.
USAF School of Aerospace Medicine, Brooks Air Force Base, USAFSAM-TR-8449, 1985; and Naylor
WP: Nongold base dental casting alloys, Vol II. Porcelain-fused-to-metal Alloys. USAF School of
Aerospace Medicine, Brooks Air Force Base, USAFSAM-TR-86-5, 1986.

*This two-part series of technical manuals assesses the physical properties and handling characteristics of
Ag-Pd, Ni-Cr-Be, Ni-Cr, and Co-Cr alloys offered as alternatives to type 3 gold (Vol. 1) and palladium-
based noble alloys (high palladium and Pd-Ag) and nickel-based (Ni-Cr-Be and Ni-Cr) and cobalt-based
(Co-Cr) base metal alloys used in the fabrication of metal-ceramic crowns and fixed partial dentures (Vol. 2).*

Prystowsky SD, Allen AM, Smith RW, et al: Allergic contact hypersensitivity to nickel, neomycin,
ethylenediamine, and benzocaine. Arch Dermatol 115:959, 1979.

*Early reports such as this found that 9% of women and 0.09% of men are allergic to nickel. Before the
review of the literature by Morris and coworkers in 1987, these values were believed to be representative of
populations at large.*

Skog E, and Thyresson N: The occupational significance of some contact allergens. Acta Dermatol
Venereol 33:65, 1953.

21 *Inlay Casting Wax*

- Types of Inlay Wax
- Composition
- Desirable Properties
- Flow
- Thermal Properties
- Wax Distortion
- Manipulation of Inlay Wax
- Other Dental Waxes

TYPES OF INLAY WAX

The first procedure in the casting of an inlay or crown for the lost-wax process is the preparation of a wax pattern. The cavity is prepared in the tooth and the pattern is carved, either directly in the tooth or on a die that is a reproduction of the tooth and the prepared cavity. If the pattern is made within the tooth, it is said to be prepared by the *direct technique*. If it is prepared within a die, the procedure is called the *indirect technique*. There are modifications of the techniques, but these two classifications are sufficient for the present purpose.

The American National Standards Institute/American Dental Association (ADA) Specification No. 4 for Dental Inlay Casting Wax covers two types of inlay wax: Type I is for *medium wax* employed in direct techniques, and Type II is for *soft waxes* used in the indirect techniques. Somewhat different properties are required for the various types, as discussed later.

However the pattern is prepared, it should be an accurate reproduction of the missing tooth structure. The wax pattern forms the outline of the mold into which the gold alloy is cast. Consequently, the casting can be no more accurate than the wax pattern, regardless of the care observed in subsequent procedures. Therefore, the pattern should be well adapted to the prepared cavity and properly carved, and the distortion should be minimized. Before the adaptation of the wax pattern within a tooth or a die, a separating medium must be used to ensure the complete separation of the wax pattern without distortion. After the pattern is removed from the prepared cavity, it is surrounded by a gypsum-containing material or other type of refractory material known as an *investment*. This process is called *investing the pattern*. Investments and investing procedures are discussed in Chapters 22 and 23.

Wax patterns are used in the casting of many complex restorations other

461

than inlays and crowns, but the present discussion is limited primarily to the construction of restorations employed in operative dentistry.

COMPOSITION

A number of formulas for inlay wax have been reported, some of which are quite complex. The essential ingredients of a successful inlay wax are paraffin wax, gum dammar, carnauba wax, and a coloring agent. All these substances are of natural origin, derived from mineral or vegetable sources. Paraffin wax is generally the main ingredient, usually in a concentration of 40 to 60 wt%. Paraffin is derived from the high-boiling fractions of petroleum. It is composed mainly of a complex mixture of hydrocarbons of the methane series, together with a minor amount of amorphous or microcrystalline phases. The wax can be obtained in a wide melting or softening range, depending on the molecular weight and distribution of the constituents. The melting range can be determined by a temperature-time cooling curve as shown in Figure 21–1 for a paraffin-based inlay wax. The temperature-time relationship during cooling indicates the successive solidification of progressively lower-molecular-weight fractions. Such a condition is desirable from a dental standpoint because it imparts a moldability to the wax below the temperature of liquefaction. Because paraffin can be obtained with almost any desired melting point, it is evident that the paraffin used for Type I waxes has a higher melting point than does the paraffin used for Type II waxes.

Paraffin wax is likely to flake when it is trimmed, and it does not present a smooth, glossy surface, which is a desirable requisite for an inlay wax. Consequently, other waxes and natural resins are added as modifying agents.

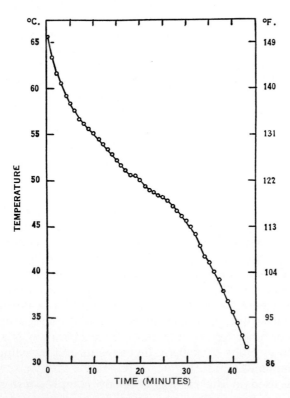

Figure 21–1. Time-temperature cooling curve for Type I inlay wax.

Gum dammar, or dammar resin, is a natural resin. It is added to the paraffin to improve the smoothness in molding and to render it more resistant to cracking and flaking. It also increases the toughness of the wax, and it enhances the smoothness and luster of the surface.

Carnauba wax occurs as a fine powder on the leaves of certain tropical palms. This wax is quite hard, and it has a relatively high melting point. It is combined with the paraffin to decrease the flow at mouth temperature. It has an agreeable odor, and it also contributes to the glossiness of the wax surface even more than does the dammar resin.

Candelilla wax can also be added to partially or entirely replace the carnauba wax. The candelilla wax provides the same general qualities as the carnauba wax, but its melting point is lower, and it is not as hard as carnauba wax. Ceresin may replace part of the paraffin to modify the toughness and carving characteristics of the wax.

In modern inlay waxes, the carnauba wax is often replaced in part with certain synthetic waxes that are compatible with paraffin wax. At least two waxes of this type can be used: one is a complex nitrogen derivative of the higher fatty acids, and the other is composed of esters of acids derived from montan wax, a petroleum derivative. For an impression compound, a synthetic wax is preferable to a natural wax because it has greater uniformity. Because of the high melting point of the synthetic waxes, more paraffin can be incorporated, and the general working qualities of the product are improved.

Control of the properties of the wax is accomplished by a combination of factors. These include the amount of carnauba wax, the melting range of the hydrocarbon wax, and the presence of resin.

DESIRABLE PROPERTIES

Some of the properties that are desirable in an inlay wax can be summarized as follows:

1. When softened, the wax should be uniform. In other words, it should be compounded with ingredients that blend with each other so that there is no graininess or hard spot when the wax is softened.

2. The color should be such that it contrasts with the die material or prepared tooth. It is necessary to carve the wax margins close to the die; therefore, a definite contrast in color facilitates proper finishing of the margins.

3. There should be no flakiness or similar surface roughening when the wax is bent and molded after softening. Such flakiness is likely to be present in paraffin wax, and this is one of the reasons modifiers are added.

4. After the wax pattern has solidified, it is necessary to carve the original tooth anatomy in the wax and, as stated before, to carve the wax at the margins so that the pattern conforms exactly to the surface of the die. The latter procedure sometimes requires that the wax be carved to a very thin layer. If the wax pulls away with the carving instrument or if it chips as it is carved, such precision cannot be attained.

5. As previously noted, after the mold has been formed, the wax is eliminated from the mold. Elimination is usually accomplished by heating the mold so as to ignite the wax. If, after burning, the wax leaves a residue that might provide an impervious coating on the walls of the mold, the final cast inlay may be adversely affected, as described in a later section. Consequently, the wax should burn out, forming carbon, which is later eliminated by oxidation to volatile

gases. ADA Specification No. 4 requires that the melted wax, when it is vaporized at 500° C (932° F), shall leave no solid residue in excess of 0.10% of the original weight of the specimen.

6. Ideally, the wax pattern should be completely rigid and dimensionally stable at all times until it is eliminated. The wax pattern is subject to flow unless it is handled carefully. It is also subject to relaxation, a factor that must be taken into consideration in its manipulation.

FLOW

One of the desirable properties of the Type I inlay wax is that it exhibits a marked plasticity or flow at a temperature slightly above that of the mouth. The temperatures at which the wax is plastic are indicated by the time-temperature cooling curve for a typical Type I wax shown in Figure 21–1. The interpretation of this curve is the same as for its counterpart—a typical time-temperature cooling curve for a solid solution alloy. The wax begins to harden at approximately 56° C (133° F), the point at which the curve first departs from a straight line, and it is solid below approximately 40° C (104° F), when it again cools at a constant rate.

Inlay waxes do not solidify with a space lattice, as does a metal. Instead the structure is more likely to be a combination of crystalline and amorphous materials, displaying limited ordering of the molecules. The wax lacks rigidity and may flow under stress even at room temperature.

ADA Specification No. 4 provides certain requirements for the flow properties of inlay waxes at specific temperatures, as seen in Table 21–1. The flow is measured by subjecting cylindrical specimens to a designated load at the stated temperature and measuring the percentage of reduction in length. The maximum flow permitted for Type I waxes at 37° C (98° F) is 1%. The low flow at this temperature permits carving and removal of the pattern from the prepared cavity at oral temperature without distortion. In addition, both Type I and Type II waxes must have a minimal flow of 70% at 45° C (113° F) and a maximum flow of 90%. At approximately this temperature, the wax is inserted into the prepared cavity. If the wax does not have sufficient plasticity, it does not flow into all of the areas in the preparation and reproduce the required detail.

THERMAL PROPERTIES

As previously noted, the inlay waxes are softened with heat, forced into the prepared cavity in either the tooth or the die, and cooled. The thermal conductivity of the waxes is low, and time is required both to heat them uniformly throughout and to cool them to body or room temperature.

Another thermal characteristic of inlay waxes is their high coefficient of

TABLE 21–1. Flow (%) Requirements for ADA Specification No. 4

Type of Inlay Wax	30° C	37° C	40° C		45° C	
	Max	Max	Min	Max	Min	Max
1	—	1.0	—	20	70	90
2	1	—	50	—	70	90

Max, maximum; Min, minimum.

thermal expansion. As shown in Figure 21-2, the wax may expand as much as 0.7% with an increase in temperature of 20° C (36° F) or contract as much as 0.35% when it is cooled from 37° C to 25° C (99° F to 77° F). The average linear coefficient of thermal expansion over such a temperature range is 350×10^{-6} per degree centigrade.

A comparison of the coefficients of thermal expansion of dental materials given in the chapter on physical properties indicates that inlay wax expands and contracts thermally more per degree temperature change than any other dental material. This is one of the disadvantages inherent in waxes, when they are used in the direct technique. This property is less significant when the wax is used in the indirect technique because the pattern is not subjected to a change from mouth to room temperature. In fact, ADA Specification No. 4 contains no requirements for thermal expansion for Type II waxes. A maximum of 0.6% linear change in dimension when they are heated from 25° C to 37° C (77° F to 99° F) is permitted for Type I waxes.

The amount of the thermal dimensional change may be affected by the previous treatment of the wax. Curve A in Figure 21-2 represents the thermal expansion of an inlay wax that has been previously cooled under pressure. As can be observed, the expansion rate increases abruptly above approximately 35° C (95° F). The temperature at which the change in rate occurs is known as the *glass transition temperature*. Some constituents of the wax probably change crystalline form at this temperature, and the wax is more plastic at higher temperatures. Not all waxes exhibit transition temperatures; the transition point shown in Figure 21-2 appears to be characteristic of a paraffin wax.

If the wax is allowed to cool without being placed under pressure, the transition temperature is not so pronounced when it is reheated, nor is the

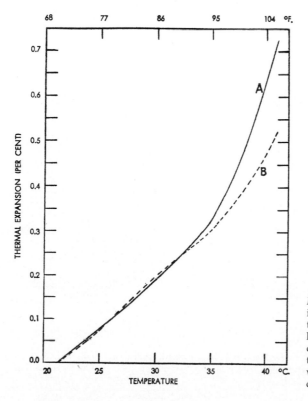

Figure 21–2. Thermal expansion of inlay wax. Curve A represents the thermal expansion when the wax was held under pressure while it was cooling from the liquid state. When the same wax was allowed to cool without pressure and again heated, curve B resulted.

change in the linear coefficient of thermal expansion so great, as shown in curve B of Figure 21–2. There is another possible explanation for the difference in behavior, on reheating, of a wax cooled under pressure and the same wax cooled without applied pressure. It is related to the behavior of dissolved or occluded air or solvents. Certain waxes have a phenomenal capacity for gas and solvent retention, which may often remain undetected. The gas trapped within the wax expands on reheating, causing a pronounced expansion as the wax becomes sufficiently plastic to flow.

Other factors, such as the temperature of the die and the method used for applying pressure to the wax as it solidifies, also influence the coefficient of thermal expansion. However, this property of inlay waxes is probably not a serious problem when they are used in the indirect technique, provided no marked variation in temperature occurs after the removal of the pattern from the die.

WAX DISTORTION

Distortion is probably the most serious problem that one can experience when forming and removing the pattern from the mouth or die. It results from thermal changes and the release of stresses that arise from contraction on cooling, occluded air, change of shape during molding, carving, removal, and time and temperature during storage.

Waxes, like other thermoplastics, tend to return to their original shape after manipulation. This is commonly known as *elastic memory*. A stick of inlay wax can be softened over a Bunsen burner, bent into a horseshoe shape, and chilled in this position. If it is then floated in room-temperature water for a number of hours, the horseshoe will open as shown in Figure 21–3A and B. This is more critical in inlay waxes than other impression materials, because the resulting metallic restorations must fit onto unyielding hard tooth tissue.

The elastic memory of waxes is further illustrated during the measurement of the thermal expansion of a wax that was held under pressure during cooling.

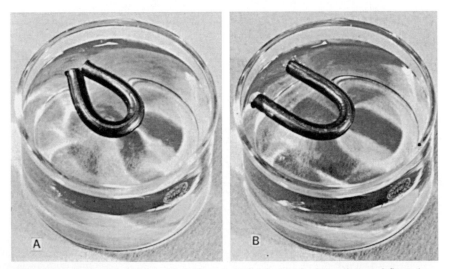

Figure 21–3. *A,* A stick of inlay wax is bent into the shape of a horseshoe and floated on water at room temperature. *B,* After 24 hours the same stick of wax tends to relax and distortion occurs.

The expansion increased above the glass transition temperature, more so than when it is cooled without pressure, as shown in Figure 21–1. Again, this illustrates the nature of wax to try to return to its normal uninhibited state. In recalling Figure 21–3A, when the wax was bent into a horseshoe, the inner molecules were under compression and the outer ones were in tension. Once the stresses were gradually relieved at room temperature, the wax tended to straighten.

The possible effect of storing the wax pattern is shown in Figure 21–4. Note that the casting fits best when the pattern is invested immediately after its removal from the preparation (Fig 21–4A).

MANIPULATION OF INLAY WAX

In the process of manipulating inlay wax, dry heat is generally preferred to the use of a water bath. The latter can result in the inclusion of droplets of water that could splatter on flaming, smear the wax surface during polishing, and distort the pattern during thermal changes.

When stick wax is softened over a flame, care should be taken not to overheat it. It should be twirled until it becomes shiny and then removed from the flame. The process is repeated until the wax is warm throughout. It is then kneaded together and shaped to the prepared cavity. Type I wax has adequate plasticity in a temperature range safely tolerated by the pulp. Pressure should be applied by the finger or by the patient biting on the wax. It is cooled gradually at mouth temperature, not by cold water.

Care should be exercised in removing the pattern. It should be hooked with an explorer point and rotated out of the cavity. A mesial-occlusal-distal (MOD) pattern can best be removed by luting a staple so that each prong is fastened above a corresponding step portion. It can then be removed with dental floss looped through the staple and withdrawn in a direction parallel to the axial walls, and with minimum distortion. After removal, touching with the fingers should be avoided as much as possible to prevent any temperature changes.

For fabricating indirect patterns, first lubricate the die, preferably with a lubricant containing a wetting agent. Any excess must be avoided, because it would prevent intimate adaptation to the die. The melted wax may be added in layers with a spatula or a waxing instrument, or it may be painted on with a brush. The prepared cavity is overfilled, and the wax is then carved to the proper contour. When the margins are being carved, extreme care should be taken to avoid abrading any surface of the stone die. A silk cloth may be used

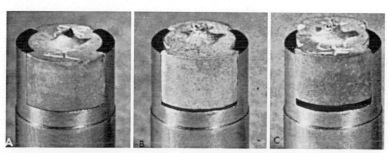

Figure 21–4. Castings made from patterns prepared with melted wax cooled under pressure. *A,* Pattern invested immediately. *B,* Pattern stored for 2 hours before investing. *C,* Pattern stored for 12 hours before investing.

for a final polishing of the pattern, rubbing toward the margins. Theoretically, applying pressure is undesirable (see Fig. 21–2). However, many clinicians prefer to apply finger pressure as the wax is cooling to help fill the cavity and to prevent distortion during cooling. The fingers also accelerate the cooling. Again, although temperature changes should be avoided, some careful operators repeatedly remelt tiny portions around the margins while carving and examine them under a low-power microscope.

Another excellent method of fabrication is to swage the pattern. The die and pattern are mounted in a closed vessel with a piston and containing water, preferably at 38° C (100° F). When a pressure is applied to the piston, a hydrostatic pressure is applied evenly over the finished pattern. This minimizes the final distortion.

Regardless of the method chosen, the most practical method for avoiding any possible delayed distortion is to invest the pattern immediately after removal from the mouth or the die, as noted earlier. Once the investment hardens, there will be no more distortion of the pattern.

Softer waxes, having higher flow, produce larger castings than harder waxes because the former expand more as the investment warms during setting. Also they offer less resistance to the expanding investment during setting.

As the emphasis on economics continues to increase, faster waxing procedures are being accentuated. In some dental laboratories, it is virtually an assembly line process. To meet this need, the use of dipping waxes that are kept molten for constant usage has evolved. Although standard types of inlay waxes may be used, the trend has included newer types that are more "rubbery," tending toward the amorphous rather than the crystalline nature. Wax pots that can be set to different temperatures are used. The properties of these "dipping" waxes have not been characterized, nor do they fall into any present specification. As these waxes become more popular and better understood, their standardization will eventually be forthcoming.

Waxes oxidize on heating, and on prolonged heating some evaporate. There will also be a darkening and a precipitation of gummy deposits. Therefore, care should be exercised to use the lowest temperature possible and to clean the pot and replace the wax periodically.

OTHER DENTAL WAXES

There are a number of other types of waxes employed for somewhat different purposes than the inlay waxes described. The composition of each type is adjusted for the particular requirements called for. One of the most common is *baseplate wax.*

As the name suggests, baseplate wax is used principally to establish the initial arch form in the construction of complete dentures. Supplied in 1- to 2-mm thick red or pink sheets, the wax is approximately 75% paraffin or ceresin, with additions of beeswax and other resins or waxes. ADA specification No. 24 includes Types I, II, and III, also designated as soft, medium, and hard, respectively. The differentiation from one type to another is by the percentage of flow of each type at room temperature, at mouth temperature, and at 45° C (113° F). The harder the wax, the less the flow at a given temperature. The difference in flow of the three types is advantageous in the particular usage. Type I, a soft wax, is used for building veneers; Type II, a medium wax, is designed for patterns to be tried in the mouth in normal climatic conditions; and Type III, a hard wax, is for trial fitting in the mouth in tropical climates. Because residual stress is present within the wax from contouring and manipulating the wax, the finished denture pattern should be flasked as soon as possible after completion.

Another group of dental waxes is composed of the impression waxes, also referred to as *bite* or *corrective waxes*. They distort if they are withdrawn from undercut areas and therefore are limited to use in edentulous portions of the mouth. Although corrective waxes are quite soft at mouth temperature, they do have sufficient body to register the detail of soft tissue, and they are rigid at room temperature.

Other waxes include the *sticky waxes,* which are quite tacky when they are melted but firm and brittle when they are cooled. These waxes are used to join and temporarily stabilize the components of a bridge before soldering or the pieces of a broken denture prior to the repair. *Boxing wax* is yet another useful material for enclosing an impression before the plaster or stone cast is poured.

SELECTED READING

Baum L, Phillips RW, and Lund MR: Textbook of Operative Dentistry, 2nd ed. Philadelphia, WB Saunders, 1985.
Techniques for manipulating wax and forming the pattern are described.
Craig RG, Eick JD, and Peyton FA: Strength properties of waxes at various temperatures and their practical application. J Dent Res 46:300, 1967.
Properties of waxes are controlled by the composition and melting range of certain components.
Steinbock AF: An overview of dental waxes. Dental Lab News, July, p 50, 1989.
An excellent review of the various types of waxes, their composition, and their properties.

22 *Investments for Small Castings*

- Gypsum-bonded Investments
- Phosphate-bonded Investments
- Ethyl Silicate–bonded Investments

The principal laboratory method used to form metal inlays, onlays, crowns, and bridges is to cast molten metal by centrifugal force or under pressure into a mold cavity that was formed by a sprued wax pattern. A *sprue* is the channel in a refractory investment mold through which molten metal flows. After the wax pattern has been made, either directly on a prepared tooth or on a die replica of the tooth, a *sprue former* is attached to it, and it is surrounded with investment. The investment material is mixed in the same manner as plaster or dental stone, placed around the pattern, and allowed to set. After the investment hardens, the sprue former is removed. The wax is also eliminated by boiling in water or by burning it out in an oven. This process is called *burnout*. The molten metal is then forced into the mold cavity left by the wax, through the *sprue* or *ingate* created by the sprue former. These procedures are described in detail in Chapter 23.

The following discussion deals with the investments used for the fabrication of small dental castings (i.e., inlays, onlays, and crowns). Generally, two types of investment—gypsum-bonded and the phosphate-bonded investment—are employed, depending on the melting range of the alloy and the preference of the clinician. The gypsum-based materials represent the type traditionally used for conventional gold alloys. The phosphate-based investments are designed primarily for alloys used in the metal-ceramic restoration (see Chapter 26). A third type is the ethyl silicate–bonded investment, which is used principally in the casting of removable partial dentures with base metal alloy.

GYPSUM-BONDED INVESTMENTS

American Dental Association (ADA) Specification No. 2 for casting investments for dental gold alloys encompasses three types of investments. The types are determined by whether the appliance to be fabricated is fixed or removable, and the method of obtaining the expansion required to compensate for the contraction of the molten gold alloy during solidification. Type I investments are those employed for the casting of inlays or crowns when the alloy casting shrinkage compensation is accomplished principally by thermal expansion of the investment. Type II investments are also used for the casting of inlays or crowns, but the major mode of compensation is by the hygroscopic expansion of the investment. Type III investments are used in the construction of partial dentures with gold alloys. This chapter is concerned only with Type I and II investments.

Composition

As already noted, the essential ingredients of the dental inlay investment employed with the conventional gold casting alloys are α-hemihydrate of gypsum and a form of silica. Most investments now contain α-hemihydrate because greater strength is obtained. This gypsum product serves as a binder to hold the other ingredients together and to provide rigidity. The strength of the investment is dependent on the amount of binder present. The investment may contain 25% to 45% of the gypsum product.

Gypsum. The α-hemihydrate form of gypsum is generally the binder for investments used in casting gold-containing alloys with melting ranges below 1000° C (1800° F). When this material is heated to the temperatures required for complete dehydration and sufficiently high to ensure complete castings, it shrinks considerably and frequently fractures.

The thermal expansion curves of the three common forms of gypsum products are shown in Figure 22–1. All forms shrink considerably after dehydration between 200° C and 400° C (392° F to 750° F). A slight expansion then occurs between 400° C and approximately 700° C (1300° F), and then a large contraction occurs. This latter shrinkage is most likely caused by decomposition, and sulfur gases, such as sulfur dioxide, are emitted. This decomposition not only causes shrinkage but also contaminates the castings with the sulfides of the non-noble alloying elements, such as silver and copper. Thus, it is imperative that gypsum investments not be heated above 700° C (1300° F). However, for gypsum products containing carbon, the maximum temperature should be 650° C (1200° F). In this way, proper fit as well as uncontaminated alloys are obtained.

Usually, castings that are made in pure gypsum molds are extremely undersized. The α-hemihydrate, which requires less mixing water and shrinks less (as shown in Figure 22–1), is now the optimum choice as a binder.

Silica. Silica (SiO_2) is added to provide a refractory during the heating of the investment and to regulate the thermal expansion. Usually, the wax pattern is eliminated from the mold by heat. During the heating, the investment is expected to expand thermally to compensate partially or totally for the casting shrinkage of the gold alloy. As shown in Figure 22–1, gypsum shrinks considerably when it is heated, regardless of whether it is set plaster or stone.

If the proper form of silica is employed in the investment, this contraction during heating can be eliminated and changed to an expansion. Silica exists in at least four allotropic forms: quartz, tridymite, cristobalite, and fused quartz. The first and third forms are of particular dental interest.

When quartz, tridymite, or cristobalite is heated, a change in crystalline form occurs at a transition temperature characteristic of the particular form of silica. For example, when quartz is heated, it inverts from a "low" form, known as α-quartz, to a "high" form, called β-quartz, at a temperature of 575° C (1067° F). In a similar manner, cristobalite undergoes an analogous transition between

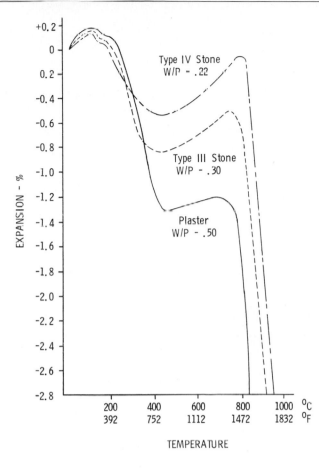

Figure 22–1. Dimensional change of three forms of gypsum when heated. (Courtesy of R. Neiman, Whip-Mix Corporation, Louisville, KY.)

200° C (392° F) and 270° C (518° F) from "low," called α-cristobalite, to "high," called β-cristobalite. Two inversions of tridymite occur at 117° C (243° F) and 163° C (325° F), respectively. The α-allotropic forms are stable only above the transition temperature noted, and an inversion to the lower or α form occurs on cooling in each case. In powdered form, the inversions occur over a range of temperature rather than instantaneously.

The density decreases as the α form changes to the β form, with a resulting increase in volume that is exhibited by a rapid increase in the linear expansion as indicated in Figure 22–2. Consequently, the shrinkage of gypsum shown in Figure 22–1 can be counterbalanced by the inclusion of one or more of the crystalline silicas.

Fused quartz is amorphous and glasslike in character, and it exhibits no inversion at any temperature below its fusion point. It has an extremely low linear coefficient of thermal expansion and is of little use in dental investments.

Quartz, cristobalite, or a combination of the two forms may be used in a dental investment. Both are now available in pure form. Tridymite is no longer an expected impurity in cristobalite. On the basis of the type of silica principally employed, dental investments are often classified as *quartz* or *cristobalite investments*.

Modifiers. In addition to silica, certain modifying agents, coloring matter, and reducing agents, such as carbon and powdered copper, are present. The reducing agents are used in some investments to provide a nonoxidizing atmosphere in the mold when the gold alloy is cast.

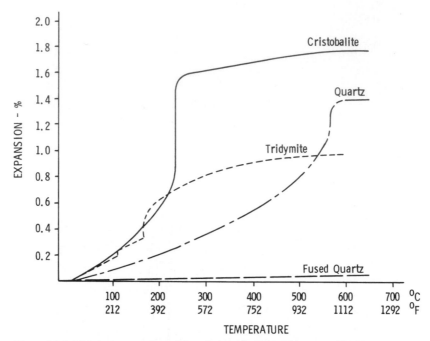

Figure 22–2. Thermal expansion of four forms of silica. (Courtesy of R. Neiman, Whip-Mix Corporation, Louisville, KY.)

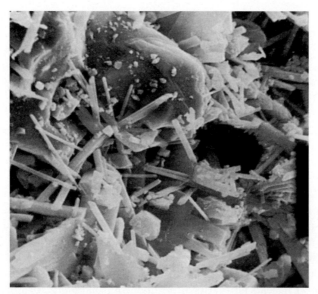

Figure 22–3. Microstructure of the surface of a set cristobalite investment. The large, irregular particles are the silica refractory, and the rodlike particles are cristobalite. ×3000. (Courtesy of R. Earnshaw.)

Unlike the dental stones, a setting expansion is usually desirable to assist in compensating for the contraction of the alloy. Some of the added modifiers, such as boric acid and sodium chloride, not only regulate the setting expansion and the setting time, but they also prevent most of the shrinkage of gypsum when it is heated above 300° C (572° F), as discussed subsequently. In some instances, the modifiers are limited to the usual *balancing agents* to regulate the setting time and setting expansion, as described for the dental stones. The microstructure of a set gypsum-bonded investment can be seen in Figure 22–3.

Setting Time

The setting time of an investment can be measured in the same manner as plaster. Furthermore, it can be controlled in the same manner. According to ADA Specification No. 2 for dental inlay casting investment, the setting time should not be shorter than 5 minutes nor longer than 25 minutes. Usually, the modern inlay investments set initially in 9 to 18 minutes. Sufficient time should be allowed for mixing and investing the pattern before the investment sets.

Normal Setting Expansion

A mixture of silica and gypsum hemihydrate results in setting expansion greater than that of the gypsum product when it is used alone. The silica particles probably interfere with the intermeshing and interlocking of the crystals as they form. Thus, the thrust of the crystals is outward during growth, and they increase expansion.

Generally, the resulting setting expansion in such a case is high. ADA Specification No. 2 for Type I investment permits a maximum setting expansion *in air* of only 0.6%. The setting expansion of such modern investments is approximately 0.4%. It can be regulated by retarders and accelerators, as described previously.

The purpose of the setting expansion is to aid in enlarging the mold to compensate partially for the casting shrinkage of the gold. There is some doubt that all of the setting expansion is effective in expanding the wax pattern. The normal setting expansion of investment has traditionally been determined in a manner similar to that for dental plaster, in which the expansion is measured as the linear dimensional change that occurs as the investment sets in a V-shaped trough. Thus, the normal setting expansion can occur essentially unrestricted. However, the trough technique does not accurately measure the actual or effective expansion of the investment while it is setting under the conditions of practical usage. For example, the effectiveness of the setting expansion in enlarging the mold containing the wax pattern may be related to the thermal expansion of the pattern caused by the heat of reaction that occurs coincidentally with the setting of the investment. It follows from such a theory that the setting expansion is effective only to the extent that the exothermic heat is transmitted to the pattern. The amount of heat present depends on the gypsum content of the investment; therefore, the setting expansion of an investment with a comparatively high gypsum content is more effective in enlarging the mold than is a product with a lower gypsum content. Likewise, manipulative conditions that increase the exothermic heat increase the effective setting expansion (e.g., the lower the water:powder ratio for the investment, the greater is the effective setting expansion).

Variables other than the exothermic heat of reaction also influence the effective setting expansion. As the investment sets, it eventually gains sufficient strength to produce a dimensional change in the wax pattern as setting expansion occurs. The inner core of the investment within a mesial-occlusal-distal (MOD) wax pattern can actually force the proximal walls outward to a certain extent. If the pattern has a thin wall, then the effective setting expansion is somewhat greater than for a pattern with thicker walls because the investment can move the thinner wall more readily. Also, the softer the wax, the greater the effective setting expansion, because the softer wax is more readily moved by the expanding investment. If a wax softer than a Type II inlay wax is used, the setting expansion may cause a serious distortion of the pattern.

Hygroscopic Setting Expansion

The theory of the hygroscopic setting expansion was previously described in connection with the setting of dental plaster and stone. It was pointed out that the hygroscopic setting expansion differs from the normal setting expansion in that it occurs when the gypsum product is allowed to set under or in contact with water and that it is greater in magnitude than the normal setting expansion.

The hygroscopic setting expansion was first discovered in connection with an investigation of the dimensional changes of a dental investment during setting. As illustrated in Figure 22–4, the hygroscopic setting expansion may be six or

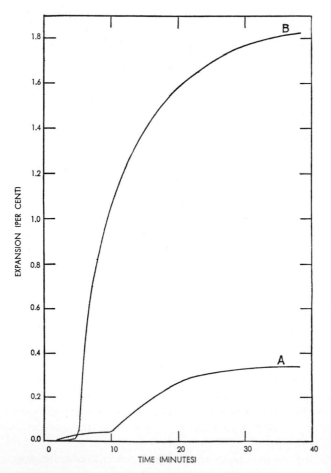

Figure 22–4. Curve A, normal setting expansion of dental investment; Curve B, hygroscopic setting expansion. Water was added 5 minutes after the beginning of mixing; the water:powder ratio is 0.30.

more times the normal setting expansion of a dental investment. In fact, when it is measured on a mercury bath, it may be as high as 5 linear percent. As discussed in Chapter 23, the hygroscopic setting expansion is one of the methods for expanding the casting mold to compensate for the casting shrinkage of the gold alloy.

Commercial investments exhibit different amounts of hygroscopic expansion. Although all investments appear to be subject to hygroscopic expansion, the expansion in some instances is not as great as in others. For this reason, certain investments are specially formulated to provide a substantial hygroscopic expansion when the investment is permitted to set in contact with water. ADA Specification No. 2 for such Type II investments requires a minimum setting expansion in water of 1.2%; the maximum expansion permitted is 2.2%. As discussed in the following sections, a number of factors are important in the control of the hygroscopic expansion.

Effect of Composition. The magnitude of the hygroscopic setting expansion of a dental investment is generally proportional to the silica content of the investment, other factors being equal. The finer the particle size of the silica, the greater the hygroscopic expansion. In general, the α-hemihydrate is apt to produce a greater hygroscopic expansion in the presence of silica than is the β-hemihydrate, particularly when the expansion is unrestricted. As previously stated in Chapter 9, the hygroscopic expansion of the stone or plaster alone is slight.

A dental investment should have enough hemihydrate binder with the silica to provide sufficient strength after hygroscopic expansion. Otherwise, a shrinkage occurs during the subsequent drying of the set investment. At least 15% of binder is necessary to prevent a drying shrinkage.

Effect of the Water:Powder Ratio. The higher the water:powder ratio of the original investment water mixture, the less the hygroscopic setting expansion. This effect is more marked in some commercially available investments than in others.

Effect of Spatulation. With most investments, as the mixing time is reduced, the hygroscopic expansion is decreased. This factor is important in connection with the control of the effective setting expansion as well.

Shelf Life of the Investment. The older the investment, the lower is its hygroscopic expansion. Consequently, the amount of investment purchased at one time should be limited.

Effect of Time of Immersion. The greatest amount of hygroscopic setting expansion is observed if the immersion takes place before the initial set. The longer the immersion of the investment in the water bath is delayed beyond the time of the initial set of the investment, the lower is the hygroscopic expansion.

Effect of Confinement. Both the normal and the hygroscopic setting expansions are confined by opposing forces, such as the walls of the container in which the investment is placed or the walls of a wax pattern. However, the confining effect on the hygroscopic expansion is much more pronounced than the similar effect on the normal setting expansion. The effective hygroscopic setting expansion is, therefore, likely to be less in proportion to the expected expansion than is the normal setting expansion.

When the dimensional change in the wax pattern itself is measured after investing, the increase in the effective setting expansion when the investment is immersed in a 38° C (100° F) water bath is apparently not primarily the result of hygroscopic expansion. Rather, it is caused mainly by the softening of the wax pattern at the water-bath temperature, permitting an increase in effective setting expansion. The latter results from a combination of thermal expansion of the wax pattern plus the softened condition of the wax, reducing its confining effect on the expansion of the setting investment. This is substantiated by the fact that immersion in room-temperature water reduces the effective expansion.

Effect of the Amount of Added Water. In the previous discussions, it has been assumed that the investment was immersed in a water bath to absorb as much water as necessary to control the expansion. However, the magnitude of the hygroscopic setting expansion can be controlled by the amount of water that is added to the setting investment.

It has been proved that the magnitude of the hygroscopic expansion is in direct proportion to the amount of water added during the setting period until a maximum expansion occurs. No further expansion is evident regardless of any amount of water added.

The effect of some of the factors previously discussed (water:powder ratio, mixing, and shelf life) on the maximum hygroscopic setting expansion is illustrated in Figure 22–5 relative to the amount of water added.

As shown in Figure 22–5, the magnitude of the hygroscopic setting expansion below the maximum expansion value is dependent only on the amount of water added and is independent of the water:powder ratio, the amount of mixing, and the age or shelf life of the investment. This finding is the basis for a mold expansion technique to be described in Chapter 23.

As discussed in connection with the hygroscopic expansion of gypsum products (see Chapter 9), the hygroscopic setting expansion is a continuation of the ordinary setting expansion because the immersion water replaces the water of hydration and thus prevents the confinement of the growing crystals by the

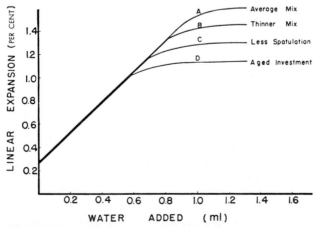

Figure 22–5. Graphic representation of the relation of the linear hygroscopic setting expansion and the amount of water added as influenced by certain manipulative factors. (From Asgar K, Mahler DB, and Peyton FA: Hygroscopic technique for inlay casting using controlled water additions. J Prosthet Dent 5:711, 1955.)

surface tension of the excess water. Because of the diluent effect of the quartz particles, the hygroscopic setting expansion in these investments is greater than that of the gypsum binder when used alone. This effect is the same as previously described for normal setting expansion.

The phenomenon is purely physical. The hemihydrate binder is not necessary for the hygroscopic expansion because investments with other binders exhibit a similar expansion when they are allowed to set under water. As a matter of fact, expansion can be detected when water is poured into a vessel containing only small, smooth quartz particles. The water is drawn between the particles by capillary action and thus causes the particles to separate, creating an expansion. The effect is not permanent after the water is evaporated, unless a binder is present.

Any water-insoluble powder that is wettable can be mixed with the gypsum hemihydrate, and hygroscopic expansion results. Consequently, the quartz is not a factor. The influence of all the factors previously described can be related to the theory presented. The greater the amount of the silica or the inert filler, the more easily the added water can diffuse through the setting material and the greater is the expansion, for the same reason as described for the normal setting expansion of investment. The water:powder ratio affects the hygroscopic expansion for the same reason that it affects the normal setting expansion. Once setting starts, the later water is added to the investment, the less is the hygroscopic setting expansion because part of the crystallization has already started in a "normal" fashion. Some of the crystals have intermeshed and inhibit further crystal growth after the water is added. On the same basis, the less water that is added, the lower is the expansion; that is, there is less counteraction of the surface tension.

Finally, the term *hygroscopic* in a strict sense is a misnomer. Although the added water may be drawn into the setting material by capillary action, the effect is not related to hygroscopy. Furthermore, on the basis of the theory, the hygroscopic setting expansion is as normal a phenomenon as that which occurs during normal setting expansion. However, the terms have gained general acceptance by usage even though they may be inaccurate on the basis of theoretical considerations.

Thermal Expansion

As noted in a previous section, the thermal expansion of a gypsum-bonded investment is directly related to the amount of silica present and to the type of silica employed. A considerable amount of quartz is necessary to counterbalance the contraction of the gypsum during heating. Even when the quartz content of the investment is increased to 60%, with the balance being hemihydrate binder, the initial contraction of the gypsum is not eliminated.

The contraction of the gypsum is entirely balanced when the quartz content is increased to 75% (Fig. 22–6). If a sufficient amount of setting expansion had been present, the casting made at 700° C (1292° F) would probably have fit the die reasonably well. The thermal expansion curves of quartz investments are influenced by the particle size of the quartz, the type of gypsum binder, and the resultant water:powder ratio necessary to provide a workable mix.

The effect of cristobalite compared with that of quartz is strikingly demonstrated in Figure 22–7. Because the much greater expansion that occurs during the inversion of the cristobalite, the normal contraction of the gypsum during heating is easily eliminated. Furthermore, the expansion occurs at a lower

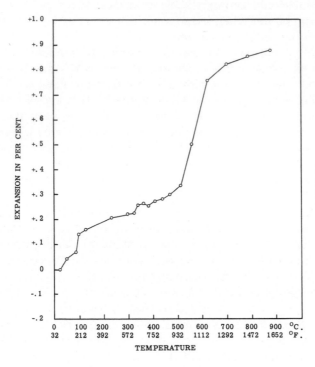

Figure 22–6. Thermal expansion of an investment that contains 25% plaster of Paris and 75% quartz. (Courtesy of G. C. Paffenbarger.)

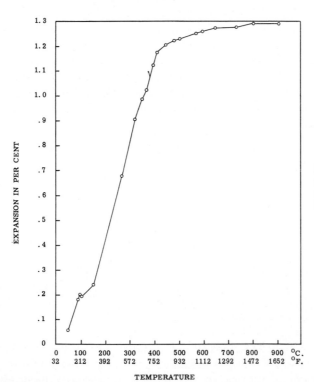

Figure 22–7. Thermal expansion of an investment that contains cristobalite instead of quartz. (Courtesy of G. C. Paffenbarger.)

temperature because of the lower inversion temperature of the cristobalite in comparison with that of quartz. As can be noted in Figure 22–7, a reasonably good fit of the castings is obtained when the gold alloy is cast into the mold at temperatures of 500° C (932° F) and higher.

The thermal expansion curves of an investment give one some idea of the form of the silica that is present. As can be seen from Figures 22–6 and 22–7, the investments containing cristobalite expand earlier and to a greater extent than those containing quartz. Some of the modern investments probably contain both quartz and cristobalite.

The desirable magnitude of the thermal expansion of a dental investment depends on its use. If the hygroscopic expansion is to be used to compensate for the contraction of the gold alloy, as for the Type II investments, ADA Specification No. 2 requires that the thermal expansion be between 0% and 0.6% at 500° C (932° F). However, for the Type I investments, which rely principally on thermal expansion for compensation, the thermal expansion must be not less than 1% nor greater than 1.6%. In addition, the specification establishes minimum and maximum values for the combined setting or hygroscopic expansion, whichever the case may be, and the respective thermal expansion.

Another desirable feature of an inlay investment is that its maximum thermal expansion be attained at a temperature not higher than 700° C (1292° F). Thus, when a thermal expansion technique is employed, the maximum mold temperature for the casting of gold alloy should be less than 700° C. As noted earlier and as shown later, the gold alloys can become contaminated at a mold temperature higher than this.

Effect of the Water:Powder Ratio. The magnitude of thermal expansion is related to the amount of solids present. Therefore, it is apparent that the more water that is used in mixing the investment, the less is the thermal expansion that is achieved during subsequent heating. This effect is demonstrated by the curves shown in Figure 22–8. Although the variations in the water:powder ratios shown are rather extreme, the curves indicate that it is imperative to measure the water and powder accurately if the proper compensation is to be realized.

Effect of Chemical Modifiers. A disadvantage of an investment that contains sufficient silica to prevent any contraction during heating is that the weakening effect of the silica in such quantities is likely to be too great. The addition of small amounts of sodium, potassium, or lithium chlorides to the investment eliminates the contraction caused by the gypsum and increases the expansion without the presence of an excessive amount of silica.

Boric acid has a similar effect. It also hardens the set investment. However, it apparently disintegrates during the heating of the investment and a roughened surface on the casting may result. Silicas do not prevent gypsum shrinkage but counterbalance it, whereas chlorides actually reduce gypsum shrinkage below temperatures of approximately 700° C (1292° F).

Thermal Contraction

When an investment is cooled from 700° C, its contraction curve follows the expansion curve during the inversion of the β quartz or cristobalite to its stable form at room temperature. Actually, the investment contracts to less than its original dimension. This contraction below the original dimension is unrelated

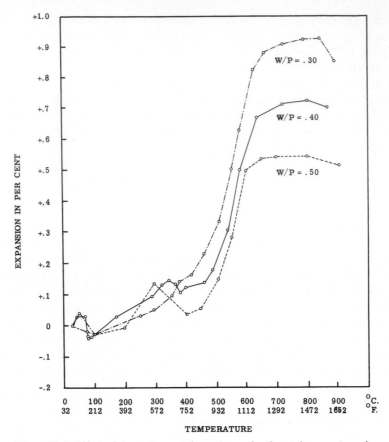

Figure 22–8. Effect of the water:powder ratio on the thermal expansion of an investment that contains 20% plaster of Paris and 80% quartz. (Courtesy of G. C. Paffenbarger.)

to any property of the silica; it occurs because of the shrinkage of gypsum when it is first heated.

If the investment is reheated, it expands thermally to the same maximum reached when it was first heated. However, in practice the investment should not be heated a second time because internal cracks may develop.

Strength

The strength of the investment must be adequate to prevent fracture or chipping of the mold during heating and casting of the gold alloy. Although a certain minimum strength is necessary to prevent fracture of the investment mold during casting, surprisingly it has been postulated that the compressive strength should not be unduly high. In several studies on the fit of castings made by various techniques, it has been found that all castings for the National Institute of Standards and Technology MOD die showed a constant pattern of distortion. The distortion apparently results from a directional restraint by the investment to the thermal contraction of the casting as the alloy cools to room temperature.

Although the total thermal contraction of the investment is similar to that of the gold alloy from the casting temperature to room temperature, the contraction of the investment is fairly constant until it cools to below 550° C (1022° F). Thus, when the alloy is still quite hot and weak, the investment can resist alloy shrinkage by virtue of its strength and constant dimension. This can cause distortion and even fracture in the casting if the hot strength of the alloy is low. Although this is rarely a factor with gypsum-bonded investments, it can be important with other types of investments (see later discussion).

Thus, it is theorized that the compressive strength of the investment mold can be a primary factor to be considered, in addition to the expansion, when evaluating the dimensional accuracy of dental castings. Ideally, the investment should have sufficient expansion to compensate for all of the thermal contraction of the alloy. However, after burn-out of the mold, the strength need be no greater than that required to resist the impact of the metal entering the mold.

The strength of an investment is usually measured under compressive stress. The compressive strength is increased according to the amount and the type of the gypsum binder present. For example, the use of α-hemihydrate instead of plaster definitely increases the compressive strength of the investment. The use of chemical modifiers as described in the previous section also aids in increasing the strength because more of the binder can be used without a marked reduction in the thermal expansion.

According to ADA Specification No. 2, the compressive strength for the inlay investments should not be less than 2.4 MPa (350 psi) when tested 2 hours after setting. Any investment that meets this requirement should possess adequate strength for the casting of an inlay. However, when larger, complicated castings are made, a greater strength is necessary, as required for Type III partial denture investment.

The strength of the investment is affected by the water:powder ratio in the same manner as any other gypsum product; the more water that is employed in mixing, the lower is the compressive strength. Heating the investment to 700° C (1292° F) may increase or decrease the strength as much as 65%, depending on the composition. The greatest reduction in strength on heating is found in investments containing sodium chloride. After the investment has cooled to room temperature, its strength decreases considerably, presumably because of fine cracks that form during cooling.

Other Gypsum Investment Considerations

Fineness. The fineness of the investment may affect its setting time, the surface roughness of the casting, and other properties. It was previously noted that a fine silica results in a higher hygroscopic expansion than when a coarser silica is present. A fine particle size is preferable to a coarse one. The finer the investment, the smaller are the surface irregularities on the casting.

Porosity. During the casting process, the molten metal is forced into the mold under pressure. As the molten metal enters the mold, the air must be forced out ahead of it. If the air is not completely eliminated, a back pressure builds up to prevent the gold alloy from completely filling the mold. The common method for venting the mold is through the pores of the investment.

Generally, the more gypsum crystals that are present in the set investment, the less is its porosity. It follows, therefore, that the lower the hemihydrate content and the greater the amount of gauging water used to mix the investment, the more porous it becomes.

The particle size of the investment is also a factor. The more uniform the particle size, the greater is its porosity. This factor is of greater importance than is the actual particle size. A mixture of coarse and fine particles exhibits less porosity than an investment composed of a uniform particle size.

Storage. The same precautions for storage of an investment should be observed as for plaster or dental stone. Under conditions of high relative humidity, the setting time may change. Under such conditions, the setting expansion and the hygroscopic expansion may be altered so that the entire casting procedure may be adversely affected. Therefore, the investments should be stored in airtight and moisture-proof containers. During use, the containers should be opened for as short a time as possible. All investments are composed of a number of ingredients, each of which possesses a different specific gravity. There is a tendency for these components to separate as they settle, according to their specific gravity, under the normal vibration that occurs in the dental laboratory. Under certain conditions this separation may influence the setting time and other properties of the investment. For this reason, as well as the danger of accidental moisture contamination, it is advisable to purchase the investment in relatively small quantities.

The selection of an investment is largely a matter of preference. Some investments are formulated for casting inlays and crowns employing thermal expansion as the main factor for casting shrinkage compensation, and some are designed for use with hygroscopic setting expansion. Consequently, the choice is dependent partly on the specific techniques for which the investment is designed. Acceptable castings for the range of typical dental cavity preparations can be made with a number of investments and techniques.

As previously noted, the investment should be weighed and the water should be measured according to the proportion of the investment mix. Only in this manner can one expect to control the setting or the thermal expansion in relation to the compensation needed for the casting shrinkage and other important properties.

Some dental manufacturers supply their investment in preweighed packages so that one need only measure the gauging water. The mixing and subsequent manipulations of the investment are described in Chapter 23.

PHOSPHATE-BONDED INVESTMENTS

The rapid growth in use of metal-ceramic restorations and the increased use of higher melting alloys have resulted in an increased use of phosphate or silica-bonded investments. Although these investments are somewhat more difficult to remove from castings than gypsum investments, that problem has been reduced recently, and they produce satisfactory results with conventional gold alloys.

As suggested by Skinner (1963), "The definite advantage of this type of investment is that there is less chance for the contamination of the gold alloy during casting. . . . So far as is known at present, such contamination is avoided with phosphate-bonded investments. On this basis, I am inclined to predict that the dental investment of the future may be phosphate-bonded and not gypsum-bonded." As predicted, the phosphate investments now enjoy a popularity even greater than that of the gypsum-bonded ones. The tremendous increase in the use of metal-ceramic restorations necessitates the use of higher melting gold alloys that do not cast well into gypsum investments. Likewise, the present trend is toward the use of less expensive base metal alloys, most of which require phosphate investments. Commercially pure titanium and titanium alloys require specially formulated investments to minimize the interaction of the molten metal with the investment.

Composition

These investments, like the gypsum investments, consist of refractory fillers and a binder. The filler is silica, in the form of cristobalite, quartz, or a mixture of the two and in a concentration of approximately 80%. The purpose of the filler is to provide high-temperature thermal shock resistance (refractoriness) and a high thermal expansion. The particle size varies from a submicron level to that of a fine sand. The sandy feel of the investment does not necessarily relate to casting smoothness or affect the ease of removing the casting from the investment.

The binder consists of magnesium oxide (basic) and a phosphate that is acid in nature. Originally phosphoric acid was used, but monoammonium phosphate has replaced it, because it can be incorporated into the powdered investment.

Because the newer gold-containing alloys and other alloys used for metal-ceramic restorations have higher melting temperature ranges than traditional gold alloys, it usually follows that their contraction during solidification is also greater. This necessitates a greater expansion of the investment. It is fortunate that the colloidal silica suspensions became available in time for use with the phosphate investments in place of water.

Because colloidal silica liquid suspensions can freeze and become useless, these suspensions and their investment powder should be ordered before winter. Some suspensions are available as *freeze-stable* products. Although they freeze solid at low temperatures, they become useful again after they have been thawed out and shaken. Some phosphate investments are made to be used with water for the casting of many alloys. For predominantly base metal alloys, a 33% dilution of the colloidal silica is required.

Carbon is often added to the powder to produce clean castings and facilitate the *devesting* of the casting from the mold. This addition is appropriate when the casting alloy is gold, but there is disagreement regarding the effects of carbon in phosphate investments used for casting silver-palladium alloys, palladium-silver alloys, or base metal alloys. It is believed that carbon embrittles the alloys, even though the investment is heated to temperatures that burn out the carbon. The latest evidence indicates that palladium does react with carbon at temperatures above 1504° C (2740° F). Thus, if the casting temperature of a high palladium alloy exceeds this critical point, a phosphate investment without carbon should be used. Also, a carbon crucible should not be employed for melting the alloy. Generally, even gold alloys used with porcelain should not be premelted or fluxed on charcoal blocks because trace elements that provide high strength are removed or are reduced below the desired level.

Setting Reactions

The chemical reaction for the binder system that causes the investment to set and harden is generally written as follows:

(1) $$NH_4H_2PO_4 + MgO + 5H_2O \longrightarrow NH_4MgPO_4 \cdot 6H_2O$$

However, phosphates are quite complex, and the reaction is not as simple as indicated here. One version is that the magnesium ammonium phosphate formed is polymeric. Although the stoichiometric quantities are equal molecules of magnesia and monoammonium phosphate, an excess of magnesia is usually present, and some of it is never fully reacted. What is thus formed is a predominantly colloidal multimolecular $(NH_4MgPO_4 \cdot 6H_2O)_n$ aggregate around excess MgO and fillers. On heating, the binder of the set investment undergoes thermal reactions as suggested in the following sequence:

(2) $MgO + NH_4H_2PO_4 + H_2O$
          $\downarrow$ Room temperature
     $(NH_4MgPO_4 \cdot 6H_2O)n$
          MgO
          $NH_4H_2PO_4$ $\longrightarrow$ Colloidal-type particles
          H_2O

          $\downarrow$ Prolonged setting at room temperature
                                      or dehydration at 50° C
     $(NH_4MgPO_4 \cdot 6H_2O)n$
          $\downarrow$ Dehydrated at 160° C
     $(NH_4MgPO_4 \cdot H_2O)n$
          $\downarrow$ Heated from 300–650° C
     $(Mg_2P_2O_7)n'$
          $\downarrow$ Noncrystalline polymeric phase
     $Mg_2P_2O_7$
          $\downarrow$ Heated above 1040° C
     $Mg_3(P_2O_4)_2$

The final products are crystalline $Mg_2P_2O_7$ and some excess MgO, along with essentially unchanged quartz, cristobalite, or both. Some $Mg_3(PO_4)_2$ may be formed if the investment is grossly overheated or when the molten metal contacts the mold cavity surfaces.

Setting and Thermal Expansion

Theoretically, the reaction should entail a shrinkage, as in gypsum products, but in practice there is a slight expansion, and this can be increased considerably by using a colloidal silica solution instead of water. This latter substitution gives phosphate investments an unusual advantage in that the expansions can be controlled from a shrinkage to a significant expansion. Figure 22–9 shows the effect of the concentration of a typical liquid, essentially colloidal silica in aqueous suspension, on increasing the setting and thermal expansion.

Figure 22–10 illustrates the thermal expansion of a typical phosphate investment when mixed with water, as compared with the same investment when mixed with its accompanying special liquid. When phosphate investments are mixed with water, they exhibit a shrinkage within essentially the same temperature range as gypsum-bonded investments (200° C to 400° C [400° F to 750° F]). This contraction is practically eliminated when a colloidal silica solution replaces the water. Some users of phosphate-bonded investment prefer to decrease expansion by increasing the liquid:powder ratio rather than by decreasing the concentration of the special liquid, or they may use a combination of these methods.

The early thermal shrinkage of phosphate investments is associated with the decomposition of the binder, magnesium ammonium phosphate, and is accompanied by evolution of ammonia, which is readily apparent by its odor. For gypsum investments the shrinkage is caused by the transformation of the calcium sulfate from the hexagonal to the rhombic configuration. However, some

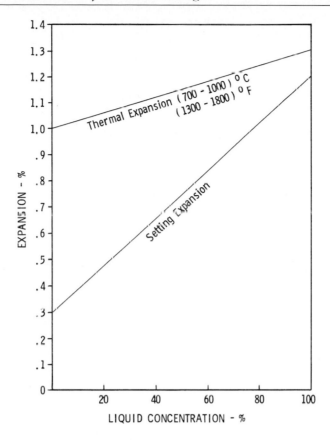

Figure 22–9. The influence of liquid concentration on the setting and thermal expansion of a phosphate-bonded investment. (Courtesy of R. Neiman, Whip-Mix Corporation, Louisville, KY.)

of the shrinkage is masked because of the expansion of the refractory filler, especially in the case of cristobalite.

Working and Setting Time

Unlike gypsum investments, phosphate investments are markedly affected by temperature. The warmer the mix, the faster it sets. The setting reaction itself gives off heat, and this further accelerates the rate of setting. Increased mixing time and mixing efficiency, as determined by the type of mixer and speed of mixing, result in a faster set and a greater rise in temperature. In general, the more efficient the mixing, the better the casting in terms of smoothness and accuracy. The ideal technique is to mix as long as possible yet have just enough time for investing. Mechanical mixing under vacuum is preferred.

A third variable that has a considerable effect on the working and setting time is the liquid:powder ratio, which is often varied considerably depending on user preference. An increase in the liquid:powder ratio increases the working time, which can be very short (2 minutes or less) when the investment is mixed at the manufacturer's recommended liquid:powder ratio, at high speed (1750 rpm) for the recommended time, and if the laboratory is warm and the liquid has not been chilled.

Miscellaneous Properties

At one time, detail reproduction and surface smoothness of a metal-ceramic gold alloy restoration cast in a phosphate-bonded investment were generally

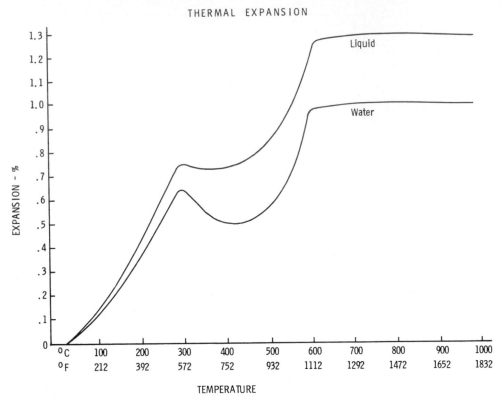

Figure 22–10. Thermal expansion of a phosphate-bond investment mixed with water as compared with the special liquid. (Courtesy of R. Neiman, Whip-Mix Corporation, Louisville, KY.)

considered inferior to those characteristic of a conventional gold alloy that had been cast in a gypsum-bonded investment. Increasing the special liquid:water ratio used for the mix markedly enhances casting surface smoothness but can lead to oversized extracoronal castings. However, improvement in the technique, and also perhaps the investment, now makes it possible to fabricate castings having few surface imperfections when the phosphate-bonded investment is used with either a low-fusing gold alloy, a high-fusing gold alloy, or a base-metal alloy. The phosphate investment now approaches that of the gypsum investments in fineness. However, their ability to improve the smoothness is dependent on the alloy and casting procedure employed.

ETHYL SILICATE–BONDED INVESTMENTS

Ethyl silicate–bonded investment is losing popularity because of the more complicated and time-consuming procedures involved, but it is still used in the construction of the high-fusing base metal partial denture alloys. In this case, the binder is a silica gel that reverts to silica (cristobalite) on heating. Several methods may be used to produce the silica or silicic acid gel binders. When the pH of sodium silicate is lowered by the addition of an acid or an acid salt, a bonding silicic acid gel forms. The addition of magnesium oxide strengthens the gel. An aqueous suspension of colloidal silica can also be converted to a gel by the addition of an accelerator, such as ammonium chloride.

Another system for binder formation is based on ethyl silicate. A colloidal silicic acid is first formed by hydrolyzing ethyl silicate in the presence of hydrochloric acid, ethyl alcohol, and water. In its simplest form, the reaction can be expressed as:

(3) $$Si(OC_2H_5)_4 + 4H_2O \rightarrow Si(OH)_4 + 4C_2H_5OH$$

Because a polymerized form of ethyl silicate is actually used, a colloidal sol of polysilicic acids is expected instead of the simpler silicic acid sol shown in the reaction.

The sol is then mixed with the quartz or cristobalite to which is added a small amount of finely powdered magnesium oxide to render the mixture alkaline. A coherent gel of polysilicic acid then forms, accompanied by a setting shrinkage. This soft gel is dried at a temperature below 168° C (334° F). During the drying process, the gel loses alcohol and water to form a concentrated, hard gel. As might be expected, a volumetric contraction accompanies the drying, which reduces the size of the mold. This contraction is known as "green shrinkage," and it occurs in addition to the setting shrinkage.

This gelation process is likely to be slow and time consuming. An alternative and faster method for the production of the silica gel can be employed. Certain types of amines can be added to the solution of ethyl silicate so that hydrolysis and gelation occur simultaneously. It follows that with an investment of this type the mold enlargement before casting must compensate not only for the casting shrinkage of the metal but also for the green shrinkage and the setting shrinkage of the investment.

Investments of this type are designed to reduce the layer of silica gel around the particles. They have a special particle-size gradation and are handled in a different manner. The powder is added to the hydrolyzed ethyl silicate liquid, mixed quickly, and vibrated into a mold that has an extra collar to increase the height. The mold, or a number of molds, are placed on a platform of a special type of vibrator that has a slow jogging, jolting, or sometimes so-called tamping action. This allows the heavier particles to settle quickly while the excess liquid and some of the fine particles rise to the top. In about 30 minutes, the accelerator in the powder hardens the settled part, and the top excess is poured off. Thus, the liquid:powder ratio in the settled part is greatly reduced, and the setting shrinkage is reduced to 0.1%.

The remaining cast is somewhat fragile because the amount of binder is quite low and is essentially composed of silica. The wax pattern is formed on the cast and invested in a manner similar to other investments. It is a little more complicated than the phosphate type in that care must be exercised in handling and burnout, because flammable alcohol is given off. If it is heated high enough, some silica converts to quartz and provides added expansion. This type of investment can be heated to 1090° C to 1180° C (2000° F to 2150° F) and is compatible with the higher fusing alloys. Its low setting expansion minimizes distortion.

SELECTED READING

Cooney JP, and Caputo AA: Type III gold alloy complete crowns cast in a phosphate-bonded investment. J Prosthet Dent 46:414, 1981.
   Marginal fit was superior for castings from the phosphate-bonded investment; surface roughness was less for the casting cast in the gypsum-bonded investment.
Earnshaw R: The effect of casting ring liners on the potential expansion of a gypsum-bonded investment. J Dent Res 67:1366, 1988.
   Total expansion, setting expansion, and thermal expansion, of the investment setting against a smooth, dry

surface was 1.7%; against a dry ceramic liner, 1.6% to 1.7%; and against wet cellulose or wet asbestos, 2.2% to 2.3%. The ceramic liner can be used wet if it is treated with a surfactant instead of water.

Finger W, and Ohsawa M: Accuracy of cast restorations produced by a refractory die-investing technique. J Prosthet Dent 52:800, 1984.

By minimizing distortion of the wax pattern, the refractory die-investing procedure can produce consistently accurate cast gold alloy restorations.

Jorgensen KD, and Okamoto A: Restraining factors affecting setting expansion of phosphate-bonded investments. Scand J Dent Res 94:178, 1986.

It is suggested that setting expansion is a most unreliable means to compensate partially for the thermal contraction of casting alloys.

Junner RE, and Stevens L: Anisotropic setting expansion of phosphate-bonded investment. Aust Dent J 31:434, 1986.

The vertical setting expansion was significantly greater than the horizontal expansion in a rigid ring with liners. A flexible ring offered little restriction to horizontal expansion, reducing mold distortion.

Kaplan J, and Newman SM: Accuracy of the divestment casting technique. Oper Dent 8:82, 1983.

Castings made using the divestment procedure fit more accurately than did castings made using a conventional stone-die/gypsum-bonded refractory investment technique.

Mahler DB, and Ady AB: An explanation for the hygroscopic setting expansion of dental gypsum products. J Dent Res 39:578, 1960.

A classic publication on the theory of hygroscopic setting expansion. Excellent reference for those interested in the mechanics of this phenomenon.

Matsuya S, and Yamane M: Decomposition of gypsum-bonded investments. J Dent Res 60:1418, 1981.

At 900° C decomposition of gypsum-bonded investments occurred, leading to the formation of $CaSiO_3$ and Ca_2SiO_4 · CaO was not formed during thermally induced decomposition.

Mueller HJ, Reyes W, and McGill S: Surfactant-containing phosphate investment. Dent Mater 2:42, 1986.

The addition of surfactants to a phosphate-bonded casting investment can increase the hygroscopic setting expansion. The surfactant also makes the unset investment more viscous and reduces the compressive strength.

Neiman R, and Sarma AC: Setting and thermal reactions of phosphate investments. J Dent Res:1478, 1980.

An explanation of the chemical reaction involved in the setting of phosphate-bonded investments.

Santos JF, and Ballester RY: Delayed hygroscopic expansion of phosphate-bonded investments. Dent Mater 3:165, 1987.

Delayed hygroscopic expansion occurs when the investment is immersed in water after setting. Increased time of immersion and increase in the special liquid concentration increased the hygroscopic setting expansion.

Skinner EW: Some recent technical advances in dental materials. J Am Dent Assoc 66:176, 1993.

Stevens L: The effect of early heating on the expansion of a phosphate-bonded investment. Aust Dent J 28:366, 1983.

The thermal expansion of a phosphate-bonded investment decreased as heating was delayed from 1 to 6 hours after mixing. The setting expansion increased as the special liquid replaced water for mixing.

Taggart WH: A new and accurate method of making gold inlays. Dent Cosmos 49:1117, 1907.

The dental "lost wax" process was developed by Taggart, opening up the opportunity to cast accurate restorations in an investment mold. A historical landmark.

Verrett RG, and Duke ES: The effect of sprue attachment design on castability and porosity. J Prosthet Dent 61:418, 1989.

Flared and straight sprue attachments optimized castability and minimized porosity.

23 *Casting Procedures for Dental Alloys*

- **Clinical Evaluation of Casting Fit**
- **Compensation for Solidification Shrinkage**
- **Preparation of the Master Die**
- **The Sprue Former**
- **Casting Ring Liners**
- **Investing Procedure**
- **Casting Procedure**
- **Technical Considerations for Phosphate-bonded Investments**
- **Causes of Defective Castings**

Although dental castings of any size (from a denture base to the smallest inlay) can be made, only the procedures employed for the construction of a small restoration, such as an inlay, onlay, crown, and endodontic post, are discussed in this chapter. The fundamental principles are the same, regardless of the size of the casting, and the techniques differ only in sprue design, type of investment, and method of melting the alloy.

CLINICAL EVALUATION OF CASTING FIT

The objective of the casting process is to provide a metallic duplication of missing tooth structure, with as much accuracy as possible. The tolerance limits for the fit and marginal adaptation of a cast restoration are not known. In a clinical study, 10 experienced dentists were asked to evaluate the marginal adaptation of a group of inlays, using an explorer and radiographs. After the cemented restorations were graded, they were microscopically measured at the marginal openings of various areas. For "acceptable" restorations, the mean opening was 21 μm at the occlusal surface and 74 μm at the gingival region, which is not as accessible visually. There was little agreement among these 10 dentists on the acceptability of the marginal openings in some areas when evaluated by either explorers or radiographs.

The difficulty in detecting small discrepancies at the margins of cemented restorations is associated with the use of explorers that have a relatively large radius of curvature at the tip compared with the width of margin gaps that are being evaluated. As shown in Figure 23–1, the tip of this unused explorer may not "catch" a 60-μm margin gap, whose width is represented by the diameter of a human hair, as it traverses along a path perpendicular to the gap. If this explorer tip substantially penetrates into a gap during probing, the fit of a crown, inlay, or onlay will not be clinically acceptable. The illustration poses the question of how readily a hairline gap can be detected by running an explorer over the margins of the restoration, especially in interdental areas that must often be probed at a small angle to the surface.

Therefore, it is obvious that the accuracy of the inlay or crown should be greater than can be detected by the eye or by the conventional methods of clinical testing. At the margins of the cemented restoration, a thin line of cement is always present, even though it may not be readily visible. With the exception of resin-based luting materials, the present dental cements are somewhat soluble and can deteriorate in the oral cavity. Thus, the less accurate the casting fit and the greater the amount of cement exposed, the more likely the restoration will fail because of cement degradation. Certainly, a high degree of accuracy in margin adaptation of 25 μm or less cannot be guaranteed for all cast restorations. It stands to reason, however, that the more accurate the fit of the casting, the less the likelihood of leakage and secondary caries.

Assuming that the wax pattern is satisfactory, the procedure then becomes a matter of enlarging the mold uniformly and sufficiently to compensate for the casting shrinkage of the gold alloy. Theoretically, if the shrinkages of the wax and the gold alloy are known, the mold can be expanded an amount equal to such shrinkages, and the problem is solved. It is unfortunate that there are variables in the behavior of the materials involved, especially the wax, that cannot be rigidly controlled. The overall dimensional accuracy possible with current techniques has never been clearly defined. Thus, neither the allowable tolerance of accuracy in the fit of the casting nor that obtainable during the casting procedure is known. In the last analysis, the casting procedure is partly empirical and a matter of routine procedure. The latter should be rigidly followed.

There are, however, many steps in the procedure for which a considerable number of facts are known, and there are also certain variations in techniques described here produce equally satisfactory results. However, any technique

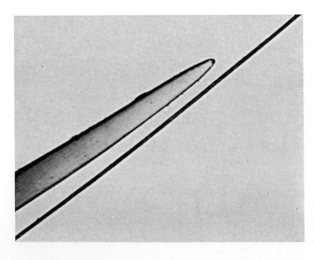

Figure 23–1. Cross section of an unused explorer tip *(top)* and a 60-μm hair. ×25. (From McLean JW, and Van Fraunhofer JA: The estimation of cement film thickness by an *in vivo* technique. Br Dent J 131:107, 1971.)

involves strict adherence to certain fundamental principles that are common to all. It is these fundamentals that are stressed in this chapter.

COMPENSATION FOR SOLIDIFICATION SHRINKAGE

The compensation for the shrinkages inherent in the dental casting procedure may be obtained by either one or both of the following two methods:

- Setting or hygroscopic expansion of the investment
- Thermal expansion of the investment

Both techniques are currently in use and are commonly termed the *hygroscopic expansion* (low-heat) and the *thermal expansion* (high-heat) methods. As their names alone might indicate, the high-heat method requires thermal expansion of the investment to increase from room temperature to a high temperature (650° C to 700° C for gypsum-bonded investments and up to 871° C for phosphate-bonded investments).

Despite these stated differences, the overall procedures involved in investing and casting are quite similar and, therefore, are described simultaneously. If not stated to the contrary, the reader can assume that the procedures mentioned are common to both the high-heat and the low-heat techniques. For best results, the manufacturer's recommendations for the specific alloy used should be followed.

Ringless Casting System. To provide maximum expansion of investment, a ringless system is available commercially. The system, called the *PowerCast Ringless System* (Whip Mix Corporation, Louisville, KY), consists of three sizes of rings and formers, preformed wax sprues and shapes, investment powder, and a special investment liquid. The tapered plastic rings allow for removal of the investment mold after the material has set. This system is suited for the casting of alloys that require greater mold expansion than traditional gold-based alloys.

PREPARATION OF THE MASTER DIE

The most commonly used die materials are Type IV (dental stone, high strength) and Type V (dental stone, high strength, high expansion) improved stones. They are relatively inexpensive, easy to use, and generally compatible with all impression materials. Certified Type IV stones have a setting expansion of 0.1% or less, whereas the harder Type V stones expand as much as 0.3% in accordance with American Dental Association (ADA) Specification No. 25. This greater expansion is useful for compensation of the relatively large solidification shrinkage of base metal alloys.

The chief disadvantage of the Type IV gypsum die is its susceptibility to abrasion during carving of the wax pattern. Gypsum dies are sometimes modified to (1) make them more abrasion resistant, (2) change the dimensions of the dies, (3) increase the refractoriness of the dies, or (4) produce a combination of these effects. Several means are used to increase the abrasion resistance including silver plating, coating the surface with cyanoacrylate, and adding a die hardener to the gypsum. However, each may also increase the die dimensions, thus reducing accuracy (Table 23–1).

Methods of Altering Die Dimensions. To reduce the setting expansion of the Type IV die stone to less than 0.1%, and therefore to reduce the diameter of the die, additional accelerator (potassium sulfate) and retarder (borax) can be added

TABLE 23–1. Dimensional Change in Dies Made from Silicone Impression Material Compared with a Standardized Die

Material	Dimensional Change (%)	
	Occlusal	*Cervical*
Type IV stone	0.06	0.00
Type IV stone + gypsum hardener A	0.16	0.08
Type IV stone + gypsum hardener B	0.10	0.10
Silica-filled epoxy resin	−0.15	−0.26
Aluminum-filled epoxy resin	−0.14	−0.19
Electroformed silver die	−0.10	−0.20

With permission from Toreskog S, Phillips RW, and Schnell RJ: J Prosthet Dent 16:119, 1966.

to the gauging water. To produce relief space for cement, it is common to use a *die spacer* with a stone die. The most common die spacers are resins. Although proprietary paint-on liquids are sold for this purpose, model paint, colored nail polish, or thermoplastic polymers dissolved in volatile solvents enjoy widespread popularity. Such spacers are applied in several coats to within 0.5 mm of the preparation finish line to provide relief for the cement luting agent and to ensure complete seating of an otherwise precisely fitting casting.

Die Stone–Investment Combination. There is yet another technique that has been developed, in which the die material and the investing medium have a comparable composition. A commercial gypsum-bonded material, called *Divestment* (Whip Mix Corporation, Louisville, KY), is mixed with a colloidal silica liquid. The die is made from this mix and the wax pattern constructed on it. Then the entire assembly (die and pattern) is invested in a mixture of Divestment and water, thereby eliminating the possibility of distortion of the pattern on removal from the die or during the setting of the investment. The setting expansion of the material is 0.9%, and thermal expansion is 0.6%, when it is heated to 677° C. Because Divestment is a gypsum-bonded material, it is not recommended for high-fusing alloys, as used in metal-ceramic restorations. However, it is a highly accurate technique for use with conventional gold alloys, especially for extracoronal preparations. Divestment phosphate is a phosphate-bonded investment that is used in the same manner as Divestment and is suitable for use with high-fusing alloys. Phosphate-bonded die-investment materials formulated for use in making ceramic restorations can also be used when casting high-fusing alloys.

Other Die Materials. With the inelastic impression materials, such as compound, amalgam may be condensed into the impression to form the die. Other nongypsum die materials are also available, such as acrylic, polyester, and epoxy resins. These materials are limited in their compatibility with impression materials that would ordinarily be nonaqueous elastomers rather than hydrocolloid or compound. Compatibility is specific and germane only to the particular brand rather than to chemical types of impression materials. Moreover, in the case of filled autopolymerizing acrylic resins, the curing contraction is excessive (0.6 linear percent for one material). Therefore, acrylic resin cannot be used when an accurate die is required. The same is true for polyester resin materials.

Various epoxy die materials are reliable with respect to the 0.1% to 0.2% dimensional change on polymerization (see Table 23–1). Even though epoxy dies are generally undersized in comparison with the prepared tooth, especially in the axial direction, they are used successfully by some commercial dental laboratories.

In some cases the resin die should be no more undersized than the stone die is oversized. However, this must be taken into consideration, because it may be necessary to adjust the investing and casting technique accordingly. A casting fabricated on a slightly undersized resin die does not seat completely on the tooth compared with one made on the slightly large stone die.

The high-strength stones (Types IV and V) appear to be the most successful die materials available. With care, abrasion during carving of the wax pattern can be avoided. However, in the construction of a porcelain jacket crown, a platinum matrix is generally swaged on a die of the preparation. Gypsum dies are readily damaged, so a less brittle material, such as resin or metal, is preferred.

In the last few years, several gypsum die stones have been compounded with resins to provide the advantage of each material. These modified die stones maintain the low expansion of stone, but they also have an increased toughness and resistance to carving imparted by the resins.

Electroformed Dies. The metal dies that are produced from electroplated impression material have high strength, hardness, and abrasion resistance. Detail reproduction of a line 4 μm or less in width is readily attainable when a nonaqueous elastomeric impression material is used.

The popularity of copper-plated compound dies began in the early 1930s and silver-plated dies became more popular in later years. There are several modifications of the fabrication technique, but the following description is typical.

The first step in the procedure is to treat the surface of the impression material so that it conducts electricity. This process is referred to as *metallizing*. In this process, a thin layer of metal, such as silver, is deposited on the surface of the impression material. This metal layer determines to a large extent the surface character of the finished die. Various metallizing agents are available, including bronzing powder and aqueous suspensions of silver powder and powdered graphite. These agents can be burnished on the surface of the impression with a camel-hair brush.

The electroplating bath itself is primarily a solution of silver cyanide. Care must be taken to avoid the addition of acids to the cyanide solution, which can cause the release of cyanide vapor, a "death chamber" gas. Chemical deposition of silver from a silver nitrate solution can be employed if greater surface detail reproduction is desired.

In the silver-plating process, the greater the concentration of silver in the bath, the faster the silver is deposited. The acid content increases the *throwing power,* a term that refers to the ionic penetration of the electrical field in a concave structure, such as an impression for a full crown. Impressions of teeth generally have walls with long depth relative to the location of the occlusal area. Therefore, a considerable amount of throwing power is desirable.

An electrical contact is made with the metallized surface of the impression, which is the cathode in the electroplating bath. A plate of silver is used as the anode. A direct current is applied for approximately 10 hours.

Hydrocolloid impressions are difficult to electroplate, and the process is not feasible for dental use. Electroformed dies made from polysulfide rubber impressions are clinically acceptable when a silver cyanide bath is used, although they are generally slightly less accurate than a properly constructed stone die.

The polysulfide rubber impression is cleaned thoroughly and dried. It is then metallized with a fine silver powder. Although other metallizing agents can be used, the silver powder results in a superior surface on the electroformed die.

An anode of pure silver, at least twice the size of the area to be plated, is employed, and the electroplating is carried out as before for approximately 10 hours using 5 to 10 mA/cm^2 of cathode surface.

The impression that contains the electroformed die surface is then filled with dental stone. When the stone hardens, it is mechanically locked to the rough interior of the electroformed metal shell. The impression material is then removed to provide a die with greater surface hardness and resistance to abrasion than one of gypsum. The model and die are prepared in the normal manner, and margins of the die are trimmed with a finishing disk.

THE SPRUE FORMER

The purpose of a *sprue former*, or sprue pin, is to provide a channel through which molten alloy can reach the mold in an invested ring after the wax has been eliminated. With large restorations or prostheses, such as removable partial denture frameworks and fixed partial dentures, the sprue formers are made of wax.

The diameter and length of the sprue former depend to a large extent on the type and size of the pattern, the type of casting machine to be used, and the dimensions of the flask or ring in which the casting is to be made. Prefabricated sprue formers are available in a wide range of gauges or diameters (Table 23–2).

Sprue former gauge selection is often empirical, yet it is based on the following five general principles:

- Select the gauge sprue former with a diameter that is approximately the same size as the thickest area of the wax pattern. If the pattern is small, the sprue former must also be small because a large sprue former attached to a thin, delicate pattern could cause distortion. However, if the sprue former diameter is too small, this area will solidify before the casting itself and localized shrinkage porosity ("suck-back" porosity) may develop. Reservoir sprues are used to help overcome this problem.
- If possible, the sprue former should be attached to the portion of the pattern with the largest cross-sectional areas. It is best for the molten alloy to flow from a thick section to surrounding thin areas (e.g., margins) and not the reverse. This design minimizes the risk for turbulence. Also, the sprue former orientation should minimize the risk of metal flow onto flat areas of the investment or small areas such as line angles.

TABLE 23–2. American (Brown & Sharpe) Wire Gauge Numbers and Wire Diameter

Gauge No. B & S	Diameter	
	cm	*Inches*
6	0.4115	0.1620
8	0.3264	0.1285
10	0.2588	0.1019
12	0.2053	0.08081
14	0.1628	0.06408
16	0.1291	0.05082
18	0.1024	0.04030

Reprinted with permission from Handbook of Chemistry and Physics, 58th ed., 1977–1978, p. F-16. Copyright CRC Press, Inc., Boca Raton, FL.

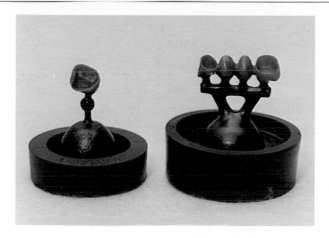

Figure 23–2. Wax patterns sprued directly (left and right). On the right is an example of indirect spruing showing a reservoir bar that is positioned near the heat center of the invested ring.

- The length of the sprue former should be long enough to properly position the pattern in the casting ring within 6 mm of the trailing end and yet short enough so the molten alloy does not solidify before it fills the mold.
- The type of sprue former selected influences the burnout technique used. Wax sprue formers are more common than plastic. It is advisable to use a two-stage burnout technique whenever plastic sprue formers or patterns are involved to ensure complete carbon elimination, because plastic sprues soften at temperatures above the melting point of inlay waxes.
- Patterns may be sprued either *directly* or *indirectly*. For direct spruing, the sprue former provides a direct connection between the pattern area and the sprue base or *crucible former* area (Fig. 23–2). With indirect spruing, a connector or *reservoir bar* is positioned between the pattern and the crucible former (see right side of Fig. 23–2). It is common to use indirect spruing for multiple single units and fixed partial dentures, although several single units can be sprued with multiple direct sprue formers.

A *reservoir* should be added to a spruing network to prevent localized shrinkage porosity (Fig. 23–3). When the molten alloy fills the heated casting ring, the pattern area should solidify first and the reservoir last. Because of its large mass of alloy and position in the heat center of the ring, the reservoir remains molten to furnish liquid alloy into the mold as it solidifies. The resulting solidification shrinkage occurs in the reservoir bar and not in the restorations, assuming that the reservoir bar is larger in volume than that of the patterns and that the sprue formers attached to those patterns were placed in the appropriate position and were of the correct gauge.

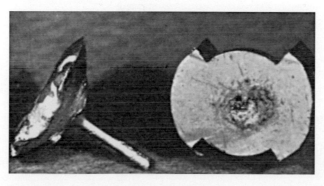

Figure 23–3. Localized shrinkage caused by using a sprue of improper diameter.

Sprue Former Attachment. The sprue former connection to the wax pattern is generally flared for higher density gold alloys but is often restricted for lower density alloys. Flaring of the sprue former may act in much the same way as a reservoir, facilitating the entry of the fluid alloy into the pattern area.

Sprue Former Position. The position of the sprue former attachment is often a matter of individual judgment, based on the shape and form of the wax pattern. Some clinicians prefer placement at the occlusal surface, whereas others choose sites such as a proximal wall or just below a nonfunctional cusp to minimize subsequent grinding of occlusal anatomy and contact areas. As indicated earlier, the ideal area for the sprue former is the point of greatest bulk in the pattern to avoid distorting thin areas of wax during attachment to the pattern and to permit a smooth flow of the alloy.

Sprue Former Direction. The sprue former should be directed away from any thin or delicate parts of the pattern, because the molten metal may abrade or fracture investment in this area and result in a casting failure. It should not be attached at a right angle to a broad flat surface. Such an orientation of the sprue former leads to turbulence within the mold cavity and severe porosity in this region (Fig. 23–4A). When this same pattern is sprued at a 45-degree angle to the proximal area, a satisfactory casting is obtained (Fig. 23–4B).

Sprue Former Length. The length of the sprue former depends on the length of the casting ring. If the sprue is too short, the wax pattern may be so far removed from the end of the casting ring that gases cannot be adequately vented to permit the molten alloy to fill the ring completely. When these gases are not completely eliminated, porosity may result. Therefore, the sprue length should

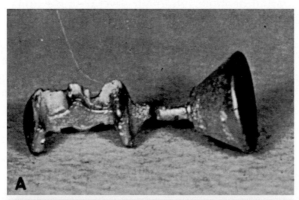

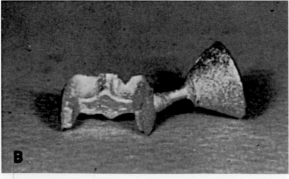

Figure 23–4. A, Detached sprue indicates severe porosity at the point of attachment because of turbulence occasioned by an improper sprue angle. *B*, Sound casting results with sprue at approximately 45 degrees to the proximal wall.

be adjusted so that the top of the wax pattern is within 6 mm of the open end of the ring for gypsum-bonded investments (Fig. 23–5). With the higher-strength phosphate-bonded investments, it may be possible to position it within 3 to 4 mm of the top of the investment. For reproducibility of casting accuracy, the pattern should be placed as close to the center of the ring as possible.

Wax Pattern Removal. The sprue former should be attached to the wax pattern with the pattern on the master die, provided the pattern can be removed directly in line with its path of withdrawal from the die. Any motion that might distort the wax pattern should be avoided during removal.

CASTING RING LINERS

With the use of solid metal rings or casting flasks, provision must be made to permit investment expansion. The mold may actually become smaller rather than larger because of the reverse pressure resulting from the confinement of the setting expansion. This effect can be overcome by using a split ring or flexible rubber ring that permits the setting expansion of the investment.

However, the most commonly used technique to provide investment expansion is to line the walls of the ring with a ring liner. Traditionally, asbestos was the material of choice, but it can no longer be used because its carcinogenic potential makes it a biohazard. Two types of nonasbestos ring liner materials have been produced: an aluminum silicate ceramic liner and a cellulose (paper) liner.

To ensure uniform expansion, the liner is cut to fit the inside diameter of the casting ring with no overlap. The dry liner is tacked in position with sticky wax and then is used either dry or wet. With a wet liner technique, the lined ring is immersed in water for a time, and the excess water is shaken away. Squeezing the liner should be avoided because this leads to variable amounts of water removal and uneven expansion. Although a ceramic liner may not absorb water like a cellulose liner, its network of fibers can retain water on the surface.

Not only does the liner afford greater normal setting expansion in the investment, but also the absorbed water causes a semihygroscopic expansion as it is drawn into the investment during setting, as shown for gypsum investments in Figure 23–6. The use of one liner (Fig. 23–6C) increases the normal setting expansion compared with no liner. A thicker liner material or two layers of liner (Fig. 23–6D) provide even greater semihygroscopic expansion and also afford a

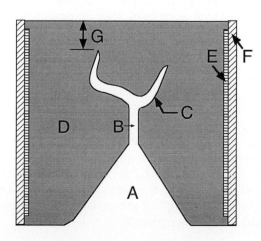

Figure 23–5. Diagrammatic representation of a dental casting mold: *A*, crucible former; *B*, sprue; *C*, cavity formed by wax pattern after burnout; *D*, investment; *E*, liner; *F*, casting ring; *G*, recommended maximum investment thickness of approximately 6 mm between the end of the mold cavity and the end of the invested ring, to provide pathways for sufficient gas escape during casting.

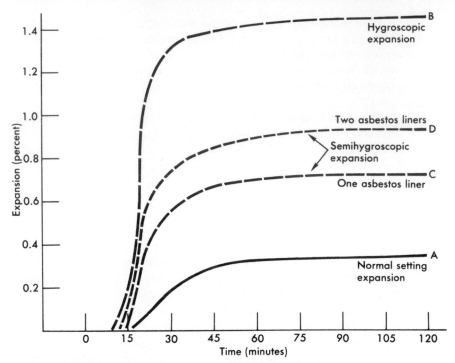

Figure 23–6. Normal setting (A) and hygroscopic expansion (B) of an investment as compared with the somewhat restricted expansion that occurs in an inlay ring lined with one (C) and two (D) asbestos liners. (Courtesy of R. Neiman, Whip-Mix Corporation.)

more unrestricted normal setting expansion of the investment. As shown in the figure, two layers of liner can be used to increase the expansion slightly compared with that obtained from one liner. In any case, the thickness of the liner should not be less than approximately 1 mm.

Cellulose liners, being paper products, are burned away during the burnout procedure, so a technique must be found to secure the investment in the ring. However, the desired length of the liner remains a matter of controversy. If the length of the liner is somewhat shorter than the ring itself, the investment is confined at one or both ends of the ring. The longitudinal setting and hygroscopic expansion are thereby restricted, as compared with an end where the liner is flush with the ends of the ring.

The expansion of the investment is always greater in the unrestricted longitudinal direction than in the lateral direction, that is, toward the ring itself. Therefore, it is desirable to reduce the expansion in the longitudinal direction. Placing the liner somewhat short (3.25 mm) of the ends of the ring tends to produce a more uniform expansion; thus, there is less chance for distortion of the wax pattern and the mold.

INVESTING PROCEDURE

The wax pattern should be cleaned of any debris, grease, or oils. A commercial wax pattern cleaner or a diluted synthetic detergent is used. Any excess liquid is shaken off and the pattern is left to air dry while the investment is being prepared. The thin film of cleanser left on the pattern reduces the surface tension of the wax and permits better "wetting" of the investment to ensure complete coverage of the intricate portions of the pattern.

While the wax pattern cleaner is air drying, the appropriate amount of distilled water (gypsum investments) or colloidal silica special liquid (phosphate investments) is measured out. The liquid is added to a clean, dry mixing bowl, and the powder is gradually added to the liquid with the same care and caution to minimize air entrapment as was discussed when mixing dental stones. Mixing is started gently until all the powder has been wet, or the unmixed powder may inadvertently be ejected from the bowl. Although hand mixing is an option, it is far more commonplace to mechanically mix all casting investments under vacuum.

Vacuum Mixing. Mechanical mixing under vacuum removes air bubbles created during mixing and evacuates any potentially harmful gases produced by the chemical reaction of the high-heat investments. Once mixing is completed, the pattern may be hand invested or vacuum invested. For investing by hand, the entire pattern is painted (inside and out) with a thin layer of investment. The casting ring is positioned on the crucible former, and the remainder of the investment is vibrated slowly into the ring. With vacuum investing, the same equipment used to mix the investment is employed to invest the pattern under vacuum.

As noted, the amount of porosity in the investment is reduced by vacuum investing. As a result, the texture of the cast surface is somewhat smoother with better detail reproduction. The tensile strength of vacuum mixed investment is also increased. In one study, it was found that 95% of vacuum-invested castings were free of nodules, whereas only 17% of castings made in hand-invested molds were entirely free of defects. Freedom of any surface imperfections is highly important, because even a small nodule on a casting may damage a fragile enamel margin when the casting is evaluated for fit in the prepared cavity. The finished casting should always be checked under magnification for such defects before fitting it on the die.

Air bubbles that remain in the mix, even with vacuum mixing, can be entrapped on flat or concave surfaces that are not oriented suitably for air evacuation. Tilting the ring slightly aids in releasing these bubbles so they can rise to the surface. Excessive vibration is to be avoided, because it can cause solids in the investment to settle and may lead to free water accumulation adjacent to the wax pattern, resulting in surface roughness. Excessive vibration may also dislodge small patterns from the sprue former, resulting in a miscast.

If the hygroscopic technique is employed, the filled casting ring is immediately placed in a 37° C water bath with the crucible former side down. For the thermal expansion or high-heat technique, the invested ring is allowed to bench set undisturbed for the time recommended by the manufacturer.

Compensation for Shrinkage. Occasionally, it may be desirable to alter the mold dimensions of a full cast crown compared with a small inlay. A number of factors influence the mold size. As previously discussed, two liners allow a greater setting and thermal expansion than does a single liner.

Also the setting, hygroscopic, and thermal expansions of investments can be controlled to a certain extent by varying the liquid:powder (L:P) ratio of the investment. The lower the L:P ratio, the greater the potential for investment expansion. Conversely, thinner mixes reduce the expansion. With some investments, however, the effect of minor adjustments to the L:P ratio is insignificant.

However, there is a limit to which the L:P ratio can be altered. If it is too thick, it cannot be applied to the pattern without a likelihood of distorting the pattern and producing air voids during investing. On the other hand, if the mixture is too thin, a rough surface on the casting may result.

The problem of too much expansion of the mold in the thermal expansion technique using a cristobalite investment may be important. As was discussed in the previous chapter, a thermal expansion of 1.3% may take place. If an effective setting expansion of 0.3% to 0.4% is added to such a thermal expansion, a total linear expansion as high as 1.7% may be obtained, higher than the average casting shrinkage of a gold alloy. As a result, a crown casting may be too large.

In addition to controlling the hygroscopic expansion by the L:P ratio, it can be regulated either by reducing the time of immersion of the setting investment or by controlling the amount of water to be added during the setting process. The longer the delay before the investment is immersed in the water bath, the less the hygroscopic expansion that occurs.

The modern hygroscopic investment technique generally provides correct expansion for most types of patterns. However, some may require a variation in expansion. Increasing the burnout temperature and the water bath temperature increases the expansion, and vice versa.

In one technique, the shrinkage compensation is controlled by the addition of water during the setting of the investment, as described in Chapter 22. This method is usually referred to as the *controlled water-added technique.*

Controlled Water-added Technique. As shown in Chapter 22, the linear hygroscopic expansion increases directly with the amount of water added until a maximal expansion is attained. The compositions of investments for use with the water-added hygroscopic casting technique ensure maximal expansion during immersion in water. The amount of hygroscopic expansion needed for compensation is then obtained by adding only enough water to provide the desired expansion.

A soft, flexible rubber ring is employed instead of the usual asbestos-lined metal ring. The pattern is invested as usual. A specified amount of water is then added on the top of the investment in the rubber ring, and the investment is allowed to set, usually at room temperature. This technique is rarely used, since the hygroscopic expansion method described earlier provides adequate expansion in most cases.

CASTING PROCEDURE

Once the investment has set for an appropriate period—approximately 1 hour for most gypsum- and phosphate-bonded investments—it is ready for burnout. The procedures for the two types of investment are similar, so the following discussion focuses on gypsum investments. The crucible former and any metal sprue former are carefully removed. Any debris from the ingate area (funneled opening at end of the ring) is cleaned with a camel-hair brush. If the burnout procedure does not immediately follow the investing procedure, the invested ring is placed in a humidor at 100% humidity. If at all possible, the investment should not be permitted to dry out. Rehydration of set investment that has been stored for an extended period may not replenish all of the lost water.

Wax Elimination and Heating. The invested rings are placed in a room-temperature furnace and heated to the prescribed maximum temperature. For gypsum-bonded investments, that temperature can be either 468° C for the *hygroscopic* *technique* or 650° C for the *thermal expansion technique*. With phosphate-bonded investments, the maximum temperature setting may range from 700° C to 870° C, depending on the type of alloy selected. The temperature setting is more critical with gypsum-bonded investments than with the phosphate type because the gypsum investments are more prone to investment decomposition. During burnout, some of the melted wax is absorbed by the investment, and residual carbon produced by ignition of the liquid wax becomes trapped in the porous investment. It is also advisable to begin the burnout procedure while the mold is still wet. Water trapped in the pores of the investment reduces the absorption of wax, and as the water vaporizes, it flushes wax from the mold. This process is facilitated by placing the ring with the sprue hole down over a slot in a ceramic tray in the burnout furnace. When the high-heat technique is used, the mold temperature generates enough heat to convert carbon to either carbon monoxide or dioxide. These gases can then escape through the pores in the heated investment.

Hygroscopic Low-Heat Technique. This technique obtains its compensation expansion from three sources: (1) the 37° C water bath expands the wax pattern; (2) the warm water entering the investment mold from the top adds some hygroscopic expansion; and (3) the thermal expansion at 500° C provides the needed thermal expansion. This low-heat technique offers the advantages of less mold degradation, a cooler surface for smoother castings, and the convenience of placing the molds directly in the 500° C furnace. The last benefit makes it possible to keep one or more furnaces at the burnout temperature so that molds may be put in as they are ready. This is particularly useful in large laboratories where molds are ready at various times. Care must nevertheless be taken to allow sufficient burnout time because the wax is more slowly oxidized (eliminated) at the low temperature. The molds should remain in the furnace at least 60 minutes, and they may be held up to 5 hours longer with little damage. Since molds placed in the furnace at intervals lower the temperature of the furnace, extra time should be given to ensure complete wax elimination. Even though the mold is usually held at this temperature for 60 to 90 minutes, sufficient residual fine carbon may be retained to reduce the venting of the mold. Because of this potential for reduced venting, back-pressure porosity is a greater hazard in the low-heat technique than in the high-heat technique, since the investments generally employed with the low-heat technique may be more dense.

Muffle furnaces may be so airtight that burnout takes place in a reducing atmosphere, thereby preventing complete oxidation of the wax residues. Keeping the door open slightly permits air to enter and provides enough oxygen for elimination of the wax. This is particularly important for the hygroscopic expansion technique when a lower burnout temperature is used.

The standardized hygroscopic technique was developed for alloys with a high gold content; thus, there may be a need for slightly more expansion for the newer noble alloys. This added expansion may be obtained by making one or more of the following changes:

1. Increasing the water bath temperature to 40° C
2. Using two layers of liner
3. Increasing the burnout temperature to a range of 600° C to 650° C.

High-Heat Thermal Expansion Technique. This approach depends almost entirely on high-heat burnout to obtain the required expansion, while at the same time eliminating the wax pattern. Additional expansion results from the slight heating of gypsum investments on setting, thus expanding the wax pattern, and the water entering the investment from the wet liner, which adds a small amount of hygroscopic expansion to the normal setting expansion.

Gypsum Investments. These casting investments are relatively fragile and require the use of a metal ring for protection during heating. The molds are usually placed in a furnace at room temperature and slowly heated to 650° C to 700° C in 60 minutes and held for 15 to 30 minutes at the upper temperature.

The rate of heating has some influence on the smoothness and, in some instances, on the overall dimensions. Initially, the rapid heating can generate steam that can cause flaking or spalling of the mold walls. Too many patterns in the same plane within the investment often cause separation of a whole section of investment, because the expanding wax creates excessive pressure over a large area.

Too rapid a heating rate may also cause cracking of the investment. In such a case, the outside layer of the investment becomes heated before the center sections. Consequently, the outside layer starts to expand thermally, resulting in compressive stress in the outside layer that counteracts tensile stresses in the middle regions of the mold. Such a stress distribution causes the brittle investment to crack from the interior outwardly in the form of radial cracks. These cracks, in turn, produce a casting with fins or spines similar to those shown in Figure 23–7. This condition is especially likely to be present with a cristobalite investment. The comparatively low inversion temperature of the cristobalite, and the rapid rate of expansion during the inversion, makes it especially important to heat the investment slowly.

Breakdown of the dental investment and the resulting contamination and brittleness of the gold alloy casting probably occur more frequently than is generally realized. The mechanism of this investment decomposition and alloy contamination is related to a chemical reaction between the residual carbon and calcium sulfate binder.

Calcium sulfate *per se* does not decompose unless it is heated above 1000° C.

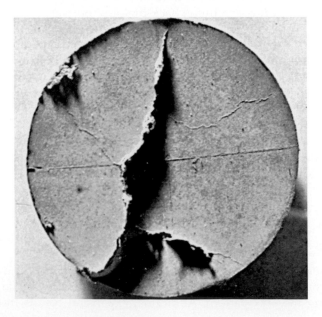

Figure 23–7. Fins on the surface of a casting that formed as a result of cracks in the investment before casting of the metal.

However, the reduction of calcium sulfate by carbon takes place rapidly above 700° C in accordance with the following reactions:

$$CaSO_4 + 4C \rightarrow CaS + 4CO$$

$$3CaSO_4 + CaS \rightarrow 4CaO + 4SO_2$$

Thus, this reaction takes place whenever gypsum investments are heated above 700° C in the presence of carbon. The sulfur dioxide as a product of this reaction contaminates gold castings and makes them extremely brittle. This fact emphasizes the need for completely eliminating the wax and avoiding burnout temperatures above 700° C, particularly if the investment contains carbon. Also, sulfur gases are generated by the gypsum investment when it is heated above 700° C.

After the casting temperature has been reached, the casting should be made immediately. Maintaining a high temperature for any considerable length of time may result in a sulfur contamination of the casting and also in a rough surface on the casting because of the disintegration of the investment.

Notwithstanding all of the these precautions and reasons for using a slow burnout technique, the inevitable human desire for instant results has reached the ears of investment manufacturers. There are now a few gypsum investments, some with a considerable amount of cristobalite, that are offered for use with a much more rapid burnout procedure. Some suggest placing the mold in a furnace at 315° C for 30 minutes and following with very rapid heating to the final burnout temperature. In addition, a few are offering investments that may be placed directly into a furnace at the final burnout temperature, held for 30 minutes, and cast. Because the design of the furnace, the proximity of the mold to the heating element, and the availability of air in the muffle may affect size and smoothness, it is advisable to examine these factors carefully before a casting is made in this manner.

Phosphate Investments. Many of the earlier statements about gypsum investments also apply to phosphate investments. There are several differences, however, because the setting mechanism and reactions on heating are quite different.

Phosphate investments obtain their expansion from the following sources:

1. The expansion of the wax pattern—this is considerable because the setting reaction raises the mold temperature considerably.
2. The setting expansion—this is usually higher than in gypsum investments, especially because special liquids are used to enhance such expansion.
3. The thermal expansion is greater when taken to temperatures higher than those used for gypsum-bonded investments.

A total expansion of 2% or more is required for porcelain-bonding alloys, since the gold and base metal alloys require higher melting and solidification temperatures when they have been designed for metal-ceramic restorations.

Although phosphate investments are usually much harder and stronger than gypsum investments, they are nevertheless quite brittle and are subject to the same unequal expansion of adjacent sections as phase changes occur during heating.

Because phosphate investments require (1) higher burnout temperatures to ensure total elimination of wax patterns, (2) the completion of chemical and physical changes, and (3) prevention of premature solidification of higher melting alloys, the usual burnout temperatures range from 750° C to 900° C. The heating rate is usually slow to 315° C and is quite rapid thereafter, reaching completion after a hold at the upper temperature for 30 minutes. Most burnout furnaces now have the capability to be programmed for heating rates and holding times.

Because the entire process involving phosphate investments takes a long time, the demand for time-saving changes is universal. Again, investment manufacturers have attempted to cooperate, and there are now some investments that can be subjected to two-stage heating more rapidly and placed directly in the furnace at the top temperature, held for 20 to 30 minutes, and then cast. To save more time, the use of a ring and a liner is also eliminated, the metal ring being replaced with a plastic ring that is tapered so that once the investment has set, it can be pushed out of the ring, held for a specified time to complete setting, and then placed directly into the hot furnace. Obviously, the expansion on setting is different than when a lined ring is used so that changes in overall fit must be considered. The required expansion may be adjusted by varying the liquid concentration.

Time Allowable for Casting. The investment contracts thermally as it cools. When the thermal expansion or high-heat technique is used, the investment loses heat after the heated ring is removed from the furnace, and the mold contracts. Because of the liner and the low thermal conductivity of the investment, a short period can elapse before the temperature of the mold is appreciably affected. Under average conditions of casting, approximately 1 minute can pass without a noticeable loss in dimension.

In the low-heat casting technique, the temperature gradient between the investment mold and the room is not as great as that employed with the high-heat technique. Also, the thermal expansion of the investment is not as important to the shrinkage compensation. However, the burnout temperature lies on a fairly steep portion of the thermal expansion curve rather than on a plateau portion as in the high-heat technique. Therefore, in the low-heat casting technique, the alloy should also be cast soon after removal of the ring from the oven or a significant variation from the desired casting dimensions may occur.

Casting Machines. Alloys are melted in one of the three following ways, depending on the available types of casting machines:

- The alloy is melted in a separate crucible by a torch flame and the metal is cast into the mold by centrifugal force (Fig. 23–8).
- The alloy is melted electrically by a resistance or induction furnace, then cast into the mold centrifugally by motor or spring action. Representative casting machines of these types are shown in Figures 23–9 and 23–10, respectively.
- The alloy is melted as in the first two ways, but it is cast by air pressure, a vacuum, or both.

The general procedure for each is described in the following sections, with certain advantages and disadvantages cited. However, it is important to follow the manufacturer's directions precisely.

Centrifugal Casting Machine. The casting machine spring is first wound from two to five turns (depending on the particular machine and the speed of casting rotation desired). The metal is melted by a torch flame in a glazed ceramic crucible attached to the "broken arm" of the casting machine. The broken-arm feature accelerates the initial rotational speed of the crucible and casting ring, thus increasing the linear speed of the liquid casting alloy as it moves into and

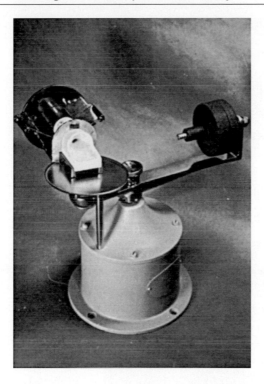

Figure 23–8. Centrifugal casting machine, spring-wound.

through the mold. Once the metal has reached the casting temperature and the heated casting ring is in position, the machine is released and the spring triggers the rotational motion.

As the metal fills the mold there is a hydrostatic pressure gradient develops along the length of the casting. The pressure gradient from the tip of the casting

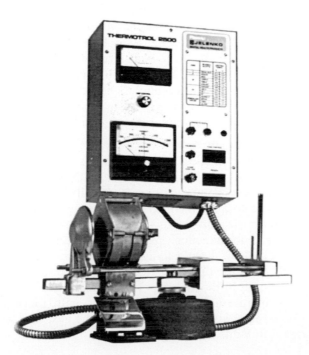

Figure 23–9. Casting machine, spring-wound, electrical resistance, melting furnace.

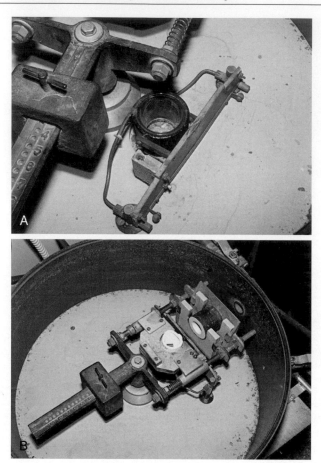

Figure 23–10. Induction melting casting machine. *A,* Water-cooled induction coil. *B,* Vertical crucible (white area) positioned within the induction coil.

to the bottom surface is quite sharp and parabolic in form, reaching zero at the button surface. Ordinarily, the pressure gradient at the moment before solidification begins reaches about 0.21 to 0.28 MPa (30 to 40 psi) at the tip of the casting. Because of this pressure gradient, there is also a gradient in the heat transfer rate such that the greatest rate of heat transfer to the mold is at the high pressure end of the gradient (i.e., the tip of the casting). Because this end also is frequently the sharp edge of the margin of a crown, there is further assurance that the solidification progresses from the thin margin edge to the button surface.

Electrical Resistance–heated Casting Machine. In this instance there is an automatic melting of the metal in a graphite crucible within a furnace rather than by use of a torch flame. This is an advantage, especially for alloys such as those used for metal-ceramic restorations, which are alloyed with base metals in trace amounts that tend to oxidize on overheating. Another advantage is that the crucible in the furnace is located flush against the casting ring. Therefore, the metal button remains molten slightly longer, again ensuring that solidification progresses completely from the tip of the casting to the button surface. A carbon crucible should not be used in the melting of high palladium or palladium-silver alloys, where the temperature exceeds 1504° C or with nickel-chromium or cobalt-chromium base metal alloys. An example of the electrical resistance casting machine is shown in Figure 23–9.

Induction Melting Machine. With this unit, the metal is melted by an induction field that develops within a crucible surrounded by water-cooled metal tubing (see Fig. 23-10). Once the metal reaches the casting temperature, it is forced into the mold by air pressure, vacuum, or both, at the other end of the ring. The device has become popular in the casting of jewelry but has not been used as much as the other two techniques for noble alloy castings. It is more commonly used for melting base metal alloys.

There is little practical difference in the properties or accuracy of castings made with any of the three types of casting machines. The choice is a matter of access and personal preference.

Casting Crucibles. Generally, three types of casting crucibles are available: clay, carbon, and quartz (including zircon-alumina). Clay crucibles are appropriate for many of the crown and bridge alloys, such as the high noble and noble types. Carbon crucibles can be used not only for high noble crown and bridge alloys but also for the higher-fusing, gold-based metal-ceramic alloys.

Quartz crucibles are recommended for high-fusing alloys of any type. They are especially suited for alloys that have a high melting range and are sensitive to carbon contamination. Crown and bridge alloys with a high palladium content, such as palladium-silver alloys for metal-ceramic copings, and any of the nickel-based or cobalt-based alloys are included in this category.

Melting Noble Metal Alloy. This type of alloy is best melted by placing it on the inner sidewall of the crucible. In this position, the operator can better observe the progress of the melting, and there a greater opportunity for any gases in the flame to be reflected from the surface of the metal rather than to be absorbed.

The fuel employed in most instances is a mixture of natural or artificial gas and air, although oxygen-air and acetylene can also be used. The temperature of the gas-air flame is greatly influenced by the nature of the gas and the proportions of gas and air in the mixture. Considerable care should be taken to obtain a nonluminous brush flame, with the different combustion zones clearly differentiated. Two types of flame can be obtained with a casting torch, as shown in Figure 23-11. The air supply for the lower flame (see Fig. 23-11) is excessive, and incomplete combustion and a lower temperature result. This type of flame is likely to be favored by the beginner because the roaring sound that accompan-

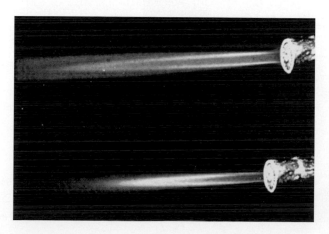

Figure 23–11. Two types of nonluminous flame showing combustion areas. The upper flame should be employed for fusing the noble metal alloy. The lower flame results from too much air in the mixture.

ies this flame adjustment "sounds" hot. The upper brush flame indicates the proper adjustment for maximal efficiency and temperature.

The parts of the flame can be identified by the conical areas in Figure 23–11 (see also Fig. 27–6). The first long cone emanating directly from the nozzle is the zone in which the air and gas are mixed before combustion. No heat is present in this zone. The next cone, which is green and immediately surrounding the inner cone, is known as the *combustion zone.* Here, the gas and air are partially burned. This zone is definitely oxidizing, and it should always be kept away from the molten metal during fusion.

The next zone, dimly blue, is the *reducing zone.* It is the hottest part of the flame and is just beyond the tip of the green combustion zone. This area should be kept constantly on the metal during melting. The outer cone (*oxidizing zone*) is the area in which combustion occurs with the oxygen in the air. Under no circumstances should this portion of the flame be employed to melt the alloy. Not only is its temperature lower than that of the reducing zone, but it also oxidizes the metal.

With a little practice, the proper zone in contact with the metal can be readily detected by the condition of the metal surface. When the reducing zone is in contact, the surface of the gold alloy is bright and mirrorlike, as indicated in Figure 23–12*A*. When the oxidizing portion of the flame is in contact with the metal, there is a dull film of "dross" developed over the surface, as seen in Figure 23–12*B*. Although care should be taken not to overheat the alloy, there is generally more likelihood of underheating when the gas-air flame is used. The alloy first appears to be spongy, and then small globules of fused metal appear.

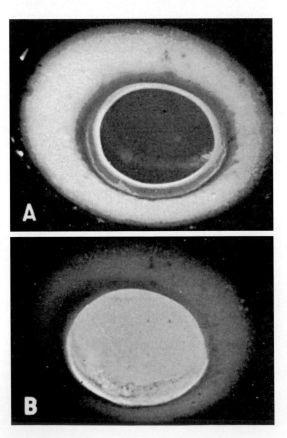

Figure 23–12. A, Mirrorlike surface of the metal indicates proper fusion. *B,* Cloudy surface indicates surface oxidation by improper positioning of the torch flame.

The molten alloy soon assumes a spheroidal shape as indicated in Figure 23–12*A*. At the proper casting temperature, the molten alloy is light orange and tends to spin or follow the flame when the latter is moved slightly. At this point, the metal should be approximately 38° C to 66° C above its liquidus temperature. The casting should be made immediately when the proper temperature is reached. As previously discussed, there are also various devices available for melting the alloy electrically.

It is desirable to use a flux for gold crown and bridge alloys to aid in minimizing porosity. When properly employed, the flux increases the fluidity of the metal and the film of flux formed on the surface of the molten alloy helps prevent oxidation. Reducing fluxes containing powdered charcoal are often used, but small bits of carbon may be carried into the mold and cause a deficiency at a critical margin. Although such reducing fluxes are excellent for cleaning old metal, a better flux for the casting procedure may be made from equal parts of fused borax powder ground with boric acid powder. The boric acid aids in retaining the borax on the surface of the metal. The flux is added when the alloy is completely melted and should be used with both old and new metal. Old sprues and buttons from the same alloy may be recast if they are not contaminated.

Cleaning the Casting. Let us first consider the gold crown and bridge alloys. After the casting has been completed, the ring is removed and quenched in water as soon as the button exhibits a dull-red glow. Two advantages are gained in quenching: (1) the noble metal alloy is left in an annealed condition for burnishing, polishing, and similar procedures, and (2) when the water contacts the hot investment, a violent reaction ensues. The investment becomes soft and granular, and the casting is more easily cleaned.

Often the surface of the casting appears dark with oxides and tarnish. Such a surface film can be removed by a process known as *pickling*, which consists of heating the discolored casting in an acid. Probably the best pickling solution for gypsum-bonded investments is a 50% hydrochloric acid solution. The hydrochloric acid aids in the removal of any residual investment as well as of the oxide coating. The disadvantage of the use of hydrochloric acid is that the fumes from the acid are likely to corrode laboratory metal furnishings. In addition, these fumes are a health hazard and should be vented via a fume hood. A solution of sulfuric acid is more advantageous in this respect. Ultrasonic devices are also available for cleaning the casting, as are commercial pickling solutions made of acid salts.

The best method for pickling is to place the casting in a test tube or dish and to pour the acid over it. It may be necessary to heat the acid, but boiling should be avoided because of the considerable amount of acid fumes involved. After pickling, the acid is poured off and the casting is removed. The pickling solution should be renewed frequently because it is likely to become contaminated with use.

In no case should the casting be held with steel tongs so that both the casting and the tongs come into contact with the pickling solution, as this may contaminate the casting. The pickling solution usually contains small amounts of copper dissolved from previous castings. When the steel tongs contact this electrolyte, a small galvanic cell is created and copper is deposited on the casting at the point where the tongs grip it. This copper deposition extends into the metal and is a future source for discoloration in the area.

It is a common practice to heat the casting and then to drop it into the pickling solution. The disadvantage of this method is that a delicate margin may be melted in the flame or the casting may be distorted by the sudden thermal shock when plunged into the acid.

Gold-based and palladium-based metal-ceramic alloys and base metal alloys are bench cooled to room temperature before the casting is removed from the investment. Castings from these alloys are generally not pickled, and when it is recommended for certain metal-ceramic alloys, it is only to selectively remove specific surface oxides.

TECHNICAL CONSIDERATIONS FOR PHOSPHATE-BONDED INVESTMENTS

When investing a wax pattern in a phosphate-bonded investment, the procedure is essentially the same as for a gypsum-bonded investment. As previously mentioned, the working time can vary depending on the L:P ratio, special liquid concentration used, temperature, mixing time, mixing rate, and operator skill and experience.

When phosphate investments were introduced in dental laboratories that were also using gypsum investments, some problems arose with faulty setting of the investments and imperfect castings. Specifically, castings made in gypsum investments following the use of phosphate investments were inferior. It was learned that traces of phosphate investments posed difficulties in the setting of gypsum investments. Any residual investment particles left in the mixing bowls, even after thorough washing, are sufficient to influence the behavior of the gypsum materials. Manufacturers now caution users to use separate mixing bowls and spatulas for the two different types of investment.

As with any investment having a high thermal expansion, and with marked changes in expansion or contraction occurring, it is necessary to use a slow heating rate during burnout to prevent possible cracking or spalling. Some furnaces have controls for slowing the rate of heating. For those that do not, it is advisable to use a two-stage burnout, holding at 200° C to 300° C for at least 30 minutes before completing the burnout. Recommendations for the rate of rise vary, so it is wise to follow the instructions for the specific investment used.

Although phosphate investments appear strong, they are still subject to a number of disrupting influences during burnout. At first the wax softens and then expands much more than does the investment. When investing, it is desirable to leave 3 to 6 mm of investment around each pattern and to stagger the patterns if several are placed in the same ring. A number of patterns in one plane can exert tremendous pressure and fracture almost any investment, but particularly the phosphate-bonded materials. The rapid expansion of cristobalite investment at approximately 300° C requires slow heating to prevent fracture. After the temperature reaches 400° C, the rate of heating can be safely increased. After burnout, usually at a final temperature of 700° C to 900° C depending on the alloy melting range, the casting is made. As previously mentioned, the permeability of the phosphate investment is low compared with that of a gypsum-bonded investment. Therefore, the required casting pressure should be greater than for a gypsum mold.

Recovery and cleaning of the casting are more difficult when a phosphate-bonded investment is used because such materials do not contain the soft gypsum products. Also, the particles usually include large grains of quartz. In some instances, such as with gold-containing alloys, the investment adheres rather tenaciously, usually requiring cleansing in an ultrasonic cleaner. Neither the phosphate binder nor the silica refractory is soluble in hydrochloric or sulfuric acid. Cold hydrofluoric acid dissolves the silica refractory quite well without damage to a gold-palladium-silver alloy but must be used carefully with other alloys. In fact, even dilute hydrofluoric acid should not be used unless the clinician is familiar with first aid techniques and the necessary neutralizing solutions are immediately at hand. However, once tissue injury has occurred it cannot be reversed with such solutions. Alternative solutions such as No-San can be used with greater safety.

Base metal alloys require a light sandblasting, usually with fine aluminum oxide. Chromium-based partial dentures are usually sandblasted to remove the investment. Acid should never be used for cleaning base metal alloys.

The selection of the appropriate phosphate-bonded investment must be made on the basis of the composition of the alloy to be used. Carbon-containing investments are well suited for gold-based crown and bridge casting alloys and metal-ceramic alloys. However, if the alloy is carbon sensitive (such as in silver-palladium, high palladium, palladium-silver, nickel-chromium-beryllium, nickel-chromium, and cobalt-chromium alloys), a noncarbon investment should be used.

CAUSES OF DEFECTIVE CASTINGS

An unsuccessful casting results in considerable trouble and loss of time. In almost all instances, defects in castings can be avoided by strict observance of procedures governed by certain fundamental rules and principles. Seldom is a defect in a casting attributable to other factors than the carelessness or ignorance of the operator. With present techniques, casting failures should be the exception, not the rule.

Defects in castings can be classified under four headings: (1) distortion; (2) surface roughness and irregularities; (3) porosity; and (4) incomplete or missing detail. Some of these factors have been discussed in connection with certain phases of the casting techniques. The subject is summarized and analyzed in some detail in the following sections.

Distortion. Any marked distortion of the casting is probably related to a distortion of the wax pattern, as described in the chapter on inlay wax. This type of distortion can be minimized or prevented by proper manipulation of the wax and handling of the pattern.

Unquestionably, some distortion of the wax pattern occurs as the investment hardens around it. The setting and hygroscopic expansions of the investment may produce an uneven movement of the walls of the pattern.

This type of distortion occurs in part from the uneven outward movement of the proximal walls. The gingival margins are forced apart by the mold expansion, whereas the solid occlusal bar of wax resists expansion during the early stages of setting. The configuration of the pattern, the type of wax, and the thickness influence the distortion that occurs, as has been discussed. For example, distortion increases as the thickness of the pattern decreases. As would be expected, the less the setting expansion of the investment, the less is the distortion. Generally, it is not a serious problem except that it accounts for some of the unexplained inaccuracies that may occur in small castings. There is probably not a great deal that can be done to control this phenomenon.

Surface Roughness, Irregularities, and Discoloration. The surface of a dental casting should be an accurate reproduction of the surface of the wax pattern from which it is made. Excessive roughness or irregularities on the outer surface of the casting necessitate additional finishing and polishing, whereas irregularities on the cavity surface prevent a proper seating of an otherwise accurate casting.

Surface roughness should not be confused with surface irregularities. Surface roughness is defined as relatively finely spaced surface imperfections whose height, width, and direction establish the predominant surface pattern. Surface irregularities refer to isolated imperfections, such as nodules, that do not characterize the total surface area.

Even under optimal conditions, the surface roughness of the dental casting is invariably somewhat greater than that of the wax pattern from which it is made. The difference is probably related to the particle size of the investment and its ability to reproduce the wax pattern in microscopic detail. With proper manipulative techniques, the normal increased roughness in the casting should not be a major factor in dimensional accuracy. However, improper technique can lead to a marked increase in surface roughness, as well as to the formation of surface irregularities.

Air Bubbles. Small nodules on a casting are caused by air bubbles that become attached to the pattern during or subsequent to the investing procedure. Such nodules can sometimes be removed if they are not in a critical area. However, for nodules on margins or on internal surfaces, as at A in Figure 23–13, removal of these irregularities might alter the fit of the casting. As previously noted, the best method to avoid air bubbles is to use the vacuum investing technique.

If a manual method is used, various precautions can be observed to eliminate air from the investment mix before the investing. As previously outlined, the use of a mechanical mixer with vibration both before and after mixing should be practiced routinely. A wetting agent may be helpful in preventing the collec-

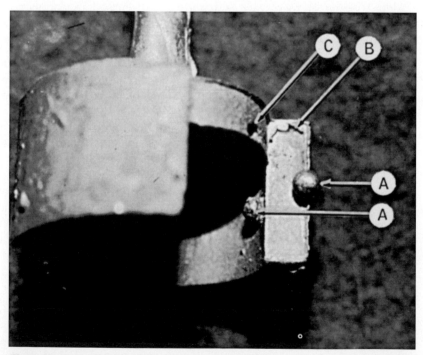

Figure 23–13. Surface irregularities on an experimental casting caused by air bubbles (A), water film (B), and inclusion of foreign body (C). (Courtesy of D. Veira.)

tion of air bubbles on the surface of the pattern, but it is by no means a certain remedy. As previously discussed, it is important that the wetting agent be applied in a thin layer. It is best to air dry the wetting agent, because any excess liquid dilutes the investment, possibly producing surface irregularities on the casting.

Water Films. Wax is repellent to water, and if the investment becomes separated from the wax pattern in some manner, a water film may form irregularly over the surface. Occasionally, this type of surface irregularity appears as minute ridges or veins on the surface, as shown at B in Figure 23–13.

If the pattern is moved slightly, jarred, or vibrated after investing, or if the painting procedure does not result in an intimate contact of the investment with the pattern, such a condition may result. A wetting agent is of aid in the prevention of such irregularities. Too high an L:P ratio may also produce these surface irregularities.

Rapid Heating Rates. This factor has been discussed in a previous section. It results in fins or spines on the casting similar to those shown in Figure 23–7, or a characteristic surface roughness may be evident because of flaking of the investment when the water or steam pours into the mold. Furthermore, such a surge of steam or water may carry some of the salts used as modifiers into the mold, which are left as deposits on the walls after the water evaporates. As previously mentioned, the mold should be heated gradually; at least 60 minutes should elapse during the heating of the investment-filled ring from room temperature to 700° C. The greater the bulk of the investment, the more slowly it should be heated.

Underheating. Incomplete elimination of wax residues may occur if the heating time is too short or if insufficient air is available in the furnace. These factors are particularly important with the low-temperature investment techniques. Voids or porosity may occur in the casting from the gases formed when the hot alloy comes in contact with the carbonaceous residues. Occasionally, the casting may be covered with a tenacious carbon coating that is virtually impossible to remove by pickling.

Liquid:Powder Ratio. The amount of water and investment should be measured accurately. The higher the L:P ratio, the rougher the casting. However, if too little water is used, the investment may be unmanageably thick and cannot be properly applied to the pattern. In vacuum investing, the air may not be sufficiently removed. In either instance, a rough surface on the casting may result.

Prolonged Heating. When the high-heat casting technique is used, a prolonged heating of the mold at the casting temperature is likely to cause a disintegration of the investment, and the walls of the mold are roughened as a result. Furthermore, the products of decomposition are sulfur compounds that may contaminate the alloy to the extent that the surface texture is affected. Such contamination may be the reason that the surface of the casting sometimes does not respond to pickling. When the thermal expansion technique is employed, the mold should be heated to the casting temperature—never higher than 700° C—and the casting should be made immediately.

Temperature of the Alloy. If an alloy is heated to too high a temperature before casting, the surface of the investment is likely to be attacked, and a surface roughness of the type described in the previous section may result. As previously noted, in all probability the alloy will not be overheated with a gas-air torch when used with the gas supplied in most localities. If other fuel is used, special care should be observed that the color emitted by the molten gold alloy, for example, is no lighter than a light orange.

Casting Pressure. Too high a pressure during casting can produce a rough surface on the casting. A gauge pressure of 0.10 to 0.14 MPa in an air pressure casting machine or three to four turns of the spring in an average type of centrifugal casting machine is sufficient for small castings.

Composition of the Investment. The ratio of the binder to the quartz influences the surface texture of the casting. In addition, a coarse silica causes a surface roughness. If the investment meets ADA Specification No. 2, the composition is probably not a factor in the surface roughness.

Foreign Bodies. When foreign substances get into the mold, a surface roughness may be produced. For example, a rough crucible former with investment clinging to it may roughen the investment on its removal so that bits of investment are carried into the mold with the molten alloy. Carelessness in the removal of the sprue former may be a similar cause.

Usually, contamination results not only in surface roughness but also in incomplete areas or surface voids. An example may be seen at C in Figure 23–13. Any casting that shows sharp, well-defined deficiencies indicates the presence of some foreign particles in the mold, such as pieces of investment and bits of carbon from a flux. Bright-appearing concavities may be the result of flux being carried into the mold with the metal.

Surface discoloration and roughness can result from sulfur contamination, either from investment breakdown at elevated temperatures or from a high sulfur content of the torch flame. The interaction of the molten alloy with sulfur produces black castings that are brittle and do not clean readily during pickling.

Impact of Molten Alloy. The direction of the sprue former should be such that the molten gold alloy does not strike a weak portion of the mold surface. Occasionally, the molten alloy may fracture or abrade the mold surface on impact, regardless of its bulk. It is unfortunate that sometimes the abraded area is smooth so that it cannot be detected on the surface of the casting. Such a depression in the mold is reflected as a raised area on the casting, often too slight to be noticed yet sufficiently large to prevent the seating of the casting. This type of surface roughness or irregularity can be avoided by proper spruing so as to prevent the direct impact of the molten metal at an angle of 90 degrees to the investment surface. A glancing impact is likely to be less damaging, and at the same time an undesirable turbulence is avoided.

Pattern Position. If several patterns are invested in the same ring they should not be placed too close together. Likewise, too many patterns positioned in the same plane in the mold should be avoided. The expansion of wax is much greater than that of the investment, causing breakdown or cracking of the investment if the spacing between patterns is less than 3 mm.

Carbon Inclusions. Carbon, as from a crucible, an improperly adjusted torch, or a carbon-containing investment, can be absorbed by the alloy during casting. These particles may lead to the formation of carbides or even create visible carbon inclusions.

Other Causes. There are certain surface discolorations and roughness that may not be evident when the casting is completed but that may appear during service. For example, various gold alloys, such as solders, bits of wire, and mixtures of different casting alloys should never be melted together and reused. The resulting mixture would not possess the proper physical properties and might form eutectic or similar alloys with low corrosion resistance. Discoloration and corrosion may also occur.

A source of discoloration often overlooked is the surface contamination of a gold alloy restoration by mercury. Mercury penetrates rapidly into the alloy and causes a marked loss in ductility and a greater susceptibility to corrosion. Thus, it is not a good practice to place a new amalgam restoration adjacent to a high noble alloy restoration. In addition, these dissimilar metals form a galvanic cell that can lead to breakdown of the anode (amalgam) relative to the cathode (noble alloy).

Porosity. Porosity may occur both within the interior region of a casting and on the external surface. The latter is a factor in surface roughness, but also it is generally a manifestation of internal porosity. Not only does the internal porosity weaken the casting but if it also extends to the surface, it may be a cause for discoloration. If severe, it can produce leakage at the tooth–restoration interface, and secondary caries may result. Although the porosity in a casting cannot be prevented entirely, it can be minimized by use of proper techniques.

Porosities in noble metal alloy castings may be classified as follows:

I. Solidification defects
   A. Localized shrinkage porosity
   B. Microporosity
II. Trapped gases
   A. Pinhole porosity
   B. Gas inclusions
   C. Subsurface porosity
III. Residual air

Localized shrinkage is generally caused by incomplete feeding of molten metal during solidification. The linear contraction of noble metal alloys in changing from a liquid to a solid is at least 1.25%. Therefore, there must be continual feeding of molten metal through the sprue to make up for the shrinkage of metal volume during solidification. If the sprue freezes in its cross section before this feeding is completed to the casting proper, a localized shrinkage void will occur in the last portion of the casting that solidifies. Four types of porosity are shown in Figure 23–14A and B: (a) localized shrinkage porosity; (b) microporosity; (c) pinhole porosity; and (d) subsurface porosity. Localized shrinkage porosity is also shown in Figure 23–14C. The porosity in the pontic area is caused by the ability of the pontic to retain heat because of its bulk and because it was located in the heat center of the ring. This problem can be solved in the future simply by attaching one or more small-gauge sprues (e.g., 18 gauge) at the surface most distant from the main sprue attachment and extending the sprue(s) laterally within 5 mm of the edge of the ring. These small chill-set sprues ensure

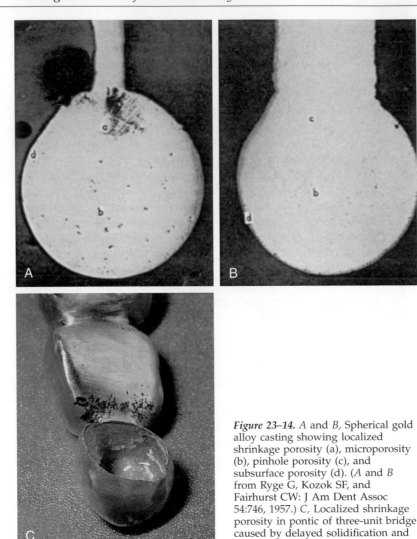

Figure 23–14. A and B, Spherical gold alloy casting showing localized shrinkage porosity (a), microporosity (b), pinhole porosity (c), and subsurface porosity (d). (A and B from Ryge G, Kozok SF, and Fairhurst CW: J Am Dent Assoc 54:746, 1957.) C, Localized shrinkage porosity in pontic of three-unit bridge caused by delayed solidification and lack of a chill-set sprue.

that solidification begins within these sprues and they act as cooling pins to carry heat away from the pontic.

Localized shrinkage generally occurs near the sprue-casting junction, but it may occur anywhere between dendrites, as shown in Figure 23–15C, where the last part of the casting that solidified was in the low melting metal that remained as the dendrite branches develop.

This type of void may also occur externally, usually in the interior of a crown near the area of the sprue, if a hot spot has been created by the hot metal impinging from the sprue channel on a point of the mold wall. This hot spot causes the local region to freeze last and result in what is called *suck-back porosity*, as shown in Figure 23–16 (left). This often occurs at an occlusoaxial line angle or incisoaxial line angle that is not well rounded. The entering metal impinges onto the mold surface at this point and creates a higher localized mold temperature in this region that is called a *hot spot.* A hot spot may retain a localized pool of molten metal after other areas of the casting have solidified. This in turn creates a shrinkage void, or suck-back porosity. Suck-back porosity can be elimin-

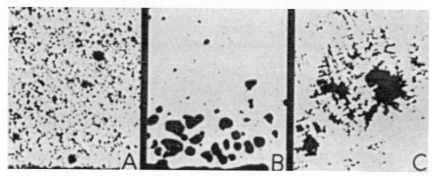

Figure 23–15. *A,* Microporosity, pinhole porosity, and gas inclusions. Microporosity voids are irregular in shape, whereas the two other types tend to be spherical; the largest spherical voids are gas inclusions. *B,* Subsurface porosity. *C,* Localized shrinkage porosity. (*A* to *C* courtesy of G. Ryge.)

ated by flaring the point of sprue attachment and by reducing the mold-melt temperature differential, that is, lowering the casting temperature by about 30° C.

Microporosity also occurs from solidification shrinkage but is generally present in fine grain alloy castings when the solidification is too rapid for the microvoids to segregate to the liquid pool. This premature solidification causes the porosity shown in Figure 23–14C and portions of Figure 23–16 in the form of small irregular voids.

Such phenomena can occur from the rapid solidification if the mold or casting temperature is too low. It is unfortunate that this type of defect is not detectable unless the casting is sectioned. In any case, it is generally not a serious defect. The effects of various factors involved in formation of microporosity, and other types of porosity, are summarized in Table 23–3.

Both the *pinhole* and the *gas inclusion porosities* are related to the entrapment of gas during solidification. Both are characterized by a spherical contour, but they are decidedly different in size. The gas inclusion porosities are usually much larger than pinhole porosity, as indicated in Figure 23–15A. Many metals dissolve or occlude gases while they are molten. For example, both copper and silver dissolve oxygen in large amounts in the liquid state. Molten platinum and palladium have a strong affinity for hydrogen as well as oxygen. On solidifica-

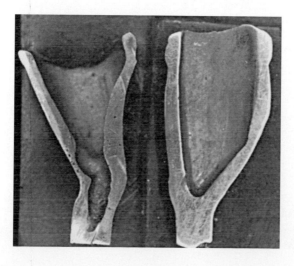

Figure 23–16. Demonstration of suck-back porosity. *Left,* The coping was cast at 1370° C (2500° F). *Right,* This coping was cast at 1340° C (2450° F). (Courtesy of J. Nielsen.)

TABLE 23–3. Effects of Technical Factors on the Porosity Resulting from Metal Solidification

Type of Porosity	Increased Sprue Thickness	Increased Sprue Length	Increased Melt Temperature	Increased Mold Temperature
Localized shrinkage porosity	Decreased	Increased	Decreased	Decreased
Subsurface porosity	Increased	Decreased	Increased	Increased
Microporosity	No effect	No effect	Decreased	Decreased

With permission from Ryge G, Kozak SF, and Fairhurst CW: J Am Dent Assoc 54:746, 1957.

tion, the absorbed gases are expelled and the pinhole porosity results. The larger voids (Fig. 23–15A) may also result from the same cause, but it seems more logical to assume that such voids may be caused by gas that is mechanically trapped by the molten metal in the mold or that is incorporated during the casting procedure. All castings probably contain a certain amount of porosity, as exemplified by the photomicrographs shown in Figure 23–17. However, the porosity should be kept to a minimum because it may adversely affect the physical properties of the casting.

Oxygen is dissolved by some of the metals, such as silver, in the alloy while

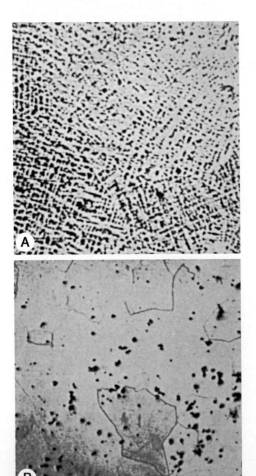

Figure 23–17. A, Grain structure of a Type III noble metal alloy as cast. B, Same alloy after a homogenization heat treatment at 725° C (1337° F) for 70 minutes. Pinhole porosity can be noted in B. (A and B courtesy of B. Hedegard.)

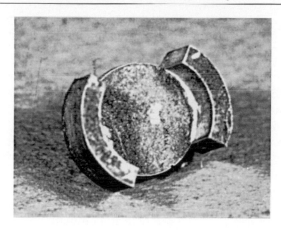

Figure 23–18. A black-coated noble metal alloy casting resulting from sulfur contamination or oxidation during melting of the alloy.

they are in the molten state. During solidification, the gas is expelled to form blebs and pores in the metal. As was pointed out earlier, this type of porosity may be attributed to abuse of the metal. Castings that are severely contaminated with gases are usually black when they are removed from the investment and do not clean easily on pickling (Fig. 23–18). The porosity that extends to the surface is usually in the form of small pinpoint holes (see Fig. 23–15A). When the surface is polished, other pinholes appear.

Larger spherical porosities can be caused by gas occluded from a poorly adjusted torch flame, or the use of the mixing or oxidizing zones of the flame rather than the reducing zone (see Fig. 23–15A). These types of porosity can be minimized by premelting the gold alloy on a graphite crucible or a graphite block if the alloy has been used before and by correctly adjusting and positioning the torch flame during melting.

Subsurface porosity occurs on occasion as is shown in Figures 23–14B and 23–15B and at other times it may be particularly evident. The reasons for such voids have not been completely established. They may be caused by the simultaneous nucleation of solid grains and gas bubbles at the first moment that the metal freezes at the mold walls. As has been explained, this type of porosity can be diminished by controlling the rate at which the molten metal enters the mold.

Entrapped air porosity on the inner surface of the casting, sometimes referred to as *back-pressure porosity,* can produce large concave depressions such as those seen in Figure 23–19. This is caused by the inability of the air in the mold to

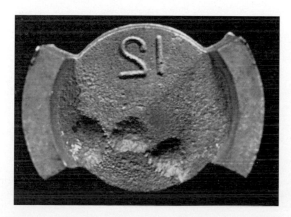

Figure 23–19. Surface irregularity on cavity side of casting caused by back-pressure porosity.

escape through the pores in the investment or by the pressure gradient that displaces the air pocket toward the end of the investment via the molten sprue and button. The entrapment is frequently found in a "pocket" at the cavity surface of a crown or mesio-occlusal-distal casting (see Fig. 23–19). Occasionally, it is found even on the outside surface of the casting when the casting temperature or mold temperature is so low that solidification occurs before the entrapped air can escape. The incidence of entrapped air can be increased by the dense modern investments, an increase in mold density produced by vacuum investing, and the tendency for the mold to clog with residual carbon when the low-heat technique is used. Each of these factors tends to slow down the venting of gases from the mold during casting.

Proper burnout, an adequate mold and casting temperature, a sufficiently high casting pressure, and proper L:P ratio can help to eliminate this phenomenon. It is good practice to make sure that the thickness of investment between the tip of the pattern and the end of the ring not be greater than 6 mm.

Incomplete Casting. Occasionally, only a partially complete casting, or perhaps no casting at all, is found. The obvious cause is that the molten alloy has been prevented, in some manner, from completely filling the mold. At least two factors that might inhibit the ingress of the liquefied metal are insufficient venting of the mold and high viscosity of the fused metal.

The first consideration, insufficient venting, is directly related to the back pressure exerted by the air in the mold. If the air cannot be vented quickly, the molten alloy does not fill the mold before if solidifies. In such a case, the magnitude of the casting pressure should be suspected. If insufficient casting pressure is employed, the back pressure cannot be overcome. Furthermore, the pressure should be applied for at least 4 seconds. The mold is filled and the metal is solidified in 1 second or less, yet it is quite soft during the early stages. Therefore, the pressure should be maintained for a few seconds beyond this point. Examples of an incomplete casting because of insufficient casting pressure are shown in Figures 23–20 and Figure 23–21. These failures are usually exemplified in rounded, incomplete margins.

A second common cause for an incomplete casting is incomplete elimination of wax residues from the mold. If too many products of combustion remain in the mold, the pores in the investment may become filled so that the air cannot be vented completely. If moisture or particles of wax remain, the contact of the molten alloy with these foreign substances produces an explosion that may produce sufficient back pressure to prevent the mold from being filled. An

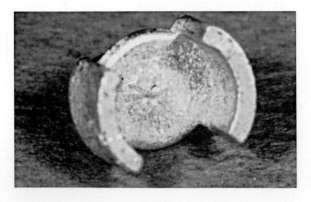

Figure 23–20. Rounded, incomplete margins are evidence of insufficient casting pressure.

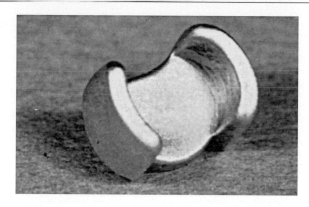

Figure 23–21. Incomplete casting resulting from incomplete wax elimination is characterized by rounded margins and shiny appearance.

example of a casting failure caused by incomplete wax elimination can be seen in Figure 23–21. Although similar to the incomplete casting in Figure 23–20, it can be noted that the rounded margins are quite shiny rather than dull. This shiny condition of the metal is caused by the strong reducing atmosphere created by carbon monoxide left by the residual wax.

The possible influence of the L:P ratio of the investment has already been discussed. A lower L:P ratio is associated with less porosity of the investment. An increase in casting pressure during casting solves this problem.

Different alloy compositions probably exhibit varying viscosities in the molten state, depending on composition and temperature. However, both the surface tension and the viscosity of a molten alloy are decreased with an increase in temperature. An incomplete casting resulting from too great a viscosity of the casting metal can be attributed to insufficient heating. The temperature of the alloy should be raised higher than its liquidus temperature so that its viscosity and surface tension are lowered and it does not solidify prematurely as it enters the mold. Such premature solidification may account for the greater susceptibility of the white gold alloys to porosity because their liquidus temperatures are higher. Thus, they are more difficult to melt with a gas-air torch flame.

SELECTED READING

Asgar K, and Peyton FA: Pits on inner surfaces of cast gold crowns. J Prosthet Dent 9:448, 1959.
  With the hygroscopic water-added technique, increases in casting pressure, the amount of gold, and the sprue former diameter reduced or eliminated casting pits and voids. Flaring the sprue former at its attachment to the wax pattern acts like a reservoir and facilitates the flow of alloy to the pattern area.
Christensen GJ: Marginal fit of gold inlay castings. J Prosthet Dent 16:297, 1966.
  In this laboratory study, 10 dentists accepted cemented gold inlays with a mean occlusal margin opening of 21 μm (range of 2 to 51 μm), a mean proximal margin opening of 26 μm (range of 9 to 34 μm), and a gingival margin opening of 74 μm (range of 34 to 119 μm). Explorer examination of visually accessible areas was superior to either explorer or radiographic examination of visually inaccessible areas.
Dootz ER, and Asgar K: Solidification patterns of single crowns and three-unit bridge castings. Quint Dent Technol 10:299, 1986.
  Solidification rates and patterns differed for Type III gold alloy and a palladium-silver alloy. The gold alloy solidified in a scattered or random pattern, whereas the palladium-silver metal-ceramic alloy solidified in a unidirectional manner.
Eames WB, O'Neal SJ, Monteiro J, et al: Techniques to improve the seating of castings. J Am Dent Assoc 96:432, 1978.
  Die spacing was the most suitable method to compensate for casting variables and ensure improved marginal adaptation yet increasing retention 25%.
Finger W: Effect of the setting expansion of dental stone upon the die precision. Scand J Dent Res 88:159, 1980.
  The addition of potassium sulfate and borax to Type IV gypsums reduced setting expansion without affecting the physical properties.

Lyon HW, Dickson G, and Schoonover IC: Effectiveness of vacuum investing in the elimination of surface defects of gold castings. J Am Dent Assoc 46:197, 1953.
Vacuum investing was found to eliminate nodules from 95 of 100 castings as compared with only 17 of 100 nodule-free castings produced from hand-invested castings. The defects in the five vacuum-invested castings occurred when nodules were trapped under horizontal or concave surfaces on the pattern.

Mackert JR Jr: An expert system for analysis of casting failures. Int J Prosthodont 1:268, 1988.
An expert system is proposed for the diagnosis of common lost-wax casting problems that is based on an interactive consultation session at a PC station during which the user answers questions about defective castings. The computer responds with conclusion on the most likely cause of the problem.

Martin KH: An investigation of the effect of the water/powder ratio on the accuracy of the fit of gold alloy castings. Aust Dent J 1:202, 1956.
Use of the correct water:powder ratio with a gypsum investment is essential to obtaining a good fit of castings, especially when using the low-heat technique.

Mumford GM, and Phillips RW: Measurements of thermal expansion of cristobalite-type investments in the inlay ring—preliminary report. J Prosthet Dent 8:860, 1958.
Thermal expansion of a gypsum investment is restricted by the ring when a single-ring liner is used. However, for areas not in direct contact with the ring, the expansion is greater.

Naylor WP, Moore BK, and Phillips RW: A topographical assessment of casting ring liners using scanning electron microscopy (SEM). Quint Dent Technol 11:413, 1987.
Three types of nonasbestos ring liners exist: ceramic, cellulose, and a ceramic-cellulose combination. A liner containing an aluminum silicate component has the potential to produce respirable-size ceramic particles.

Naylor WP: Spruing, Investing, and Casting Techniques. Section 4. Non-gold Base Dental Alloys: Volume 11. Porcelain Fused to Metal Alloys. USAFSAM-TR-5, 1986, pp 75–99.
This section of the technical manual reviews the principles of spruing (direct and indirect), the laws of casting, and the buttonless casting technique.

Nielsen JP: Pressure distribution in centrifugal dental casting. J Dent Res 57:261, 1978.
This article discusses the factors that contribute to the pressure gradient that develops along the length of a casting when cast in a centrifugal casting machine.

Nielsen JP, and Ollerman R: Suck-back porosity. Quint Dent Technol 1:61, 1976.
Using a gold-palladium-silver alloy with different sprue former lengths, diameters, and angles of attachment, lower casting temperature and flaring of the sprue former reduced suck-back porosity. The authors postulated that a "hot spot" is created in the mold that causes this type of porosity.

Nomura GT, Reisbick MH, and Preston JD: An investigation of epoxy resin dies. J Prosthet Dent 44:45, 1980.
In a comparison of three epoxy die materials with a Type IV stone, full crown epoxy dies were undersized, MOD onlay resin dies were accurate, and detail reproduction was found to be comparable to the Type IV gypsum. However, only one epoxy material had a hardness approaching that of the dental stone.

O'Brien WJ, and Nielsen JP: Decomposition of gypsum investments in the presence of carbon. J Dent Res 38:541, 1959.
The reduction of calcium sulfate by carbon or carbon monoxide takes place rapidly above 700° C, releasing calcium sulfide and sulfur dioxide.

Tombasco T, and Reilly RP: A comparison of burnout temperatures and their effects on elimination of plastic sprues. Trends Techniques 4:36, 1987.
In assessing the effect of different burnout temperatures on wax and plastic elimination, the authors found that a two-stage burnout technique using a first stage of 427° C (800° F) for 30 minutes was better than a one-stage burnout at 260° C (500° F), 316° C (600° F), or 427° C (700° F).

Vaidyanathan TK, Schulman A, Nielsen JP, and Shalita S: Correlation between macroscopic porosity location and liquid metal pressure in centrifugal casting technique. J Dent Res 60:59, 1981.
Radiographic analysis of uniform cylindrical castings revealed that the porosity is dependent on the location at which the sprue is attached to the casting. The location of the macroscopic porosity, at portions of the casting close to the free surface of the button, is dependent on the pressure gradient and, therefore, different heat transfer rates in different portions of the casting.

24 *Dental Cements for Restorations and Pulp Protection*

- Uses and Classification of Dental Cements
- Silicate Cement
- Anticariogenic Properties of Fluoride
- Glass Ionomer Cement
- Properties of Glass Ionomer Cement
- Critical Procedures for Glass Ionomer Restorations
- Metal-modified Glass Ionomer Cement
- Resin-modified Glass Ionomer Cement
- Zinc Oxide–Eugenol Cement
- Agents for Pulp Protection
- Cavity Varnishes
- Cavity Liners
- Cement Bases

USES AND CLASSIFICATION OF DENTAL CEMENTS

Dental cements used as restorative materials have low strengths compared with those of resin-based composites and amalgams, but they can be used for low-stress areas. Regardless of their inferior strength, they possess many desirable characteristics that justify their use in up to 60% of all restorations.

Although restorative cements are used for temporary and longer-term restorations, they are also required for other applications. For example, before placement of a restoration, the pulp may have been irritated or damaged from a variety of sources, such as caries and cavity preparations. To protect the pulp against further trauma, thermal-insulating bases are often placed under metallic restorations, and pulp-capping agents and cavity liners are placed on prepared tooth surfaces that are close to the pulp chamber. Cavity liners such as cavity varnish and dentin bonding agents can also protect pulp tissue against the effects of certain components of restorative materials and against microleakage.

Some fluoride-containing cements can be used as fissure sealants, root canal sealants, and core buildups for restoration of broken-down teeth.

Other major applications of dental cements include cementation *(luting)* of prostheses and orthodontic appliances and securing posts and pins placed for retention of restorations. These applications are discussed in Chapter 25.

Some dental cements are supplied in two components: a powder and a liquid. They are generally classified according to their chemical formulation, as presented in Table 24–1. With the exception of calcium hydroxide and resin products, most cements set by an acid-base reaction. The liquids are usually acidic solutions, and the powders are basic formulations that consist of either glass or metallic oxides. As indicated in Table 24–1, many of the cements have multiple uses. The basic formulations are modified by the manufacturer to adjust the handling characteristics (*e.g.,* setting time) or properties (*e.g.,* film thickness and strength) to adapt them for the performance of specific tasks.

Cements for Restorations. Cements are employed for temporary or short-term (days to weeks), intermediate-term (weeks to months), and "permanent" or long-term (years) restorations and for the aesthetic restoration of anterior teeth. Glass ionomers and resin-modified glass ionomers are designed for the latter purpose. Both are translucent and resemble porcelain in appearance. Glass ionomer cement (GIC) is the direct descendent of silicate cement, which served as a primary aesthetic material in years past. Although fluoride release from silicate cement was highly effective for caries inhibition, the longevity of silicate restorations was unimpressive because of their high solubility rates, loss of anatomic contour, and degradation of margin quality. Less is known concerning the longevity of glass ionomer restorations, because this material system is relatively new. However, glass ionomer restorations perform adequately over periods of 10 years or

TABLE 24–1. Classification and Uses of Dental Cements

Cement	Principal Uses	Secondary Uses
Zinc phosphate	Luting agent for restorations and orthodontic appliances	Intermediate restorations; thermal-insulating bases
Zinc oxide–eugenol	Temporary and intermediate restorations Temporary and permanent luting agent for restorations; thermal-insulating bases; cavity liner; pulp capping	Root canal restorations Periodontal surgical dressing
Polycarboxylate	Luting agent for restorations; thermal-insulating bases	Luting agent for orthodontic appliances; intermediate restorations
Silicate	Anterior restorations	
Silicophosphate	Luting agent for restorations	Intermediate restorations; luting agent for orthodontic appliances
Glass ionomer	Anterior restorations; luting agent for restorations and orthodontic appliances; cavity liners	Pit and fissure sealant; thermal-insulating bases
Metal-modified glass ionomers	Conservative posterior restorations; core buildups	
Resin	Luting agent for restorations and orthodontic appliances	Temporary restorations
Calcium hydroxide	Pulp capping agent; thermal-insulating bases	

longer. Recently, metal-modified and resin-modified GICs have become available, and clinical applications for these materials have been expanded, including the restoration of conservative cavity preparations in posterior teeth.

SILICATE CEMENT

The use of silicate cement diminished markedly with the advent of resin-based composites for restoration of anterior teeth and, later, with the development of the GIC. However, the silicate cement warrants some discussion because it possesses anticariogenic properties and a mechanism that has been well defined.

Composition and Chemistry. The cement powder is a glass consisting of silica (SiO_2); alumina (Al_2O_3); fluoride compounds, such as NaF, CaF_2, and Na_3AlF_6; and some calcium salts, such as $Ca(H_2PO_4)_2 \cdot H_2O$ and CaO. The ingredients are fused at approximately 1400° C to form a glass. The purpose of the fluoride compounds is to lower the fusing temperature of the glass.

The silicate glass powder is an acid-soluble glass. The liquid is an aqueous solution of phosphoric acid with buffer salts. When the powder and liquid are mixed, the surface of the powder particles is attacked by the acid, releasing Ca^{2+}, Al^{3+}, and F^- ions. The metal ions precipitate as phosphates that form the cement matrix with inclusions of fluoride salts. The chemistry of this material system is virtually the same as that for the glass ionomers, which are described in greater detail later in this chapter. The primary difference is associated with the acid component of the liquid.

Physical Properties. The properties of commercial brands of silicate cement are given in Table 24–2. Like most brittle materials, silicate cement is relatively strong in compression but weak in tension. The solubility and disintegration data were obtained by determining the amount of nonvolatile material leached from cement specimens during the first 24 hours when they were immersed in water, as prescribed by American Dental Association (ADA) Specification No. 9. As discussed in Chapter 25, the data obtained by this test do not correlate with the disintegration rates of various cements in the oral cavity. Thus, these values should be treated as quality control indicators to compare cements of the same type.

TABLE 24–2. Properties of Filling Cements

	Silicate Cement	Glass Ionomer (Type II)	Metal-Modified Glass Ionomer (Cermet)	Resin-Modified Glass Ionomer
Compressive strength (24 hr)				
MPa	180	150	150	105
psi	26,000	22,000	22,000	15,000
Diametral tensile strength (24 hr)				
MPa	3.5	6.6	6.7	20
psi	500	960	970	2,900
Hardness (KHN)	70	48	39	40
Pulp response	Severe	Mild	Mild	Mild
Anticariogenic	Yes	Yes	Yes	Yes
Solubility (ADA test)	0.7	0.4	—	—

KHN, Knoop hardness number; ADA, American Dental Association.

Biologic Properties. With respect to biologic properties, the pH of silicate cement is less than 3 at the time of insertion into the cavity, and it remains below 7 even after 1 month. Relative to pulpal response, it is classified as a severe irritant and often serves as the reference material to judge the potential of other materials to elicit a relatively severe reaction. Thus, a silicate cement restoration requires a greater need for pulp protection than the other two cements listed in Table 24–2.

ANTICARIOGENIC PROPERTIES OF FLUORIDE

It is commonly recognized that the incidence of secondary caries is markedly less adjacent to the silicate cement restoration than that associated with all other filling materials. For example, a study of approximately 20,000 existing restorations revealed a 12% incidence of secondary caries occurring over time adjacent to amalgam restorations, whereas the incidence was only 3% for silicate restorations. Also, the incidence of proximal surface caries adjacent to silicate cement restorations is less than that of proximal surfaces adjacent to amalgam restorations. Thus, although silicate cement has many weaknesses, its anticariogenic potential has been impressive. This behavior is somewhat surprising when one considers that gross leakage often occurs at the margins of silicate restorations.

Laboratory studies show that fluoride is released from silicate and other fluoride-containing cements into an aqueous medium in small but significant amounts for an indefinite period, as shown in Figure 24–1. The release of fluoride apparently can last throughout the life of the restoration, but the rate of release is expected to decrease over time.

Fluoride contributes to caries inhibition in the oral environment by means of both physicochemical and biologic mechanisms. From a physicochemical viewpoint, fluoride inhibits demineralization through formation of an acid-resistant phase and it enhances remineralization of carious (demineralized),

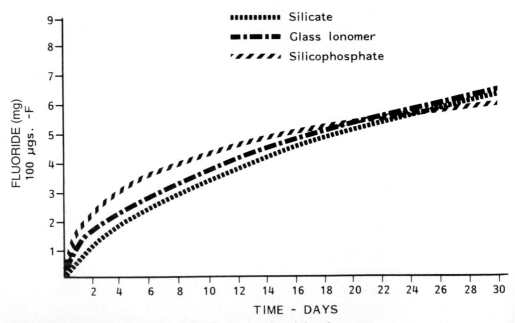

Figure 24–1. Fluoride release from three silicate glass–based dental cements.

noncavitated enamel. On the other hand, the fluoride also inhibits carbohydrate metabolism by the acidogenic plaque microflora.

Physicochemical Mechanism of Caries Inhibition. A logical explanation for this unique effect is that the fluoride ions released from the restorative material become incorporated in hydroxyapatite crystals of adjacent tooth structure to form a structure such as fluorapatite that is slightly more resistant to acid-mediated decalcification. Thus, in effect, the mechanism is analogous to that of topically applied fluoride solutions. The increase in the fluoride content of the surface layer of enamel adjacent to a fluoride-containing silicate restoration and the reduction in the enamel acid solubility are given in Table 24–3. When similar experiments were performed with a silicate cement prepared with a nonfluoride flux, there was no appreciable change in fluoride content of the enamel. In fact, the enamel solubility actually increased.

The ionic fluoride in the aqueous solution, in plaque, and within enamel and dentin shifts the equilibrium balance between demineralization and remineralization toward remineralization. Fluoride acts as a catalyst for uptake of calcium and phosphate ions. Compared with sound enamel, carious enamel is more porous. This porosity allows greater penetration of fluoride ions. Thus, the presence of fluoride ions in low concentrations contributes to the formation of acid-resistant crystals and reduces the risk of caries development. Several studies have shown that remineralized enamel, including lesions treated with fluoride, remains significantly resistant to secondary acid attack and more acid resistant than intact enamel.

Measurements of fluoride in enamel before and after restoration of teeth with fluoride-containing cements also show that the fluoride in the surface enamel is increased at sites on the treated tooth remote from the restoration. This suggests that the beneficial effects of the fluoride leached from silicate cement are not confined only to the margins of the restoration.

Biologic Mechanism of Caries Inhibition. Fluoride accumulates in dental plaque. The sources of plaque fluoride include saliva, gingival fluid, diet, topically applied fluoride gel, and demineralizing enamel. It is well established that fluoride inhibits carbohydrate metabolism by acidogenic plaque microflora. Fluoride enters micro-organisms against a concentration gradient and accumulates intracellularly as the extracellular pH decreases. The transport of hydrogen fluoride into cells leads to dissociation into H^+ and F^- ions within the more alkaline intracellular fluid. Ionic fluoride then induces enzyme inhibition, leading to a slower rate of acid production. Meanwhile the fluoride increases cell permeability, and it can rapidly diffuse out of the bacterium, contributing again to the fluoride content within the plaque matrix.

TABLE 24–3. Changes in Fluoride Content and Acid Solubility of Enamel Induced by Cements

Cement	Percentage Change in F Content	Percentage Change in Acid Solubility
Silicate (without F)	0	+ 20
Silicate (with F)	+ 3500	40
Zinc silicophosphate	+ 5000	− 50
Glass ionomer	+ 3000	− 30

Values encompassed by the straight line are not significantly different from each other.

High concentrations of fluoride eliminate sensitive bacterial populations. Sublethal concentrations alter carbohydrate metabolism in such a way as to reduce acidogenicity; alter the production of extracellular, insoluble polysaccharides; and possibly reduce adhesion. In addition, sublethal concentrations of fluoride may alter the acid tolerance of *Streptococcus mutans* and other organisms, leading to a less acidogenic plaque flora. In fact, chemical analyses of plaque collected at the margins of resin, amalgam, and cast gold restorations reveal a difference in composition, as compared with the plaque that accumulates at the margins of silicate cement restorations.

Fluoride in Dental Materials

Silicate, glass ionomer, and silicophosphate cements acquire fluoride through the addition of fluoride salts that lower the fusion temperature of the glass. Our understanding of the caries prevention mechanism of silicate cement has led to numerous investigations designed to capture this anticariogenic characteristic by the addition of fluoride compounds to resins, amalgam, zinc phosphate cement, zinc oxide–eugenol (ZOE), pit and fissure sealants, cavity varnishes, and even chewing gums. Addition of fluoride can be achieved by physically incorporating soluble fluoride salt within the bulk material or by adding virtually insoluble fluoride–containing minerals as a filler. Another alternative for fluoride release is chemical in nature and uses monomers with fluorine in pendant groups as the matrix former. These monomers release fluorine ions by mean of ion exchange, in which hydroxyl groups replace fluorine ions that have been released.

There are two principal concerns regarding the efficacy of fluoride additions to restorative materials. First, the amount and longevity of fluoride release can be quite variable, as shown in Figure 24–1. Second, because fluorides are part of the material structure, the degradation of pertinent material properties is also a concern.

One *in vivo* study has shown that fluoride release from amalgams loaded with soluble fluoride salts was detectable within the first month and thereafter fluoride was not released in measurable amounts. Another *in vitro* study showed that fluoride release can continue as long as 2 years but at a much lower rate than that from GIC. Whether such short-term, low levels of release are effective in combating caries remains to be determined. Furthermore, the leaching of fluoride makes the amalgam more susceptible to corrosion. A fluoride-releasing zinc phosphate cement was developed, but its solubility was extremely high. Some restorative resins containing fluoride have exhibited a sustained release of fluoride *in vitro* for more than 18 months, but at a level much lower than that released from GIC. The question of fluoride efficacy on the control of the demineralization-remineralization balance based on variable concentrations and release rates from restorations is still unanswered.

GLASS IONOMER CEMENT

Glass ionomer is the generic name of a group of materials that use silicate glass powder and an aqueous solution of polyacrylic acid. This material acquires its name from its formulation of a glass powder and an ionomeric acid that contains carboxyl groups. It is also referred to as *polyalkenoate cement.*

Originally, the cement was designed for the aesthetic restoration of anterior teeth and it was recommended for use in restoring teeth with Class III and V cavity preparations. Some representative products, with their delivery systems,

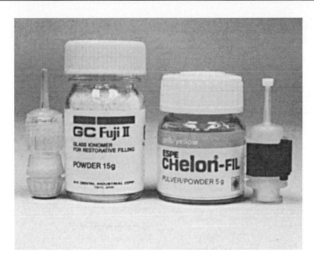

Figure 24–2. Representative Type II restorative glass ionomer cements. Only the powder is shown for the bulk. The capsules contain both powder and liquid.

are shown in Figure 24–2. Also, because the cement produces a truly adhesive bond to tooth structure, it is particularly useful for the conservative restoration of eroded areas. The need for mechanical retention via a cavity preparation is eliminated or reduced.

The use of GICs has broadened to encompass formulations as luting agents, liners, restorative materials for conservative Class I and II restorations and core buildups, and a pit and fissure sealant. However, GIC is not recommended for Class II or IV restorations because current formulations lack fracture toughness and appear to be more susceptible to wear by enamel when compared with composites.

There are three types of GIC based on their formulations and their potential uses. These are designated as follows: Type I for luting applications (see Chapter 25), Type II as a restorative material, and Type III for use as a liner or base. Light-curable versions of GICs are also available. Because of the need for incorporating light-curable resin in the formulation, this type of product is also called a *resin-modified GIC*. Discussion at this point focuses on the Type II GIC.

Composition. The glass ionomer powder is an acid-soluble calcium fluoroaluminosilicate glass. The composition of two commercial glass ionomer powders is given in Table 24–4. The raw materials are fused to a uniform glass by heating them to a temperature of 1100° C to 1500° C. Lanthanum, strontium, barium, or zinc oxide additions provide radiopacity. The glass is ground into a powder having particles in the range of 20 to 50 μm. Originally, the liquids for GIC were

TABLE 24–4. Composition of Two Glass Ionomer Cement Powders

Species	Weight (%)	
	A	B
SiO_2	41.9	35.2
Al_2O_3	28.6	20.1
AlF_3	1.6	2.4
CaF_2	15.7	20.1
NaF	9.3	3.6
$AlPO_4$	3.8	12.0

From Wilson AD, and McLean JW: Glass Ionomer Cement. Chicago, Quintessence, 1988, p. 40.

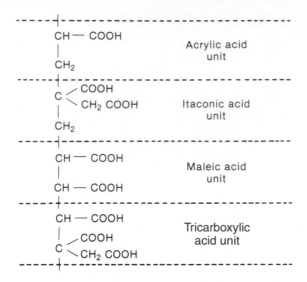

Figure 24–3. Structure of various types of alkenoic acids that make up polyacids of glass ionomer cements.

aqueous solutions of polyacrylic acid in a concentration of about 50%. The liquid was quite viscous and tended to gel over time. In most of the current cements, the acid is in the form of a copolymer with itaconic, maleic, or tricarboxylic acid. These acids tend to increase the reactivity of the liquid, decrease the viscosity, and reduce the tendency for gelation.

The copolymeric acids (Fig. 24–3) used in modern glass ionomer liquids are more irregularly arranged than in the homopolymer of acrylic acid. This configuration reduces hydrogen bonding between acid molecules and thus reduces the degree of gelling. Tartaric acid is also present in the liquid. It improves the handling characteristics and increases the working time; however, it shortens the setting time (Fig. 24–4). The viscosity of the tartaric acid–containing cement does not change over time, but it later exhibits a sharp increase in viscosity.

To extend the working time, one glass ionomer formulation consists of freeze-dried acid powder and glass powder in one bottle and water or water with tartaric acid in another bottle as the liquid component. When the powders are mixed with water, the acid dissolves to reconstitute the liquid acid. The chemical reaction then proceeds in the same manner as that demonstrated by a traditional

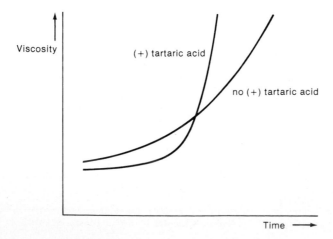

Figure 24–4. The effect of tartaric acid on the viscosity vs. time curve for a glass ionomer cement during setting. (From Wilson AD, and McLean JW: Glass Ionomer Cement. Chicago, Quintessence, 1988, p 37.)

powder-liquid system. These cements have a longer working time with a shorter setting time. They are referred to occasionally as *water settable GICs* and erroneously as *anhydrous GICs*.

Chemistry of Setting. When the powder and liquid are mixed to form a paste, the surface of the glass particles is attacked by the acid. Calcium, aluminum, sodium, and fluorine ions are leached into the aqueous medium. The polyacrylic acid chains are cross-linked by the calcium ions and form a solid mass. Within the next 24 hours a new phase forms in which aluminum ions become bound within the cement mix. This leads to a more rigid set cement. Sodium and fluorine ions do not participate in the cross-linking of the cement. Some of the sodium ions may replace the hydrogen ions of carboxylic groups, whereas the rest combine with fluorine ions, forming sodium fluoride uniformly dispersed within the set cement. During the maturing process, the cross-linked phase is also hydrated by the same water used as the medium. The unreacted portion of glass particles are sheathed by silica gel that develops during removal of the cations from the surface of the particles. Thus, the set cement consists of an agglomeration of unreacted powder particles surrounded by a silica gel in an amorphous matrix of hydrated calcium and aluminum polysalts. This is illustrated in the diagram shown in Figure 24–5 and is seen in the micrograph of the set cement shown in Figure 24–6.

Role of Water in the Setting Process. Water is a most important constituent of the cement liquid. It serves as the reaction medium initially, and it then slowly hydrates the cross-linked matrix, thereby increasing the material strength. During the initial reaction period, this water can readily be removed by desiccation and is called *loosely-bound water*. As the setting continues, the same water hydrates the matrix and cannot be removed by desiccation and is then called *tightly-bound water*. This hydration is critical in yielding a stable gel structure and building the strength of the cement. If freshly mixed cements are kept

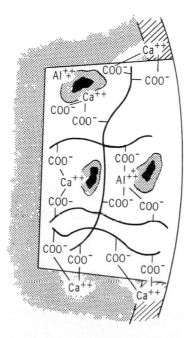

Figure 24–5. Structure of the glass ionomer cement. The solid black particles represent unreacted glass particles surrounded by the gel *(shaded structure)* that form when Al^{3+} and Ca^{2+} ions are leached from the glass as a result of attack by the polyacrylic acid. The Ca^{2+} and Al^{3+} form polysalts with the COO groups of the polyacrylic acid to form a cross-linked structure. The carboxyl groups react with the calcium of the enamel and dentin.

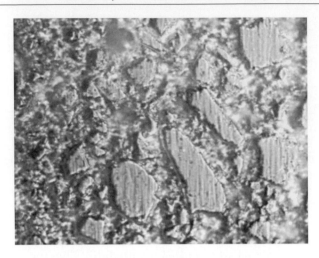

Figure 24–6. Micrograph of a set glass ionomer cement showing unreacted particles surrounded by the continuous matrix.

isolated from the ambient air, the loosely held water will slowly become tightly bound water over time. This phenomenon results in a cement that is stronger and less susceptible to moisture.

If the same mixes are exposed to ambient air without any covering, the surface will craze and crack as a result of desiccation. Any contamination by water that occurs at this stage can cause a dissolution of the matrix-forming cations and anions to the surrounding areas. This process results in a weak and more soluble cement. Although the dissolution susceptibility tends to decrease over time, the minimum time at which the danger of cracking from exposure to air no longer exists has not been established. As discussed, the ionomer cement must be protected against water changes in the structure during placement and for a few weeks after placement if possible.

PROPERTIES OF GLASS IONOMER CEMENT

Physical Properties. The pertinent properties of the GICs are listed in Table 24–2. The initial solubility is associated with leaching of intermediate products or those not involved in matrix formation. However, when the GIC is tested under *in vitro* conditions, it tends to be more resistant to attack by acids. Its *in vivo* solubility is compared with that of other cements in Chapter 25.

Another property that is particularly pertinent to the use of GIC as a restorative material is its fracture toughness (Table 24–5), a measure of the energy required to produce fracture. Type II GICs are much inferior to composites in this respect. They also are more vulnerable to wear than are composites when

TABLE 24–5. Fracture Toughness of Materials Relative to Amalgam*

	Toughness (Amalgam)
	Toughness (Material)
Posterior composites	0.83–1.3
A-Type II glass ionomer	0.29
cermet	0.27
B-Type II glass ionomer	0.11
silver alloy admix	0.16

*The fracture toughness of amalgam was assigned the value of 1, and the values presented for other materials are fractions thereof. The higher the value, the tougher the material.

subjected to *in vitro* toothbrush abrasion tests and simulated occlusal wear tests. However, GICs are attractive in that they are reasonably biocompatible, they bond to enamel and dentin, and they provide an anticariogenic benefit.

Mechanism of Adhesion. The mechanism by which the glass ionomer bonds to tooth structure has not been clearly elucidated. However, there seems little doubt that it primarily involves chelation of carboxyl groups of the polyacids with the calcium in the apatite of the enamel and dentin (see Fig. 24–5). (Another illustration of this reaction can be seen in Figure 25–10.) Although this deals with a polycarboxylate cement, the adhesive mechanism for a glass ionomer would be comparable, as both are based on polyacids. The bond to enamel is always higher than that to dentin, probably because of the greater inorganic content of enamel and its greater homogeneity from a morphologic standpoint.

Biologic Properties. Although long-term controlled clinical studies are lacking, there is every indication that GIC possesses the same anticariogenic properties as does silicate cement. As can be seen in Figure 24–1, Type II glass ionomers release fluoride in amounts comparable with those released initially from silicate cement and continue to do so over an extended period. Likewise, enamel adjacent to GIC (see Table 24–3) and also in more remote areas undergoes a comparable uptake of fluoride. There is a considerable range in the amounts of fluoride released from the various types of GICs. Although the minimal amount of fluoride release and subsequent uptake necessary to inhibit caries has not been defined, an assumption has always been made that release in amounts comparable with that released by silicate is effective. In fact, results from controlled clinical studies and surveys of practicing dentists are inconclusive. For example, several controlled clinical studies of GIC for restoration or fissure sealants over a 2- to 5-year period show that the number of secondary caries lesions that developed ranged between zero and a number as high as that associated with composite restorations that were placed in the same study. Surveys of dentists show that the frequency of secondary caries in teeth with glass ionomer fillings compared with that of teeth with posterior composites was lower for one group of dentists but higher for another group of dentists.

Most histologic studies indicate that Type II glass ionomers are relatively biocompatible. They elicit a greater pulp reaction than ZOE but generally less than that from zinc phosphate cement. Polyacids are relatively weak acids. However, the powder:liquid (P:L) ratio influences the degree of acidity and the duration of a low pH environment. As might be expected, the luting agents (Type I cements) pose a greater hazard in this regard because of a lower P:L ratio and a slower setting reaction than that for Type II glass ionomers. Nonetheless, with any GIC, it is wise to place a thin layer of a protective cement, such as $Ca(OH)_2$, on areas close to the pulp in a deep preparation.

CRITICAL PROCEDURES FOR GLASS IONOMER RESTORATIONS

To achieve a long-lasting restoration, several conditions must be satisfied. They include appropriate cavity surface preparation to achieve the bonding, proper mixing to obtain a workable mixture, and surface finishing and protection during the maturing of the cement. These areas of concern are discussed in the following sections.

Surface Preparation. As stated in Chapter 2, clean surfaces are essential to promote adhesion. A pumice wash can be used to remove the smear layer that is produced during cavity preparation. On the other hand, organic acids, such as polyacrylic acid of various concentrations, can remove the smear layer but still leave the collagenous tubule plug in place. These plugs inhibit the penetration of the cement constituents and affect the hydrodynamic fluid pressure within dentin.

One workable method is to apply a 10% polyacrylic acid solution to the surface for 10 to 15 seconds, followed by a 30-second water rinse. Figure 24–7 shows the result of a 10-second swabbing on a cut dentin surface with a 10% solution. It shows that the smear layer has been removed, but the tubules remain plugged. This procedure of removing the smear layer is called *conditioning*. In restoring eroded areas with no cavity preparation, the dentin and cementum should first be cleaned with a pumice slurry, followed by a 5-second or longer swabbing with polyacrylic acid. The purpose of the pumice débridement is to remove the fluoride-rich surface layer that may compromise the surface-conditioning process.

After conditioning and rinsing of the preparation, the surface should be dried but it should not be unduly desiccated. It must remain clean because any further contamination by saliva or blood impairs bonding of the cement.

Preparation of the Material. The P:L ratio recommended by the manufacturer should be followed. As noted, any reduction in that ratio adversely affects the properties of the set cement and its susceptibility to degradation in the oral environment. With a hand-mixed product, a paper pad is sufficient. A cool, dry

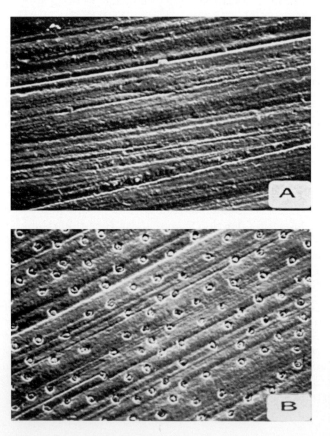

Figure 24–7. A, Prepared dentin surface showing the presence of the smear layer. *B,* After cleansing with polyacrylic acid, the smear layer is removed yet the tubules remain plugged.

glass slab may be used to slow down the reaction and extend the working time. It is important that the slab not be used if its temperature is below the dew point, that is, at temperatures that enhance moisture condensation on the glass slab that can alter the acid:water balance needed for a proper reaction. By waiting a few minutes, the temperature of the slab will rise sufficiently until water vapor no longer condenses on its surface.

The powder and liquid should not be dispensed onto the slab until just before the mixing procedure is to be started. Prolonged exposure to the office atmosphere alters the precise acid:water ratio of the liquid. The powder should be incorporated rapidly into the liquid using a stiff spatula. The mixing time should not exceed 45 to 60 seconds. At this time, the mix should have a glossy surface. The shiny surface indicates the presence of polyacid that has not participated in the setting reaction. This residual acid ensures adhesive bonding to the tooth. If the mixing process is prolonged, a dull surface develops, and adhesion will not be achieved. Because the exact time for mixing differs among various products, it is critical that the suggested mixing time be followed.

Type II glass ionomers are also supplied in capsules containing preproportioned powder and liquid (see Fig. 24–2). The mixing is accomplished in an amalgamator after the seal that separates the powder and liquid is broken. Note that the capsule contains a nozzle, so the mix can be injected directly into the cavity without any delay. The mixing speed of the amalgamator is critical, and again, the instructions of the manufacturer should be followed.

The main advantages of capsules are convenience, consistent control of the P:L ratio, and elimination of the variations associated with hand spatulation. However, a hand-mixing P:L system provides greater latitude in controlling the amount of cement needed for a specific situation and ensures a better shade-matching ability by adjusting the existing powder to achieve the desired aesthetic result.

Placement of the Material. The mixed cement is immediately packed by means of a plastic instrument or injected into the cavity. Any delay in placement leads to a dull appearance, denoting that the setting reaction has progressed to an extent that free carboxyl groups are inadequate to produce adhesion to the tooth structure.

Immediately after placement, a preshaped matrix is applied. There are two main reasons for the matrix. First, it provides maximum contour, so minimal finishing is required. In addition, the matrix ensures the best possible surface integrity. Second, the matrix protects the setting cement from losing or gaining water during the initial set. The matrix is left in place for at least 5 minutes, although this time varies with the product, based on the setting rate.

On removal of the matrix, the surface must *immediately* be protected while the excess material is trimmed from the margins. For some products, a special varnish supplied by the manufacturer can be used. If a varnish is used, it should be dried under ambient conditions, not with compressed air. Compressed air may displace the varnish and dehydrate the surface of the exposed fresh cement, producing cracks. A single-component, unfilled light-cured resin bonding agent, which is a more impermeable coating, may be a better choice. Hand instruments are preferred to rotary tools for trimming the margins to avoid ditching while the cement is still somewhat soft.

Surface Finishing of the Set Cement. Further finishing procedures, if needed, should be delayed for at least 24 hours. With some of the faster-setting cements, finishing times of 10 minutes are recommended. However, the longer one waits, the more mature the cement becomes and the risks of surface dyscrasias or tendency for the restoration to become slightly more opaque are reduced.

Postoperative Procedures. Before dismissing the patient, the restoration should be coated again with the protective agent, because the trimmed areas expose cement that is still vulnerable to the environment until it reaches full maturity. If these recommended procedures for providing protection to the setting cement are not followed, inevitably a chalky or a crazed surface will result, as seen in the failures shown in Figure 24–8. Such surfaces are usually associated with lack of protection via a matrix, varnish, or resin bonding agent or improper manipulation (*e.g.,* low P:L ratio).

It is also probable that glass ionomer restorations are vulnerable to some degree of dehydration throughout their lifetime. Therefore, it is wise to protect existing glass ionomer restorations with a coat of varnish or resin when other dental procedures are to be carried out.

Summary. There are essentially three parameters that must be controlled to ensure the successful use of restorative glass ionomers: (1) conditioning of the tooth surface, (2) proper manipulation, and (3) protection of the cement during setting and in potential situations when desiccation might occur. When these parameters are controlled, the result should be high-quality restorations such as those shown in Figure 24–9.

METAL-MODIFIED GLASS IONOMER CEMENT

GICs lack toughness and, hence, they cannot withstand high-stress concentrations. Neither are they as wear resistant as other aesthetic materials, such as composites and ceramics. GICs have been modified by the inclusion of metal filler particles in an attempt to improve the strength, fracture toughness, and resistance to wear. Two methods of modification have been employed. The first approach is that of mixing spherical silver amalgam alloy powder with the Type II glass ionomer powder. This cement is referred to as a *silver alloy admix.* The second system involves fusing glass powder to silver particles through high-temperature sintering of a mixture of the two powders. This cement is commonly

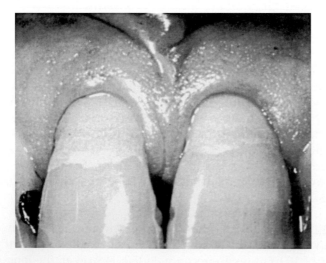

Figure 24–8. Crazed, chalky surface on glass ionomer restorations resulting from inadequate protection of the cement during its maturation. (Courtesy of G. Mount.)

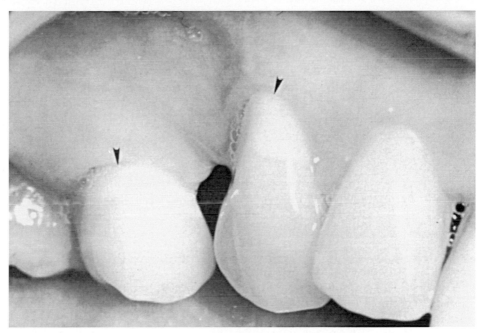

Figure 24–9. Six-year-old glass ionomer restorations *(arrows).* A conservative and aesthetic treatment for the eroded area lesion. (Courtesy of G. Mount.)

referred to as a *cermet.* The scanning electron micrograph of a cermet powder (Fig. 24–10) shows the silver powder particles attached to the surface of the cement powder particles. Modified metal cements based on each of these two systems are commercially available. Examples of representative commercial products are shown on the left and right sides of Figure 24–11. A conventional GIC is shown in the center.

General Properties. Table 24–2 shows general properties of the cermet type of GIC compared with that of the conventional type. Table 24–5 provides a relative comparison of the fracture toughness of a cermet and a silver alloy admix cement compared with that of the respective parent Type II GICs, a resin, and

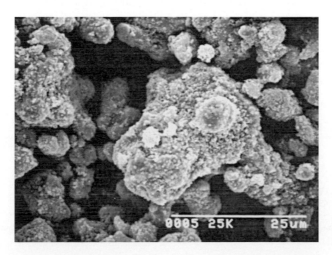

Figure 24–10. Cermet powder showing the silver particles attached. ×2000. (Courtesy of R. Guggenberger, ESPE Company, Munich, Germany.)

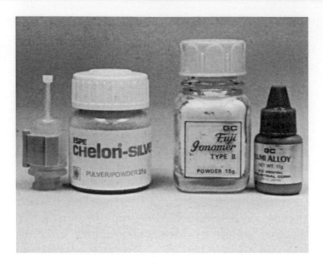

Figure 24–11. Representative commercial metal-modified glass ionomer cements. Cermet products are shown on the left, and on the right is an admix of amalgam alloy added to Type II ionomer cement (Miracle Mix).

amalgam. Both tables indicate that metallic fillers have little or no influence on the mechanical properties of Type II GICs.

Flat specimens of the restorative materials were subjected to the sliding action of a cylinder of synthetic hydroxyapatite under a simulated occlusal load for a given number of cycles, and the volume of restorative material removed during the test was measured. The measured wear values are presented in Table 24–6. The cermet material is far more resistant to sliding wear than is the Type II GIC. The improvement in wear resistance is attributed to the metal filler as evidenced by the burnished appearance that occurs when metals are subjected to this wear test.

Fluoride Release. Fluoride leaches out from both metal-modified systems in appreciable amounts (Table 24–7). However, less fluoride is released from the cermet cement than from its Type II counterpart. This is not surprising, because a portion of the original glass particle that contains the fluoride is metal coated. The admix cement releases more fluoride than does its Type II cement counterpart initially. However, the magnitude of release decreases over time. The explanation for this effect may be that the metal filler particles are not bonded to the cement matrix; thus, the filler-cement interfaces become pathways for fluid exchange. This greatly increases the surface area available for leaching of fluoride.

Clinical Considerations. With the increased wear resistance and the anticariogenic potential, these metal-modified cements have been suggested for limited use as an alternative to amalgam or composites for posterior restorations. How-

TABLE 24–6. Material Loss During Simulated Occlusal Wear

	Volumetric Change* (Cm³)
Amalgam	0.2
Conventional composite	0.4
Glass ionomer	6.0
Cermet	0.3

*Volume of material removed when specimens are rotated against synthetic hydroxyapatite cyclinder for 2500 cycles.

TABLE 24–7. Fluoride Release From Various Glass Ionomer Formulations

	μg-F	
	14 Days	30 Days
Type II glass ionomer	440	650
Cermet	200	300
Silver alloy admix	3350	4040
Type I glass ionomer	470	700
Glass ionomer liners		
Conventional	1000	1300
Light cured	1200	1600

ever, these materials must still be classified as brittle materials. For this reason their use should be restricted to conservative and, generally, Class I restorations. They appear to perform relatively well in such situations and are particularly suited for use in young patients who are prone to caries.

These cements harden rapidly so they can be finished in a relatively short time. Coupled with their potential for adhesion and caries resistance, these characteristics have prompted their use as a core buildup for teeth to be restored with cast crowns. However, because of their low fracture toughness and brittle nature, a conservative approach should be taken. It is recommended that they not be used wherever the cement constitutes more than 40% of the total core buildup. Likewise, the auxiliary use of pins or other retention forms is desirable.

RESIN-MODIFIED GLASS IONOMER CEMENT

Moisture sensitivity and low early strength of GICs are the results of slow acid-base setting reactions. Some polymerizable functional groups have been added to the formulations to impart additional curing processes that can overcome these two inherent drawbacks and allow the bulk of the material to mature through the acid-base reaction. Both chemical-curing and light-curing products are available (Fig. 24–12). This group of materials has been identified with several names, including *light-cured GICs, dual-cure GICs* (for light-cured and acid-base reaction), *tri-cure GICs* (dual cure plus chemical cure), *resin-ionomers, compomers,* and *hybrid ionomers.* None of the terms can truly describe this group of materials. We can use the term *resin-modified GIC* until a universal term is adopted. The glass ionomers that set solely by an acid-base reaction are identified as *conventional GICs.*

Composition and Setting Reactions. The powder component of a typical light-cured material consists of ion-leachable glass and initiators for light or chemical curing, or both. The liquid component usually contains water, polyacrylic acid, or polyacrylic acid with some carboxylic groups modified with methacrylate and hydroxyethyl methacrylate monomers. The last two ingredients are responsible for polymerization. The initial setting reaction of the material is by the polymerization of methacrylate groups. The slow acid-base reaction is ultimately responsible for the unique maturing process and the final strength. To accommodate the polymerizable ingredients, the overall water content is less for this type of material. A slower-setting reaction of cements with an acid-base reaction is expected compared with that for the resin-modified GIC acid-base reaction. A one-component light-curing material is also available. As a one-component material, it does not have an immediate self-curing mechanism.

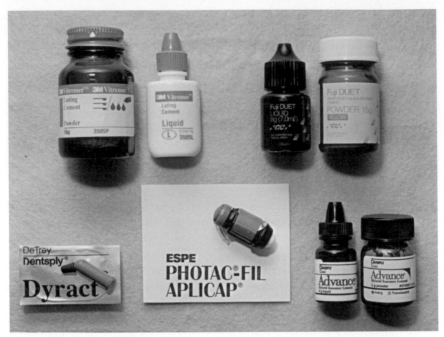

Figure 24–12. Representative commercial resin-modified glass ionomer cements.

Physical Properties. Variation of properties from conventional glass ionomers can be attributed to the presence of polymerizable resins and lesser amount of water and carboxylic acids in the liquid. The most notable one is probably the reduction of translucency of resin-modified material because of a significant difference in the refractive index between the powder and set resin matrix. Based on *in vitro* analyses, these materials release levels of fluoride comparable to those of the conventional GICs. Other relevant properties are discussed in the following sections.

Strength of Resin-modified Glass Ionomers. The diametral tensile strengths of resin-modified glass ionomers are higher than those of conventional GICs. This increase in strength is mainly attributable to the greater amount of plastic deformation that can be sustained before fracture occurs. Other properties are difficult to compare because of differences in materials and testing protocols. Other properties and characteristics are also shown in Table 24–2.

Adhesion to Tooth Structure. Bond strength values measured by shear bond strength tests generally are higher than those for resin-modified materials, but these differences are not significant. Analysis of the cement-tooth interface reveals that the bonding mechanism is similar to that of conventional GIC.

Adhesion to Other Restorative Materials. Resin-modified glass ionomers are used primarily as liners and bases, although they also can be used for restorations. Bonding of these liners or bases to the final restorative materials, normally composites, is critically important. Compared with conventional GICs, resin-modified GICs have a higher bond strength to composite resin. This is likely controlled by the residual unpolymerized functional groups within conventional GIC.

Marginal Adaptation. This group of materials should exhibit a greater degree of shrinkage on setting as the result of polymerization. Lower water and carboxylic acid content also reduces the ability of the cement to wet the tooth substrates, which can greatly increase microleakage compared with that of conventional GICs. Studies have shown that resin-modified GICs used as liners have a higher P:L ratio and exhibit greater microleakage than conventional GIC liners.

Water Sensitivity. A rationale for modifying polyacrylic acids with methacrylate functional groups is to reduce the water sensitivity of GIC. Studies have shown that the liner version of this group of GICs is still susceptible to dehydration and that this material can also absorb water, which produces significant dimensional changes. On the other hand, polishing and finishing of this material are possible on completion of the light-curing procedure.

Clinical Considerations. The biocompatibility of resin-modified GICs should be comparable to that of conventional GICs. Although one study shows that the pulp healing process is not impaired when exposed to resin-modified GIC, the same precautions that are followed for conventional GICs should be followed, such as the use of calcium hydroxide for deep preparations. The transient temperature increase associated with the polymerization process may also be a concern.

Depending on the manufacturer's formulation and P:L ratios, clinical applications of resin-modified GICs include its use as a liner, fissure sealant, base, core buildup, restoration, adhesive for orthodontic brackets, repair material for damaged amalgam cores or cusps, and retrograde root filling material. For these applications, surface conditioning with a mild acid is still essential for bond formation.

Glass Ionomer Cement as a Fissure Sealant. A cariostatic effect is a desirable property of any material used for patients who are highly likely to develop caries. Thus, GICs are viable candidates as fissure sealants. However, the traditional ionomer cement is somewhat viscous, which prevents penetration to the depth of the fissure. The use of glass ionomers in sealant therapy should increase as less viscous formulations are developed (*e.g.*, light-cured products), especially if they are marketed specifically as a sealant. One clinical study shows that the retention rate of glass ionomer sealant is poor after 1 year, but no sign of caries was observed. Close examination of the occlusal surface showed that patches of GIC remained within the fissures.

ZINC OXIDE–EUGENOL CEMENT

These cements are usually dispensed in the form of a powder and liquid or sometimes as two pastes. A wide variety of ZOE formulations are available for temporary and intermediate restorations, cavity liners, thermal-insulating bases, and temporary and permanent luting cements, as indicated in Table 24–1. They also serve as root canal sealants and periodontal dressings. Their pH is approximately 7 at the time they are inserted into the tooth. As discussed previously, ZOE cement is one of the least irritating of all dental materials and provides an excellent seal against leakage.

The various formulations and uses are reflected in ADA Specification No. 30 for ZOE restorative materials, which lists four types. Type I ZOE cement is used for temporary cementation. Type II cement is intended for permanent cementation of restorations or appliances fabricated outside of the mouth. Type III cement is used for temporary restorations and thermal-insulating bases, whereas Type IV is used as a cavity liner. The latter suggests the use of the material as a coating on the pulpal wall to provide protection against chemical irritation from the restorative material. However, the thickness is inadequate in providing thermal protection to the pulp.

In this chapter, the cements used for temporary and intermediate restorations, bases, and liners are discussed. Those formulations used for cementation are discussed in Chapter 25.

Composition and Chemistry. The principal components of the cements are zinc oxide and eugenol. Hence, the setting reaction and microstructure are essentially the same as those of the impression pastes discussed in Chapter 8. However, there are numerous means by which the handling characteristics and physical properties of ZOE preparations can be altered. As a result, cements suitable for a wide range of uses are produced. The particle size also affects their setting rate. All other variables being equal, cements prepared from smaller particles of zinc oxide powder set more rapidly than those prepared with larger particles.

Physical Properties. As with all cements, the P:L ratio of ZOE cement affects its setting time. The higher the P:L ratio, the faster the set. Cooling the mixing slab slows the setting reaction unless the temperature is below the dew point. Below the dew point, condensate is incorporated into the mix and the setting reaction is accelerated.

Particle size affects strength. In general, smaller particle sizes increase the strength. Substitution of a portion of the eugenol with ortho-ethoxybenzoic acid results in an appreciable increase in strength, as does the incorporation of polymers.

ZOE formulations designed for various uses range in strength from 3 to 55 MPa. The strength of ZOE cements depends on the intended use of the material and thus the formulation designed for these purposes.

Temporary Restorations. Materials used for temporary restorations are expected to last for only a short period, for example, a few days or a few weeks at most. They may serve as a temporary restorative treatment while the pulp heals or until a more long-lasting restoration can be fabricated and inserted. Type I ZOE cements are employed almost universally for sedative treatments, temporary coverage, and temporary cementation. Because the restorations will ultimately be removed, the maximum allowable strength, according to ADA Specification No. 30, is 35 MPa.

Intermediate Restorations. The need sometimes arises for an intermediate restoration, particularly in pedodontics. For example, in patients with rampant caries, it is desirable to remove all of the demineralized tissue from cavitated lesion sites as soon as possible to reduce the concentration of cariogenic bacteria and thus arrest the caries process. Once the initial caries removal has been accomplished and the patient has been shifted to a low-caries-risk status, the dentist can then proceed with placement of long-term restorations. The interval between removal of the caries and completion of the restorative work may be several months or longer. During this time, the teeth must be protected by some type of a durable restoration.

The strength and abrasion resistance of ZOE cement can be improved by incorporating 20 to 40 wt% of fine polymer particles and treating the surface of zinc oxide particles with carboxylic acid. The liquid component in the formulation is eugenol. Clinical experience with this type of material indicates that it can serve effectively as a restorative material for at least 1 year. To achieve the properties necessary for this use, sufficient powder must be added to achieve a stiff puttylike or filling consistency.

AGENTS FOR PULP PROTECTION

Before placement of the restoration, the pulp may have undergone irritation or damage from a variety of sources, such as caries and cavity preparation. Furthermore, the physical and chemical properties of the permanent restorative materials are such that the restoration itself can cause irritation or exacerbate an existing condition. The metallic restorations, being excellent thermal conductors, can cause thermal sensitivity during the intake of hot and cold foods or beverages. Other restorative materials, such as the phosphoric acid–containing cements, direct-filling resins, and, in some instances, GIC can produce chemical irritation. In addition, interfacial leakage as the result of setting contraction of amalgam and resin composite restorations may also cause pulpal irritation.

Cavity varnishes, liners, and bases are designed as adjuncts to the restorative materials to protect the pulp against chemical and thermal trauma. In addition to serving as barriers against thermal change, irritants within the material, and interfacial leakage with associated bacterial invasion, some of these agents may have beneficial effects on the pulp. Technically, both varnishes and liners can be classified as cavity-lining agents, because both are used as protective coatings for freshly cut tooth structure of the prepared cavity. On the other hand, bases also have to serve as thermal insulators for metallic restorations. Varnishes and liners usually form a coating by evaporation of the solvent, whereas bases and some newly introduced liners set by chemical reactions, including light-curing processes.

CAVITY VARNISHES

The typical cavity varnish is principally a natural gum (such as copal), rosin, or a synthetic resin dissolved in an organic solvent (such as acetone, chloroform, and ether). They are not generally applied in a sufficient thickness to provide the required thermal insulation. Figure 24–13 shows the increase in temperature on the side of an amalgam test specimen with various types of varnish, liners and bases, and a constant heat source on the other side. There is no difference in the amount of heat transfer through the control (curve A) and the amalgam-varnish specimen (curve B).

Effect on Leakage and Acid Penetration. The literature generally shows that varnish produces a positive effect on the reduction of pulpal irritation. This suggests that the effect may be attributed to the reduced infiltration of irritating fluids through marginal areas.

The protective effect of the varnish has been demonstrated *in vitro* by the radioactive phosphoric acid tracer in sections of dentin underlying silicate cement restorations that were prepared with radioactive liquids placed in extracted teeth and in the teeth of monkeys. The results of these experiments are shown in Figure 24–14. There is a marked reduction in the radioactive counts of the

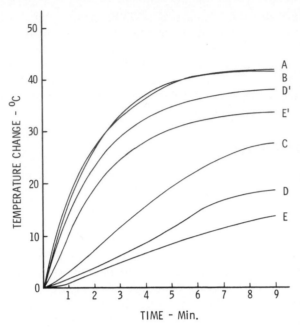

Figure 24–13. Rate of thermal diffusion through model amalgam restorations as influenced by the presence of a cavity varnish and bases. A constant heat source was applied to the surface of the amalgam and the change in temperature on the underside of the specimen (cavity floor) over time was monitored. A, Amalgam control; B, amalgam plus cavity varnish; C, zinc phosphate cement base, 1.5-mm thick; D, calcium hydroxide base, 1.5-mm thick; D', calcium hydroxide base, 0.15-mm thick; E, zinc oxide-eugenol base, 1.5-mm thick; and E', zinc oxide–eugenol base, 0.15-mm thick.

underlying dentin where the cavity walls were coated with a varnish, as compared with those of unlined dentin. Comparable results are obtained when zinc phosphate and silicophosphate cements were employed.

The varnish can also prevent penetration of corrosion products of amalgams into the dentinal tubules, and it thereby reduces the unsightly tooth discoloration often associated with amalgam restorations.

Application of the Varnish. To attain a uniform and continuous coating on all surfaces of the prepared cavity, several thin layers should be applied. When the first layer dries, small pinholes usually develop. A second or third application fills in most of these voids and thereby produces a more continuous coating. The varnish must be applied in a thin consistency using a brush or a small

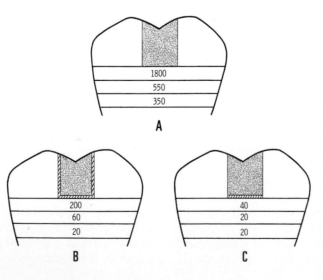

Figure 24–14. Penetration of radioactive phosphoric acid liquid into dentin from silicate cement restorations. The numbers represent the radioactive counts made on three 0.5-mm sections of dentin underlying the restoration. Obviously, the higher the number, the greater the acid penetration. *A,* Silicate cement—cavity unprotected; *B,* restoration placed over a cavity varnish; and C, restoration over a 0.2-mm thick layer of either a zinc oxide–eugenol or calcium hydroxide cement.

pledget of cotton. It is advisable that a disposable applicator be used and discarded after each use to prevent introduction of micro-organisms into the varnish bottle.

Conventional cavity varnishes should not be employed under composite restorations, because the solvent in the varnish may soften the resin and the coating prevents proper wetting of the prepared cavity by the bonding agents. However, if sufficient time is allowed for evaporation of the organic solvent, such degradation of a subsequent composite may not occur.

A varnish is not indicated when a GIC is used. The coating would eliminate the potential for adhesion. Research in current dentin bonding agents has shown that they can be used in areas that traditionally require varnish. By virtue of their desirable features, discussed in Chapter 13, dentin bonding agents will fill the role of varnish in the future.

CAVITY LINERS

The main purpose of cavity liners is to use the beneficial effects of calcium hydroxide in accelerating the formation of reparative dentin. Traditionally, it is formulated by dispersing calcium hydroxide in aqueous or resin carrier solutions to facilitate application to the walls of a cavity preparation. The carrier evaporates and leaves a thin layer of calcium hydroxide on the cavity walls. In addition, a film of calcium hydroxide with a pH of 11 can neutralize or react with acid released from adjacent phosphoric acid–containing cements. Because calcium hydroxide is soluble in oral fluids regardless of the type of carrier used, it is mandatory that this type of liner not be left on the margins of the cavity preparation.

Instead of using a suspension formulation, several other hard-setting materials are available. They include calcium hydroxide materials, low-viscosity ZOE (Type IV) and glass ionomer liner. These materials are placed in a thin layer on the pulpal floor. Although the ZOE and glass ionomer liner does not contain calcium hydroxide, they are used for the benefits described earlier.

Glass Ionomer Liners. There are two types of glass ionomer liners. Representative products of the two types can be seen in Figure 24–15. The first is a conventional powder-liquid system. The handling characteristics of the formulation have been adjusted so that it is amenable for use as a liner. For example, these materials tend to set a little faster initially than do the restorative cements and are more free-flowing.

The second type is a light-cured GIC. The chemical makeup and setting mechanism are similar to that of resin-modified GICs. The liquid of at least one product also contains hydroxyethyl methacrylate and additional light-activated accelerators. The two components are mixed, placed in the prepared tooth, and then exposed to a resin-curing light. With the light-cured ionomer liners, conditioning of the dentin surface, such as with polyacrylic acid, is not required. However, thicknesses greater than 2 mm do not cure adequately.

The compressive and tensile strengths of both types of liners, as listed in Table 24–8, are lower than those of the restorative cements (see Table 24–2).

Procedure for Use of the Glass Ionomer Liner. The primary purpose of the ionomer liner is to serve as an intermediate bonding material between the tooth and a composite restoration. In actuality, it serves as a dentin bonding agent. As a result of the adhesion to dentin, it tends to reduce the gap formation at

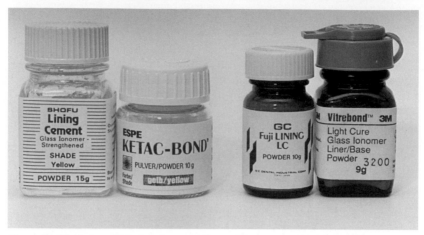

Figure 24–15. Commercial glass ionomer liners. The two on the left are based on the conventional powder-liquid system, whereas the two on the right are light cured.

gingival margins located in dentin, cementum, or both caused by the polymerization shrinkage of the resin. The advantage of the GIC over resin bonding agents lies in the proven adhesive bond, reduced technique sensitivity, and an established anticariogenic mechanism by fluoride release (see Table 24–7). When it is used in this context, this procedure is often referred to as the *sandwich technique* in that it is a resin laminate bonded to the ionomer liner. The technique takes advantage of the desirable qualities of an ionomer system yet provides the aesthetics of the composite restoration. This sandwich technique is recommended for the Class II composite restoration in particular.

The details of the procedure may be found in textbooks cited in the Selected Reading section at the end of the chapter or in operative dentistry textbooks. Briefly, the dentin is conditioned if a conventional liner is used. The dentin is coated with the cement which is extended to the margins located in dentin or cementum. The ionomer must be exposed to the oral environment to achieve fluoride release. However, if any such margin is visible, the cement must be removed from this area because of the aesthetic problem created by the mismatch in color between the radiopaque cement and the resin. However, even in such situations, the ionomer can be feathered down to a thin line that is not readily detected.

The beveled enamel margins are etched with phosphoric acid to enhance bonding to the composite. Traditionally, the surface of the set cement is also

TABLE 24–8. Properties of Glass Ionomer Liners

	Compressive Strength*		Diametral Tensile Strength*		Hardness (KHN)
	MPa	*psi*	*MPa*	*psi*	
Polyacid liquid	76	11,000	4	600	41
Water settable	83	12,000	7	1000	59
Light cured—A	97	14,000	18	2600	46
Light cured—B	69	10,000	10	1400	40

*Courtesy of H. Albers
KHN, Knoop hardness number.

etched to produce a roughened surface that ensures adhesion of the resin bonding agent, which is then applied, to be followed by the restorative composite. There is controversy as to whether etching of the lining cement is actually necessary, because the set surface may provide sufficient roughness to ensure a bond of the resin and excessive acid etching may destroy the cement. It is important to realize that the cement liner is likely to be etched somewhat during micromechanical etching. If the cement is willfully etched, the maximum time is 15 to 20 seconds. That surface is then thoroughly washed for 25 to 30 seconds to remove the debris caused by etching. The surface of a light-cured ionomer cement is *not* etched. After the application of the bond agent to the cement and to the etched enamel, the composite is inserted in the usual manner.

CEMENT BASES

The function of bases, which are thicker protective layers of cement that are placed under restorations, is to encourage recovery of the injured pulp and to protect it against the numerous types of insult to which it may be subjected. These insults include thermal shock and chemical irritation, depending on the particular restorative materials that are used. The base essentially serves as a replacement or substitute for the protective dentin that has been destroyed by caries, cavity preparation, or both.

There are a variety of materials that have been used as bases. Zinc phosphate cement has been used for this purpose for many years, as have numerous ZOE formulations. In addition, both polycarboxylate and glass ionomer cements have properties that make them suitable for use as bases. Several fast-setting ionomer cements are available for this purpose.

Thermal Properties. As shown in Table 24–9, the thermal conductivity values of zinc phosphate and ZOE cements are similar to those of recognized insulators, such as cork and asbestos. The insulation ability of other cements such as polycarboxylate, glass ionomer, and calcium hydroxide also falls within this range.

The thermal-insulating characteristics of various types of bases, as indicated by the rates of heat conduction through specimens composed of amalgam placed over 1.5- and 0.15-mm-thick bases, are shown in Figure 24–13. A constant heat source was applied to the surface of the amalgam, and the temperature change induced on the underside of the base (cavity floor) was monitored.

The reduction in the rate of temperature change of amalgam/base specimens, as compared with the control, is indicative of the thermal-insulating properties of the bases. It is apparent that the rate of heat transfer through the amalgam specimen (A) in Figure 24–13 is rapid in comparison with that through combina-

TABLE 24–9. Thermal Conductivity of Various Cement Base Materials as Compared with Two Commonly Recognized Insulators

Material	Thermal conductivity $(cal \cdot s^{-1}cm^{-2}[^\circ C/cm]^{-1}) \times 10^{-4}$
Zinc phosphate cement (dry)	3.11
Zinc phosphate cement (wet)	3.88
Zinc oxide–eugenol	3.98
Asbestos	1.90
Cork	7.00

tions of amalgam and zinc phosphate (C), amalgam and calcium hydroxide (D), and amalgam and ZOE (E).

Clinical experience has shown that temperature changes in the mouth have a more acute effect on the pulp when the amalgam restoration is not insulated by a base. As was discussed in Chapter 3, heat transfer through a material is, of course, dependent not only on the coefficient of thermal conductivity and diffusivity of the substance but also on its thickness. As shown in Figure 24–13, the thermal insulation ability of calcium hydroxide base and ZOE cement decreases substantially when the thickness of the base is reduced to 0.15 mm (curves D′ and E′).

The minimal thickness required for adequate thermal insulation is estimated to be 0.75 mm. For example, *in vivo* measurements of thermal diffusion made by placing thermocouple on the floor of Class V tooth preparations restored with amalgam revealed that, within 2 seconds after application of a thermal stimulus, the temperature on the cavity floor was only 20% less than that of the surface of the restoration. When a 0.5-mm base was present, the temperature was reduced by approximately one half and to about one third the value associated with a 1-mm-thick base.

Protection Against Chemical Insult. As would be expected, bases of calcium hydroxide and ZOE provide effective barriers against the penetration of irritating constituents from restorative materials. The hard-setting calcium hydroxide and the ZOEs designed for this purpose flow readily and therefore can be applied to the cavity floor in a relatively thin layer.

Bases of carboxylate and ionomer cements can also be used as chemical barriers. There is some concern that if zinc phosphate is employed as a base for thermal insulation, the low pH may require pulp protection. However, if the zinc phosphate cement is mixed as a thick nontacky, puttylike mass, this risk is negligible. In the case of a glass ionomer, any deep areas should be protected by a thin layer of a calcium hydroxide paste.

Strength. Dental cements used as bases must exhibit sufficient strength to withstand the forces of condensation so that the base is not fractured during insertion of the restorative material. Fracture or displacement of the base permits the amalgam to penetrate the base, contact the dentin, and thus eliminate the thermal protection provided by the base. Likewise, in a deep cavity, the amalgam may be forced into the pulp through microscopic exposures in the dentin. Accordingly, the amalgam should be placed only after the base has attained the initial set. The base should also resist fracture or distortion under any masticatory stresses transmitted to it through the restoration.

Table 24–10 shows the compressive strength of representative ZOE cement, calcium hydroxide base, and zinc phosphate cement at intervals of 7 minutes, 30 minutes, and 24 hours. Materials A, B, and C are proprietary ZOE cements. Material A is designed primarily for use as a base and is furnished in paste form. The calcium hydroxide materials, D and E, are hard-setting systems. The duration of 7 minutes represents the initial *set* of most of these materials, under controlled test conditions. Therefore, the 7-minute strengths are analogous to the strength of the material at the time when amalgam condensation pressure would be exerted clinically on the base.

To examine the minimum strength required to support amalgam condensation, bases were placed with experimental ZOE materials with 7-minute compressive strengths lower than those shown in Table 24–10. Dental amalgam restorations

TABLE 24–10. Compressive Strength of Cement Base Materials

Material	7 Minutes		30 Minutes		24 Hours	
	MPa	*psi*	*MPa*	*psi*	*MPa*	*psi*
Zinc oxide–eugenol						
A	2.8	400	3.5	500	5.2	750
B	15.9	2300	20.7	3000	24.1	3500
C	6.2	900	6.9	1000	12.4	1800
Calcium hydroxide						
D	7.6	1100	6.2	900	8.3	1200
E	3.8	550	4.8	700	10.3	1500
Zinc phosphate						
F	6.9	1000	86.9	12,600	119.3	17,300

were immediately condensed over the bases. Sections of the restored teeth show that a compressive strength of only 1.2 MPa can withstand amalgam condensation without detectable damage, but bases with strengths of 0.5 MPa were either fractured or displaced, as shown in Figures 24–16 and 24–17. Thus, the minimum strength requirement lies somewhere between 0.5 and 1.2 MPa. Based on this study, all the materials shown in Table 24–10 should perform adequately as bases.

Similar tests conducted with direct-filling gold indicate that bases of greater strength, and perhaps with somewhat different properties, are required to resist the stress developed during condensation. For example, material A (see Table 24–10) was sometimes displaced when gold foil was condensed against it. The surfaces of bases prepared from materials A and D also flaked off, and the particles were incorporated into the body of the restoration. Zinc phosphate and the stronger ZOE cements, such as B, supported the condensation of the gold foil, as undoubtedly would zinc polycarboxylate or GICs.

The exact strength required to resist masticatory forces has not been determined. Unquestionably, the design of the cavity is a factor. In the simple Class I preparation in which the base is supported on all sides by tooth structure, less strength may be necessary than in the Class II preparation, for example. Actually, there are insufficient clinical data available on this subject to make specific

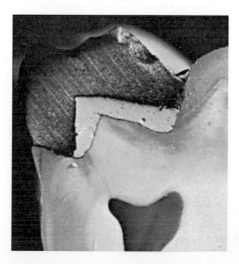

Figure 24–16. Section through an amalgam restoration condensed with a heavy condensation force against a base having 7-minute compressive strength of 1.2 MPa.

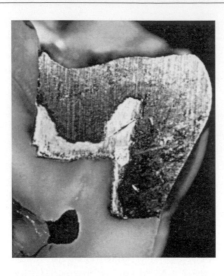

Figure 24–17. Section through an amalgam restoration condensed with the same technique used in Figure 24–16 but against a base having a 7-minute compressive strength of 0.5 MPa. Note the displacement and fracture of the ZOE base near the pulpoaxial line angle of the prepared tooth.

conclusions. A report involving more than 350 amalgam restorations that had bases of a hard-setting calcium hydroxide reported a minimal percentage of failure.

Clinical Considerations. The selection of a base is governed to an extent by the design of the cavity preparation, the type of direct restorative material used, and the proximity of the pulp in relation to the cavity wall. With amalgam, one of the hard-setting calcium hydroxide materials or ZOE usually serves effectively as the sole base. In other situations, such as with a direct-filling gold, it may be necessary to use a stronger material for the base, such as zinc phosphate, polycarboxylate, or a GIC. Thus, in those instances in which it is desirable to place a calcium hydroxide or ZOE cement on the floor of the cavity, the liner should be overlaid with a stronger cement.

With resin restorations, calcium hydroxide is the material of choice as a thin base over ZOE, which may interfere with polymerization, as noted earlier. Some of the fast-setting, stronger GICs are also satisfactory for this purpose.

Use of a base in conjunction with amalgam or gold foil does not prevent microleakage and acid penetration. If a cavity varnish or dentin bonding agent is selected to assist sealing of the restoration, the type of base governs the respective order of applying the materials. If a zinc phosphate cement base is to be used, then the sealing material should be applied to the cavity walls before placement of the base. On the other hand, if the base cement is biocompatible, such as calcium hydroxide, ZOE, polycarboxylate, and GIC, the cement should be placed first, to be followed by the sealing after the base material has hardened.

In summary, cavity varnishes and cement bases generally serve somewhat different functions, as has been described. In the deep cavity, where maximum protection against all types of insult is required, both a varnish and a base may be needed.

SELECTED READING

Duke ES, Phillips RW, and Blumershine R: Effects of various agents in cleaning cut dentine. J Oral Rehabil 12:295, 1985.
  The effectiveness of various dentin-conditioning agents was evaluated by SEM observations. The results

document that polyacrylic acid removes the smear layer yet leaves the tubules plugged, assuming an appropriate concentration and treatment time.

Goldman M: Fracture properties of composite and glass ionomer dental restorative materials. J Biomed Mater Res 19:771, 1985.
The investigation found lower fracture toughness for metal-modified glass ionomer cements as compared with composite resins—a reflection of the brittleness of the material.

Harper RH, Schnell RJ, Swartz ML, and Phillips RW: In vivo measurements of thermal diffusion through restorations of various materials. J Prosthet Dent 43:180, 1980.
Thermocouples placed on the floor of Class V cavities were used to measure thermal diffusion through amalgam restorations as a function of the thickness of the underlying cement base. The data suggested that a minimal thickness of at least 0.5 mm is needed to protect the pulp against thermal changes.

Hinoura K, Moore BK, and Phillips RW: Tensile bond strength between glass ionomer cement and composite resin. J Am Dent Assoc 114:167, 1987.
The bond strength of dentin bond agents improved when the glass ionomer surface was etched. The matter still remains somewhat controversial when viewed under clinical conditions (see Welburg et al).

Jendresen MD, and Phillips RW: A comparative study of four zinc oxide and eugenol formulations as restorative materials. II. J Prosthet Dent 21:300, 1969.
The laboratory and clinical data support the use of a specific reinforced zinc oxide–eugenol as a temporary restorative for periods of at least 1 year.

Maldonado A, Swartz M, and Phillips RW: An *in vitro* study of certain properties of a glass ionomer cement. J Am Dent Assoc 96:785, 1978.
Acid solubility of enamel in contact with glass ionomer cement was reduced, even more than that for silicate cement.

McKinney JE, Antonucci JM, and Rupp NW: Wear and microhardness of a silver-sintered glass ionomer cement. J Dent Res 67:831, 1988.
The investigation showed reduced wear with a cermet ionomer, as compared with an unfilled cement, by test procedures designed to replicate masticatory wear patterns. It was also suggested that the incorporation of silver may provide a lubricating effect.

McLean JW: Limitations of posterior composite resins and extending their use with glass ionomer cements. Quint Int 18:517, 1987.
The advantages and disadvantages of composite resins versus glass ionomer cements in posterior situations are reviewed.

Mount GJ: An Atlas of Glass Ionomer Cements. London, Martin Dumitz, 1990; and Wilson AD, and McLean JW: Glass Ionomer Cements. Chicago, Quintessence, 1988.
Both of these texts are a must for the serious student of the glass ionomer cement, and their publication attests to the growth of, and interest in, the system. The first is an excellent step-by-step presentation of the clinical usage of the various formulations. The second text also includes an in-depth discussion of the evolution and chemistry of the different formulations.

Mount GJ: The tensile strength of the union between various glass ionomer cements and various composite resins. Aust Dent J 34:136, 1989.
Bond strengths vary with different combinations of ionomer cements and resin bond agents, greatly influenced by the viscosity of the bond agent.

Phillips RW (Guest Editor): J Am Dent Assoc January 1990.
This special issue is devoted to glass ionomer cements. Articles by the leading authorities in the world cover all aspects of the chemistry, properties, biologic characteristics, and usage in all aspects of clinical dentistry.

Phillips RW, Crim G, Swartz ML, and Clark HE: Resistance of calcium hydroxide preparations to solubility in phosphoric acid. J Prosthet Dent 52:358, 1984.
Newer formulations of "hard-setting" calcium hydroxide base materials are decidedly less soluble in acid than earlier versions.

Powis DR, Folleras T, Merson SA, and Wilson AD: Improved adhesion of a glass ionomer cement to dentin and enamel. J Dent Res 61:1416, 1982.
The first of a number of studies showing improvement in the bond strength of a glass ionomer cement to tooth structure when the smear layer is removed with polyacrylic acid.

Reinhardt JW, Swift EJ, and Bolden AJ: A national survey on the use of glass ionomer cements. Oper Dent 18:56, 1993.
A review of glass ionomer use in the United States.

Sidhu SK, and Watson TF: Resin-modified glass ionomer materials—a status report for the *American Journal of Dentistry*. Am J Dent 8:59, 1994.
A comprehensive review of the current development of glass ionomers with polymerizable functional groups. It covers nomenclature, physical and mechanical properties, and clinical applications.

Sipahier M, and Ulusu T: Glass-ionomer-cermet cements applied as fissure sealants. II. Clinical evaluation. Quint Int 26:43, 1995.
Based on clinical evaluations of a glass-ionomer-silver-cermet cement used as a fissure sealant, 30% and 43% of the cermet sealants were lost after 6 and 12 months, respectively compared with corresponding losses of 14% and 12%, respectively, for a conventional resin sealant. Although no significant difference in occlusal caries was found for the sealant materials, the large percentage of cermet sealants lost suggests that they should not be used for this purpose.

Swartz ML, Phillips RW, and Clark HE: Long-term fluoride release from glass ionomer cements. J Dent Res 63:158, 1984.

One of several reports showing the fluoride release pattern of glass ionomer cements. The amount released was similar to that for a silicate cement and greater than a silicophosphate cement, whereas that from a polycarboxylate cement was negligible.

Taleghani M, and Leinfelder KF: Evaluation of a new glass ionomer cement with silver as a core build-up under a cast restoration. Quint Int 19:19, 1988.

The in vitro *study supports use of an ionomer cermet as a build-up material, with posts, in endodontically treated teeth. However, it was recommended that use of the metal-modified cement not be employed for restoring the entire coronal portion of the tooth.*

ten Cate JW, and Featherstone JD: Mechanistic aspect of the interactions between fluoride and dental enamel. Crit Rev Oral Biol Med 2:283, 1991.

This article critically reviews the current information about tooth-fluoride interactions from laboratory and clinical studies.

Walls AWG: Glass polyalkenoate (glass ionomer) cements: A review. J Dent 14:231, 1986.

The article nicely reviews the history and development of glass ionomer cements from their inception in the 1960s to the present.

Welburg RR, McCabe JF, Murray JJ, and Rusby S: Factors affecting the bond strength of composite resin to etched glass ionomer cement. J Dent 16:188, 1988.

Omission of the etching process did not produce a significantly inferior bond, but the results were less dependable.

Wilson AD, and McLean JW: Glass Ionomer Cements. Chicago, Quintessence, 1988.

Excellent reference on the evolution and chemistry of different GICs and step-by-step protocols for each cement type.

25 *Dental Cements for Bonding Applications*

- Principles of Cementation
- Zinc Phosphate Cement
- Zinc Silicophosphate Cement
- Zinc Polycarboxylate Cement
- Glass Ionomer Cement
- Zinc Oxide–Eugenol Cement
- Resin-based Cement
- *In Vivo* Solubility and Disintegration of Cements
- Summary

PRINCIPLES OF CEMENTATION

As pointed out in Chapter 24, numerous dental treatments necessitate attachment of indirect restorations and appliances to the teeth by means of a cement. These include metal, resin, metal-resin, metal-ceramic, and ceramic restorations; provisional or interim restorations; laminate veneers for anterior teeth; orthodontic appliances; and pins and posts used for retention of restorations. The word *luting* is often used in textbooks to describe the use of a moldable substance to *seal* a space or to *cement* two components together; hence the term is descriptive cements. Since *luting agent* is not a term that is commonly used by dental students and practicing dentists, we will adopt the term *cement* in subsequent sections. These cements are differentiated from cement bases, liners, and restorations, which were discussed in Chapter 24.

As shown in Figure 25–1, a number of materials are available for cementation purposes. These include zinc phosphate, silicophosphate, polycarboxylate, glass ionomer, zinc oxide–eugenol (ZOE), and resin-based cements. Listed in Table 25–1 are the mechanical and physical properties of the different types of cements, in addition to the requirements set forth in American Dental Association Specification No. 8 for zinc phosphate cement. The values for all the cements listed in this table are taken from a variety of sources; therefore, they are representative of typical cements. Although variation occurs from one brand to another, the differences induced by manipulative variables are usually considerably greater than those inherent between brands.

As shown in Table 25–1, the properties of various cements differ from each

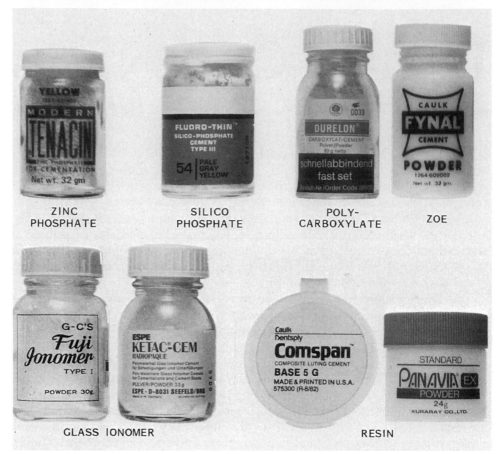

Figure 25–1. Commercial products representative of zinc phosphate, silicophosphate, polycarboxylate, reinforced zinc oxide–eugenol, glass ionomer, and resin luting cements.

other. Hence, the choice of cement is mandated to a large degree by the functional and biologic demands of the particular clinical situation. If optimal performance is to be attained, the physical and biologic properties, and the handling characteristics, such as the working and setting times and ease of removing excess materials, must be considered in selecting a cement for a specific task.

Characteristics of Abutment-Prosthesis Interface. When two relatively flat surfaces are brought into contact, analogous to a fixed prosthesis being placed on a prepared tooth, a space exists between the substrates on a microscopic scale. As shown in Figure 25–2*A*, typical prepared surfaces on a microscopic scale are rough, that is, there are peaks and valleys. When two surfaces are placed against each other, there are only point contacts along the peaks (Fig. 25–2*B*). The areas that are not in contact then become open space. The space created is substantial in terms of oral fluid flow and bacterial invasion. One of the main purposes of a cement is to fill this space completely. One can seal the space by placing a soft material, such as an elastomer, between the two surfaces that can conform under pressure to the "roughness." This is how O-rings work for water-tight or air-tight seals, but they are not applicable to dental situations. The current approach is to use the technology of adhesives. Adhesive bonding involves the placement of a third material, often called a *cement*, that flows within the rough surfaces

TABLE 25–1. Properties of Dental Cements for Bonding Applications

	Time of Setting (min)	Film Thickness (μm)	Compressive Strength—24 h (MPa)	Diametral Tensile Strength—24 h (MPa)	Modulus of Elasticity (GPa)	Solubility and Disintegration in Water (wt %)	Pulp Response
ADA Specification No. 8 Type I	5 min 9 max	25 max	68.7	No specification	No specification	0.2 max	*
Zinc phosphate	5.5	20	104	5.5	13.5	0.06	Moderate
ZOE, Type I	4–10	25	6–28	—	—	0.04	Mild
ZOE + alumina + EBA (Type II)	9.5	25	55	4.1	5.0	0.05	Mild
ZOE + polymer (Type II)	6–10	32	48	4.1	2.5	0.08	Mild
Silicophosphate	3.5–4	25	145	7.6	—	0.4	Moderate
Resin cement	2–4	<25	70–172	—	2.1–3.1	0.0–0.01	Moderate
Polycarboxylate	6	21	55	6.2	5.1	0.06	Mild
Glass ionomer	7	24	86	6.2	7.3	1.25	Mild to moderate

*Based on comparison with silicate cement, a severe irritant.
ADA, American Dental Association; ZOE, zinc oxide–eugenol; EBA, ortho-ethoxybenzoic acid.

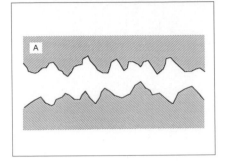
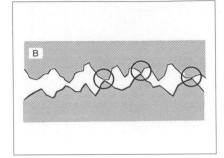
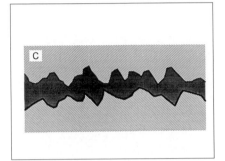
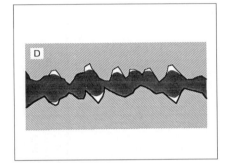

Figure 25–2. Microscopic appearances of the abutment-prosthesis interfaces. *A,* Irregular surface morphology of the two surfaces to be bonded together. *B,* Two surfaces pressed against each other without an intermediate layer, and a small number of points of contact illustrated by the circle. *C,* Continuous interface when a third material, either cement or adhesive, is used as the intermediate layer. *D,* Existence of voids as the result of the inability of the intermediate layer to wet the surfaces.

and sets to a solid form within a few minutes (Fig. 25–2C). The solid matter not only seals the space but also retains the prosthesis. Materials used for this application are classified as Type I cements. If the third material is not fluid enough or is incompatible with the surfaces, voids can develop around deep, narrow valleys (Fig. 25–2D) and undermine the effectiveness of the cement.

Procedure for Cementation of Prostheses. To be effective, a Type I cement must be fluid and be able to flow into a continuous film of 25-μm thick or less without fragmentation. The procedure consists of placing the cement on the internal surface of the prosthesis and extending slightly over the margin, seating it on the preparation, and removing the excess cement at an appropriate time. Cementation of a single crown as an example (Fig. 25–3A) is described in the following sections.

Placement of Cement. The cement paste should coat the entire inner surface of the crown and extend slightly beyond the margin. It should fill about half of the interior crown volume (Fig. 25–3B). The clinician should make certain that the occlusal aspect of the tooth preparation is free of voids to ensure that there is no air entrapment in the critical area during the early stage of the seating.

Seating. Moderate finger pressure should be used to displace excess cement and to seat the crown or other prosthesis on the preparation. An alternative method is to use a vibrational instrument to facilitate the seating of the prosthesis

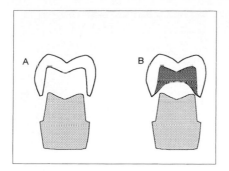
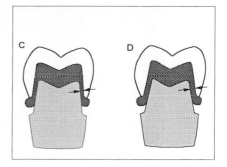

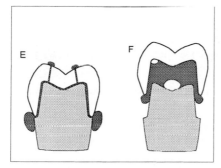
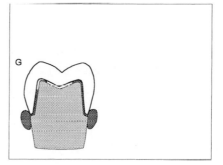

Figure 25–3. Mechanics of cementing a prosthesis. *A*, Assembly of a fixed prosthesis and respective tooth preparation. *B*, Cement placed in the prosthesis should cover the entire surface and extend slightly. *C*, The space for expelling the excess cement decreases as the prosthesis reaches its final position. The *arrows* show the thickness of space for expelling excess cement. *D*, Higher degree of abutment taper provides a greater space for expelling excess cement. *E*, Vent holes toward the occlusal surface of the prosthesis also facilitate the seating of the prosthesis. *F*, Two areas that are likely left uncoated with the cement. *G*, Discontinuous cement layer resulting from failure to coat the surfaces involved.

without creating excess pressure. After the marginal gap area is evaluated for closure with an explorer, the patient may be asked to complete the seating by biting on a soft piece of wood. During this stage, the last increment of excess cement is expelled through the space between the prosthesis and the tooth. As the prosthesis reaches its final position on the preparation, the space for expelling the excess cement becomes smaller, making the seating more difficult (Fig. 25–3C). Variables that can facilitate seating include using a cement of lower viscosity, increasing the taper and decreasing the height of the crown preparation (Fig. 25–3D), vibration, and introducing escape vents on the occlusal aspect of the prosthesis (Fig. 25–3E). Increasing the degree of taper can compromise retention, however. The escape vents can be filled with gold foil or cast gold plugs. If the occlusal surface contacts the axial wall of the tooth during insertion, air pockets may be introduced (Fig. 25–3F and G).

The effect of increased viscosity of the cement on the ability to seat a cast restoration is illustrated in Figure 25–4. A crown cemented with a zinc phosphate mix that was prepared on a cool slab and seated properly on the prepared tooth is shown in Figure 25–4A. However, because of the high viscosity of the mix prepared on a warm slab, the crown in Figure 25–4B failed to seat completely, and a thick layer of cement is exposed at the cervical margin.

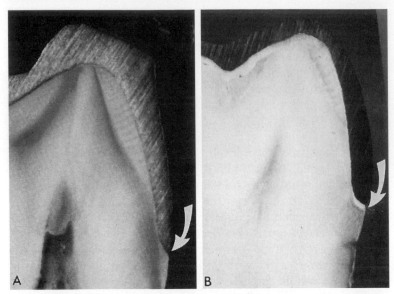

Figure 25–4. Section through gold crowns cemented with the same mix of zinc phosphate cement. The crown shown in *A* was cemented 2.5 minutes after the start of the mix, whereas that shown in *B* was cemented at 5 minutes. Because of the increase in viscosity of the cement with time, the casting in *B* failed to seat completely, leaving a thick layer of cement exposed at the margins *(arrow).*

Removal of Excess Cement. The excess cement accumulates around the marginal area at the completion of seating. Its removal depends on the properties of the cement used. If the cement sets to a brittle state and does not adhere to the surrounding surfaces, the tooth, and the prosthesis, it is best removed after it sets. This applies to zinc phosphate, silicophosphate, and ZOE cements. For glass ionomer cements, polycarboxylate cements, and resin-based cements that are potentially capable of adhering both chemically and physically to the surrounding surfaces, the protocol of excess cement removal varies. One can coat the surrounding surface with a separating medium such as petroleum jelly, thereby inhibiting the material's adherence to the surfaces, and remove the excess after the cement sets. Another technique involves the removal of excess cement as soon as the seating is completed, thus preventing the material from adhering to the adjacent surfaces.

The viscosity of the cement increases as it sets, and eventually it becomes a solid. Attempts to remove the excess cement shortly before it turns into a solid may create certain unnecessary risks. At this stage the cement is so thick that any attempt to remove the excess may inadvertently pull the cement from the marginal area. The most likely material to do this is polycarboxylate cement, which transforms to a rubbery stage before setting.

Postcementation. Aqueous-based cements continue to mature over time well after they have passed the defined setting time. If they are allowed to mature in an isolated environment, that is, free of contamination from surrounding moisture and free from loss of water through evaporation, the cements will acquire additional strength and become more resistant to dissolution. It is recommended that coats of varnish or a bonding agent should be placed around the margin before the patient is discharged. Further details are discussed later in the chapter.

Mechanism of Retention. A prosthesis can be retained by mechanical or chemical means or a combination of mechanical and chemical factors. On the microscopic level, the interface region is similar to that in Figure 25–5. Both surfaces are rough, and the cement fills the roughness of both surfaces. The entire interface region then appears continuous, and the cement layer can resist shear stress acting along the interface. This situation represents a typical mechanical retention, and the strength of retention depends on the strength of the cement, which resists applied forces that may act to dislodge a prosthesis. For certain situations, mechanical retention alone is insufficient, and incomplete wetting can also leave voids on the surface that may allow an influx of oral fluids. Because of these deficiencies, chemical bonding as a means of retention is the ultimate goal. Theoretically, chemical bonds can resist interfacial separation and thus improve retention. Aqueous cements based on polyacrylic acids do provide chemical bonding through the use of acrylic acids. Resin based cements using some specialty functional groups also have exhibited chemical bonding. Details are presented later.

Dislodgment of Prostheses. Fixed prostheses can debond because of biologic or physical reasons or a combination of the two. Recurrent caries results from a biologic origin. Disintegration of the cements can result from fracture or erosion of the cement. For brittle prostheses, such as glass-ceramic crowns, fracture of the prosthesis also occurs because of physical factors, including intraoral forces, flaws within the crown surfaces, and voids within the cement layer.

In the oral environment cementation agents are immersed in an aqueous solution. In this environment the cement layer near the margin can dissolve and erode leaving a space (Fig. 25–6). This space can be susceptible to plaque accumulation and recurrent caries; therefore, the margin should be protected with a coating (if possible) to allow continuous setting of the cement. There are two basic modes of failure associated with cements: cohesive fracture of the cement (Fig. 25–7A) and separation along the interfaces (Fig. 25–7B). Because the cement layer is the weakest link of the entire assembly, one should favor higher

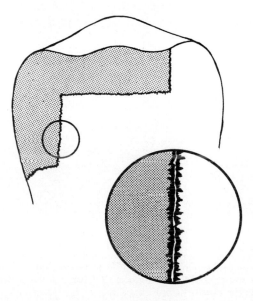

Figure 25–5. Diagram of the suggested mechanism whereby a dental cement provides mechanical retention of a gold inlay. The cement penetrates into irregularities in the tooth structure and the casting and, on hardening, aids in securing the restoration in place. The enlargement shows fracture of these tiny cement projections and loss of retention, possibly resulting in dislodgment of the inlay. (From Phillips RW, Swartz ML, and Norman RD: Materials for the Practicing Dentist. St. Louis, CV Mosby, 1969.)

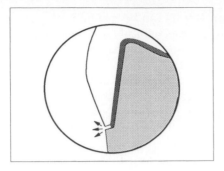

Figure 25–6. Loss of cement at the marginal area resulting from exposure to oral fluid.

strength cements to enhance retention and prevent prosthesis dislodgment by providing a firm support base against applied forces.

Several factors have an influence on the retention of these fixed prostheses. First, the film thickness beneath the prosthesis should be thin. It is believed that a thinner film has fewer internal flaws compared with a thicker one. Second, the cement should have high strength values. Generally, greater forces are required to dislodge appliances cemented with cements that have higher tensile strength than with cements of low tensile strength. It is also well established that the stresses developed during mastication are exceedingly complex. Undoubtedly, properties other than tensile strength may be involved. These include compressive and shear strength of the cement, fracture toughness, and film thickness, as discussed earlier. Third, the dimensional changes occurring in the cement during setting should be minimized. Sources include gain or loss of water and differences in the coefficients of thermal expansion among the tooth, the prosthesis, and the cement. It is, therefore, important to isolate the cement immediately after removal of the excess. Fourth, a cement with the potential of chemically bonding to the tooth and prosthetic surfaces or bond-enhancing intermediate layers may be used to reduce the potential of separation at the interface and maximize the effect of the inherent strength on the retention.

When a mechanical undercut is the mechanism of retention, the failure often occurs along the interfaces. If chemical bonding is involved, the failure often occurs cohesively through the cement itself. The prosthesis becomes loose only when the cement fractures or dissolves.

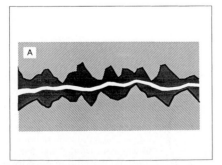
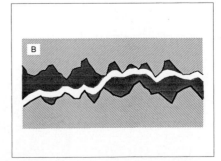

Figure 25–7. Failure modes of the interface. *A,* Cleavage through the cement layer. This is unlikely because of the dimension of the cement involved. *B,* The most likely failure that occurs at the cement-prosthesis and cement-tooth interfaces. Remnants of the cement often remain on the opposing surface.

ZINC PHOSPHATE CEMENT

General Description

Zinc phosphate is the oldest of the cementation agents and thus is the one that has the longest track record. It serves as a standard by which newer systems can be compared. It consists of powder and liquid in two separate bottles.

Composition and Chemistry. The main ingredients of the powder are zinc oxide (90%) and magnesium oxide (10%). The ingredients of the powder are sintered at temperatures between 1000° C and 1400° C into a cake that is subsequently ground into fine powders. The powder particle size influences setting rate. Generally, the smaller the particle size, the faster the set of the cement.

The liquids contain phosphoric acid, water, aluminum phosphate, and, in some instances, zinc phosphate. The water content of most liquids is 33% ± 5%. The water controls the ionization of the acid, which in turns influences the rate of the liquid-powder (acid-base) reaction.

When the powder is mixed with the liquid, the phosphoric acid attacks the surface of the particles and releases zinc ions into the liquid. The aluminum, which already forms a complex with the phosphoric acid, reacts with the zinc and yields a zinc aluminophosphate gel on the surface of the remaining portion of the particles. Thus, the set cement is a cored structure consisting primarily of unreacted zinc oxide particles embedded in a cohesive amorphous matrix of zinc aluminophosphate.

It is obvious that because water is critical to the reaction, the composition of the liquid should be preserved to ensure a consistent reaction. Changes in composition and reaction rates may occur either because of self-degradation or by water evaporation from the liquid. This means that changes in the composition can affect the reaction. Self-degradation effects are best detected as a clouding of the liquid over time. The result is often an inferior material. In addition, it is inadvisable to interchange brands of powder and liquid, because sufficient differences may exist to impair the handling and the physical properties of the resultant cement.

Working and Setting Times. Working time is the time measured from the start of mixing during which the viscosity (consistency) of the mix is low enough to flow readily under pressure to form a thin film. It is obvious that the rate of matrix formation dictates the length of working time. On the other hand, setting time means that the matrix formation has reached a point where external physical disturbance will not cause permanent dimensional changes. It can be measured with a 4.5-N (1-pound) Gillmore needle at a temperature of 37° C and relative humidity of 100%. It is defined as the elapsed time from the start of mixing until the point of the needle no longer penetrates the cement as the needle is lowered onto the surface. Practically, it is the time at which the zinc phosphate cement flash (excess cement) should be removed from the margins of the restoration. A reasonable setting time for a zinc phosphate cement is between 5 and 9 minutes, as specified in ADA Specification No. 8.

Factors Influencing Working and Setting Times. Working and setting times of a commercial product are inherent properties controlled by the manufacturing process. Generally, it is desirable to extend the setting time of the cement to provide sufficient working time for manipulation. The following are means to extend the setting time at chairside.

Powder:Liquid Ratio. Working and setting times can be increased by reducing the powder:liquid (P:L) ratio. This procedure, however, is not an acceptable means of extending setting time because it impairs the physical properties and results in a lower initial pH of the cement. The reduction in compressive strength, along with the decrease in the P:L ratio, is clearly demonstrated in Figure 25–8. The initial pH of the mixture also decreases with the increasing P:L ratio.

Rate of Powder Incorporation. Introduction of a small quantity of powder into the liquid for the first few increments increases working and setting times by reducing the amount of heat generated and permits more powder to be incorporated into the mix. Therefore, it is the recommended procedure for zinc phosphate cement.

Spatulation Time. Operators who prolong the spatulation time are effectively destroying the matrix that was forming. Fragmentation of the matrix means extra time is needed to rebuild the bulk of the matrix. This is different from that observed in the case of dental stones where a fragmented matrix represents new nuclei for crystallization that are needed for structure formation.

Temperature of Mixing Slab. The most effective method of controlling the working and setting times is to regulate the temperature of the mixing slab. Cooling the slab markedly retards the chemical reaction between the powder and the liquid so that matrix formation is retarded. This permits incorporation of the optimum amount of powder into the liquid without the mix developing an unduly high viscosity.

Figure 25–9 shows the effects of slab temperature with respect to the consistency of the resultant mixes that were made using the same P:L ratio and mixing technique. The cement prepared on the cool slab (Fig. 25–9A) is still fluid and suitable for cementation of cast restorations. The mix made on the slab at room temperature (Fig. 25–9B) is much too viscous for use in seating precision castings, especially those with a large surface area such as fixed partial dentures (bridges). Although this procedure is performed routinely by dental assistants on a room-

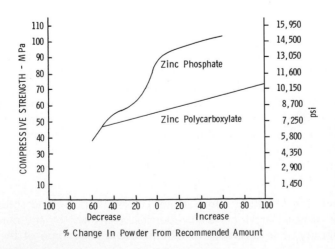

Figure 25–8. Effect of powder:liquid ratio on the strength of two cements. Cement specimens were prepared with greater and lesser amounts of powder (higher and lower powder:liquid ratios) than recommended by the manufacturers, which is represented by a 0% change.

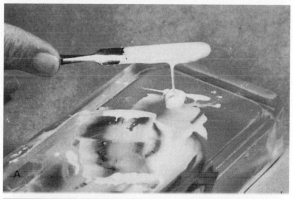

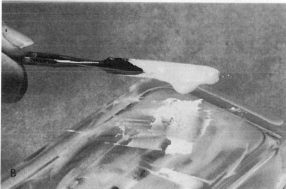

Figure 25–9. Two mixes of cement prepared with identical powder:liquid ratios. The temperature of the mixing slab in *A* was 18° C; the temperature of the slab in *B* was 29.5° C. (From Phillips RW, Swartz ML, and Norman RD: Materials for the Practicing Dentist. St. Louis, CV Mosby, 1969.)

temperature slab, it is not recommended because a lower P:L ratio and lower strength result.

Physical and Biologic Properties

Two physical properties of the cement that are relevant to the retention of fixed prostheses are the mechanical properties and the solubilities. The prosthesis can become dislodged if the underlying cement is stressed beyond its strength. High solubility can induce loss of the cement needed for retention and may create plaque retention sites.

Zinc phosphate cements, when properly manipulated, exhibit a compressive strength of 104 MPa and a diametral tensile strength of 5.5 MPa (see Table 25–1). Zinc phosphate cement has a modulus of elasticity approximately 13 GPa. Thus, it is quite stiff and should be resistant to elastic deformation even when it is employed for cementation of restorations that are subjected to high masticatory stress.

As illustrated in Figure 25–8, the compressive strength (and perhaps tensile strength values) vary with the P:L ratio. The recommended P:L ratio for this zinc phosphate cement is about 1.4 g to 0.5 mL. The increase in strength attained by addition of powder in excess of the recommended amount is modest as compared with the reduction incurred by decreasing the amount of powder in the mix. A reduction in the P:L ratio of the mix produces a markedly weaker cement. A loss or gain in the water content of the liquid reduces the compressive and tensile strengths of the cement.

Zinc phosphate cements show relatively low solubility in water when they are tested in accordance with the ADA specification. However, as was noted in Chapter 24, this test is for quality control and does not reflect the relative rates of disintegration of various types of cement in the oral cavity. *In vivo* disintegration is discussed later. In addition, the solubility rate of zinc phosphate cement is appreciably greater in dilute organic acids (*e.g.,* lactic, acetic, and particularly citric).

Retention. Setting of the zinc phosphate cement does not involve any reaction with surrounding hard tissue or other restorative materials. Therefore, primary bonding occurs by mechanical interlocking at interfaces and not by chemical interactions.

Biologic Properties. As might be expected from the presence of the phosphoric acid, the acidity of the cement is quite high at the time when a prosthesis is placed on a prepared tooth. Two minutes after the start of the mixing, the pH of zinc phosphate cement is approximately 2, as indicated in Table 25–2. The pH then increases rapidly but still is only about 5.5 at 24 hours. The pH is lower and remains lower for a longer period when thin mixes are employed.

From these data it is evident that any damage to the pulp from acid attack by zinc phosphate cement probably occurs during the first few hours after insertion. However, studies of zinc phosphate cements prepared with liquids containing radioactive phosphoric acid indicate that in some teeth the acid from the cement can penetrate a dentin thickness as great as 1.5 mm. Thus, if the underlying dentin is not protected against the infiltration of acid via the dentinal tubules, pulpal injury may occur.

Manipulation

In summary, the following points should be observed in the manipulation of zinc phosphate cements.

1. It is probably not necessary to use a measuring device for proportioning the powder and liquid, because the desired consistency may vary to some degree with the clinical situation. However, the maximal amount of powder possible for the operation at hand should be used to ensure minimum solubility and maximum strength.

2. A cool mixing slab should be employed. The cool slab prolongs the working and the setting times and permits the operator to incorporate the maximum amount of powder before the matrix formation proceeds to the point at which

TABLE 25–2. pH of Cements for Bonding Applications

Time (minutes)	Zinc Phosphate	Silicophosphate	Polycarboxylate	Glass Ionomer	
				Polyacid Liquid	*Water Settable*
2	2.14	1.43	3.42	2.33	1.76
5	2.55	1.74	3.94	3.26	1.98
10	3.14	2.15	4.42	3.78	3.36
15	3.30	2.46	4.76	3.91	3.88
20	3.62	2.56	4.87	3.98	4.19
30	3.71	2.79	5.03	4.18	4.46
60	4.34	3.60	5.08	4.55	4.84
1440 (24 h)	5.50	5.55	5.94	5.67	5.98

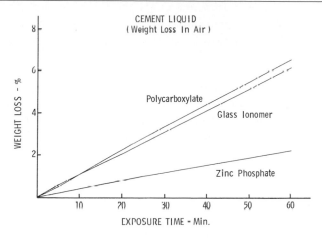

Figure 25–10. Loss of water from cement liquids when they are exposed to air.

the mixture stiffens. The liquid should not be dispensed onto the slab until mixing is to be initiated, because water will be lost to the air by evaporation, as shown in Figure 25–10.

3. Mixing is initiated by the addition of a small amount of powder, as shown in Figure 25–11. Small quantities are incorporated initially with brisk spatulation. A considerable area of the mixing slab should be used. A good rule to follow is to spatulate each increment for 15 seconds before adding another increment. The mixing time is not unduly critical. Completion of the mix usually requires approximately 1 minute and 30 seconds. As stated previously, the appropriate consistency varies according to the purpose for which the cement is to be used. However, the desired consistency is always attained by adding more powder and never by allowing a thin mix to stiffen. For a fixed partial denture, additional time is required to apply the cement. Therefore, a slightly decreased viscosity should be used.

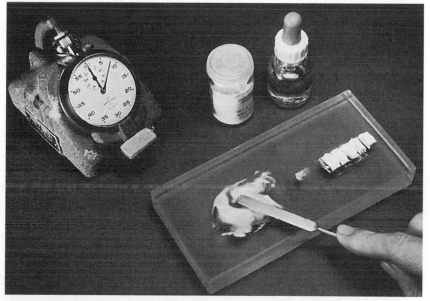

Figure 25–11. When mixing zinc phosphate cement, a small amount of powder is used at the start. A rotary motion is used with the spatula, covering a large portion of the slab.

4. The casting should be seated immediately with a vibratory action if possible, before matrix formation occurs. After the casting has been seated, it should be held under pressure until the cement sets to minimize the air spaces. The field of operation should be kept dry during the entire procedure.

5. Excessive cement can be removed after it has set. It is recommended that a layer of varnish or other nonpermeable coating should be applied to the margin. The purpose of the varnish coating is to allow the cement more time to mature and develop an increased resistance to dissolution in oral fluid.

ZINC SILICOPHOSPHATE CEMENT

Zinc silicophosphate (ZSP) cements consist of a mixture of silicate glass, a small percentage of zinc oxide powder, and phosphoric acid. The clinical indications for this cement are similar to those of zinc phosphate cement. Its strength is somewhat superior; the other major difference is that set ZSP cement appears somewhat translucent and releases fluoride by virtue of the silicate glass. Aesthetically, it is superior to the more opaque zinc phosphate cement for cementation of ceramic restorations. The use of ZSP cement is declining, as practitioners have choices of other more aesthetically pleasing materials, such as resin and glass ionomer cements.

ZINC POLYCARBOXYLATE CEMENT

General Description

In the quest for an adhesive cement that can bond strongly to tooth structure, zinc polycarboxylate was the first cement system that developed an adhesive bond to tooth structure.

Composition and Chemistry. The polycarboxylate cements are powder-liquid systems. The liquid is an aqueous solution of polyacrylic acid or a copolymer of acrylic acid with other unsaturated carboxylic acids, such as itaconic acid. The molecular weight of the polyacids ranges from 30,000 to 50,000. The acid concentration may vary to some degree from one cement to another but usually is about 40%.

The composition and manufacturing procedure for the powder are similar to those of zinc phosphate cement. The powder contains mainly zinc oxide with some magnesium oxide. Stannic oxide may be substituted for magnesium oxide. Other oxides, such as bismuth and aluminum, can be added. The powder may also contain small quantities of stannous fluoride, which modify setting time and enhance manipulative properties. It is an important additive because it increases strength. However, the fluoride released from this cement is only a fraction (15% to 20%) of the amount released from silicophosphate and glass ionomer cements.

The setting reaction of this cement involves particle surface dissolution by the acid that releases zinc, magnesium, and tin ions, which bind to the polymer chain via the carboxyl groups, as illustrated in Figure 25–12A. These ions react with carboxyl groups of adjacent polyacid chains so that a cross-linked salt is formed as the cement sets. The hardened cement consists of an amorphous gel matrix in which unreacted particles are dispersed. The microstructure resembles that of zinc phosphate cement in appearance.

Water-settable versions of this cement are available, as described in Chapter

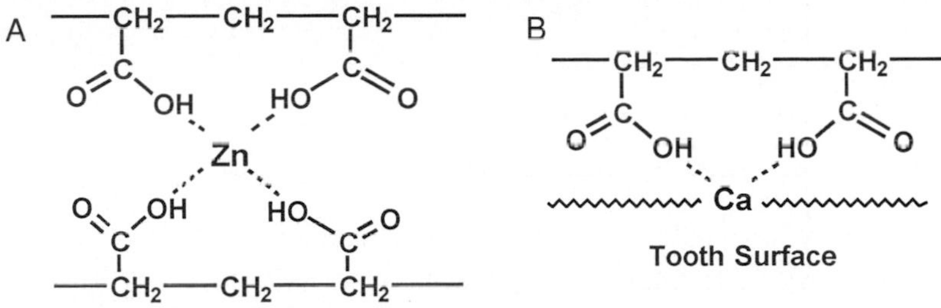

Figure 25–12. The role of carboxylate functional groups in polycarboxylate cements. *A,* Yielding matrix through cross-linking by zinc ions. *B,* Bonding to tooth structure through calcium hydroxyapatite.

24 for glass ionomer cements. The polyacid is a freeze-dried powder that is then mixed with the cement powder. The liquid is water or a weak solution of NaH_2PO_4. However, the setting reaction is the same whether the polyacid is freeze dried and subsequently mixed with water or if the conventional aqueous solution of polyacid is used as the liquid.

Bonding to Tooth Structure. As noted previously, an outstanding characteristic of zinc polycarboxylate cement is that the cement bonds chemically to the tooth structure. The mechanism is not entirely understood but is probably analogous to that of the setting reaction. As shown in Figure 25–12*B,* the polyacrylic acid is believed to react via the carboxyl groups with calcium of hydroxyapatite. As discussed in Chapter 24 in reference to glass ionomer cement, the inorganic component and the homogeneity of enamel are greater than those of dentin. Thus, the bond strength to enamel is greater than that to dentin. This is illustrated in Figure 25–13, in which the bond strengths of a polycarboxylate cement to enamel and to dentin are compared.

General Properties

The properties typical of polycarboxylate cements are presented in Table 25–1.

Film Thickness. When carboxylate cements are mixed at the recommended P:L ratio, they appear to be much more viscous than is a comparable mix of zinc phosphate cement. However, the polycarboxylate mix is classified as pseudoplastic, and it undergoes thinning at an increased shear rate (see Chapter 3). Clinically, this means that the action of spatulation and seating with a vibratory action reduce the viscosity of the cement, and those procedures yield a film thickness of 25 μm or less.

Working and Setting Times. The working time for polycarboxylate cement is much shorter than that for zinc phosphate cement, that is, approximately 2.5 minutes as compared with approximately 5 minutes for zinc phosphate. This is illustrated in Figure 25–14 in which the viscosities of zinc phosphate, polycarboxylate, and glass ionomer cements are plotted as a function of time. The flat plateaus of the curves represent the working times. Lowering the temperature of the reaction can increase the working time that may be necessary for fixed bridges. Unfortunately, the temperature of the cool slab can cause the polyacrylic acid to thicken. This increased viscosity makes the mixing procedure more difficult. It has been suggested that only the powder should be refrigerated before mixing. The rationale for this procedure is that the reaction occurs on the

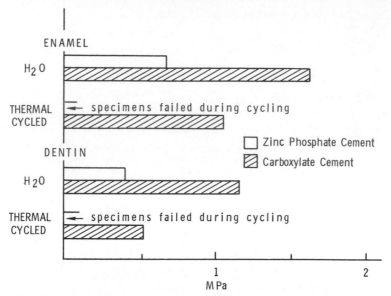

Figure 25–13. The tensile strength required to separate specimens of a polycarboxylate cement, as compared with zinc phosphate cement, from enamel and dentin surfaces after storage in water for 1 week. Thermally stressed specimens were subjected to 2500 cycles between water baths maintained at 10° C and 50° C.

surface and the cool temperature retards the reaction without thickening the liquid. The setting time ranges from 6 to 9 minute, which is within the acceptable range for a luting cement.

Mechanical Properties. The compressive strength of polycarboxylate cement is approximately 55 MPa; hence, the cement is inferior to zinc phosphate cement in this respect. However, the diametral tensile strength is slightly higher. It is not as stiff as zinc phosphate cement. Its modulus of elasticity is less than half that of zinc phosphate cement. In addition, it is not as brittle as zinc phosphate cement. Thus, it is more difficult to remove the excess after the cement has set.

Solubility. The solubility of the cement in water is low, but when it is exposed to organic acids with a pH of 4.5 or less, the solubility markedly increases. Also, a reduction in the P:L ratio results in significantly higher solubility and disintegration rate in the oral cavity.

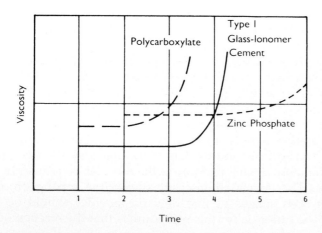

Figure 25–14. Development of viscosity of freshly mixed cements. The viscosity is related to the relative ability to allow complete seating of restoration. Zinc phosphate cement is more viscous initially but provides a longer working time for seating than either polycarboxylate or glass ionomer cements. (From Mount GJ: An Atlas of Glass-Ionomer Cements. London, Martin Dunitz, 1990.)

Biologic Considerations. The pH of the cement liquid is approximately 1.7. However, the liquid is rapidly neutralized by the powder. Thus, the pH of the mix rises rapidly as the setting reaction proceeds, as can be seen in Table 25–2. The pH of a polycarboxylate cement is higher than that of a zinc phosphate cement at various time intervals. Despite the initial acidic nature of the polycarboxylate cements, these products produce minimal irritation to the pulp.

Several theories have been advanced to explain the difference in the reaction of the pulp to polycarboxylate and zinc phosphate cements. The pH of polycarboxylate cement rises more rapidly than that of zinc phosphate cement. In addition, it is possible that the larger size of the polyacrylic acid molecule compared with phosphoric acid may limit its diffusion through the dentinal tubules. The excellent biocompatibility with the pulp is a major factor in the popularity of this cement system. In this regard, polycarboxylate cements are equivalent to ZOE cements. Postoperative sensitivity effects are negligible for both cements.

Manipulation

Characterization of the material provides indications of how the material may perform in a clinical setting. To obtain satisfactory results, the operator must follow instructions carefully and take every precaution to avoid undesirable complications. Areas of major concern are the mixing of the cements, the surface preparation of the prosthesis, the nature of the tooth surfaces receiving the prosthesis, and the time at which the excess cement is removed.

Mixing. The cement liquids are quite viscous. The viscosity is a function of the molecular weight and concentration of the polyacrylic acid and thereby varies from one brand of cement to another. Thus, the P:L ratios required to produce a cement of suitable cementing consistency may vary from product to product. Generally, they are in the range of 1.5 parts of powder to 1 part of liquid by weight.

This cement should be mixed on a surface that does not absorb liquid. A glass slab affords the advantage over paper pads supplied by manufacturers, because once it is cooled it maintains the temperature longer. As stated previously, cooling the slab and the powder provides a somewhat longer working time, but under no circumstance should the liquid be cooled in a refrigerator.

The liquid should not be dispensed before the time when the mix is to be made. It loses water to the atmosphere rapidly, as shown in Figure 25–10. The loss of water from the liquid results in a marked increase in its viscosity.

The powder is rapidly incorporated into the liquid in large quantities. Shown in Figure 25–15 is the consistency of the cement immediately after completion of the 30-second mix as compared with the consistency after a longer mixing time or an additional time on the mixing slab. If good bonding to tooth structure is to be achieved, the cement must be placed on the tooth surface before it loses its glossy appearance. The glossy appearance indicates a sufficient number of free carboxylic acid groups on the surface of the mixture that are vital for bonding to tooth structure. A dull-looking mixture, on the other hand, means that an insufficient number of unreacted carboxyl groups are available to bond to the calcium in the tooth surface.

Surface Preparation and Retention. Despite the adhesion of the cement to tooth structure, polycarboxylate cements are not superior to zinc phosphate cement in the retention of cast noble metal restorations. A comparable force is required

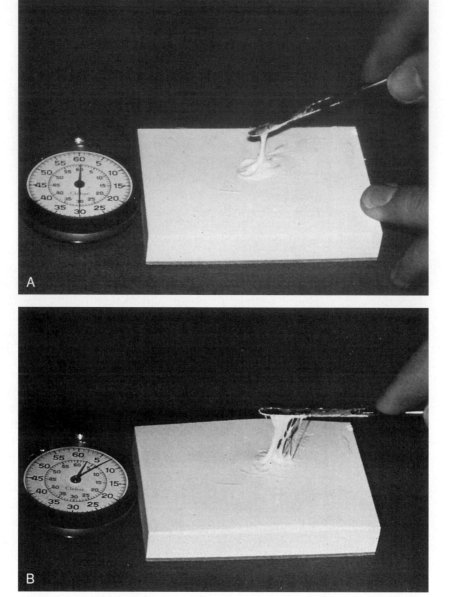

Figure 25–15. *A,* Consistency of polycarboxylate cement on completion of a 30-second mix. *B,* If mixing time is prolonged or the mix is allowed to remain on the slab, the cement becomes dull in appearance and the consistency becomes tacky. (*A* and *B* courtesy of M. Jendresen.)

to remove gold inlays cemented either with zinc phosphate cement or with polycarboxylate cement. Examination of the fractured surface shows that failure usually occurs at the cement-tooth interface with zinc phosphate cement. In the case of the polycarboxylate cements, the failure occurs usually at the cement-metal interface rather than at the cement-tooth interface.

The cement does not bond to the metal in the chemically contaminated as-cast or pickled condition. Thus, it is essential that this contaminated surface on the casting be removed to improve wettability and the mechanical bond at the cement-metal interface. The surface can be carefully abraded with a small stone, or it can be sandblasted with high pressure air and alumina abrasive, for example. After exposure of the fresh metal, the casting should be thoroughly washed to remove debris.

Because this type of cement affords an opportunity to obtain adhesion to tooth structure, a meticulously clean cavity surface is necessary to ensure intimate contact and interaction between the cement and the tooth. A recommended procedure is to apply a 10% polyacrylic acid solution for 10 to 15 seconds followed by rinsing with water, as described in Chapter 24 for removal of the smear layer before placement of glass ionomer restorations.

After cleansing, the tooth is isolated to prevent further contamination by oral fluids. Blotting the surface before cementation is considered sufficient as a drying procedure.

Removal of Excess Cement. During setting, the polycarboxylate cement passes through a rubbery stage that makes the removal of the excess cement quite difficult. The excess cement that has extruded beyond the margins of the casting should not be removed while the cement is in this stage, because there is danger that some of the cement may be pulled out from beneath the margins, leaving a void. The excess should not be removed until the cement becomes hard. The outer surface of the prosthesis must be coated carefully with a separating medium, such as petroleum jelly, to prevent excess cement from adhering. Care should be taken not to allow the medium to touch the margin of the prosthesis. Another approach is to start removing excess cement as soon as seating is completed. The goal of these two methods is to avoid removing the excess during the rubbery stage.

GLASS IONOMER CEMENT

Type I glass ionomer cements are designed for cementation of castings. The powder is finely ground with a particle size of 15 μm or less. The composition and chemistry are the same as those described in Chapter 24 for the Type II glass ionomer cements. The cements are also available in the conventional polyacid liquid-powder system and the water-added versions. The glass ionomer cements bond to tooth structure just as other glass ionomer cements and polycarboxylate cements, that is, via a reaction of the carboxyl groups of the polyacid with the calcium in the tooth, as diagrammed in Figure 25–12B.

General Properties. The properties of a typical Type I glass ionomer cement are listed in Table 25–1. The as-mixed cement is capable of forming films of 25 μm or less. The working time is usually less than that for zinc phosphate cement (see Fig. 25–14) but varies with the system. The range is from about 3 to 5 minutes. The water-settable systems tend to have somewhat longer working times. The setting time for the different brands of cement is usually between 5 and 9 minutes. The water-added cements have a more rapid initial set than those that use the polyacid liquid.

The compressive strength of Type I glass ionomer cement is comparable with that of zinc phosphate, and its diametral strength is slightly higher. The modulus of elasticity is only about one half that of zinc phosphate cement. Thus, the glass ionomer cement is less stiff and more vulnerable to elastic deformation.

Solubility in water during the first 24 hours is high. It is important that the cement should be protected from any moisture contamination during this period. After the cement has been allowed to mature fully, it becomes one of the most resistant of the nonresin cements to solubility and disintegration in the oral cavity, as shown in the following discussion.

Biologic Properties. The glass ionomer cements bond adhesively to tooth structure, and they inhibit infiltration of oral fluids at the cement-tooth interface. This particular property plus the less irritating nature of the acid should reduce the frequency of postoperative sensitivity. However, there are occasional reports of postcementation sensitivity. These reports seem to be associated most frequently with water-settable formulations.

There are several factors that contribute to the potential for irritation. One is the pH and the length of time that this acidity persists. The pH values of a water-settable and a traditional powder-polyacid cement over time are listed in Table 25–2. Although the pH values of the two formulations are virtually the same at 10 minutes, the pH of the water-settable cement is considerably lower than that of the polyacid-liquid powder mix at 2 and 5 minutes. Another factor may be the viscosity of the cement. Remember that these pH values are related to the thinner mixes used for cementation and do not apply to the higher P:L ratios used in the restorative ionomers discussed in Chapter 24. Postoperative sensitivity is seldom if ever mentioned in their use.

Regardless of the type of ionomer cement formulation, when postoperative sensitivity does occur, it is likely that one or more conditions may exist. These conditions include a pre-existing pulpitus, a particularly deep cavity preparation and associated minimal dentin thickness that reduces the time for diffusion of irritants to reach the pulp, and bacterial invasion along the tooth-cement interface.

Precautions should be taken to protect the pulp when cementing restorations with glass ionomer cements. The biologic considerations take precedence over other matters, such as the potential for adhesion that ensures a strong bond to tooth structure. The smear layer on the cut surface of the cavity preparation should not be removed but should be left intact to act as a barrier to the penetration of the tubules by the acid component of the cement. All deep areas of the preparation should be protected by a thin layer of a hard-setting calcium hydroxide cement.

Manipulation. As described in the section on polycarboxylate cements, surface preparation, cement mixing, cementation, and excess cement removal are areas of concern.

The prepared tooth structure should be cleaned with a slurry of pumice, rinsed, and then dried but not dehydrated. Undue desiccation opens up the tubules, again enhancing penetration of the acidic liquid.

The mixing procedure is similar to that described for zinc polycarboxylate cement. The powder is introduced into the liquid in large increments and spatulated rapidly for 30 to 45 seconds. As for all cements, the properties of a Type I glass ionomer cement are markedly influenced by manipulative factors. The recommended P:L ratio varies with different brands, but it is in the range of 1.25 to 1.5 g of powder per 1 mL of liquid.

The retention of the casting can be improved if the inside surface is cleaned, as described for the polycarboxylate cement. Cementation should be carried out before the cement loses its glossy appearance. Glass ionomer cement, like zinc phosphate cement, becomes brittle once it has set. When the cement hardens, the excess can be removed by flicking or breaking the cement away at the margins. Like polycarboxylate cement, it is important to prevent excess cement from spreading to the tooth structure or the prosthesis. This cement is particularly susceptible to attack by water during setting. Therefore, the accessible margins of the restoration should be coated to protect the cement from premature exposure to moisture.

ZINC OXIDE–EUGENOL CEMENT

Type I ZOE cements are designed for temporary cementation of indirect restorations, whereas Type II cements are designed for long-term applications. The chemistry is the same as for formulations employed for impression pastes and temporary and intermediate restorations. Just as for the formulations employed for temporary and intermediate restorations, the mixing technique, rate of powder addition, and spatulation time are not crucial.

Type I ZOE Cements. As noted previously, ZOE cement has a pH of 7 and is biocompatible with the pulp. In addition, it seals the cavity surprisingly well against the ingress of oral fluids, at least for a brief period; hence, irritation caused by microleakage is minimized.

The strength of a temporary cement must be low to permit removal of the restoration without trauma to the teeth and damage to the restoration itself. These cements are available with a relatively wide range of strengths. To facilitate removal of the restorations, it is desirable to employ a formulation that has a lower strength.

Type II ZOE Cements. The biologic properties of ZOE also make it attractive as a final cement, if its lower strength can be accepted. Commercial cements largely have been based on two systems. One is based on the addition of alumina to the powder and ortho-ethoxybenzoic acid to the eugenol liquid, and the second is based on the use of a polymer, as is employed in the ZOE formulations designed for intermediate restorations (see Chapter 24).

As can be seen in Table 25–1, the compressive strength of these *improved* ZOE cements is acceptable, but overall the mechanical properties are inferior to those of other cements. In addition, the cements are somewhat difficult to manipulate in the oral cavity. The film thickness of some products tends to be high and the set cement excess is quite difficult to remove. For these reasons, the use of ZOE cements for long-term applications has been confined primarily to those situations in which it was anticipated that sensitivity might be a problem. Currently, however, zinc polycarboxylate cement, which is equally kind to the pulp and has far better handling characteristics, has virtually replaced the improved ZOE cements in the dentist's armamentarium.

RESIN-BASED CEMENT

General Description

A variety of resin-based cements have now become available because of the development of the direct-filling resins with improved properties, the acid-etch technique for attaching resins to enamel, and molecules with a potential to bond to dentin conditioned with organic or inorganic acid. Some are designed for general use and others for specific uses such as attachment of orthodontic brackets or resin-bonded bridges.

Composition and Chemistry. The composition of most modern resin-based cements is similar to that of resin-based composite filling materials (*i.e.*, a resin matrix with silane-treated inorganic fillers). Because most of a prepared tooth surface is dentin, monomers with functional groups that have been used to induce bonding to dentin are often incorporated in these resin cements. They include organophosphonates, hydroxyethyl methacrylate (HEMA), and the 4-methacrylethyl trimellitic anhydride (4-META) system. The chemical structures of these groups are shown in Chapter 13. Bonding of the cement to enamel can be attained through the acid-etch technique.

Polymerization can be achieved by the conventional peroxide-amine induction system or by light activation. Several systems use both mechanisms and are referred to as *dual-cure systems.* The fillers are those used in composites (silica or glass particles, 10 to 15 μm in diameter) and the colloidal silica is that used in microfilled resins.

Properties. Resin-based cements as a group are virtually insoluble in oral fluids, but, as indicated in Table 25–1, there is a wide variation in the range of other properties from one product to another. These variations, as discussed in Chapter 12, undoubtedly are associated with compositional differences, the amounts of diluent monomers, and filler levels.

Resin-based cements are often designed for specific applications rather than general uses. They are formulated to provide the handling characteristics required for the particular application. For example, cements recommended for cementation of indirect restorations have film thicknesses of 25 μm or less. A cement that is indicated for direct bonding of orthodontic brackets would not have the same handling characteristics or properties desired for a crown and bridge cement.

With respect to bonding to dentin, the so-called adhesive cements, which incorporate the phosphonate, HEMA, or 4-META adhesion systems, generally develop reasonably good bond strengths to dentin. Just as with the dentin bonding agents, they have not been in use long enough to define their long-term efficacy. Some of the other commercial resin-based cements furnish a bonding agent as a separate component of the cement system. Bonding to tooth structure may be more critical for resin-based cements than for some other types of cement, because they possess no anticariogenicity potential.

Biologic Properties. Resin-based cements, just like the composite restorative resins, are irritating to the pulp. Thus, pulp protection via a calcium hydroxide or glass ionomer liner is important when one is cementing an indirect restoration that involves bonding to dentin. Obviously, if the bonding area involves only enamel, or if the remaining dentin thickness is sufficient, the irritating properties of the monomers are not significant.

Manipulation. The chemically activated versions of these cements are supplied as two-component systems: a powder and liquid, or two pastes. The peroxide initiator is contained in one component, and the amine activator is contained in the other. The two components are combined by mixing on a treated paper pad for 20 to 30 seconds. The time of excess removal is critical. If it is done while the cement is in a rubbery state, the cement may be pulled from beneath the margin of the restoration, leaving a void that increases the risk of plaque buildup and secondary caries. Removal of the excess cement is difficult if it is delayed until the cement has polymerized. It is best to remove the excess cement immediately after the restoration is seated.

Light-cured cements are single-component systems just as are the light-cured filling resins. They are widely used for cementation of porcelain and glass-ceramic restorations and for direct bonding of ceramic orthodontic brackets. The time of exposure to the light that is needed for polymerization of the resin cement is dependent on the light transmitted through the ceramic restoration or bracket and the layer of polymeric cement. However, the time of exposure to the light should never be less than 40 seconds.

The dual-cure cements are two-component systems and require mixing that is similar to that for the chemically activated systems. The chemical activation is slow and provides extended working time until the cement is exposed to the curing light, at which point the cement solidifies rapidly. It then continues to gain strength over an extended period because of the chemically activated polymerization.

Applications

Several dental procedures for which a resin-based cement is the material of choice are described in the following sections.

Resin-bonded Bridges. These prostheses are widely employed as alternatives to metal-ceramic bridges. In this procedure, the preparation of the abutment teeth is minimal and is confined to enamel of the lingual surface and proximal surfaces. Such an appliance is shown in Figure 25–16. The tissue surfaces of the abutments are roughened by electrochemical etching or other means, and the surfaces of the prepared tooth enamel are acid etched to provide mechanical retention areas for the resin cement.

Orthodontic Brackets. The enamel surface is acid etched, and the tissue side of the brackets is designed to provide some means of mechanical retention (*e.g.*, a metal mesh). Ceramic brackets are becoming increasingly popular, because they

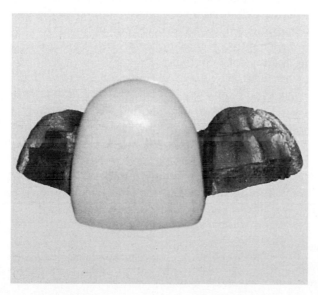

Figure 25–16. Resin-bonded bridge. Note that the metal has been etched for retention. (Courtesy of Rose Marie Jones.)

are tooth colored and hence are more aesthetic. Bonding resin to ceramic brackets is achieved either by mechanical retention within the bracket or by coating the back of the bracket with an organosilane analogous to the coupling agents employed to bond the inorganic fillers to the resin matrix of resin-based composite. A problem is sometimes encountered in removal of the bracket. In this case, the bond of the cement to the bracket and etched enamel is strong and the cement is tough. When an attempt is made to pry the bracket off the tooth, the brittle ceramic bracket sometimes fractures and it may become necessary to remove remnants by grinding.

Glass-Ceramic Restorations. These restorations often are translucent and require specific shades of cementation agent to maximize their aesthetic appearance. Resin cements have been the cementation agent of choice recently for all-ceramic inlays, crowns, and bridges because of their ability to reduce fracture of the ceramic structures. To achieve the best retention, the undersurface of the glass-ceramic restoration usually is etched, and a silane coating is applied before cementation.

IN VIVO SOLUBILITY AND DISINTEGRATION OF CEMENTS

An important property of a bonding cement is that it should be resistant to solubility and disintegration in the oral cavity. With the exception of resin cements, all the cements that have been discussed have the potential for significant degradation in oral fluids. If the cement is dissolved or deteriorates so that fragments are lost from beneath a restoration, leakage and bacterial invasion ensue with subsequent problems of sensitivity, caries, or both.

However, the complexity of the oral environment is such that it is virtually impossible to duplicate in a test tube. Cements are continually exposed to a variety of acids produced by micro-organisms and the breakdown of food. Some acids are taken into the mouth in the form of foods and drinks. Both pH and temperature of the oral cavity fluctuate. This complexity of the oral environment, coupled with the fact that different cements behave in different ways, has hindered development of a standard laboratory test that will accurately predict the relative resistance to degradation of various cements in the mouth.

Because of problems with *in vitro* tests, the most reliable data on the durability of the various cementing agents have been obtained *in vivo* by placing small specimens of the cements in intraoral appliances that can be removed from the mouth to measure the loss of material.

The results of such tests are shown in Table 25–3. These data were obtained by inserting the cements in tiny wells placed in the proximal surfaces of cast crown restorations. The crowns were cemented with a temporary ZOE cement. At 1 year, they were removed and the cement loss was measured. As shown in Table 25–3, the relative disintegration rates of the cements bear no relationship

TABLE 25–3. *In Vivo* **Solubility and Disintegration of Cementation Agents***

Least Disintegration	Most Disintegration
Glass ionomer	Polycarboxylate (recommended powder:liquid ratio)
Silicophosphate	Zinc phosphate
	Polycarboxylate (low powder:liquid ratio)

*Cements connected by vertical lines are not significantly different from each other.

to the solubility data presented in Table 25–1 that were obtained in water via the ADA test. Silicophosphate and glass ionomer cement are significantly more resistant to the rigors of the oral environment than other cements. The solubility of zinc polycarboxylate cement, when it was mixed at the recommended P:L ratio of 1.5:1, and that of zinc phosphate cement were not significantly different. However, a reduction in the amount of powder in the polycarboxylate mixture produced a mixture that disintegrated rapidly.

Another study that employed this test procedure revealed that the permanent ZOE cements show more rapid disintegration than either zinc phosphate or polycarboxylate cement.

SUMMARY

Zinc phosphate has long served as the universal cementation agent. It has the advantage of good handling characteristics and a proven longevity in the oral cavity when it is used for cementation of well-designed and well-fitting restorations. On the other hand, it has the disadvantages of being a pulp irritant, lacks adhesiveness to tooth structure, and has no anticariogenic properties.

The advantage of the "improved" ZOE cements is biocompatibility. The physical and mechanical properties and the handling characteristics generally are inferior to other permanent luting cements.

Polycarboxylate cements are moderately good as compared with zinc phosphate cement. The outstanding characteristics are their blandness to the pulp and formation of an adhesive bond to tooth structure. Disadvantages include the short working time, the sensitivity of the cement to disintegration as related to the P:L ratio, and the lack of significant release of fluoride.

Glass ionomer cements bond to tooth structure and release fluoride in amounts comparable with cements known to be anticariogenic. Compared with zinc phosphate cements, glass ionomer cements show greater resistance to disintegration in the oral cavity and comparable mechanical properties, with the exception of elastic modulus. A primary disadvantage of these cements is the slow maturing process that is required to develop the ultimate properties. They are used for cementing glass-ceramic restoration because of their translucency. However, their low stiffness values may allow excessive elastic deformation of the ceramic prosthesis that may result in fracture of the brittle prosthesis. Generally, these cements are relatively biocompatible, but sensitivity of the pulp to cemented restorations sometimes occurs, so it is judicious to employ pulp-protective measures.

Certainly, the established anticariogenic nature of the silicate cement is a strong argument for the use of the glass ionomer system when protection against secondary caries is the major consideration in cement selection. This would include patients with a high caries index, those with eating disorders, and those with poor oral hygiene. It also includes those who need replacement of restorations that have failed because of secondary caries and those who live in areas where fluoride protection, as by fluoridation of the water supply, is unavailable.

Resin-based cements are virtually insoluble, and their fracture toughness is higher than that of other cements. They bond to dentin by mean of a dentin bonding agent, and all can form a strong attachment to enamel via the acid-etch technique. A primary problem of modern resin-based cements centers on their handling characteristics. It is critical to remove the cement flash before the onset or immediately after seating of the restoration or orthodontic attachment device. From a biologic standpoint, the cements are irritating to the pulp.

Thus, it is readily apparent that no single type of cement satisfies all the ideal characteristics desired. One system may be better suited to one task than another. It is prudent for the dentist to have several types available. Each situation should be appraised on the basis of the pertinent environment and the biologic and mechanical factors involved. The previous discussion has established the basis for making the appropriate decision as to the cement system best suited for each specific case.

SELECTED READING

Ady AB, and Fairhurst CW: Bond strength of cement to gold alloy. J Prosthet Dent 29:217, 1973.
This study found that mechanical cleansing of the chemically dirty surface of a noble metal alloy casting left after pickling provides a satisfactory metal-cement bond.

Berekally TL, Makinson OF, and Pietrobon RA: A microscopic examination of bond surfaces in failed electrolytically etched cast metal fixed prostheses. Aust Dent J 38:229, 1993.
This article examined the patterns of resin cement failure between debonded Maryland bridges and their respective abutment teeth. The results showed that most of the failures (27/28) occurred within the cement layer close to the enamel-resin interface.

Christensen GJ: Marginal fit of gold inlay castings. J Prosthet Dent 16:297, 1966.

Nelsen RJ, Wolcott RB, and Paffenbarger GC: Fluid exchange at the margins of dental restorations. J Am Dent Assoc 44:288, 1952.
These authors demonstrated that under oral conditions the marginal discrepancy that can be detected at the margins of a cemented restoration is approximately 50 μm. It is much greater at the cervical area.

Crowell WS: Physical chemistry of dental cement. J Am Dent Assoc 14:1030, 1927.
This early publication is a landmark on the chemistry and properties of zinc phosphate cement. The clinical relationship, particularly to the pH of the setting cement, is also discussed.

Dilorenzo SC, Duke ES, and Norling BK: Influence of laboratory variables on resin bond strength of an etched chrome-cobalt alloy. J Prosthet Dent 55:27, 1986.
Shear bond strengths of resin to etched enamel exceeded 10 MPa, with higher values at the resin-metal interface were reported.

Knibbs PJ, and Walls AWG: A laboratory and clinical evaluation of three dental luting cements. J Oral Rehabil 16:467, 1989.
A number of studies such as this one have found a poor correlation between in vitro and in vivo disintegration of different luting cements. The possible explanations are discussed.

Krabbendam CA, ten Harkel HC, Duijsters PPE, and Davidson CL: Shear bond strength determinations on various kinds of luting cements with tooth structure and cast alloys using a new testing device. J Dent 15:77, 1987.
A glass ionomer and two resin cements were investigated for shear strength among enamel, dentin, and three casting alloy systems. The roles of acid etching and sandblasting the substrates were also studied.

Maijer R, and Smith DC: A comparison between zinc phosphate and glass ionomer cements in orthodontics [Abstract No. 781]. J Dent Res 65:182, 1986.
A clinical study that demonstrated decalcification beneath some orthodontic bands cemented with zinc phosphate cement, but none under those cemented with glass ionomer.

Pameijer CH, and Nilner K: Long-term clinical evaluation of three luting materials. Swed Dent J 18:59, 1994.
Three cements—a zinc phosphate, a glass ionomer, and a resin cement—were tested for their reaction to periodontal tissues, pulpal response and other clinical parameters. The choice of a final luting agent should be based on anticipated postoperative pulpal reactions, rather than exclusive reliance on physical properties.

Phillips RW, Swartz ML, Lund MS, et al: *In vivo* disintegration of luting agents. J Am Dent Assoc 114:489, 1987.
The in vivo solubility of a glass ionomer cement was superior to that of either zinc phosphate or polycarboxylate cement. Only silicophosphate cement approached the performance characterization of glass ionomer cement.

Sasanaluckit P, Albustany KR, Doherty PJ, and Williams DF: Biocompatibility of glass ionomer cements. Biomaterials 14:906, 1993.
This article details a comprehensive biocompatibility evaluation of a number of glass ionomer cements. These include conventional materials, novel formulations, and a new light-cured material.

Servais GE, and Cartz L: Structure of zinc phosphate dental cement. J Dent Res 50:613, 1971.
The structure of zinc phosphate cement was established as zinc oxide particles in a noncrystalline amorphous phosphate matrix. Pores and surface layers of crystals affect the properties.

Simonsen R, Thompson VP, and Barrack G: Etched Cast Restorations: Clinical and Laboratory Techniques. Chicago, Quintessence, 1983.
The technology of resin-bonded bridges is described.

Smith DC: A new dental cement. Br Dent J 125:381, 1968.

The first report of a new luting cement, the carboxylate system. This research opened up the entire field of polyacrylic acid cements.

Smith DC, and Ruse ND: Acidity of glass ionomer cements during setting and its relation to pulp sensitivity. J Am Dent Assoc 112:654, 1986.

The pH of various types of luting agents is reported. The relatively low pH of glass ionomer luting cements and their slow setting times may be causative factors in reported postoperative sensitivity.

Smith DC, Norman RD, and Swartz ML: Dental cements: Current status and future prospects. In: Reese JA, and Valega TM (eds): Restorative Dental Materials: An Overview. London, Quintessence, 1985, pp 33–74.

A comprehensive and thorough review of all dental cement systems.

Smith DC: Dental cements: Current status and future prospects. Dent Clin North Am 6:763, 1983.

A comprehensive survey of the various types, advantages, and disadvantages of cementation agents. Various manipulative factors that control performance are discussed, as well as criteria for selection of a particular system.

Swartz ML: Luting cements: A review of current materials. Dent Annu 1988, p 232.

A comprehensive and up-to-date review of the recent literature on cementation agents, critiqued by one of the internationally respected authorities in this field.

Swartz ML, Phillips RW, and Clark HE: Long-term F release from glass ionomer cements. J Dent Res 63:158, 1984.

Fluoride release from a glass ionomer cement over a prolonged period is comparable to that of a silicate cement. There is no appreciable leaching of carboxylate cements containing fluoride.

Wilson AD: The chemistry of dental cements. Chem Soc Rev 7:625, 1978.

The introduction of the glass ionomer cement, which was based on Smith's (1968) research of polyacrylic acid systems.

Wolff MS, Barretto MT, Gale EN, et al: The effect of the powder-liquid ratio on *in vivo* solubility of zinc phosphate and polycarboxylate cements. J Dent Res 64:316, 1985.

Cements with low powder:liquid ratios undergo significantly more rapid disintegration than mixes made with recommended ratios (see also Phillips et al, 1987).

26 *Dental Ceramics*

- Historical Perspective on Ceramics
- Classes of Dental Ceramics for Fixed Prosthetics
- Dental Porcelains
- Methods of Strengthening Ceramics
- Factors Affecting the Color of Ceramics
- Metal-Ceramic Restorations
- All-Ceramic Restorations
- Chemical Attack of Dental Ceramics by Acidulated Phosphate Fluoride

TERMINOLOGY

Alumina core–a ceramic containing sufficient crystalline alumina (Al_2O_3) to achieve adequate strength and opacity when used for the production of a core for ceramic jacket crowns.

Aluminous porcelain–a ceramic composed of a glass matrix phase and 35 vol% or more of Al_2O_3.

CAD-CAM ceramic–a machinable ceramic material formulated for the production of inlays and crowns through the use of a computer-aided design, computer-aided machining process.

Castable dental ceramic–a dental ceramic specially formulated to be cast using a lost-wax process.

Ceramic–a compound of metallic and nonmetallic elements.

Ceramic, dental–a compound of metals (such as aluminum, calcium, lithium, magnesium, potassium, sodium, tin, titanium, and zirconium) and nonmetals (such as silicon, boron, fluorine, and oxygen) that may be used as a single structural component, such as when used in a CAD-CAM inlay, or as one of several layers that are used in the fabrication of a ceramic-based prosthesis. Dental ceramics are formulated to provide one or more of the following properties: castability, moldability, injectability, color, opacity, translucency, machinability, abrasion resistance, strength, and toughness. *Note:* all porcelains and glass-ceramics are ceramics, but not all ceramics are porcelains or glass-ceramics.

Ceramic jacket crown (CJC)–an all-ceramic crown without a supporting metal substrate that is made from a ceramic with a substantial crystal content (>50 vol%) from which its higher strength and/or toughness is derived. These crowns are distinguished from *porcelain jacket crowns* that are made with a lower-strength core material, usually aluminous porcelain or feldspathic porcelain. (See porcelain jacket crown.)

Copy-milling–a process of machining a structure using a device that traces the surface of a master metal, ceramic, or polymer pattern and transfers the traced spatial positions to a cutting station where a blank is cut or ground in a manner similar to a key-cutting procedure.

Core ceramic–a dental ceramic material that provides a mechanically strong base onto which a body ceramic (also called *dentine* or *gingival ceramic*) can be veneered.

Cracking–the formation of large or minute fissures (microcracks).

Crazing–the formation of one or more minute cracks as an immediate or delayed result of thermally induced stresses.

Feldspathic porcelain–a ceramic composed of a glass matrix phase and one or more crystal phases. An important crystal phase is leucite ($K_2O \cdot Al_2O_3 \cdot 4SiO_2$), which is used to create a high-expansion porcelain that is thermally compatible with gold-based, palladium-based, and nickel-based alloys. A more technically correct name for this class of dental ceramics is *leucite porcelain,* because feldspar is not present in the final processed porcelain nor is it necessary as a raw material to produce leucite crystals.

Glass-ceramic–a solid consisting of a glassy matrix and one or more crystal phases produced by the controlled nucleation and growth of crystals in the glass.

Glass-ceramic core–the substructure of a restoration, typically made by casting glass containing a nucleating agent into a mold, devesting the cast structure, removing the sprue extensions, and ceramming to produce a specific volume fraction of crystals. If necessary for color and opacity control, the core may then be veneered with a specially formulated porcelain or other ceramic at an elevated temperature. An example is Dicor glass-ceramic.

Glass-infiltrated dental ceramic–a minimally sintered Al_2O_3 or $MgAl_2O_4$ core with a void network that has been sealed by the capillary flow of molten glass. Examples include In-Ceram (Al_2O_3) and In-Ceram Spinell ($MgAl_2O_4$) core.

Injection-molded ceramic–a glass or other ceramic material that is used to form the ceramic core of an inlay, veneer, or crown by heating and compressing a heated ceramic into a mold under pressure. An example is IPS Empress.

Metal-ceramic restoration–a crown, fixed partial denture, or other prosthesis made with a metal substrate (usually cast) to which porcelain is bonded for aesthetic enhancement via an intermediate metal oxide layer. The terms *porcelain-fused-to-metal* (PFM), *porcelain-bonded-to-metal* (PBM), *porcelain-to-metal* (PTM), and *ceramometal* are also used to describe these restorations, but *metal-ceramic* is the preferred descriptor term for these restorations.

Porcelain jacket crown (PJC)–one of the first types of all-ceramic crown, made from a low-strength aluminous core porcelain and veneering porcelain (with matching thermal contraction coefficient) without the use of a supporting metal substrate except, in some instances, for a thin platinum foil. (See ceramic jacket crown.)

Shade guide, ceramic–a series of ceramic tooth-shaped tabs mounted on metal or plastic strips that is designed for comparison of hue, value, and chroma characteristics with those of natural teeth or existing ceramic restorations. The letter and number code on the metal strip allows the dentist to communicate the perceived appearance properties to a dental technologist who may not be able to observe the teeth to be restored.

Shoulder porcelain–a porcelain that is formulated to be sintered at a lower temperature than that of opaque porcelain and higher than that of body porcelain to produce an aesthetic porcelain margin as an alternative to a metal margin on a metal-ceramic crown.

Sintering–the process of heating closely packed particles to achieve interparticle bonding and sufficient diffusion to decrease the surface area or increase the density of the structure. For products such as In-Ceram and In-Ceram Spinell, surface contact sintering and minimal density change are required.

Spinel or spinelle–a hard crystalline mineral ($MgAl_2O_4$) consisting of magnesium and aluminum. Also, any of a group of mineral oxides of ferrous iron, magnesium, manganese, or zinc.

Stain–a mixture of one or more pigmented metal oxides and usually a low-fusing glass that when dispersed in an aqueous slurry or monomer medium, applied to the surface of porcelain or other specialized ceramic, dried or light cured, and fired will modify the shade of the ceramic-based restoration. One product is supplied in a light-curable binder. These stain products are also called surface colorants or characterization porcelains.

Thermal compatibility–the desirable condition of low transient and residual tensile stress in porcelain adjacent to a metal coping that is associated with a small difference in the thermal contraction coefficients between the metal and the veneering porcelains. The contraction coefficient of the metal should be slightly greater than that of the porcelains so that residual axial and hoop compressive stresses are produced. This condition will ensure the cooling of metal-ceramic prostheses without immediate crack formation or delayed fracture caused by residual tensile stresses in porcelain.

HISTORICAL PERSPECTIVE ON CERAMICS

Ceramics were the most sophisticated material of the Stone Age more than 10,000 years ago, and they have retained their importance in human societies ever since. Most all ceramics are characterized by their refractory nature, hardness, susceptibility to brittle fracture, and chemical inertness. For dental applications a hardness of a ceramic similar to that of enamel is desirable to minimize the wear of resulting ceramic restorations and reduce the wear damage that can be produced on enamel by the ceramic restoration. The susceptibility to brittle fracture is a drawback, particularly when flaws and tensile stress coexist in the same region of a ceramic restoration. Chemical inertness is an important characteristic because it ensures that the surface of dental restorations does not release potentially harmful elements, and it reduces the risk for surface roughening and an increased susceptibility to bacterial adhesion over time. Two other important attributes of dental ceramics are their potential for matching the appearance of natural teeth and their insulating properties (low thermal conductivity, low thermal diffusivity, and low electrical conductivity). Because the metal atoms transfer their outermost electrons to the nonmetallic atoms and thereby stabilize their highly mobile electrons, ceramics are excellent thermal and electrical insulators.

Feldspathic porcelains with reliable chemical bonding have been used in metal-ceramic restorations for more than 35 years. Recent developments such as opalescence, specialized internal staining techniques, greening-resistant porcelains, and porcelain shoulder margins have significantly enhanced the overall appearance and "vitality" of metal-ceramic crowns and bridges and the clinical survivability of these restorations. Unfortunately, feldspathic porcelains have been too weak to use reliably in the construction of all-ceramic crowns without a cast-metal core or metal-foil coping. Furthermore, their firing shrinkage causes significant discrepancies in fit and adaptation of margins unless correction bakes are made.

Since the introduction of aluminous porcelain jacket crowns in the early 1900s, recent improvements in both the composition of ceramics and the method of forming the core of all-ceramic crowns have greatly enhanced our ability to produce more accurate and fracture-resistant jacket crowns made entirely of ceramic material. This chapter describes the new generation of ceramics, including Dicor glass-ceramic, Dicor MGC, Optec HSP, IPS Empress, and In-Ceram.

Dental ceramic technology is one of the fastest growing areas of dental materials research and development. The past 2 decades have seen the development of shoulder porcelains for butt-joint porcelain margins on porcelain-fused-to-metal (PFM) crowns and all-ceramic inlay and crown materials, including high-leucite porcelain, shrink-free core ceramic, injection-molded core ceramic, castable ceramic, computer-aided design, computer-aided machinable (CAD-CAM) ceramics, and high-strength glass-infiltrated alumina core ceramic. Most of these materials can be formed into inlays, onlays, veneers, and crowns, and they can be resin-bonded to tooth structure. The future of dental ceramics is bright because the increased demand for tooth-colored restorations will lead to an increased demand for ceramic-based and polymer-based restorations and the reduced use of amalgam and traditional cast metals.

CLASSES OF DENTAL CERAMICS FOR FIXED PROSTHETICS

There are several categories of dental ceramics: conventional leucite-containing porcelain, leucite-enriched porcelain, ultra-low-fusing porcelain that may contain leucite, glass-ceramic, specialized core ceramics (alumina, glass-infiltrated alumina, magnesia, and spinel), and CAD-CAM ceramics. Dental ceramics can be classified by type (feldspathic porcelain, leucite-reinforced porcelain, aluminous porcelain, alumina, glass-infiltrated alumina, glass-infiltrated spinel, and glass-ceramic), by use (denture teeth, metal-ceramics, veneers, inlays, crowns, and anterior bridges), by processing method (sintering, casting, or machining), or by substructure material (cast metal, swaged metal, glass-ceramic, CAD-CAM porcelain, or sintered ceramic core). Methods of fabricating ceramic restorations include condensation and sintering, pressure molding and sintering, casting and ceramming, slip-casting, sintering and glass infiltration, and milling by computer control. A classification according to the substructure or core material is shown in Figure 26–1.

The single-unit crowns may be a metal-ceramic crown, also called a *PFM crown*, a traditional porcelain jacket crown (PJC) based on a core of aluminous porcelain, or the newer ceramic jacket crowns (CJCs) based on a core of leucite-reinforced porcelain, injection- or pressure-molded leucite-based ceramic, glass-ceramic, sintered aluminous porcelain, sintered aluminum oxide, pressure-molded aluminum oxide, glass-infiltrated aluminum oxide, or glass-ceramic processed from cast glass. Each type of restoration, with its variations, is discussed in detail in the succeeding sections. These materials are summarized in Figure 26–1, together with their specialized veneering porcelains and typical commercial names.

DENTAL PORCELAINS

Composition. Conventional dental porcelain is a vitreous ceramic based on a silica (SiO_2) network and potash feldspar ($K_2O \cdot Al_2O_3 \cdot 6SiO_2$) or soda feldspar ($Na_2O \cdot Al_2O_3 \cdot 6SiO_2$) or both. Pigments, opacifiers, and glasses are added to

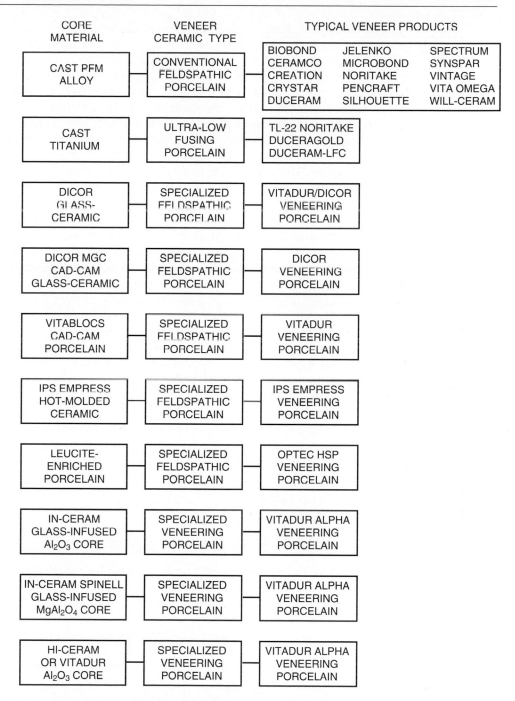

CORE MATERIAL	VENEER CERAMIC TYPE	TYPICAL VENEER PRODUCTS		
CAST PFM ALLOY	CONVENTIONAL FELDSPATHIC PORCELAIN	BIOBOND CERAMCO CREATION CRYSTAR DUCERAM	JELENKO MICROBOND NORITAKE PENCRAFT SILHOUETTE	SPECTRUM SYNSPAR VINTAGE VITA OMEGA WILL-CERAM
CAST TITANIUM	ULTRA-LOW FUSING PORCELAIN	TL-22 NORITAKE DUCERAGOLD DUCERAM-LFC		
DICOR GLASS-CERAMIC	SPECIALIZED FELDSPATHIC PORCELAIN	VITADUR/DICOR VENEERING PORCELAIN		
DICOR MGC CAD-CAM GLASS-CERAMIC	SPECIALIZED FELDSPATHIC PORCELAIN	DICOR VENEERING PORCELAIN		
VITABLOCS CAD-CAM PORCELAIN	SPECIALIZED FELDSPATHIC PORCELAIN	VITADUR VENEERING PORCELAIN		
IPS EMPRESS HOT-MOLDED CERAMIC	SPECIALIZED FELDSPATHIC PORCELAIN	IPS EMPRESS VENEERING PORCELAIN		
LEUCITE-ENRICHED PORCELAIN	SPECIALIZED FELDSPATHIC PORCELAIN	OPTEC HSP VENEERING PORCELAIN		
IN-CERAM GLASS-INFUSED Al_2O_3 CORE	SPECIALIZED VENEERING PORCELAIN	VITADUR ALPHA VENEERING PORCELAIN		
IN-CERAM SPINELL GLASS-INFUSED $MgAl_2O_4$ CORE	SPECIALIZED VENEERING PORCELAIN	VITADUR ALPHA VENEERING PORCELAIN		
HI-CERAM OR VITADUR Al_2O_3 CORE	SPECIALIZED VENEERING PORCELAIN	VITADUR ALPHA VENEERING PORCELAIN		

Figure 26–1. Core ceramic and ceramic veneer products for metal-ceramic and all-ceramic restorations.

control the fusion temperature, sintering temperature, thermal contraction coefficient, and solubility. The feldspars used for dental porcelains are relatively pure and colorless. Thus, pigments must be added to produce the hues of natural teeth or the color appearance of tooth-colored restorative materials that may exist in adjacent teeth.

Silica (SiO_2) can exist in four different forms: crystalline quartz, crystalline cristobalite, crystalline tridymite, and noncrystalline fused silica. Fused silica is a high-melting material whose high-melting temperature is attributed to the three-dimensional network of covalent bonds between silica tetrahedra, which are the basic structural units of the glass network. Fluxes (low-fusing glasses) are often included to reduce the temperature that is required to sinter the porcelain powder particles together at low enough temperatures so that the alloy to which it is fired does not melt or sustain sag (flexural creep) deformation.

Glass Modifiers. The sintering temperature of crystalline silica is too high for use in veneering aesthetic layers onto dental casting alloys. At such temperatures the alloys would melt. In addition, the thermal contraction coefficient of crystalline silica is too low for these alloys. Bonds between the silica tetrahedra can be broken by the addition of alkali metal ions such as sodium, potassium, and calcium. These ions are associated with the oxygen atoms at the corners of the tetrahedra and interrupt the oxygen-silicon bonds. As a result, the three-dimensional silica network contains many linear chains of silica tetrahedra that are able to move more easily at lower temperatures than the atoms that are locked into the three-dimensional structure of silica tetrahedra. This ease of movement is responsible for the increased fluidity (decreased viscosity), lower softening temperature, and increased thermal expansion conferred by glass modifiers. Too high a modifier concentration, however, reduces the chemical durability (resistance to attack by water, acids, and alkalies) of the glass. In addition, if too many tetrahedra are disrupted, the glass may crystallize (devitrify) during porcelain firing operations. Hence, a balance between a suitable melting range and good chemical durability must be maintained.

Manufacturers employ glass modifiers to produce dental porcelains with different firing temperatures. Dental porcelains are classified according to their firing temperatures. A typical classification is as follows:

High fusing	1300° C (2372° F)
Medium fusing	1101–1300° C (2013–2072° F)
Low fusing	850–1100° C (1562–2012° F)
Ultra-low fusing	<850° C (1562° F)

The medium-fusing and high-fusing types are used for the production of denture teeth. The low-fusing and ultra-low-fusing porcelains are used for crown and bridge construction. Some of the ultra-low-fusing porcelains are used for titanium and titanium alloys because of their low-contraction coefficients that closely match those of the metals and because the low firing temperatures reduce the risk for growth of the metal oxide. However, some of these ultra-low-fusing porcelains contain enough leucite to raise their thermal contraction coefficients as high as those of conventional low-fusing porcelains.

Because commercial dental laboratories do not fabricate denture teeth for complete dentures or removable partial dentures, it has become more common to classify crown and bridge porcelains as high fusing (850–1100° C) and low fusing (<850° C). This change in classification has not been universally adopted. Thus, to avoid confusion, the sintering temperature range should be identified (at least initially) in discussions between dentists and dental technologists.

To ensure adequate chemical durability, a self-glaze of porcelain is preferred to an add-on glaze. A thin external layer of glassy material is formed during a self-glaze firing procedure at a temperature and time that cause localized softening of the glass phase and settling of crystalline particles within the surface region. The add-on glaze slurry material that is applied to the porcelain surface for an applied glaze procedure contains more glass modifiers and thus has a lower firing temperature. However, a higher proportion of glass modifiers tends to reduce the resistance of the applied glazes to leaching by oral fluids.

Another important glass modifier is water, although it is not an intentional addition to dental porcelain. The hydronium ion, H_3O^+, can replace sodium or other metal ions in a ceramic that contains glass modifiers. This fact accounts for the phenomenon of "slow crack growth" of ceramics that are exposed to tensile stresses and moist environments. It also may account for the occasional long-term failure of porcelain restorations after several years of service.

Feldspar in Dental Porcelains. Potassium and sodium feldspar are naturally occurring minerals composed of potash (K_2O), soda (Na_2O), alumina (Al_2O_3), and silica (SiO_2). It is used in the preparation of many dental porcelains designed for metal-ceramic crowns and many other dental glasses and ceramics. When potassium feldspar is mixed with various metal oxides and fired to high temperatures, it can form leucite and a glass phase that will soften and flow slightly. The softening of this glass phase during porcelain firing allows the porcelain powder particles to coalesce together. For dental porcelains, the process by which the particles coalesce is called *liquid-phase sintering*, a process controlled by diffusion between particles at a temperature sufficiently high to form a dense solid. The driving force for sintering is the decrease in energy caused by a reduction in surface area. As explained in the terminology section, two dental products (In-Ceram and In-Ceram Spinell) are slightly sintered to produce interconnected pore channels that are necessary for subsequent glass infiltration. The driving force for sintering is the energy associated with a reduction in surface area.

Another important property of feldspar is its tendency to form the crystalline mineral leucite when it is melted. Leucite is a potassium-aluminum-silicate mineral with a large coefficient of thermal expansion (20 to 25 $\times$ $10^{-6}/°$ C) compared with feldspar glasses (that have coefficients of thermal expansion somewhat less than $10 \times 10^{-6}/°$ C). When feldspar is heated at temperatures between 1150° C and 1530° C, it undergoes incongruent melting to form crystals of leucite in a liquid glass. Incongruent melting is the process by which one material melts to form a liquid plus a different crystalline material. This tendency of feldspar to form leucite during incongruent melting is used to advantage in the manufacture of porcelains for metal bonding. Further information is given in the section on metal-ceramic restorations.

Many dental glasses do not contain leucite as a raw material. Since feldspar is not essential as a precursor to the formation of leucite, as described earlier, these glasses are modified with additions of leucite to control their thermal contraction coefficients.

Other Additions to Dental Porcelains. Other metallic oxides also can be introduced, as indicated in Table 26–1. Boric oxide (B_2O_3) can behave as a glass modifier, that is, it decreases viscosity, lowers the softening temperature, and forms its own glass network. Because boric oxide forms a separate lattice interspersed with the silica lattice, it still interrupts the more rigid silica network and lowers the softening point of the glass. The role of alumina (Al_2O_3) in glass formation is complicated. Alumina cannot be considered a true glass former by itself because of the dimensions of the ion and the oxygen:aluminum ratio.

TABLE 26–1. Chemical Composition of Some Dental Porcelains

	Low-Fusing Vacuum Porcelain			Metal-bonded Porcelain	
	Aluminous Core	D	E	D	E
SiO_2	35.0	66.5	64.7	59.2	63.5
Al_2O_3	53.8	13.5	13.9	18.5	18.9
CaO	1.12		1.78		
Na_2O	2.8	4.2	4.8	4.8	5.0
K_2O	4.2	7.1	7.5	11.8	12.3
B_2O_3	3.2	6.6	7.3	4.6	0.12
ZnO				0.58	0.11
ZrO_2				0.39	0.13
Firing temp. (C)	980	980	950	900	900

Chemical composition in percentages.
D, dentin; E, enamel.
From Yamada H, and Grenoble P: Dental Porcelain—The State of the Art. University of Southern California Proceedings, 1977, p 26.

Nevertheless, it can take part in the glass network to alter the softening point and viscosity.

Pigmenting oxides are added to obtain the various shades needed to simulate natural teeth. These coloring pigments are produced by fusing metallic oxides together with fine glass and feldspar and then regrinding to a powder. These powders are blended with the unpigmented powdered frit to provide the proper hue and chroma. Examples of metallic oxides and their respective color contributions to porcelain include iron or nickel oxide (brown); copper oxide (green); titanium oxide (yellowish brown); manganese oxide (lavender); and cobalt oxide (blue). Opacity may be achieved by the addition of cerium oxide, zirconium oxide, titanium oxide, or tin oxide.

METHODS OF STRENGTHENING CERAMICS

It is possible to predict the strength of a substance based on the strengths of the individual bonds between the atoms in the material. The values of strength obtained by such a prediction are typically 10% of the modulus of elasticity (0.1 E). Hence, a material with a modulus of elasticity of 20 GPa* has a predicted strength of 2 GPa (2000 MPa) based on the strength of its interatomic bonds. Based only on the strengths of the primary interatomic bonds (ionic, metallic, or covalent), a ceramic (MgO), a metal (iron), and a polymer (polyethylene) should each have a modulus of elasticity of 20 GPa and a strength of 2 GPa. However, the measured strengths of most materials are more than 100 times lower than this theoretical value.

Why do materials fail to exhibit the strengths that would be expected from the bonds between atoms? As explained in Chapter 4, the answer is found in the minute scratches and other defects that are present on the surfaces of nearly all materials. These surface defects behave as sharp notches whose tips may be as narrow as the spacing between atoms in the material. A phenomenon known as *stress concentration* at the tips of these minute scratches or flaws causes the localized stress to increase to the theoretical strength of the material at a relatively low average stress throughout the structure. When the theoretical strength

---

*1 gigapascal (GPa) = 1 billion pascals (Pa) = 10^9 Pa.

of the material is exceeded at the tip of the notch, the bonds at the notch tip break and initiate crack formation. As the crack propagates through the material, the stress concentration is maintained at the crack tip until the crack moves completely through the material or until it meets another crack, a pore, or a crystalline particle. This phenomenon of stress concentration explains how materials can fail at stresses far lower than their theoretical strength.

The brittle behavior of ceramics and their low tensile strengths compared with those predicted from bonds between atoms can be understood by considering the stress concentration around surface flaws. While metals can yield to high stress by deforming plastically, ceramics tend to have no mechanism for yielding to stress without fracture as do metals, and thus, cracks may propagate through a ceramic material at low-average stress levels. As a result, ceramics and glasses have tensile strengths that are much lower than their compressive strengths.

Because of the many desirable properties of ceramics—such as good aesthetic qualities, high hardness and compressive strength, good chemical durability, and excellent biocompatibility—a great effort has been expended to overcome their principal deficiencies—brittleness, low fracture toughness, and low tensile strength. Methods used to overcome the deficiencies of ceramics fall into two general categories: (1) methods of strengthening brittle materials and (2) methods of designing components to minimize stress concentrations and tensile stresses. Methods of strengthening brittle materials such as dental porcelains are discussed in this section, whereas methods of designing dental restorations to minimize stress concentration and tensile stresses are discussed briefly in the section on the design of dental restorations involving ceramics. In the oral environment, tensile stresses are usually created by bending forces, and the maximum tensile stress created by the bending forces occurs at the surface of a restoration or prosthesis. It is for this reason that surface flaws are of particular importance in determining the strength of ceramics. The removal of surface flaws or the reduction of their size and number can produce a large increase in strength. Smoothing and reducing flaws on the surface is one of the reasons for the glazing of dental porcelain. Strengthening of brittle materials occurs through one or both of two mechanisms: (1) *development of residual compressive stresses* within the surface of the material; and (2) *interruption of crack propagation* through the material. These two approaches to the strengthening of brittle materials, as well as specific methods based on these strategies, are discussed in the following sections.

Development of Residual Compressive Stresses. As previously mentioned, the propagation of cracks from surface flaws is responsible for the poor mechanical behavior of ceramics in tension, although it is also possible that flaws within the interior of the material can also cause fracture initiation under certain conditions. One widely used method of strengthening glasses and ceramics is the introduction of residual compressive stresses within the surface of the object. Strengthening is gained by virtue of the fact that these residual stresses must first be negated by developing tensile stresses before any net tensile stress develops. For example, if the net compressive stress within a surface of ceramic A is -40 MPa and the normal tensile strength of the stress-free ceramic is 60 MPa, it would take a total induced tensile stress of $+100$ MPa in this region to cause a fracture of the material.

Consider two strips of ceramic A, one that was subjected to a treatment that introduced a residual compressive stress of -100 MPa into its surface and the other that was not treated. As the two strips are flexed equal amounts, the untreated strip develops tensile stresses in its convex surface, whereas the treated strip merely experiences a decrease in the residual compressive stress. When the tensile stress in the untreated strip reaches $+60$ MPa, for example, the untreated strip fractures but the treated strip has a residual compressive stress of -40 MPa remaining within its surface. If the untreated strip breaks at $+60$ MPa, the treated strip subjected to the same force will still have -40 MPa of residual compressive stress remaining. It would take an additional applied tensile stress of $+100$ MPa to bring the surface tensile stress of the treated strip to $+60$ MPa. This increase in applied tensile stress from 60 to 160 MPa represents a 200% increase in strength over the untreated strip. There are several techniques for introducing these residual compressive stresses into the surfaces of ceramic articles. Three of these methods are discussed below.

Ion Exchange. The technique of ion exchange, sometimes called chemical tempering, is one of the more sophisticated and effective methods of introducing residual compressive stresses into the surfaces of ceramics. This process involves the exchange of larger potassium ions for the smaller sodium ions, a common constituent of a variety of glasses. If a sodium-containing glass article is placed in a bath of molten potassium nitrate, potassium ions in the bath exchange places with some of the sodium ions in the surface of the glass article. The potassium ion is about 35% larger than the sodium ion. The squeezing of the potassium ion into the place formerly occupied by the sodium ion creates large residual compressive stresses (roughly 700 MPa [100,000 psi]) in the surfaces of glasses subjected to this treatment. These residual compressive stresses produce a pronounced strengthening effect. However, this process is best used on the internal surface of a crown, veneer, or inlay because this surface is protected from grinding and exposure to acids. One study has shown that grinding of only 100 μm from an external surface reduces the strength of the treated structure to its original value. Furthermore, contact with acidulated phosphate fluoride over a cumulative time of 3 hours removes most of the ion-exchanged layer as well. Not all ceramics are amenable to ion exchange. For example, alumina core materials, Dicor glass-ceramic core material, and some conventional feldspathic porcelains that are highly enriched with potash feldspar ($K_2O \cdot Al_2O_3 \cdot 6SiO_2$) cannot be sufficiently ion exchanged with potassium to warrant this treatment.

Thermal Tempering. Perhaps the most common method for strengthening glasses is by thermal tempering. Thermal tempering creates residual surface compressive stresses by rapidly cooling (quenching) the surface of the object while it is hot and in the softened (molten) state. This rapid cooling produces a skin of rigid glass surrounding a soft (molten) core. As the molten core solidifies, it tends to shrink, but the outer skin remains rigid. The pull of the solidifying molten core, as it shrinks, creates residual tensile stresses in the core and residual compressive stresses within the outer surface.

Thermal tempering is used to strengthen glass for uses such as automobile windows and windshields, sliding glass doors, and diving masks. Often, the rapid cooling of the outer skin is accomplished by jets of air directed at the molten glass surface. If one observes the rear window of an automobile through polarized sunglasses, it is usually possible to discern a regular pattern of spots over the entire window. This pattern of spots corresponds to the arrangement of the air jets employed by the manufacturer in the tempering process. For dental applications, it is more effective to quench hot glass-phase ceramics in silicone oil or other special liquids rather than using air jets that may not uniformly cool the surface.

Thermal Compatibility. Most metals expand linearly with temperature up to the melting range. Thus, a metal expands approximately the same amount when heated from 50° C to 60° C as it does from 200° C to 210° C. Dental porcelains behave differently; they have different values in different temperature ranges, and, as a result, the thermal expansion or contraction of the porcelain cannot be precisely matched to that of the alloy. Instead, the thermal behavior of the metal and porcelain must be adjusted by the manufacturer in such a way that during the cool-down period after firing, the transient and residual stresses are sufficiently low and properly directed so that the porcelain is not subject to immediate or delayed failure. Ideally, the porcelain should be under slight compression in the final restoration. This objective is accomplished by selecting an alloy that contracts slightly more than the porcelain on cooling to room temperature.

The fabrication of glass or ceramic articles usually involves forming or processing at high temperature, and the process of cooling to room temperature affords the opportunity to take advantage of potential mismatches in coefficients of thermal contraction of adjacent materials in the ceramic structure. For example, consider three layers of porcelain: the outer two of the same composition and thermal contraction coefficient and the middle layer of a different composition and a higher thermal contraction coefficient. Suppose that the layers are bonded together and the bonded structure is allowed to cool to room temperature. The inner layer has a higher coefficient of thermal contraction and thus contracts more as it cools. Hence, on cooling to room temperature, the inner layer produces compressive stresses in the outer layers as previously described for thermal tempering. This three-layer laminate technique is used by Corning Glass Works to manufacture their dinnerware.

A similar rationale applies to porcelains and alloys for metal-ceramic restorations. The metal and porcelain should be selected with a slight mismatch in their thermal contraction coefficients (the metal thermal contraction coefficient is slightly larger), so that the metal contracts slightly more than the porcelain on cooling from the firing temperature to room temperature. This mismatch leaves the porcelain in residual compression and provides additional strength for the restoration. Shown in Figure 26–2 is a metal-ceramic bridge for which the metal contraction coefficient is less than that of the porcelain. Two of the three stress components represent a state of tension in this case. For the case in which the metal has a greater contraction coefficient, the axial and hoop stresses would be compressive and the radial stress would be tensile, thus representing a more thermally compatible condition because the compressive stresses are dominant.

Disruption of Crack Propagation. A further, yet fundamentally different, method of strengthening glasses and ceramics is to reinforce them with a dispersed phase of a different material that is capable of hindering a crack from propagating through the material. There are two different types of dispersions used to interrupt crack propagation. One type relies on the toughness of the particle to absorb energy from the crack and deplete its driving force for propagation. The other relies on a crystal structural change under stress to absorb energy from the crack. These methods of strengthening are described later.

Dispersion of a Crystalline Phase. When a tough, crystalline material such as alumina (Al_2O_3) in particulate form is added to a glass, the glass is toughened and strengthened because the crack cannot penetrate the alumina particles as easily as it can the glass. This technique has found application in dentistry in the development of aluminous porcelains (Al_2O_3 particles in a glassy porcelain

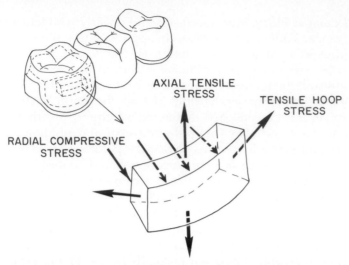

Figure 26–2. Schematic illustration of residual stresses in the porcelain veneer of a metal-ceramic crown for a case in which the coefficient of thermal contraction for the metal is less than that of the porcelain.

matrix) for PJCs. Another ceramic dental material that uses reinforcement of a glass by a dispersed crystalline substance is Dicor glass-ceramic. The cast glass crown is subjected to a heat treatment that causes micron-sized mica crystals to grow in the glass. When glass-ceramic restorations are subjected to high tensile stresses, these microscopic crystals will disrupt crack propagation, thereby strengthening the crown. In most instances, the use of a dispersed crystalline phase to disrupt crack propagation requires a close match between the thermal contraction coefficients of the crystalline material and the surrounding glass matrix.

Transformation Toughening. A newer technique for strengthening glasses involves the incorporation of a crystalline material that is capable of undergoing a change in crystal structure when placed under stress. The crystalline material usually used is termed *partially stabilized zirconia* (PSZ). The energy required for the transformation of PSZ is taken from the energy that allows the crack to propagate. Experimental work has shown that transformation toughening may be a viable method for strengthening dental porcelains. One drawback of PSZ is that its index of refraction is much higher than that of the surrounding glass matrix. As a result, the particles of PSZ scatter light as it passes through the bulk of the porcelain, and this scattering produces an opacifying effect that may not be aesthetic in most dental restorations.

Design of Dental Restorations Involving Ceramics. Dental restorations containing ceramics should be designed in such a way as to overcome their weaknesses. The design should avoid exposure of the ceramic to high tensile stresses. It should also avoid stress concentration at sharp angles or marked changes in thickness.

Minimizing Tensile Stress. Conventional PJCs are contraindicated for restoring posterior teeth because occlusal forces can subject them to large tensile stresses, which are usually concentrated near the interior surface of the crown. PJCs can be subjected to large tensile stresses even on anterior teeth when there is a great amount of vertical overlap (overbite) with only a moderate amount of horizontal overlap (overjet).

Metal-ceramic crowns use a metal coping as the foundation of the restoration to which the porcelain is fused. In an attempt to overcome these stresses, the strong, yet ductile metal coping minimizes flexure of the porcelain structure of the crown that is associated with tensile stresses. Both the bonded platinum foil PJC technique and the swaged gold alloy foil technique (Captec, Leach and Dillon) are also based on this same concept. Descriptions of these materials are presented in the following sections.

Reducing Stress Raisers. Stress raisers are discontinuities in ceramic structures and in other brittle materials that cause stress concentration. The design of ceramic dental restorations should also avoid stress raisers in the ceramic. Abrupt changes in shape or thickness in the ceramic contour can act as stress raisers and make the restoration more prone to failure.

In PJCs, several conditions can cause stress concentration. Creases or folds of the platinum foil substrate that become embedded in the porcelain leave notches that act as stress raisers. Sharp line angles in the preparation also create areas of stress concentration in the restoration. Large changes in porcelain thickness, a factor also determined by the tooth preparation, can create areas of stress concentration.

A small particle of porcelain along the internal porcelain margin of a crown also induces locally high tensile stresses. A stray particle that is fused within the internal porcelain margin of a metal-ceramic crown can also cause localized tensile stress concentrations in porcelain when the crown is placed on the prepared tooth with an applied force.

Even though a metal-ceramic restoration is stronger than a PJC, care must be taken to avoid subjecting the porcelain in a PFM to loading that produces large stress changes. If the occlusion is not adjusted properly on a porcelain surface, contact points rather than contact areas will greatly increase the localized stresses in the porcelain surface as well as within the internal surface of the crown.

FACTORS AFFECTING THE COLOR OF CERAMICS

The principal reason for the choice of porcelain as a restorative material is its aesthetic qualities in matching the adjacent tooth structure in translucence, color, and chroma. Color phenomena and terminology are discussed in Chapter 3. Perfect color matching is extremely difficult, if not impossible. The structure of the tooth influences its color. Dentin is more opaque than enamel and reflects light. Enamel is a crystalline layer over the dentin and is composed of tiny prisms or rods cemented together by an organic substance. The indices of refraction of the rods and the cementing substance are different. As a result, a light ray is scattered by reflection and refraction to produce a translucent effect and a sensation of depth as the scattered light ray reaches the eye. As the light ray strikes the tooth surface, part of it is reflected, and the remainder penetrates the enamel and is scattered. Any light reaching the dentin is either absorbed or reflected to be again scattered within the enamel. If dentin is not present, as in the tip of an incisor, some of the light ray may be transmitted and absorbed in the oral cavity. As a result, this area may appear to be more translucent than that toward the gingival area. Thus, because the law of energy conservation must apply, the following relationship shows the four energy components that are derived from the energy (E) of the incident light:

$$E_{incident} = E_{scattered} + E_{reflected} + E_{absorbed} + E_{transmitted} + E_{fluoresced}$$

Although some of the absorbed light may be converted into heat, some may be transmitted back to the eye as fluorescent energy. When the ultraviolet rays of daylight or of nightclub lighting contact teeth or restorations, some of the radiant energy is converted into light of one or more colors, for example, red, orange, and yellow.

Light rays can also be dispersed, giving a color or shade that varies in different teeth. The dispersion can vary with the wavelength of the light. Therefore, the appearance of the teeth may vary according to whether they are viewed in direct sunlight, reflected daylight, tungsten light, or fluorescent light. This phenomenon is called *metamerism.* It is impossible to imitate such an optical system perfectly. The dentist and/or laboratory technician can, however, reproduce the aesthetic characteristics sufficiently such that the difference is conspicuous only to the trained eye.

Dental porcelains are pigmented by the inclusion of oxides to provide desired shades, as discussed earlier. Specimens of each shade (collectively called a *shade guide,* as shown in Chapter 3) are provided for the dentist, who, in turn, attempts to match the tooth color as nearly as possible. Shade guides made of solid porcelain are used most often by dentists to describe a desired appearance of a natural tooth or ceramic prosthesis. However, there are several deficiencies of shade guides. Shade guide tabs are much thicker than the thickness of ceramic that is used for dental crowns or veneers, and they are more translucent than teeth and ceramic crowns that are backed by a nontranslucent dentin substructure. Much of the incident light is transmitted through a tab. In contrast, most of the incident light on a crown is reflected back except at the incisal edge and at incisoproximal areas. Furthermore, the necks of shade tabs are made from a deeper hue, that is, higher chroma, and this region tends to distract the observer's matching ability of the observer of the gingival third of the tab. To avoid this situation, some clinicians grind away the neck area of a set of shade tabs (see Fig. 3–7).

The production of color sensation with a pigment is a physically different phenomenon from that obtained by optical reflection, refraction, and dispersion. The color of a pigment is determined by selective absorption and selective reflection. For example, if white light is reflected from a red surface, all the light with a wavelength different from that of red is absorbed and only the red light is reflected. It follows, then, that if a red hue is present in a PJC, but the red wavelength is not present in the light beam, the tooth will appear as a different shade. If the tooth or restoration surface is rough, most of the light will be scattered and little will penetrate the structure. In some instances, almost no color can be seen.

Shade Matching Guidelines. The selection of tooth or restoration shades should be done at the start of a clinical session before the operator's eyes become fatigued. Have the patient remove all lipstick, heavy make-up, or large jewelry that may influence color perception. Pumice the teeth involved if extrinsic stains are present. Do not use the operatory light for shade selection. Use cool, color-corrected fluorescent lighting or sunlight near a window. To avoid confusion, use an orderly method of shade selection. If your eyes seem fatigued to yellow, look at a blue napkin or blue wall to desensitize your eyes. Avoid metamerism (differences in color when viewed under various light sources) by viewing the restoration under a second light source—outside in natural light or in incandescent light. Since an exact match is not always possible, select a shade slightly lower in value (darker) than the tooth being matched. A slightly darker shade is less conspicuous than a lighter shade.

Try to select the basic hue of the tooth by matching the shade of the patient's canine, usually the most highly chromatic tooth in the mouth. With the correct hue group selected, work within that group on the shade guide to obtain the proper match. Although metallic oxides are fairly heat stable, some color change occurs on firing. The opaque white loses chroma fairly consistently after firing.

Ideally, the dentist should match the color of teeth with the shade guide under the illumination of northern light from a blue sky, because this light usually contains the most uniform balance of light wavelengths. If the sky is cloudy, the shade may appear to be grayer than if the surface reflected incident sunlight. If the light is reflected from a red brick wall, for example, the shade takes on a pink hue. Thus, if possible, the color matching should be done under two or more different light sources. One source should be northern exposure daylight, and the shade matching would best be done during the middle portion of a day that is slightly overcast, if possible. Porcelain restorations exhibit their best aesthetic qualities in an illumination of the same wavelength as that employed for the original color matching if the technician uses the same lighting conditions during fabrication.

Another factor that is important to the aesthetic qualities is the cementing medium. For example, an opaque material, such as zinc phosphate cement, can change the shade of a translucent crown because of its light absorption and its color. Thus, the more translucent silicophosphate and, more recently, glass ionomer cements are preferred for such restorations. Many cements designed for the cementation of all-ceramic crowns are specifically tinted to aid in achieving a proper color match with the adjacent tooth, and some types of restorations actually depend on the cement to provide a portion of the color for the crown.

METAL-CERAMIC RESTORATIONS

Porcelain Condensation. Porcelain for PJCs and metal-ceramic restorations, as well as for other applications, is supplied as a fine powder that is designed to be mixed with water or another vehicle and condensed into the desired form. The powder particles are of a particular size distribution to produce the most densely packed porcelain when they are properly condensed. If the particles were of the same size, the density of packing would not be nearly as high. Proper and thorough condensation is also crucial in obtaining dense packing of the powder particles. Dense packing of the powder particles provides two benefits: lower firing shrinkage and less porosity in the fired porcelain. This packing, or *condensation*, may be achieved by various methods, including the vibration, spatulation, and brush techniques.

The first method uses mild vibration to pack the wet powder densely on the underlying framework. The excess water is blotted away with a clean tissue, and condensation occurs toward the blotted area. In the second method, a small spatula is used to apply and smooth the wet porcelain. The smoothing action brings the excess water to the surface, where it is removed. The third method employs the addition of dry porcelain powder to the surface to absorb the water. The dry powder is placed by a brush to the side opposite from an increment of wet porcelain. As the water is drawn toward the dry powder, the wet particles are pulled together. Whichever method is used, it is important to remember that the surface tension of the water is the driving force in condensation and that the porcelain must never be allowed to dry out until condensation is complete.

Firing Procedure. The thermochemical reactions between the porcelain powder components are virtually completed during the original manufacturing process. Therefore, the purpose of firing is simply to sinter the particles of powder together properly to form the restoration. Some chemical reactions do occur during prolonged firing times or multiple firings. Of particular importance are the observed changes in the leucite content of the porcelains designed for fabrication of metal-ceramic restorations. Leucite is a high-expansion (or high-contraction) crystal phase whose volume fraction in the glass matrix can greatly affect the thermal contraction coefficient of the porcelain. Changes in the leucite content can cause the development of a thermal contraction coefficient mismatch between the porcelain and the metal and thus can produce stresses during cooling that are sufficient to cause crack formation in the porcelain.

The condensed porcelain mass is placed in front of or below the muffle of a preheated furnace (approximately 650° C [1200° F] for low-fusing porcelain). This preheating procedure permits the remaining water vapor to dissipate. Placement of the condensed mass directly into even a moderately warm furnace results in a rapid production of steam, thereby introducing voids or fracturing large sections of the veneer. After preheating for approximately 5 minutes, the porcelain is placed into the furnace, and the firing cycle is initiated.

The size of the powder particles influences not only the degree of condensation of the porcelain but also the soundness or apparent density of the final product. At the initial firing temperature, the voids are occupied by the atmosphere of the furnace. As sintering of the particles begins, the porcelain particles bond at their points of contact. As the temperature is raised, the sintered glass gradually flows to fill up the air spaces. However, air becomes trapped in the form of voids because the fused mass is too viscous to allow all the air to escape. An aid in the reduction of porosity in dental porcelain is *vacuum firing*.

Vacuum firing reduces porosity in the following way. When the porcelain is placed into the furnace, the powder particles are packed together with air channels around them. As the air pressure inside the furnace muffle is reduced to about one tenth of atmospheric pressure by the vacuum pump, the air around the particles is also reduced to this pressure. As the temperature rises, the particles sinter together, and closed voids are formed within the porcelain mass. The air inside these closed voids is isolated from the furnace atmosphere. At a temperature about 55° C (99° F) below the upper firing temperature, the vacuum is released and the pressure inside the furnace increases by a factor of 10, from 0.1 to 1 atm. Because the pressure is increased by a factor of 10, the voids are compressed to one tenth of their original size, and the total volume of porosity is accordingly reduced. The reduction in number and size of the air voids by vacuum firing is shown in Figure 26–3. Not all the air can be evacuated from the furnace. Therefore, a few bubbles are present in Figure 26–3*B*, but they are markedly smaller than the ones obtained with the usual air-firing method shown in Figure 26–3*A*.

Add-on Glazing and Shading Materials. Porcelains for PFMs, PJCs, porcelain veneers, or even denture teeth may be characterized with stains and glazes to provide a more lifelike appearance. As previously described, the fusing temperatures of glazes are reduced by the addition of glass modifiers that lower the

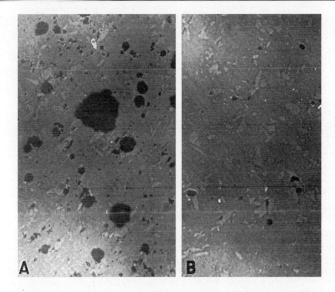

Figure 26–3. A, Air-fired porcelain. B, Vacuum-fired porcelain. (From Vine RF, and Semmelman JO: Densification of dental procelain. J Dent Res 36:950, 1957.)

chemical durability of glazes somewhat. Stains are simply tinted glazes and are therefore subject to the same chemical durability problems. However, most of the currently available glazes have adequate durability if they are as thick as 50 μm or more.

One method for ensuring that the applied characterizing stains will be permanent is to use them internally. *Internal staining* and characterization can produce a lifelike result, particularly when simulated enamel craze lines and other features are built into the porcelain rather than merely applied to the surface. The disadvantage of internal staining and characterization is that the porcelain must be stripped completely if the color or characterization is unsuitable.

As shown in Table 26–2, autoglazed feldspathic porcelain is much stronger than unglazed porcelain, particularly if the surface is rough. As previously stated, the glaze is effective in reducing crack propagation. If the glaze is removed by grinding, the transverse strength may be only half that of the sample with the glaze layer intact. However, the results of recent studies indicate that porcelains with highly polished surfaces have strength values comparable to those of specimens that were polished and glazed. This observation is of clinical importance. After the porcelain restoration is cemented in the mouth, it is common practice for the dentist to adjust the occlusion by grinding the surface

TABLE 26–2. Modulus of Rupture of Various Dental Porcelains

Classification	Firing Atmosphere	Surface Condition	Modulus of Rupture	
			MPa	*psi*
Porcelain*	Air	Ground	75.8	11,000
		Glazed	141.1	20,465
	Vacuum	Ground	79.6	11,547
		Glazed	132.3	19,187
Aluminous porcelain	Air	Ground	135.9	19,709
		Glazed	138.9	20,142
Fused alumina			519.3	75,310

*Feldspathic porcelains. The air-fired and vacuum-fired porcelains are of the medium-fusing variety.
Adapted from McLean JW, and Hughes TH: The reinforcement of dental porcelain with ceramic oxides. Br Dent J 119:251, 1965.

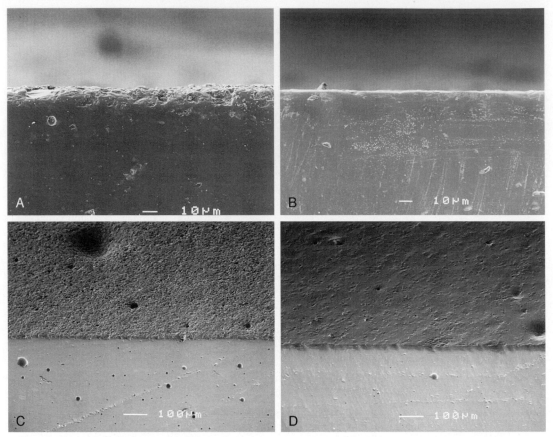

Figure 26–4. Scanning electron microscopic image of body (gingival) porcelain prepared by abrasive blasting with 50 μm of alumina abrasive for 30 seconds (*A,* side view; *C,* oblique view) followed by self-glazing *(B and D).*

of the porcelain with a diamond bur. It is unfortunate that this procedure weakens the porcelain markedly if the glaze is removed and the surface is left in a rough condition. For this condition, the best solution is to polish the surface with Sof-Lex (3M, Minneapolis, MN) finishing disks, a Shofu (Shofu, Kyoto, Japan) porcelain laminate polishing kit, or other abrasive system. A smoother surface also reduces the abrasion damage caused to opposing teeth or restorations.

It is widely believed that glazing of feldspathic porcelain eliminates all flaws from the surface. However, an optimum method of producing the smoothest surface in the shortest time has not been established. It is logical to assume that fine polishing of a roughened surface followed by glazing produces smoother surfaces than polishing alone, sandblasting followed by glazing, or diamond grinding followed by glazing. Shown in Figure 26–4 are scanning electron microscopic (SEM) images of body (gingival) porcelain prepared by abrasive blasting with 50 μm alumina abrasive for 30 seconds (*A,* side view and *C,* oblique view) followed by self-glazing *(B and D).* Similar views are shown after roughening the surface with a coarse "Two-Striper" diamond *(E and G)* followed by self-glazing for 30 seconds *(F and H).* A highly polished surface (0.05 μm) is also shown after polishing *(I)* and after self-glazing for 30 seconds *(J).* Note that the highly polished and glazed surface *(J)* is smoother than the surfaces of glazed specimens that had been sandblasted *(D)* or roughened with a diamond followed by glazing *(H).*

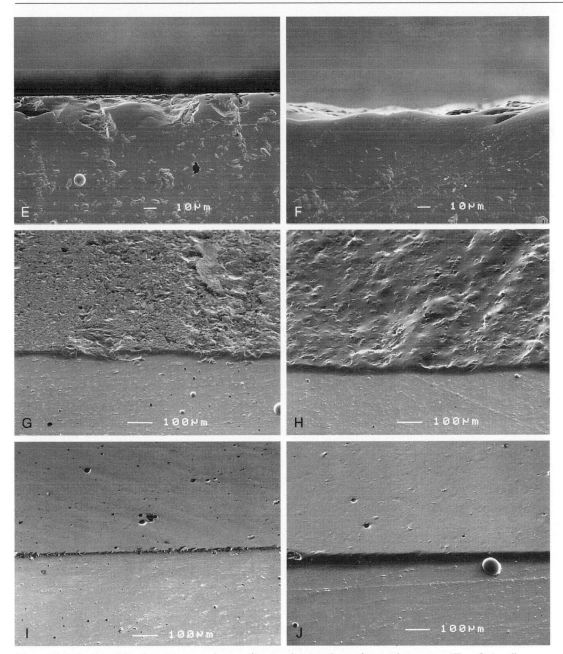

Figure 26–4 Continued Similar views are shown after roughening the surface with a coarse "Two-Striper" diamond *(E and G)* followed by self-glazing for 30 seconds *(F and H)*. A highly polished surface (0.05 μm) is also shown after polishing *(I)* and after self-glazing for 30 seconds *(J)*. Note that the highly polished and glazed surface *(J)* is smoother than the glazed specimens that had been sandblasted *(D)* or roughened with a diamond *(H)* before glazing.

Cooling. The proper cooling of a porcelain restoration from its firing temperature to room temperature is the subject of considerable controversy. The catastrophic fracture of glass that has been subjected to sudden changes in temperature is a sufficiently familiar experience that most clinicians are cautious about exposing dental porcelain to rapid cooling after firing. The cooling of dental porcelain, however, is a complex matter, particularly when the porcelain is fused to a metallic substrate. Multiple firings of a metal-ceramic restoration can cause the coefficient of thermal contraction of the porcelain to increase and can actually make it *more* likely to crack or craze because of tensile stress development.

The chief limitation to the use of an all-porcelain crown in fixed prosthodontics is its lack of tensile and shear strength. A method for minimizing this disadvantage is to fuse the porcelain directly to a metal coping that fits the prepared tooth. Such a metal-ceramic restoration is shown schematically in Figure 26–5. The metal on the facial side is approximately 0.3- to 0.5-mm thick. It is veneered with opaque porcelain approximately 0.3 mm in thickness. The body porcelain is about 1-mm thick.

If a stronger material is used as an inner core of a PJC, then cracks can develop only when the stronger material is deformed or broken, assuming that the porcelain is firmly bonded to the reinforcing substrate. With proper design and physical properties of the porcelain and metal, the porcelain is reinforced so that brittle fracture can be avoided or at least minimized when these crowns are restricted to anterior teeth. Although most metal-ceramic restorations involve cast metal copings, several novel noncast approaches (sintering, machining, swaging, and burnishing) to coping fabrication have been developed in recent years.

Cast Coping. The development of the metal-ceramic restoration was the result of advances in the formulation of both alloys and porcelains. To bond to alloys suitable for the copings, porcelains must be sufficiently low fusing and they also must have a coefficient of thermal contraction that is closely matched to that of the alloys.

The gold alloys developed for porcelain bonding have higher melting ranges than typical Type III gold alloys; the higher melting ranges are necessary to prevent sag, creep, or melting of the coping during porcelain firing. These gold alloys contain small amounts (about 1%) of base metals such as iron, indium, and tin, as discussed in Chapter 20. The base metals form a surface oxide layer during the "degassing" treatment, and this surface oxide is responsible for development of a bond with porcelain. This porcelain-metal bond is primarily chemical in nature and is capable of forming even when the metal surface is smooth and little opportunity exists for mechanical interlocking.

The alloys and porcelains used for the construction of such restorations have a number of rather stringent requirements. For example, both the metal and the

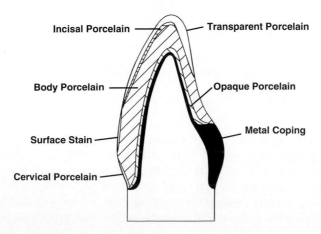

Figure 26–5. Porcelains used in the construction of a metal-ceramic crown.

ceramic must have coefficients of thermal contraction that are closely matched such that the metal has a slightly higher value, if undesirable residual tensile stresses in the porcelain are to be avoided. If the contraction coefficients are not nearly equal, stresses may occur that weaken both the porcelain and the bond. For example, a difference in the coefficients of thermal contraction of $1.7 \times 10^{-6}/° C$ can produce a shear stress of 280 MPa (39,800 psi) in porcelain next to the gold-porcelain interface when the porcelain is cooled from 954° C (1750° F) to room temperature. Because the shear resistance to failure is far less than 280 MPa, these thermal stresses would cause spontaneous bond failure.

High tensile stresses would also develop from a contraction coefficient mismatch between alloy and porcelain. The tensile stresses induced within the restoration by occlusal forces would, of course, be added to residual thermal tensile stresses. However, for metal-porcelain systems that have an average contraction coefficient difference of $0.5 \times 10^{-6}/° C$ or less (between 600° C and room temperature), fracture is unlikely to occur except in cases of extreme stress concentration or extremely high intraoral forces. These are known as *thermally compatible systems*. However, many restorations made from metal and porcelain combinations having contraction coefficient differences between 0.5 and $1.0 \times 10^{-6}/° C$ are known to survive for many years. These results are explainable by survival probability analyses that assume that the maximum biting forces on anterior crowns rarely exceed 890 N (200 lb) and the maximum force on posterior crowns rarely exceed 2224 N (500 lb). In fact, the *Guinness Book of Records (1993)* cites the maximum clenching force ever recorded for posterior teeth as 4337 N (975 lb) sustained for 2 seconds. The second highest bite force ever recorded was 2447 N (550 lb). Most patients generate typical bite forces of 400 to 800 N (90 to 180 lb) between molar teeth and much lower forces between premolars and between anterior teeth. Thus, there exists a rather small number of patients with bite force capabilities that are likely to cause fracture of metal-ceramic crowns or bridges even when residual thermal incompatibility stresses are present. As a general rule, lower forces are generated by younger children versus older children, female patients versus male patients, a more closed bite versus a raised bite table, occlusion between natural teeth and a denture versus natural teeth and natural teeth, and between quadrants containing a fixed partial denture versus between those with only natural teeth.

Another equally important property of metal-ceramic systems is that the alloy should have a high proportional limit and, particularly, a high modulus of elasticity. Alloys with a high modulus of elasticity also share a greater proportion of stress compared with the adjacent porcelain. The metal framework must not melt during porcelain firing and also must resist high-temperature "sag" deformation. Sag or flexural creep can occur only at high temperatures. It does not occur at oral temperatures.

Composition of Metal-Ceramic Alloys and Ceramics. The composition of the noble and base metal alloys used in metal-ceramic restorations was discussed in Chapter 20. The reader is referred to that description of these systems and of the effects and purposes of the constituent metals.

The composition of the ceramic generally corresponds to that of the glasses in Table 26–1, except for an increased alkali content. The addition of greater quantities of soda, potash, and/or leucite is necessary to increase the thermal expansion to a level compatible with the metal coping. The opaque porcelains also contain relatively large amounts of metallic oxide opacifiers to conceal the underlying metal and to minimize the thickness of the opaque layer.

Those high-contraction porcelains have a greater tendency to devitrify because of their alkali content. They should not be subjected to repeated firing, because this increases the risk of cloudiness within the porcelain, as well as changes in the thermal contraction. Thus, it is obvious that a proper matching of the properties of the alloy and porcelain is imperative to success. Criteria and test methods for determining that compatibility have been suggested. These criteria include measurements of the compatibility of coefficients of thermal contraction, thermal conductivity (to determine resistance to thermal shock), and the nature and strength of the bond, which are discussed later.

Technical Aspects of Metal-Ceramic Restorations. This type of restoration is generally fabricated by a dental technician. The casting procedures are similar to those described for the casting of inlays and crowns. Because of the high melting temperature of the alloys, gypsum-bonded investments cannot be used and a phosphate-bonded investment must be used.

The casting should be carefully cleaned to ensure a strong bond to the porcelain. For example, an alloy such as Olympia (J. F. Jelenko & Company, Armonk, NY), a gold-palladium, silver-free alloy, is heated in the porcelain furnace to a temperature of 1038° C (1900° F) to burn off any remaining impurities and to form a thin oxide layer. In many alloy systems, this so-called degassing treatment does not actually degas the interior structure of the alloy, but it does produce an oxide layer on the alloy surface that is essential for the formation of the porcelain-metal bond.

The need for a clean metal surface cannot be overemphasized. Degassing is necessary for all gold-porcelain systems. The number of bubbles formed at the interface decreases as the time and temperature of degassing are increased. Oil from fingertips also can be a possible contaminant. The surface may be cleansed adequately by finishing with clean ceramic-bonded stones or sintered diamonds, which are used exclusively for finishing. Final sandblasting with high-purity alumina abrasive ensures that the porcelain is bonded to a clean and mechanically retentive surface.

Opaque porcelain is condensed with a thickness of approximately 0.3 mm and is then fired to its maturing temperature. Translucent porcelain is then applied, and the tooth form is built. Porcelain powder is applied by the condensation methods previously described. The unit is again fired. Several cycles of porcelain application and firing may be necessary to complete the restoration. A final glaze is then obtained.

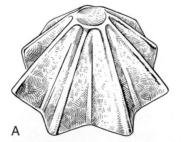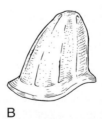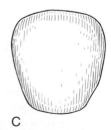

A   B   C

Figure 26–6. Renaissance laminated gold alloy foil *(A)* used to form a coping *(B)* before flame sintering and firing that is required to achieve bonding to porcelain and build-up of porcelain to form the final crown *(C)*.

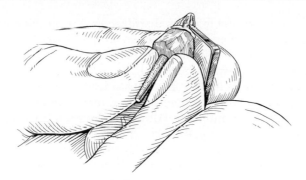

Figure 26–7. Burnishing the margin of a swaged gold alloy foil coping.

Creep or Sag. It is unfortunate that high-temperature *creep* or *sag* of some high noble and noble alloys occurs when the temperature approaches 980° C (1800° F). The creep can be reduced if the metal has the proper composition so that a dispersion strengthening effect occurs at the high temperature, as discussed in Chapter 20. When such a gold alloy is heated to 980° C, a second phase is precipitated that can harden or strengthen the alloy. Such creep has been reduced in some of the commercial alloys, but it apparently cannot be eliminated. The solidus temperature (the lower end of the melting range) of base metal alloys, such as nickel-chromium, is higher than that of gold alloys; hence, base metal alloys are less susceptible to sag than are gold-based alloys.

Metal-Ceramic Crowns Based on Swaged Foil Copings. Renaissance (Unikorn Ltd., Tel Aviv, Israel) and Captek are products designed to fabricate the metal coping of a metal-ceramic crown without the use of a melting and casting process. It is a laminated gold alloy foil that is delivered to the user in a fluted shape reminiscent of a miniature coffee filter (Fig. 26–6A). This pleated foil is swaged with a swaging instrument, burnished with a hand instrument on the die (Fig. 26–7), and then flame sintered (Fig. 26–8) to form a coping with moderate strength. An "interfacial alloy" powder is applied and fired, the coping is then veneered with condensed porcelain, and the porcelain is sintered at typical porcelain firing temperatures.

Bonding Porcelain to Metal. The primary requirement for the success of a metal-ceramic restoration is the development of a durable bond between the porcelain and the alloy. Once such a bond is achieved, there is an opportunity to introduce bending stresses in the biomaterial system during the porcelain

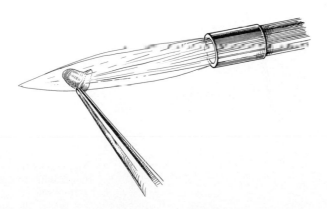

Figure 26–8. Flame sintering of a swaged foil coping.

firing procedures. An unfavorable stress distribution during the cooling process can result in cracking of the porcelain, and delayed fracture can also occur. Thus, for a successful metal-ceramic restoration to be realized, both a strong interface bond and thermal compatibility are required.

Theories of metal-ceramic bonding have historically fallen into two groups: (1) mechanical interlocking between porcelain and metal, and (2) chemical bonding across the metal-porcelain interface. Although chemical bonding is generally regarded to be responsible for metal-porcelain adherence, evidence exists that, for a few systems, mechanical interlocking may provide the principal bond. The oxidation behavior of these alloys largely determines their potential for bonding with porcelain. Research into the nature of metal-porcelain adherence has indicated that those alloys that form adherent oxides during the degassing cycle also form a good bond to porcelain, whereas those alloys with poorly adherent oxides form poor bonds. Some palladium-silver alloys form no external oxide at all but rather oxidize internally. It is for these alloys that mechanical bonding is needed.

A variety of tests have been advocated for measuring the bond strength. None can be regarded as an exact measure of the adhesion of porcelain to metal except in cases in which the metal-porcelain couple is matched thermally so that porcelain adjacent to the interface is essentially stress free. This is a situation virtually impossible to attain because the metal exhibits a linear contraction behavior as a function of temperature and the porcelain exhibits a curved contraction plot.

Clinical fractures of metal-ceramic restorations, although rare, still occur, especially when a new alloy or porcelain is being used or when a new coping technology has been adopted. As is generally true for all dental materials, there is a *learning curve* associated with the initial use of new products. When fractures occur, it is a good idea to make a vinyl polysiloxane impression of the fracture site for future fractographic analysis. All information on the crown or bridge should be recorded, including the visual appearance of the fracture site. Although there are an infinite number of fracture paths that may occur, three types are of particular importance in diagnosing the cause of fracture. Shown in Figure 26–9 are fracture paths that have occurred primarily at three sites: (1) along the interfacial region between opaque porcelain (P) and the interaction zone (I) between porcelain and the metal substrate *(top)*; (2) within the interaction zone *(center)*; and (3) between the metal and the interaction zone *(bottom)*. For conventional metal-ceramic crowns made from cast copings, the interaction zone is

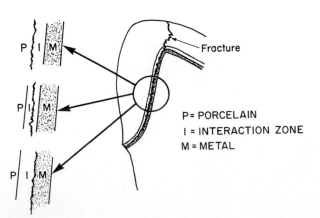

Figure 26–9. Types of interfacial bond failures in metal-ceramic restorations.

usually synonymous with the metal oxide layer. For copings made using atypical methods such as the technologies associated with the Captek system, the Renaissance system, the Ceplatec system (Ceplatec, Krefeld, Germany), and electroforming processes, bonding to porcelain is achieved though the formation of an intermediate layer of material such as the Capbond metal-ceramic "bonder" (bonding agent) for the Captek foil crown system or some other bonding agent. To characterize the principal site of fracture, magnification of 3 to 100 times is required because a thin layer of retained porcelain may not be visible without magnification. Each of the three principal fracture paths in Figure 26–9 is indicative of excessive stress development, a material deficiency, or a processing deficiency.

Bonding of Porcelain to Metal Using Electrodeposition. Ceramic bonding to metals in certain cases requires the electrodeposition of metal coatings and heating to form suitable metal oxides. Deposition of a layer of pure gold onto the cast metal, followed by a short "flashing" deposition of tin, has been shown to improve the wetting of porcelain onto the metal and to reduce the amount of porosity at the metal-porcelain interface. In addition, the electrodeposited layer acts as a barrier between the metal casting and the porcelain to inhibit diffusion of atoms from the metal into the porcelain, within the normal limits of porcelain firing cycles.

The gold color of the oxide film enhances the vitality of the porcelain when compared with the normal dark oxides that require heavy opaque layers. Because the activated surface can be controlled from golden, reddish-brown to gray, an additional dimension is available for color control of the porcelain.

Alloys and metals such as cobalt-chromium, stainless steel, palladium-silver, high- and low-gold-content alloys, and titanium all have been successfully electroplated and tin coated to achieve satisfactory ceramic bonding. Various proprietary agents are also available that are intended for application to the metal surface before condensation of the opaque porcelain layer. These are applied as a thin liquid to the metal surface and are fired in a manner similar to that of the opaque porcelain.

The function of these agents is twofold: (1) they are intended to improve metal-ceramic bonding by limiting the build-up of an oxide layer on the base metal surface during firing, and (2) they can improve aesthetics by helping to block the color of the dark metal oxide.

Benefits and Drawbacks of Metal-Ceramics. The properly made crown is stronger and more durable than the ordinary PJC. However, a long-span bridge of this type may be subject to bending strains, and the porcelain may crack or fracture because of its low ductility. These difficulties can be partly overcome with proper restoration design, as discussed earlier. Proper occlusal relationships are also particularly important for this type of restoration.

The most outstanding advantages of metal-ceramic restorations are the permanent aesthetic quality of the properly designed reinforced ceramic unit and their resistance to fracture. Unlike similar acrylic resin veneered structures, there is almost no wear of the porcelain by abrasion or change in color because of microleakage between the veneer and the metal. Furthermore, as shown in one clinical study, the fracture rate of metal-ceramic crowns as well as bridges is as low as 2.3% after 7.5 years.

A slight advantage of PFM restorations over the all-ceramic restoration is that less tooth structure needs to be removed to provide the proper bulk for the crown, especially if metal only is used on occlusal and lingual surfaces. As previously noted, high rigidity of the structure is needed to prevent fracture of the porcelain. Although the modulus of elasticity of the porcelain is moderately high (e.g., 69 GPa compared with values of 99.3 GPa for a Type IV gold alloy, 22.4 GPa for amalgam, and 16.6 GPa for a resin-based composite), its low tensile and shear strengths indicate a low maximal flexibility because, in brittle fracture, the breaking strength and proportional limit coincide. As a result, only limited elastic deformation of the porcelain can be tolerated. It follows, therefore, that even with a high modulus of elasticity, considerable bulk of metal is also necessary to provide the proper rigidity. The shape of the crown cannot be conspicuously out of line with the anatomic form of adjacent teeth. Therefore, the bulk of the natural tooth may need to be sacrificed to provide adequate space to ensure adequate fracture resistance and aesthetics.

In spite of several disadvantages, the metal-ceramic restorations are the most widely used system in fixed prosthodontics today.

ALL-CERAMIC RESTORATIONS

Ceramic Jacket Crowns (CJCs). Based on a 1994 survey, metal-ceramic crowns and bridges were used for approximately 90% of all fixed restorations. However, recent developments in ceramic products with improved fracture resistance and excellent aesthetic capability have led to a slight increase in the use of all-ceramic products. PJCs have been in widespread use since the beginning of the twentieth century. The ceramics employed in the conventional PJC were high-fusing feldspathic porcelains. The relatively low strength of this type of porcelain prompted McLean and Hughes (1965) to develop an alumina-reinforced porcelain core material for the fabrication of PJCs.

The alumina-reinforced PJCs are generally regarded as providing slightly better aesthetics for anterior teeth than are the metal-ceramic crowns that employ a metal coping. However, the strength of the core porcelain used for PJCs is inadequate to warrant the use of these restorations for posterior teeth. Thus, the newer high-strength ceramics are preferred for the production of CJCs.

Bonded Platinum-Foil Coping. Another method of bonding porcelain to metal makes use of tin oxide coatings on platinum foil. The objective of this technique is to improve the aesthetics by a replacement of the thicker metal coping with a thin platinum foil, thus allowing more room for porcelain. The method consists of bonding aluminous porcelain to platinum foil copings. Attachment of the porcelain is secured by electroplating the platinum foil with a thin layer of tin and then oxidizing it in a furnace to provide a continuous film of tin oxide for porcelain bonding. The rationale is that the bonded foil would act as an inner skin on the fit surface to reduce subsurface porosity and formation of micro-cracks in the porcelain, thereby increasing the fracture resistance of the unit. The clinical performance of these crowns has been excellent for anterior teeth, but approximately 15% of these crowns fractured within 7 years after they were cemented to molar teeth with a glass ionomer cement.

Glass-Ceramic Crown. A *glass-ceramic* is a material that is formed into the desired shape as a glass, then subjected to a heat treatment to induce partial devitrification (*i.e.,* loss of glassy structure by crystallization of the glass). The crystalline particles, needles, or plates formed during this ceramming process serve to interrupt the propagation of cracks in the material when an intraoral force is applied, thereby causing increased strength and toughness. The use of glass-ceramics in dentistry was first proposed by MacCulloch in 1968. He used a continuous glass-molding process to produce denture teeth. He also suggested that it should be possible to fabricate crowns and inlays by centrifugal casting of molten glass.

The first commercially available castable ceramic material for dental use, Dicor, was developed by Corning Glass Works and marketed by Dentsply International. Dicor is a castable glass that is formed into an inlay, facial veneer, or full-crown restoration by a lost-wax casting process similar to that employed for metals. After the glass casting core or coping is recovered, the glass is sandblasted to remove residual casting investment and the sprues are gently cut away. The glass is then covered by a protective "embedment" material and subjected to a heat treatment that causes microscopic platelike crystals of crystalline material (mica) to grow within the glass matrix. This crystal nucleation and crystal growth process is called *ceramming*. Once the glass has been cerammed, it is fit on the prepared dies, ground as necessary, and then it is coated with veneering porcelain (as shown in Fig. 26–10) to match the shape and appearance of adjacent teeth. Dicor glass-ceramic is capable of producing surprisingly good aesthetics, perhaps because of the "chameleon" effect, where part of the color of the restoration is picked up from the adjacent teeth as well as from the tinted cements used for luting the restorations.

When used for posterior crowns, ceramic crowns are most susceptible to fracture. Shown in Figure 26–11 (see also the color section in the front of the book) is the stress distribution computed by finite element analysis in a 0.5-mm-thick molar Dicor crown loaded on the occlusal surface, just within the marginal ridge area. The maximum tensile stress (73 MPa) is located within the internal surface directly below the point of applied force and just above the 50-μm-thick layer of resin cement (see the arrow in Fig. 26–11). An SEM image of a fractured clinical crown of Dicor glass-ceramic is shown in Figure 26–12. Note the site of crack initiation indicated by the arrow. This site represents the critical flaw responsible for crack initiation under an applied intraoral force. The location of initial crack formation consistent with the location of maximum tensile stress predicted by the finite element calculations is shown in Figure 26–11.

Leucite-reinforced Porcelain (Optec HSP). Optec HSP (Jeneric/Pentron) is a leucite-reinforced feldspathic porcelain that is condensed and sintered like aluminous porcelain and traditional feldspathic porcelain. Its advantages and

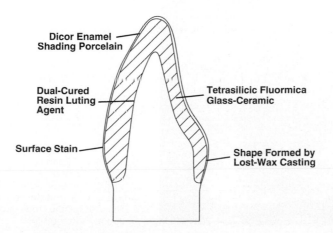

Figure 26–10. Typical materials used in the construction of a Dicor glass-ceramic crown.

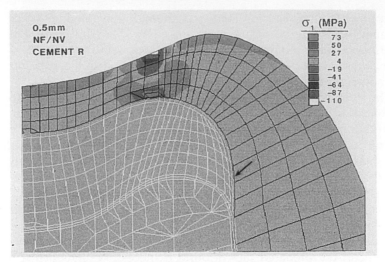

Figure 26–11. Stress distribution computed by finite element analysis in a 0.5-mm-thick molar Dicor glass-ceramic crown loaded on the occlusal surface, just within the marginal ridge area. The maximum tensile stress of 73 MPa is located directly below the point of applied force along the internal surface of the crown adjacent to the 50-μm-thick layer of resin luting agent *(arrow)*. (See also color section.)

disadvantages are summarized below. Because it has only a moderately opaque core compared with a metal or aluminous porcelain core, it is more translucent than alumina core crowns or glass-infiltrated alumina core crowns. To differentiate among these ceramic materials, refer to the classification in Figure 26–1. Because it is a feldspathic porcelain that is reinforced with leucite crystals, the strength of Optec HSP is higher than that of feldspathic porcelains made for PFM applications. Its advantages are the lack of a metal or opaque substructure, good translucency, moderate flexural strength, and its ability to be used without special laboratory equipment. Its disadvantages are potential marginal inaccuracy caused by porcelain sintering shrinkage and its potential to fracture in posterior teeth. Leucite-reinforced porcelain that is condensed and sintered shrinks when fired because of the volumetric decrease caused by sintering, and

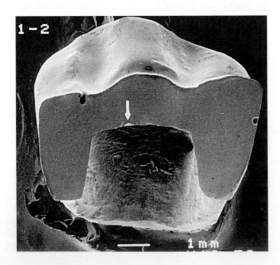

Figure 26–12. Scanning electron microscopic image of fractured clinical Dicor glass-ceramic crown. The *arrow* indicates the site of the critical flaw responsible for the crack initiation under an applied intraoral load.

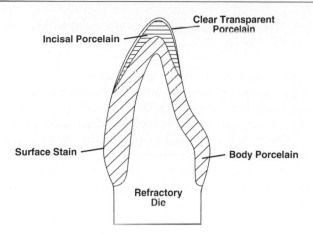

Figure 26-13. Schematic illustration of an Optec HSP crown.

the fit of crowns made from this ceramic is not as good as that of PFM crowns with metal margins.

Optec HSP contains a higher concentration of leucite crystals compared with the feldspathic porcelain used for PFM restorations. Only body and incisal porcelain are used because the opacity provided by the leucite crystals does not require the use of a core porcelain. Sandblasting is generally recommended to achieve bonding with resin cement. Reinforced porcelain of this type is recommended for inlays, onlays, low-stress crowns, and veneers. Shown in Figure 26–13 is a schematic illustration of an Optec HSP crown.

Injection-molded Glass-Ceramic (IPS Empress). IPS Empress is a precerammed glass-ceramic that is heated in a cylinder form and injected under pressure and high temperature into a mold. Like Optec HSP, it contains a higher concentration of leucite crystals that increase the resistance to crack propagation (fracture). The material is injection molded over a 45-minute period at a high temperature to produce the ceramic substructure. This crown form can be either stained and glazed or built up using a conventional layering technique. A schematic illustration of an IPS Empress crown is shown in Figure 26–14.

The advantages of this ceramic are its lack of metal or an opaque ceramic core, moderate flexural strength (similar to that of Optec HSP), excellent fit, and

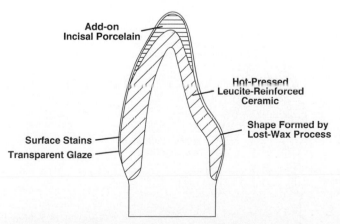

Figure 26–14. Schematic illustration of an IPS Empress crown.

excellent aesthetics. The disadvantages are its potential to fracture in posterior areas and the need for special laboratory equipment.

Glass-infiltrated Alumina Core Ceramic (In-Ceram). In-Ceram is a ceramic for single anterior and posterior crowns and anterior three-unit bridges. The slightly sintered aluminous porcelain core is infiltrated with glass at 1100° C for 4 hours to eliminate porosity and to strengthen the slip-cast core (see subsequent procedural steps). The initial sintering process for the alumina core produces a minimal volume decrease because the temperature and time are sufficient only to cause bonding between particles at small areas. Thus, the marginal adaptation and fit of this core material should be excellent because little shrinkage occurs. The flexural strength of this core material is about 450 MPa compared with strengths of 100 to 150 MPa for Dicor, Optec HSP, and IPS Empress. Despite its high strength, failures can still occur in single crowns as well as fixed partial dentures. Although its primary indication is for anterior and posterior crowns, the manufacturer's recommendations include its use for anterior three-unit bridges. As suggested in Chapter 4, it is essential that the area at the tissue side of embrasure spaces of all-ceramic bridges be thick and that it be designed with a large radius of curvature to minimize the stress-raiser effect in areas of moderate to high tensile stress.

Before In-Ceram was introduced, aluminous porcelain had not been used successfully to produce fixed partial dentures because of its low flexural strength and high sintering shrinkage. Thus, the principal indications for the use of aluminous PJCs are (1) for the restoration of maxillary anterior crowns when aesthetics is critically important; (2) for patients with allergies to metals; and (3) when aesthetics of PFMs would not be acceptable.

The advantages of the glass-infiltrated core material are its lack of metal, its very high flexural strength, and its excellent fit. The disadvantages include the opacity of the core, the unsuitability for conventional acid etching, and the need for specialized equipment. A schematic drawing of an In-Ceram crown is shown in Figure 26–15.

The steps for fabricating an In-Ceram prosthesis are as follows:

1. Prepare teeth with heavy circumferential chamfer (>1 mm).

2. Make the impression and pour two dies or duplicate one die in refractory die material.

3. Apply Al_2O_3 on duplicate die using the slip-cast method. This involves the

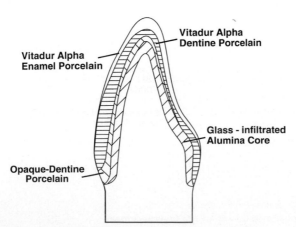

Vitadur Alpha Dentine Porcelain

Vitadur Alpha Enamel Porcelain

Glass - infiltrated Alumina Core

Opaque-Dentine Porcelain

Figure 26–15. Schematic illustration of an In-Ceram crown.

placement of a low-viscosity slurry of the powder onto a porous refractory die that draws water from the slurry, thus depositing a layer of solid Al_2O_3 on the die. The capillary action of the die continues as other layers are added. Heat the die and material at 120° C for 2 hours to dry the Al_2O_3.

4. Sinter coping for 10 hours at 1100° C.

5. Apply slurry of glass infiltration material.

6. Fire for 3 to 5 hours at 1120° C to allow infiltration of glass.

7. Trim excess glass from coping with diamond burs.

8. Build up the core with dentin and enamel porcelain (Vitadur Alpha).

9. Fire in the oven, grind in anatomy and occlusion, finish, and glaze before delivery.

A more translucent ceramic called *In-Ceram Spinell* has been introduced as an alternative to In-Ceram. This ceramic has a lower flexural strength, but its increased translucency provides improved aesthetics in clinical situations in which the adjacent teeth or restorations are quite translucent. The core of In-Ceram Spinell is $MgAl_2O_4$ infiltrated with glass, and it is fabricated similarly to In-Ceram.

Ceramic Veneers, Inlays, and Onlays. The success rate of etched and bonded porcelain veneers has been well established since acid etching of porcelain was established in 1981. Data accumulated for 5 years indicate success rates as high as 100%. Ceramic veneers represent a more conservative approach than the use of full crowns. The control of aesthetics is technique sensitive because the conventional acid-base cements or resin-based luting cements play a key role in the overall appearance. In addition, resin-bonded veneers and crowns that extend into the root area of patients with poor gingival health have occasionally been associated with recurrent caries caused by bacterial and nutrient penetration within the marginal gap.

The discovery that many dental porcelains and glass-ceramics can be etched with hydrofluoric acid or other acids to create retentive channels similar to those in acid-etched enamel has led to the development of resin-bonded, acid-etched ceramic restorations. Be extremely careful when handling hydrofluoric acid—even short-term contact can cause catastrophic injury to affected tissues. An emergency management plan for laboratories that use hydrofluoric acid should be established.

Ceramic veneers are used primarily for cosmetic improvement of stained or hypoplastic anterior teeth. Resin-bonded, acid-etched ceramic inlays and onlays are also being used as posterior restorations. A resin cement is used for bonding to the etched metal and enamel.

The long-term clinical performance of ceramic veneers and resin-bonded inlays and onlays has not been well documented, although initial short-term data appear promising. The aesthetics are excellent; however, the porcelain inlay or onlay is expensive as compared with amalgam, or even a composite restoration. Because ceramics abrade opposing teeth, the surface of the ceramic restorations should be polished after they are ground during occlusal adjustment.

CAD-CAM Ceramics. As shown in the ceramic classification chart in Figure 26–1, all-ceramic copings or cores can be produced by processes of condensation and sintering, casting and ceramming, injection molding and sintering, sintering and glass infiltration, and CAD-CAM processing. For the Cerec CAD-CAM system the internal surface of inlays, onlays, or crowns are ground with diamond disks or other instruments to the dimensions obtained from a scanned image of

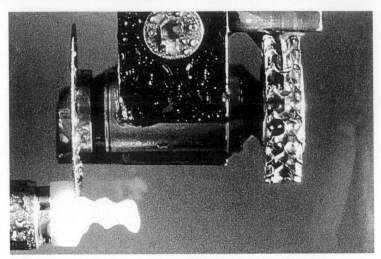

Figure 26–16. Milling operation on a CAD-CAM ceramic block by a diamond-coated disk within the Cerec CAM station.

the preparation. The external surface must be ground manually, although some recent CAD-CAM systems are capable of grinding the external surface as well.

Shown in Figure 26–16 is a milling operation within a Cerec CAD-CAM unit (Siemens Aktiengesellschaft, Bensheim, Germany). The ceramic block is being ground by a diamond-coated disk whose translational movements are guided by computer-controlled signals. A Cerec CAD-CAM ceramic block is shown in Figure 26–17 before milling, at an intermediate milling stage, and after completion of the milling operation for an inlay.

These ceramics are supplied as small blocks that can be ground into inlays and veneers in a computer-driven CAD-CAM system. Vitablocs MK II are feldspathic porcelains that are used in the same way as is Dicor MGC (machinable glass-ceramic). The disadvantages of CAD-CAM restorations include the need for costly equipment, the lack of computer-controlled processing support

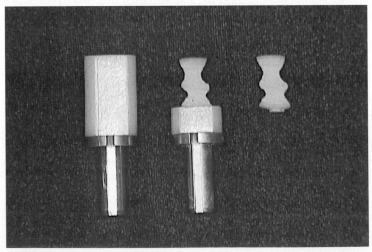

Figure 26–17. CAD-CAM ceramic block before milling *(left)*, at an intermediate stage of milling *(center)*, and after milling and removal of the inlay from the mounting stub *(right)*.

for occlusal adjustment, and the technique-sensitive nature of surface imaging that is required for the prepared teeth. Advantages include negligible porosity levels in the CAD-CAM core ceramics, the freedom from making an impression, reduced assistant time associated with impression procedures, the need for only a single appointment (with the Cerec system), and good patient acceptance.

Production of Alumina Core and Glass-infiltrated Alumina Core Ceramics Using Copy-milling Technology. Recently, a copy-milling technique has been introduced that is capable of milling porcelain, In-Ceram, and In-Ceram Spinell copings as well as In-Ceram substructures for fixed partial dentures. This technology is made possible by means of the Celay system (Mikrona Technologies, Spreitenbach, Switzerland). This system is based on a mechanical device that is used to trace the surface of a prefabricated pattern of the designed restoration made from a blue resin-based composite (Celay-Tech, ESPE, Seefeld-Oberbay, Germany). The resin pattern can be produced directly on prepared teeth or indirectly on dies made from impressions. As the tracing tool passes over the pattern, a milling machine duplicates these movements as it grinds a copy of the pattern from a block of alumina or other ceramic material. Currently, it is possible to machine Celay In-Ceram or In-Ceram Spinell material and then infiltrate the pattern with a sodium-lanthanum glass in a manner similar to that used for conventional In-Ceram crown cores or bridge frameworks. Both types of glass-infiltrated alumina are veneered with Vitadur Alpha porcelain. No long-term clinical data are yet available for Celay restorations.

Porcelain Denture Teeth. The manufacture of denture teeth constitutes virtually the sole current use for high-fusing or medium-fusing dental porcelains. Denture teeth are made by packing two or more porcelains of differing translucencies for each tooth into metal molds. They are fired on large trays in high-temperature ovens. Porcelain teeth are designed to be retained on the denture base by mechanical interlocking. The anterior teeth are made with projecting metal pins that become surrounded with the denture base resin during processing, whereas the posterior teeth are molded with diatoric spaces into which the denture base resin may flow.

Either porcelain denture teeth or acrylic resin denture teeth can be employed in the fabrication of complete and partial dentures. Porcelain teeth are generally considered to be more aesthetic than acrylic teeth. They are also much more resistant to wear, although the development of new polymers has improved the wear resistance of acrylic teeth. Porcelain teeth also have the advantage of being the only type of denture teeth that allow the denture to be rebased (replacement of all the acrylic denture base).

The disadvantages of porcelain teeth are their brittleness and the clicking sound produced on contact with the opposing teeth. Porcelain teeth also require a greater interridge distance because they cannot be ground as thin in the ridge lap area as acrylic teeth without destroying the diatoric channels that provide their only means of retention to the denture base.

CHEMICAL ATTACK OF DENTAL CERAMICS BY ACIDULATED PHOSPHATE FLUORIDE

Topical fluorides are routinely used for caries control. The effect of such agents on the surface of ceramic restorations has been studied. Acidulated phosphate

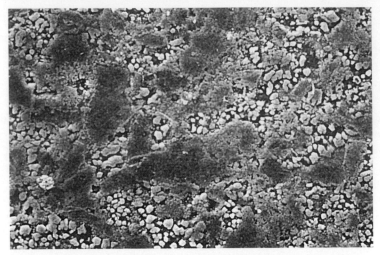

Figure 26–18. Surface of feldspathic gingival (body) porcelain after a 30-minute exposure to 1.23% acidulated phosphate fluoride.

fluoride (APF), one of the most commonly used fluoride gels, is known to etch glass, probably by selective leaching of sodium ions, thereby disrupting the silica network. When glazed feldspathic porcelain is contacted by 1.23% APF or by 8% stannous fluoride, a surface roughness is produced within 4 minutes. As can be seen in Figure 26–18, a 30-minute exposure to 1.23% APF gel appears to preferentially attack the glass phase (areas with white precipitate particles) of a gingival (body) porcelain. When the exposure time is increased to 300 minutes, a generalized severe degradation of the porcelain surface has occurred (Fig. 26–19). Obviously, this roughness could lead to staining, plaque accumulation, and further breakdown of the structure. However, the use of lower concentrations, such as 0.4% stannous fluoride and 2% sodium fluoride, has no significant effect on the ceramic surface. Dentists should be aware of these long-term clinical effects of fluorides on ceramic and composite restorations (because of their glass filler particles) and avoid the use of APF gels when composites and ceramics

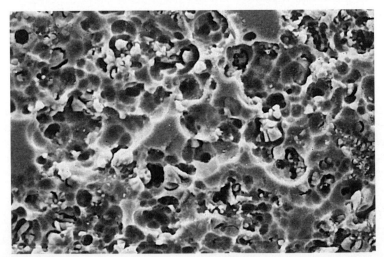

Figure 26–19. Surface of feldspathic gingival (body) porcelain after a 300-minute exposure to 1.23% acidulated phosphate fluoride.

are present. APF gels should not be used on glazed porcelain surfaces. If such a gel is used, the surface of the restoration should be protected with petroleum jelly, cocoa butter, or wax.

Acknowledgments

The authors gratefully acknowledge the critical review and constructive comments provided by Dr. Ed Reetz and the recommendation of Dr. Greg Boyajian to identify ultra-low fusing as a new porcelain classification.

SELECTED READING

Anusavice KJ, DeHoff PH, Hojjatie B, and Gray A: Influence of tempering and contraction mismatch on crack development in ceramic surfaces. J Dent Res 68:1182, 1989.
A study of the application of thermal tempering to strengthen dental porcelain.
Anusavice KJ, Shen C, Vermost B, and Chow B: Strengthening of porcelain by ion exchange subsequent to thermal tempering. Dent Mater 8:149, 1992.
The influence of ion exchange and tempering on strengthening of porcelain.
Binns DB: Some physical properties of two phase crystal-glass solids. In: Stewart GH (ed): Science of Ceramics, Vol 1. London, Academic Press, 1962, p 315.
A classic paper on the reinforcement of glasses with crystalline particles.
Dorsch P: Thermal compatibility of materials for porcelain-fused-to-metal (PFM) restorations. Ceramic Forum International/Ber Dt Keram Ges 59:1, 1982.
Considerable insight into the factors involved in porcelain-metal compatibility.
Duret F, Blouin J-L, and Duret B: CAD-CAM in dentistry. J Am Dent Assoc 117:715, 1988.
A clinician-oriented description of the computer-aided designed and machining of a ceramic restoration.
Fairhurst CS, Anusavice KJ, Hashinger DT, et al: Thermal expansion of dental alloys and porcelains. J Biomed Mater Res 14:435, 1980.
Thermal expansion data are provided for a number of alloys and porcelains, and the changes in porcelain thermal expansion that can be caused by multiple firings are described.
Jones DE: Effects of topical fluoride preparations on glazed porcelain surfaces. J Prosthet Dent 53:483, 1985.
MacCulloch WT: Advances in dental ceramics. Br Dent J 124:361, 1968.
This is the first description of the use of glass ceramics for dental applications.
Mackert JR Jr, Butts MB, and Fairhurst CW: The effect of the leucite transformation on dental porcelain expansion. Dent Mater 2:32, 1986.
A description of the importance of the mineral leucite in regulating the expansion of dental porcelain.
Mackert JR Jr, Butts MB, Morena R, and Fairhurst CW: Phase changes in a leucite-containing dental porcelain frit. J Am Ceram Soc 69:C-69, 1986.
The susceptibility of dental porcelains to phase changes during heat treatment is described.
Mackert JR Jr, Ringle RD, Parry EE, et al: The relationship between oxide adherence and porcelain-metal bonding. J Dent Res 67:474, 1988.
Evidence that the quality of the porcelain bond is dependent on the adherence of the oxide formed during the degassing treatment of the alloy is documented.
McLaren EA, and Sorensen JA: High-strength alumina crowns and fixed partial dentures generated by copy-milling technology. Quint Dent Technol 18:310, 1995.
A technique article on the Celay system that is used for copy-milling of In-Ceram cores for all-ceramic restorations.
McLean JW: The Science and Art of Dental Ceramics, Vol 1. Chicago, Quintessence, 1979; and McLean JW: The Science and Art of Dental Ceramics, Vol 2. Chicago, Quintessence, 1980.
For the serious student of dental ceramics there are no better texts. They cover the entire state of the art in the field up to that time.
McLean JW (ed): Proceedings of the First International Symposium on Ceramics. Chicago, Quintessence, 1983.
A collection of papers from the First International Symposium on Ceramics, containing valuable insights and information on all aspects of dental ceramics.
McLean JW, and Hughes TH: The reinforcement of dental porcelain with ceramic oxides. Br Dent J 119:251, 1965.
A description of the development of alumina-reinforced porcelain, which is the ceramic used as the core of porcelain jacket crowns.
Morena R, Lockwood PE, Evans AL, and Fairhurst CW: Toughening of dental porcelain by tetragonal ZrO_2 additions. J Am Ceram Soc 69:C75, 1986.
The use of partially stabilized zirconia to increase the toughness of dental porcelains is explored via a process termed transformation toughening.

Naleway CA: Laboratory methods of assessing fluoride dentifrices and other topical fluoride agents. In: Wei SH (ed): Clinical Uses of Fluorides. Philadelphia, Lea & Febiger, 1985, p 147.
A group of publications showing the deleterious effects of topical fluorides on the surface of glazed porcelain.

Nassau K (ed): The fifteen causes of color. In: The Physics and Chemistry of Color. New York, John Wiley & Sons, 1983, pp 1–454.
An excellent review of the principles of color and color perception.

Preston JD (ed): Perspectives in Dental Ceramics. In: Proceedings of the 4th International Symposium on Ceramics. Chicago, Quintessence, 1988, p 53.
This collection of papers presented at the 4th International Symposium on Ceramics contains a wealth of information on materials, aesthetics, fabrication, and communication among the members of the clinical team.

Rekow ED: A review of the developments in dental CAD-CAM systems. Curr Opin Dent 2:25, 1992.
An overview of various CAD-CAM systems, their limitations, and success rates.

Ringle RD, Mackert JR Jr, and Fairhurst CW: An x-ray spectrometric technique for measuring porcelain-metal adherence. J Dent Res 62:933, 1983.
This paper, together with the one by Mackert and associates (1988), describes a test for evaluating the quality of porcelain-metal adherence by measuring the extent of cohesive failure, versus adhesive failure, of the porcelain.

Shoher I, and Whiteman A: Captek—a new capillary casting technology for ceramo-metal restorations. Quint Dent Technol 18:9, 1995.
A technique article that describes the Captek technology and techniques.

Traini T: Electroforming technology for ceramo-metal restorations. Quint Dent Technol 18:21, 1995.
A technique article that describes a method for electroforming metal copings for metal-ceramic restorations and the method of preparing the metal for bonding to porcelain.

Vergano PJ, Hill DC, and Uhlmann DR: Thermal expansion of feldspar glasses. J Am Ceram Soc 50:59, 1967.
A classic paper on thermal expansion of feldspar glasses. It is the first report to demonstrate the influence of the high-expanding leucite phase on the thermal expansion of feldspar glasses.

Vrijhoef MMA, Spanauf AJ, Renggli HH, et al: Electroformed gold crowns and bridges. Gold Bull 17:13, 1983.
Gold electroforming technology is presented with data on the mechanical properties as influenced by the conditions of the electrodeposition bath.

Weinstein M, Katz S, and Weinstein AB: Fused porcelain-to-metal teeth. US Patent No. 3,052,982, September 11, 1962; and Weinstein M, and Weinstein AB: Porcelain-covered metal-reinforced teeth. US Patent No. 3,052,983, September 11, 1962.
These two patents describe the development of high-expanding porcelains suitable for fusing with dental alloys. The materials developed by Weinstein and colleagues form the basis for all modern metal-ceramic restorations.

Wunderlich R, and Yaman P: In vitro effect of topical fluoride on dental porcelain. J Prosthet Dent 55:385, 1986.

27 *Soldering*

- Substrate Metal
- Flux
- Soldering (Brazing) Filler Metal
- Heat Source
- Technique Considerations
- Radiographic Analysis of Solder-Joint Quality
- Laser Welding of Commercially Pure Titanium
- Cast-Joining

METAL JOINING TERMINOLOGY

The following definitions are modified versions of those given in the *Metals Handbook, Desk Edition* (1992). The term *soldering* is used commonly in dentistry to describe most metal joining processes that involve the flow of a filler metal between two or more metal components. Technically, the correct term is *brazing* if the liquidus temperature of the filler metal is above 450° C (840° F). The terms and definitions that follow serve as a reference to differentiate among *brazing, soldering,* and *welding.* Because the liquidus temperature of the filler metal is the only difference between the terms *brazing* and *soldering,* the term *soldering* is used subsequently as a general term to describe both processes.

Brazing–the process of joining closely approximated solid metal parts by heating them to a suitable temperature below the solidus temperature(s) of the parts and allowing a filler metal having a liquidus temperature above 450° C to melt and flow by capillary attraction between the parts without appreciably affecting the dimensions of the joined structure. Sufficient filler metal is provided to slightly overfill the space between the closely fitted surfaces of the joint to permit grinding and finishing of the brazed joint.

Cast-joining–a process of joining two components of a fixed partial denture by means of casting molten metal into an interlocking region between the invested components. This procedure is sometimes preferred for base metal alloys because of the technique sensitivity of brazing or soldering these alloys.

Liquidus (metal)–in an equilibrium phase diagram, the temperatures at which metals of an alloy system begin to solidify on cooling or become totally liquid on heating.

Soldering–a group of processes that join metals by heating them to a suitable temperature below the solidus of the substrate metals and applying a filler metal having a liquidus not exceeding 450° C that melts and flows by capillary attraction between the parts without appreciably affecting the dimensions of the joined structure. In dentistry, many metals are joined by brazing, although the term *soldering* is commonly used.

Soldering flux–a material used to prevent the formation of, or to dissolve and facilitate removal of, oxides and other undesirable substances that may reduce the quality or strength of the soldered metal structure.

Solidus (metal)–in a phase diagram, the temperatures at which metals of an alloy system become completely solidified on cooling or start to melt on heating.

Welding–the joining of two or more metal pieces by applying heat, pressure, or both, with or without a filler metal, to produce a localized union across the interface through fusion or diffusion. The thickness of the filler metal, if used, may be much greater than the capillary dimensions encountered in brazing.

This chapter refers to the joining of metals. Metal joining operations are usually divided into three categories: brazing, soldering, and welding. The definitions seem remarkably similar, because the primary difference between soldering and brazing is the specified temperature. The difference between these two terms and welding is the possible absence of filler metal and partial fusion of the parts joined by welding.

The soldering process involves the substrate or parent metal(s) to be joined, soldering filler metal (usually called solder), a flux, and a heat source. All are equally important, and the role of each must be taken into consideration to solder metal components successfully.

SUBSTRATE METAL

The substrate metal, sometimes known as the *basis metal,* is the original pure metal or alloy that is prepared for joining to another substrate metal or alloy. When this book was first written, most substrate metals used in dentistry were gold-based alloys that were used either in cast form or in wrought form. Before casting became the popular method of producing metal prosthetic structures, many appliances were constructed by forming shapes from wrought plate and wire and then soldering these pieces together to produce the required configuration.

Metal compositions now range from gold-copper to gold-silver, gold-palladium, silver-palladium, palladium-silver, palladium-copper, palladium-gallium, nickel-chromium, cobalt-chromium, titanium-aluminum-vanadium, and commercially pure titanium. Note that the soldering operation is the same for any substrate metal; that does not mean, however, that the ease of soldering is the same for any substrate metal. Therefore, the person who performs the soldering procedure should have some information about the substrate metals before attempting the soldering procedure.

The composition of the substrate metal determines its melting range. As noted, the soldering should take place below the solidus temperature of the substrate metal. The composition determines the oxide that forms on the surface during heating, and the flux used must be able to reduce this oxide, inhibit further oxidation, or facilitate its removal. The composition of the substrate metal determines the wettability of the substrate by the molten solder alloy. The solder chosen must wet the metal at as low a contact angle as possible to ensure wetting of the joint area.

Although composition determines the melting range, knowing the composition of the alloy is not particularly helpful in determining the melting range. No technician (or metallurgist, either) can guess the melting range or the wettability from the alloy composition. However, a metallurgist or chemist might be able to predict the nature of the oxide to be formed. The manufacturer or supplier is responsible for guidance in eliminating the oxide layer during the joining process. The instructions for every alloy should include a recommendation for filler metal (solder) and flux. For alloys to be used for porcelain, this recommendation should include both prefiring and postfiring soldering filler metals and fluxes. The technical term for joining metals before porcelain veneering is *presoldering* (or *prebrazing*). The technical term for joining metals after porcelain veneering is *postsoldering* (or *postbrazing*).

FLUX

The Latin word *flux* means flow. Soldering filler metals are designed to wet and flow across clean metal surfaces; they cannot wet oxide surfaces. The purpose of a flux is to remove any oxide coating on the substrate metal surface when the filler metal is fluid and ready to flow into place. Fluxes may be divided into the following three types, according to their primary purpose:

1. Surface protection—this type of flux covers the metal surface and prevents access to oxygen so that no oxides can form
2. Reducing agent—this type of flux reduces any oxides present and exposes clean metal
3. Solvent—this type of flux dissolves any oxides present and carries them away

The composition of most commercial fluxes is formulated to accomplish two or more of these purposes. Fluxes have temperature ranges for optimum activity as well, and thus a flux that is designed for presoldering may not do well for postsoldering, and vice versa. For instance, a borax flux is usually too fluid to remain in place for presoldering, and a fluoride flux may not have sufficient chemical activity at the lower postsoldering temperatures. In addition, fluoride-containing fluxes are likely to attack the porcelain if they are used for postsoldering.

Fluxes for use with noble metal alloys usually are based on boric or borate compounds such as boric acid, boric anhydride, and borax. They act as protective fluxes (Type I) by forming low-temperature glass. They are also reducing fluxes (Type II) for low-stability oxides such as copper oxide.

Because the oxides that form on base metal alloys are more stable, fluorides are used to dissolve chromium, nickel, and cobalt oxides. They usually contain borates as glass formers (protective), and the fluoride dissolves any metal oxide with which it comes in contact, acting as a solvent.

The flux may be used by painting it on the substrate metal at the junction of the pieces to be joined, or it may be fused onto the surface of the filler metal strip. One product is furnished as a filler metal in a tube form, and the flux is contained inside the tube. This type is called *prefluxed solder*.

Whatever technique is used, it is of primary importance to minimize the amount of flux used. Excess flux remains trapped within the filler metal and causes a weakened joint. Residual flux that is covered with porcelain can cause discoloration and bubbling of the porcelain. Flux, combined with metal oxides, forms a glass during the soldering process that is difficult to remove completely. A two-step method for removing residual flux glass is to blast the joint immediately after removal from the investment with alumina abrasive particles followed by boiling in water for about 5 minutes.

SOLDERING (BRAZING) FILLER METAL

Soldering filler metal compositions are as diverse as the compositions of the substrate metals. The filler metal must be compatible with the oxide-free substrate metal, but it does not necessarily have a similar composition. Compatibility consists of three primary properties: (1) an appropriate flow temperature; (2) the ability to wet the substrate metal; and (3) sufficient fluidity at the flow temperature. Other properties that should be considered include strength, color, and tarnish and corrosion resistance.

Flow temperature is that temperature at which the filler metal wets and flows on the substrate metal and produces a bond. It does not relate to any physical property of the alloy, such as the liquidus temperature. The flow temperature is usually higher than the liquidus temperature. However, it must be determined in the laboratory by experimentation. The flow temperature of a filler metal varies, depending on the combination of substrate metal, flux, and ambient atmosphere. The value should be furnished by the filler metal manufacturer. It is one of the requirements of a standard established by the International Organization for Standardization (ISO 9333). The standard also provides a method for its determination.

The flow temperature of the filler metal should be lower than the solidus temperature of the metals being joined. A rule of thumb is that the flow temperature of the filler metal should be 56° C (100° F) lower than the solidus temperature of the substrate metal. For a presoldered alloy substrate that will be veneered with porcelain, a higher-melting-range solder is usually needed to avoid remelting the solder when the porcelain is fired, e.g., to prevent sag deformation of a bridge framework during subsequent porcelain firing.

Wetting of the substrate metal by the filler metal is essential to produce a bond. The wetting phenomenon is discussed in Chapter 2. Let us review it again briefly. Wetting may be understood by comparing the placement of a drop of water on a piece of wax and on a piece of soap. The drop of water "balls up" on the wax and contacts the wax over a smaller area. On the soap, it spreads as far as the amount of water allows. The water wets the soap, whereas it does not wet the wax.

Similarly, if pure silver is melted on nickel or nickel-based alloys, it stands up

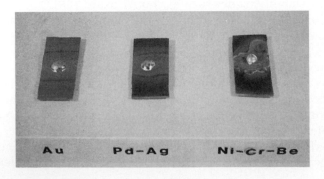

Figure 27–1. Pure silver melted on three different alloys. It wets the gold (Au) alloy and palladium-silver (Pd-Ag) alloy but does not flow onto the surface of the base metal (Ni-Cr-Be) alloy. (Courtesy of C. Ingersoll.)

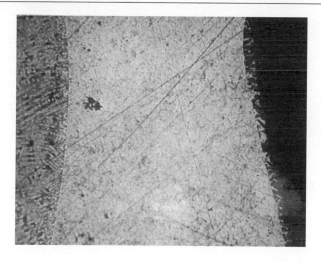

Figure 27–2. Joining of two different substrate metals with the filler metal (in center). The structure on the left represents good bonding with no alloying between the filler metal and substrate metal. Shown at the right is the same alloy at the interface between the filler metal and another substrate alloy. (Courtesy of C. Ingersoll.)

in a ball, as seen on the right side of Figure 27–1. In contrast, when pure silver is melted on gold and palladium-silver alloys, it spreads out over the surface. However, none of this holds true if an oxide layer is present on the surface of the substrate metal, because oxides have poor wettability characteristics.

When two different substrate metals are joined, such as a cast gold alloy crown to a metal-ceramic bridge, the filler metal represents a compromise. If the flow point of the filler metal is close to or above the solidus of either substrate metal, alloying can take place through a welding process. Figure 27–2 shows such a soldered joint. Two different substrate metals are joined. In one case, the filler metal-substrate metal interface is a distinct line. In the other case, the interface region is indistinct because of alloying between the substrate metal and filler metal. Diffusion of filler atoms into the substrate metal and diffusion of substrate metal atoms into the soldering metal are controlled by temperature and time. Even if the flow point of the filler metal is not too high, alloying can take place by diffusion if the temperature remains high for a sufficiently long time. An alloy formed through diffusion can have properties different from those of both the soldering filler metal and the substrate metal. As shown in Figure 27–3, for a nickel-based alloy with a gold filler metal, the resultant diffusion process can form an alloy of gold and nickel that can begin to melt at

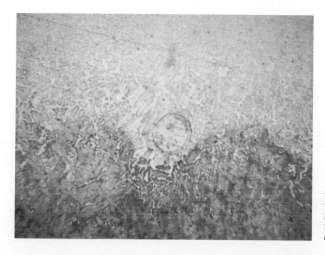

Figure 27–3. Micrograph showing alloying at interface between a gold-alloy solder metal and a base metal substrate. ×100. (Courtesy of C. Ingersoll.)

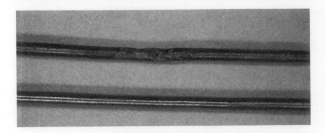

Figure 27–4. A sag test in which soldering (brazing) of a nickel-based alloy with a gold-based soldering alloy *(top)* produced a gold-nickel diffusion zone. The soldered rod has sagged as compared with the nonsoldered rod *(bottom)*. (Courtesy of C. Ingersoll.)

950° C (1740° F). Such an alloy could then melt during the firing of porcelain if the soldered metals are used to produce a metal-ceramic restoration. The result of this process is distortion of the prosthesis, as demonstrated in Figure 27–4. For this reason, gold-based filler metals should not be used as a presolder for base metal alloys.

HEAT SOURCE

The heat source is an important part of the soldering process. The most common instrument for the application of heat is a gas-air or gas-oxygen torch and the type of torch should be chosen according to the fuel being used. (Refer to Table 27–1 in the following discussion.)

Flame Temperature. There is a tendency to choose fuel based on its flame temperature, but flame temperature tells only half the story. Although an alloy cannot be melted if its melting range is higher than the flame temperature, all the gases shown in Table 27–1 have flame temperatures high enough to melt any dental casting alloy currently in use. The flame must provide enough heat to raise the temperature of both the substrate metal and the filler metal to the soldering temperature (the flow temperature of the filler metal). One must also compensate for heat loss to the surroundings. Heat comes from the heat of combustion of the fuel, and the heat content is measured in calories per cubic meter (British thermal units per cubic foot) of the fuel. The lower the heat content of the fuel, the more cubic feet of fuel must be burned to provide the required total heat. A lower heat content of fuel requires a longer period for heating to the desired temperature and is associated with more danger of oxidation during the soldering process.

Hydrogen. The low heat content value for hydrogen indicates that heating would be slow with hydrogen as a fuel. The loss of heat to the air, to the soldering investment, and to the other parts of the casting might be enough to take up all of the heat generated by the flame. Using hydrogen, it might be

TABLE 27–1. Fuel Gas Characteristics

	Flame Temperature		Heat Content
Fuel (with oxygen)	° C	° F	(BTU/cubic foot)
Hydrogen	2660	4820	275
Natural gas	2680	4855	1000
Propane	2850	5160	2385
Acetylene	3140	5685	1448

impossible to bring the joining area of a large bridge up to the temperature required for presoldering.

Natural Gas. The heat content of natural gas is about four times that of hydrogen gas and can be expected to raise the temperature of the soldered joint four times as fast. However, the value in this instance is an average value for dry natural gas. The gas that is normally available is nonuniform in composition and frequently has water vapor in it. Water vapor cools the flame and uses some of the heat content of the gas. This explains why some technicians have had trouble with this fuel when melting alloys for the casting process.

Acetylene. Acetylene has the highest flame temperature, and its heat content is greater than that of either hydrogen or natural gas. Acetylene, however, has certain problems. The variation in temperature from one part of the flame to another may be more than 100° C. With this variation, the positioning of the torch is critical so that the proper zone of the flame is used. It is also a chemically unstable gas and therefore decomposes readily to carbon and hydrogen. Carbon can be incorporated into both nickel and palladium alloys, and hydrogen can be taken up by palladium-based alloys. Improper adjustment of the flame may extinguish the torch with an associated release of carbon from the torch tip. Only individuals with extensive experience with this gas should consider its use for metal joining procedures.

Propane. Of the fuel gases in the chart in Table 27–1, the best choice is propane. It has a good flame temperature, and its heat content is the highest of the readily available gases. Butane, which is more readily available in some parts of the world, has a similar flame temperature and a similar heat content value. Both propane and butane have the advantage of being relatively pure compounds; therefore, they are uniform in quality and virtually water free and burn clean (provided that the torch flame is properly adjusted).

Oven (Furnace) Soldering. For oven soldering, a furnace should be chosen with enough wattage to provide the heat required to raise the temperature of the filler metal to its flow point. The furnace will also provide high-temperature surroundings, so less heat is lost to other parts of the bridge or to the ambient atmosphere than with torch soldering.

The success of furnace soldering depends on the heat transmission from the heating elements to the substrate metals. For best success in furnace soldering, the technician should be familiar with the three modes of heat transmission: *convection* (transmission by means of air currents), *conduction* (transmission by conductance through the furnace structure), and *radiant heat* (transmission by radiation from the heating coils).

Before the metal substrate to be soldered is placed into the oven, a uniform coating of a paste flux should be applied to the surface to be soldered. Care should be taken to avoid the use of an excessive amount of flux, because some residue may be incorporated into the solder joint, thereby weakening the structure.

TECHNIQUE CONSIDERATIONS

Operator skill, an important element of successful soldering, is a composite of psychomotor ability, knowledge of soldering principles, technique, and experience. This skill is especially important in torch soldering.

Other than to join two bridge units, soldering generally represents an emergency procedure to repair a metal appliance that contains major casting defects or that has distorted during previous fabrication procedures. Technicians may experience technical problems simply because they do not solder metals routinely, and because skill cannot be maintained, particularly in torch soldering, without practice. The problem is amplified when alloys of nickel-chromium or cobalt-chromium are involved because of the difficulty in removing oxides.

Technical Procedures. The soldering technique involves several critical steps: (1) cleaning and preparing the surfaces to be joined; (2) assembling the parts to be joined; (3) preparation and fluxing of the gap surfaces between the parts; (4) maintaining the proper position of the parts during the procedure; (5) control of the proper temperature; and (6) control of the time to ensure adequate flow of solder and complete filling of the solder joint.

Gap. The optimum gap between parts of substrate metal to be joined has never been defined. If the gap is too great, the joint strength will be controlled by the strength of the filler metal. If the gap is too narrow, the strength will probably be limited by flux inclusions, porosity caused by incomplete flow of the filler metal, or both. Inclusions or porosity can lead to distortion if any heating, such as porcelain application, takes place after the soldering operation.

The two bars shown in Figure 27–5 are of the same nickel-based alloy. They were cut in the same manner and prepared for soldering exactly in the same way except for the gap. The gap in the upper bar was 1.0 mm, whereas the gap in the lower was 0.3 mm. Both were soldered with the same filler metal. The upper bar failed in the filler metal. The lower bar failed in the substrate metal even though the tensile strength of the substrate metal was greater than that of the filler metal.

Flame. The flame can be divided into four zones (Fig. 27–6), and the portion of the flame that is used to heat the soldering assembly should be the neutral or slightly reducing part, because this produces the most efficient burning process and the most heat. An improperly adjusted torch or improperly positioned flame can lead to oxidation of the substrate or filler metal and result in a poorly soldered joint. It is also possible to introduce carbon into substrate and filler metal by using the unburned gas portion of the flame. To prevent oxide forma-

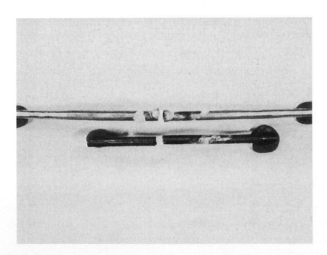

Figure 27–5. The upper bar was soldered with an excessive gap. When it was tested to failure under tension, the failure occurred in the filler metal. The lower bar, with a proper gap, failed in the substrate metal. (Courtesy of C. Ingersoll.)

COLD MIXING ZONE (UNBURNED GAS)

PARTIAL COMBUSTION ZONE (OXIDIZING)

REDUCING ZONE

OXIDIZING ZONE (BURNED GAS)

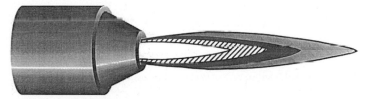

Figure 27–6. Mixing, combustion, reducing, and unburned gas zones in a propane-oxygen torch flame.

tion, the flame should not be removed once it has been applied to the joint area until the soldering process has been completed. The flame provides protection from oxidation, especially at the soldering temperature.

Temperature. The temperature used to solder should be the minimum one required to complete the soldering operation. Heat should be applied to the substrate metal so as to heat it to the flow temperature of the filler metal. Thus, the substrate metal will be hot enough to melt the filler metal as soon as it contacts the area to be joined.

Higher temperatures of the substrate metal increase the possibility of diffusion between substrate metal and filler metal. Lower temperatures of the substrate metal do not allow the filler metal to wet the substrate metal, and thus little or no bonding occurs.

Time. The flame should be maintained in place until the filler metal has flowed completely into the connection and a moment longer to allow the flux or oxide to separate out from the fluid filler metal. This longer time increases the possibility of diffusion between substrate metal and filler metal, while a shorter time increases the possibility of incomplete filling of the joint and of flux inclusion in the joint. Both of these conditions result in weaker solder joints.

RADIOGRAPHIC ANALYSIS OF SOLDER-JOINT QUALITY

When a fixed partial denture is delivered to a dental office from the dental laboratory, the processing history of the prosthesis is usually unknown to the dentist. Of particular importance is the need to identify whether the fixed partial denture was cast in one piece or whether it was soldered or cast-joined. The flexure strength of a joined metal structure decreases in the following order: cast structure, soldered structure, cast-joined structure. If one is certain that the fixed partial denture was cast in one piece, there should be little concern for its fracture potential. If the structure was soldered at one site, the fracture resistance will be decreased, especially when the joint is positioned more posteriorly in the fixed partial denture. If the framework was cast-joined (see the following section), the structure should be carefully examined for evidence of defects and for potential mechanical slippage during bending under an applied small load in one's hands. If any noticeable displacement can be detected, the fixed partial denture should be discarded or returned to the laboratory.

For either the soldered or cast-joined structures, as well as the cast connection, a radiographic examination of the joined area can be performed. The simplest method is to lay the structure on an unexposed piece of intraoral x-ray film and expose the film with an x-ray beam with an accelerating voltage of 90 kV and a current of 10 mA for 1 second. Another film should be exposed after rotating the fixed partial denture at a 90-degree angle to the initial orientation. Shown in Figure 27–7 are radiographic images of a metal-ceramic framework. One can clearly see the radiolucent flaws at the buccal and lingual aspects of the posterior presoldered connector, whereas the cast metal in the other embrasure area is sound.

LASER WELDING OF COMMERCIALLY PURE TITANIUM

Commercially pure titanium (cpTi) that is used in dentistry for crowns, bridges, and partial denture frameworks is a highly reactive metal in air. The thin oxide film that forms instantaneously on a cleaned surface converts this metal from an active to a passive state. At temperatures that are used for soldering procedures, the thickness of the titanium oxide layer increases and may spontaneously debond from the parent metal surface at temperatures exceeding 850° C. Thus, the process of soldering this metal using traditional torch-soldering or oven-soldering procedures is technique sensitive, and the quality of the soldered joint would be quite variable.

To effectively join titanium components of dental crowns, bridges, and partial denture frameworks, laser welding and plasma welding in an argon gas atmosphere can be performed. Since laser welding is associated with a lower thermal influence on the parts being joined than is plasma welding, it is the preferred method for dental applications. An advantage of welding is that the welded joint will be composed of the same pure titanium as the substrate components, thereby preserving the excellent biocompatibility potential of cpTi and avoiding the risk of galvanic corrosion effects within the prosthesis.

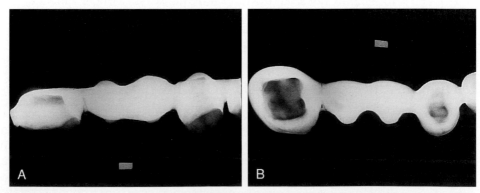

Figure 27–7. A, Buccolingual radiographic image of metal framework designed for a metal-ceramic fixed partial denture (bridge). *B*, Occlusogingival view. Note the radiolucencies at the buccal and lingual aspects of the posterior soldered connector.

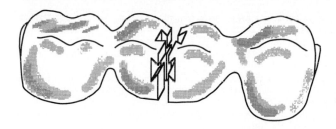

Figure 27-8. Mechanical interlocking design of a cast-joined framework for a metal-ceramic fixed partial denture (bridge).

A few commercial laser welding units are available for joining cpTi. These are usually based on a pulsed high-power neodymium laser with a very-high-power density. The first successful units of this type include the Dentaurum Dental-Laser DL 2002 (Dentaurum, Pforzheim, Germany), the Haas Laser LKS (Haas-Laser GmbH, Schramberg, Germany), and the Heraeus Haas Laser 44 P (Heraeus Kulzer GmbH, Hanau, Germany). The units consist of a small type of glove-box that contains the laser tip, an argon gas source, and a stereomicroscope with lens crosshairs for precise alignment of the laser beam with the cpTi components. The maximum penetration depth of these laser welding units is 2.5 mm. Since only a small amount of heat is generated, the parts can be hand-held during the welding procedure, and welding can be performed close to ceramic or polymeric veneers without causing damage to these materials.

CAST-JOINING

Because of the technique sensitivity of soldering predominantly base metal alloys and the variation in solder-joint quality associated with presoldering of these alloys, the cast-joining technique (see the terminology section) was proposed by Weiss and Munyon (1980) as an alternative method for joining cast components of a fixed partial denture. Cast-joined components are held together purely by mechanical retention (Fig. 27–8). Because of this situation, poorly adapted cast secondary metal within the retentive areas may cause a noticeable displacement when a bending force is manually applied. Under this condition, a porcelain veneer over this region is likely to fracture. Thus, a radiographic examination should be made of all metal frameworks to minimize this risk.

SELECTED READING

Agarwal DP, and Ingersoll CE: High-temperature soldering alloy. US Patent No. 4,399,096.
A particularly important patent, because it involved the development of a palladium-silver-nickel soldering filler metal for presoldering.

Anusavice KJ, Okabe T, Galloway SE, Hoyt DJ, and Morse PK: Flexure test evaluation of presoldered base metal alloys. J Prosthet Dent 54:507, 1985.
Wide variability in the strength of brazed joints in Ni-Cr-Mo-Be and Ni-Cr-Mo alloys was reported. The strength of the brazed joint ranged from 20% to 90% of that of a solid bar of the same metals and was not affected by gap widths of 0.25 or 0.51 mm.

Anusavice KJ, and Shafagh I: Inert gas presoldering of nickel-chromium alloys. J Prosthet Dent 55:3137, 1986.
An argon gas environment did not improve the strength of presoldered joint strength of nickel-chromium-molybdenum and nickel-chromium-molybdenum-beryllium alloys. Most of the fractures appeared to originate within the solder filler alloy. Entrapped flux particles and gases were the most likely cause of these failures.

DeHoff PH, Anusavice KJ, Evans J, and Wilson HR: Effectiveness of cast-joined structures. Int J Prosthodont 3:550, 1990.
A study of the load transfer effectiveness of five cast-joined connector designs. Compared with a solid nickel-chromium alloy bar, the percent effectiveness in sustaining an applied bending load ranged from 4.4% to 21.3%.

Kaylakie WG, and Brukl CE: Comparative tensile strengths of nonnoble dental alloy solders. J Prosthet Dent 53:455, 1985.

Tensile strengths and failure sites of a large number of base metal solders were measured. In addition, various soldering technique variables were studied, and a radiographic method for evaluating soldered joints was described.

Metals Handbook, Desk Edition. Metals Park, OH, American Society for Metals, 1992.

Monday JL, and Asgar K: Tensile strength comparison of presoldered and postsoldered joints. J Prosthet Dent 55:23, 1986.

No significant differences in the tensile strength of presoldered and postsoldered joints were found when the same technique was used. It is interesting that torch soldering yielded significantly stronger joints than the vacuum oven technique employed.

Rasmussen EJ, Goodkind RJ, and Gerberich WW: An investigation of tensile strength of dental solder joints. J Prosthet Dent 41:418, 1979.

Higher strengths reported for Type III gold alloy as gap distance was increased, but that trend was not noted for a gold-palladium alloy. These and other observations are partially explained in terms of the competing effects of yield strength, wettability, and voids at the various gap distances.

Rogers OW: The gold solder–gold alloy interface. Aust Dent J 22:168, 1977.

A discrete study of the diffusion mechanics at the grain boundaries of the substrate gold alloy and gold alloy soldering filler

Ryge G: Dental soldering procedures. Dent Clin North Am Nov.:747–757, 1958.

A thorough treatment of the various factors involved in the soldering of dental structures, with particular attention to gap distance.

Weiss PA, and Munyon RE: Repairs, corrections, and additions to ceramo-metal frameworks. II. Quint Dent Technol 7:45, 1980.

Cast-joining is proposed as an alternative to soldering of cast metal components of a fixed partial denture.

28 *Wrought Base Metal and Gold Alloys*

- Deformation of Metals
- Effects of Annealing Cold-worked Metal
- Carbon Steels
- Stainless Steels
- Corrosion Resistance
- Cobalt-Chromium-Nickel Alloys
- Nickel-Titanium Alloys
- β-Titanium Alloys
- Gold Alloys

DEFORMATION OF METALS

Wrought base metal alloys are used in dentistry, mainly as wires for orthodontic treatment and also as clasp arms for removable partial dentures. The metallurgy of these alloys is complex. The primary alloy used for orthodontic wire is stainless steel, an iron-chromium-nickel alloy. Other major systems for orthodontic and partial denture applications include cobalt-chromium-nickel, nickel-titanium, and β-titanium alloys. Before considering each of these systems in detail, a brief discussion of their application in orthodontics is appropriate.

Many of the dental structures placed in the mouth are castings. However, wires are used by the orthodontist for correction of tooth displacement and by prosthodontists and general practitioners for retention and stabilization of removable partial dentures. Wires are made from castings by drawing a cast metal through a die. Many accessory dental materials and instruments have been fabricated from cast metal that has been rolled to form a sheet or rod, drawn into wire or tubing, or forged (plastically deformed in a die under compressive force, usually at an elevated temperature) into a finished shape. Of the many metallic articles encountered in everyday life, most are wrought metal and not castings.

Whenever a casting is plastically deformed in any manner, it is considered a *wrought metal* and exhibits properties and microstructure that are not associated with a cast structure. The differences are so marked that dentists should assess benefits and limitations of cast and wrought wires before proceeding with their selection and use and they should be knowledgeable about the potential effects of plastic deformation adjustments on the properties of cast metal prostheses.

Orthodontic wires are formed into various configurations or appliances to apply forces to teeth and move them into a more desirable alignment. The force system is determined by the appliance design and the material properties of the wire. For a given design and deflection of a wire, the force applied to the tooth is proportional to the modulus of elasticity. Low, constant forces are biologically desirable, although a threshold force level is necessary for tooth movement. Large elastic deflections are clinically desirable, because they produce a more constant force during the time of tooth movement and allow for greater activation, or *working range*. The maximum elastic deflection of an orthodontic wire is usually proportional to its ratio of yield strength to modulus of elasticity. The maximum force that can be applied is a function of the yield strength.

Other material properties are also important in orthodontic treatment. A ductile wire can be formed into various shapes, although there are applications that do not require permanent bends. Ease of joining is important, and most wires can be either soldered or welded together. Finally, the wire must demonstrate biocompatibility and corrosion resistance, that is, chemical stability in the oral environment.

In Chapter 4, principles of elastic and plastic deformation are described. At stresses below the proportional limit, the atoms in the crystal lattice are displaced elastically a small amount so that when the stress is relieved, they can return to their original positions. However, once the proportional limit is exceeded, both elastic and plastic deformation have occurred, and the structure does not return to its original dimensions when the load is released. Only the elastic strain can be recovered. As the applied force increases, this displacement eventually becomes so great that the atoms are separated completely and either plastic deformation or fracture results.

An atomic model illustrating plastic deformation of a perfect lattice under an applied shear stress is illustrated in Figure 28–1. Notice that the deformation or slip process requires the simultaneous displacement of the plane A atoms relative to the plane B atoms below it. If the elastic modulus in shear for a given metal is known, this model can be used to calculate the maximum theoretic shear strength of the metal.

When this is done, the observed shear strength values are not even close to the calculated ultimate shear strength values for bulk polycrystalline materials. As can be seen in Table 28–1, the calculated values are about 40 to 150 times larger than those actually observed. In fact, values approaching the theoretic shear strengths are found only in measurements made on whisker specimens. Such tiny single-crystal filaments (approximately 2.5 μm in diameter) have been used as reinforcing agents in commercial composite materials. Their use has also been investigated for other dental applications.

The key difference in behavior of the whiskers and bulk polycrystalline specimens of the same material is the presence of lattice imperfections in the bulk material. Whiskers have nearly perfect lattice structures.

Lattice Imperfections. Crystallization from the nucleus does not occur in a regular fashion, lattice plane by lattice plane. Instead, the growth is likely to be more random, with some lattice positions left vacant and others overcrowded with atoms deposited interstitially between neighboring atoms and out of line with the principal lattice planes. These imperfections may be of many types, but they can be generally classified as *point defects* or *line defects*.

The defects just described are point defects; the simpler types are diagrammed

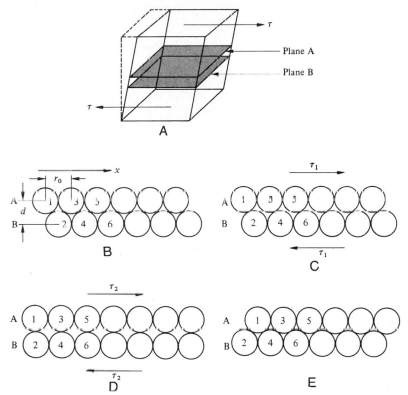

Figure 28–1. Slip between adjacent planes of atoms. *A*, A solid subjected to a shear stress. Planes A and B are adjacent. *B*, The configuration of planes A and B when the solid is not stressed. *C*, Application of a shear stress τ_1 causes plane A to move with respect to plane B. *D*, Increasing the shear stress increases the relative displacement of the two planes. This configuration corresponds to the maximum storage of elastic energy. *E*, The two planes have been displaced by a distance r_0 with respect to each other. This configuration will be maintained if the load is removed. If the load remains, the planes will continue to slip past each other. (From INTRODUCTION TO MECHANICAL PROPERTIES OF MATERIALS by Eisenstadt, M., © 1971. Reprinted by permission of Prentice-Hall, Inc., Upper Saddle River, NJ.)

TABLE 28–1. Theoretical and Observed Shear Strength

Material	Shear Modulus (GPa)	Observed Ultimate Shear Strength (Polycrystalline) (MPa)	Calculated Ultimate Shear Strength (MPa)	Observed Ultimate Shear Strength (Whisker) (MPa)*
Copper	48.3	221	7724	2093
Iron	80.0	290	12,448	9517
Nickel	75.9	476		2724
A$_2$O$_3$	170		12,069	14,621
BeO	136	276 (tension)	21,724	9241
SiC	202	172 (tension)	32,345	14,621

*The shape of the whiskers is not conductive to shear testing. The tabulated values were calculated from tensile strength data given by Broutman IJ, and Krock RH: Modern Composite Materials. Reading, MA, Addison-Wesley, 1967. (From INTRODUCTION TO MECHANICAL PROPERTIES OF MATERIALS by Eisenstadt, M., © 1971. Reprinted by permission of Prentice-Hall, Inc., Upper Saddle River, NJ.)

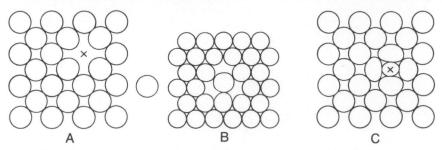

Figure 28–2. Point defects: *A,* Vacancy; *B,* divacancy (two missing atoms); and *C,* interstitial (extra atom). (From Van Vlack, ELEMENTS OF MATERIALS SCIENCE AND ENGINEERING, 4th Edition. © 1980 Addison-Wesley Publishing Company Inc. Reprinted by permission of Addison-Wesley Publishing Company Inc.)

in Figure 28–2. A vacancy representing a vacant lattice site may occur in the space lattice, as shown in Figure 28–2*A,* or two or more vacancies may condense as a divacancy or trivacancy, as shown in Figure 28–2*B.* An interstitial point defect is illustrated in Figure 28–2*C.*

Each defect results in a change in energy in the space lattice at its point of occurrence. The ultimate result is a weakening effect with regard to cleavage strength but a strengthening relative to further deformation.

Vacancies are sometimes referred to as *equilibrium defects,* because a crystal lattice that is in equilibrium contains a certain number of these defects. The vacancy concentration depends on the temperature of the lattice and increases with increasing temperature. The presence of vacancies is necessary for the process of diffusion in a solid metal.

Dislocations. The chief difference in physical properties between a perfect single crystal and a polycrystalline material is associated with the formation of line defects or dislocations in the latter.

The simplest type of dislocation, known as an *edge dislocation,* is illustrated diagrammatically in Figure 28–3*A.* It can be noted that the lattice is regular except for the one plane of atoms that is discontinuous, forming a *dislocation line* at the edge of the half plane. Dislocations are not equilibrium defects, and the formation of a dislocation requires significant energy, which is stored in the strained crystal lattice surrounding the defect. If a shearing force is applied to the crystal, the atoms in the plane above the dislocation easily break old bonds and establish new bonds with the lower atoms, and the dislocation shifts one lattice spacing, as indicated in Figure 28–3*B.* A continued application of shear stress causes successive slipping of the atomic "edge" until finally the dislocation reaches the boundary of the crystal and disappears, leaving one unit of slip at the surface of the crystal, as shown in Figure 28–3*C.* The plane along which a dislocation moves is known as a *slip plane.*

The final result is the establishment of equilibrium from a condition of energy concentration at the dislocation. Because of the dislocation, the force necessary to cause plastic lattice deformation is much less than it would be if a *perfect crystal* existed because only one line of atomic bonds has actually been disrupted.

However, as has been shown previously, in a perfect crystal a whole plane of bonds must be ruptured to cause atomic slip to occur. A simple analogy is the process of moving a large carpet a small distance closer to one wall of a room. One can grip the edge of the carpet and pull with a relatively large force or one can create a wrinkle in the carpet and "walk" the wrinkle across the floor. The

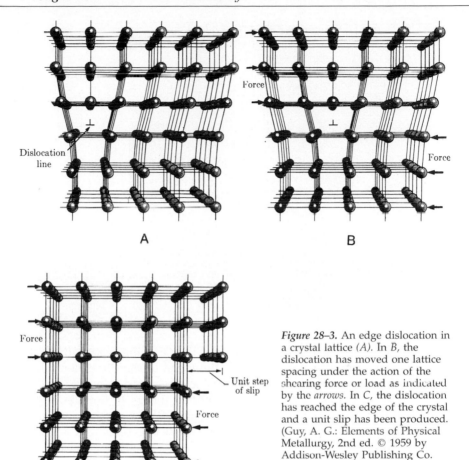

Figure 28–3. An edge dislocation in a crystal lattice (*A*). In *B*, the dislocation has moved one lattice spacing under the action of the shearing force or load as indicated by the *arrows*. In *C*, the dislocation has reached the edge of the crystal and a unit slip has been produced. (Guy, A. G.: Elements of Physical Metallurgy, 2nd ed. © 1959 by Addison-Wesley Publishing Co. Reprinted by permission of Addison-Wesley Publishing Co., Reading, MA.)

latter obviously requires much less force. The net result is the same in either case; the entire carpet is displaced a small distance. Thus, the difference between the tensile strength of a whisker and of a structure containing dislocations can be explained on the basis of lattice imperfections. Whiskers do not contain dislocations because their physical dimensions are too small to accommodate the strain field that surrounds a dislocation.

In addition to edge dislocations, there are other types of dislocations, but the mechanism of slip is essentially the same. When the slip planes occur in groups, the metal surface may become sufficiently irregular to cause diffuse reflection of light, when viewed through a metallurgical microscope, revealing slip bands as shown in Figure 28–4.

Strain Hardening. So far, it has been assumed that slip can occur in any given lattice plane unimpeded so that the dislocation can be relieved. However, as might be deduced from Figure 28–3, if the dislocation during translation meets some other type of lattice discontinuity, its gliding movement under stress might be inhibited. Such discontinuities might be (1) point defects; (2) collision of one dislocation with a different type; (3) a foreign atom or group of atoms of different lattice characteristics as in an alloy; and (4) grain boundaries in a polycrystalline metal. In addition, the process of slip consumes dislocations, as can be seen in

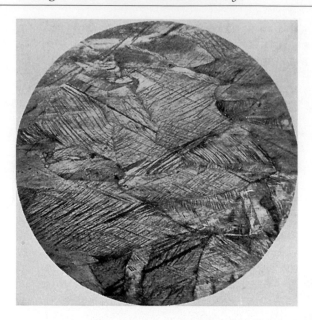

Figure 28–4. Photomicrograph of gold after cold working, showing slip bands. ×100 (Courtesy of S. D. Tylman.)

Figure 28–3. If plastic deformation is to continue at relatively high strain rates, sources must be present within the metal to rapidly generate new dislocations.

In polycrystalline metal, the dislocations tend to build up at the grain boundaries. Also, the barrier action to slip at the grain boundaries causes the slip to occur on other intersecting slip planes. Point defects increase, and the entire grain may eventually become distorted. Greater stress is required to produce further slip, and the metal becomes stronger, harder, and less ductile. The process is known as *strain hardening* or *work hardening*. The latter term is derived from the fact that the process is a result of cold work (*i.e.,* deformation at room temperature) in contrast with the effect of working at a higher temperature, such as occurs in a forging operation. In the latter case, the increase in rate of atomic diffusion caused by the increase in temperature may prevent strain hardening entirely. The ultimate result of strain hardening, with a further increase in cold work, is fracture.

The phenomenon of cold work and strain hardening is familiar to everyone. For example, one way of fracturing a wire is to bend it back and forth rapidly between your fingers. When all the possible slip has occurred, the wire fractures. When a nail is flattened with a hammer, the first few blows are quite effective. However, as the blows are continued, they are not so effective until finally no further deformation occurs. Instead, the metal cracks or fractures. The same phenomenon can occur when a patient bends a clasp arm back and forth several times to relieve discomfort caused by a partial denture.

The surface hardness, strength, and proportional limit of the metal are increased with strain hardening, whereas the ductility and resistance to corrosion are decreased. However, the elastic modulus is not changed appreciably.

The changes in physical properties of a metal produced by strain hardening often serve as the basis of a practical method in dentistry for the control of such properties. For example, it was shown in an earlier chapter on direct filling gold that strain hardening of a gold foil restoration is necessary to provide proper strength and hardness. Likewise, stainless steel wires used in dentistry are dependent on their wrought metal characteristics to produce a sufficient yield strength for their clinical applications.

An illustration of the effect on the grain structure of the flattening of a copper-zinc alloy (brass) between rollers is shown in the first row of photomicrographs at the top of Figure 28–5. The rolling took place in a direction perpendicular to the plane of the photomicrographs, and it can be observed that the thinner the specimen, as designated above each photomicrograph, the flatter or thinner the grains appear to be. If the specimens were observed in a plane 90 degrees to that shown (*i.e.*, parallel to the direction of rolling), the area of the grains would be greater. Although brass was used in this example, the same effect would occur with wrought gold alloys.

An interesting side effect of cold working or strain hardening is the tendency for preferred orientation in the distorted grain structure. The slip planes tend to line up with the shear planes of the deformation process. Thus, the strength of deformed metal, such as a rolled sheet, is usually greater in the transverse direction than in the direction of the rolling.

Fracture. If the cold work is continued, the structure eventually fractures. However, as previously noted, the stress required for fracture, that is, its tensile strength, is much less in the polycrystalline metal, than would be expected

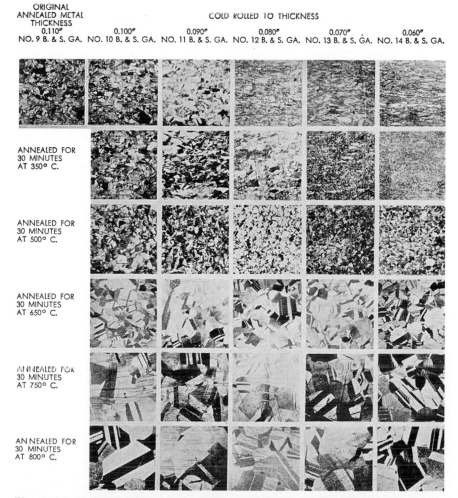

Figure 28–5. Grain size of brass (copper 66%, zinc 34%), after cold working and annealing. ×40. (Prepared by L. H. DeWald.)

theoretically. The reason generally given for this difference is that submicroscopic cracks are present in the polycrystalline metal that cause stress concentrations. Such stresses, in turn, cause propagation of the crack until rupture occurs. Such microcracks may be the result of solidification faults or a concentration of dislocations.

The observed tensile strength of a structure may increase with the rate of stress application because there is less time for plastic flow to occur near the microcrack and thus to relieve the stress concentration. Such a fracture is known as a *brittle fracture* in contrast with a *ductile fracture,* in which plastic deformation of the grains can occur before fracture because of lower loading rate. A brittle fracture has the appearance of a more granular structure at the fracture surface than does a ductile fracture, with little necking or reduction in area at the site of the fracture. Some materials also exhibit a ductile to brittle transition in behavior as the temperature is reduced below a critical value. Certain steels behave in this manner, and spectacular disasters have resulted when they were used structurally at temperatures below the ductile to brittle transition. As pointed out in Chapter 4, brittle materials do not withstand the high tensile or bending stresses that are often encountered in structural applications.

Fracture is generally *transgranular* when it occurs at room temperature rather than *intergranular,* such as occurs at elevated temperatures. Wire should never be annealed into the recrystallization stage, but only heat treated within the *recovery* range, which is discussed in the following section.

EFFECTS OF ANNEALING COLD-WORKED METAL

The effects associated with cold working, such as strain hardening, low ductility, and distorted grains, can be reversed by simply heating the metal. This process is called *annealing.* The more severe the cold working, the more rapidly the effects can be reversed by annealing.

Annealing in general comprises three stages: *recovery, recrystallization,* and *grain growth.* The effects of each of these three stages on the tensile strength and ductility of a metal are shown in Figure 28–6. The microstructural changes that accompany annealing were shown in Figure 28–5. The benefits of annealing are

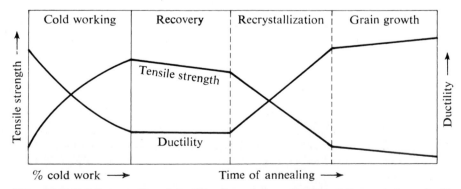

Figure 28–6. Tensile strength and ductility of a metal as a function of the percentage of cold work and annealing time. Tensile strength increases and ductility decreases during cold working. These properties change only slightly during recovery. During recrystallization the tensile strength decreases and the ductility increases rapidly. Only slight changes occur during grain growth. (From Richman MH: Introduction to the Science of Metals. Waltham, MA, Blaisdell, 1967.)

dependent on the melting range of an alloy and the annealing temperature that is used. Annealing is a relative process: the higher the melting range of the alloy, the higher the temperature needed for annealing. A rule of thumb is to use a temperature that is approximately one half that necessary to melt the metal on the absolute temperature scale (degrees Kelvin).

Recovery. Recovery is considered the stage at which the cold-work properties begin to disappear before any significant visible changes are observed under the microscope. As can be seen in Figure 28–6, there is a slight decrease in tensile strength and no change in ductility in the recovery stage. Although not shown, there is a rather pronounced change in the recovery of the electrical conductivity. Also, a cold worked metal contains residual stresses. Machining such material frequently results in warping as the stresses are relaxed. This tendency for warping on machining disappears in the recovery stage. Orthodontic appliances fabricated by bending wrought wires are often subjected to a stress relief anneal before their placement; such a process stabilizes the configuration of the appliance and allows an accurate determination of the force the appliance will be able to deliver in the mouth.

Recrystallization. When a severely cold-worked metal is annealed, recrystallization occurs after the recovery stage. This involves a rather radical change in the microstructure, as can be seen in Figure 28–5. The old grains disappear completely and are replaced by a new set of strain-free grains. These recrystallization grains nucleate in the most severely cold-worked regions in the metal, usually at grain boundaries, or where the lattice was most severely deformed. This process occurs because the strain-free nuclei consume the severely distorted matrix faster than the matrix recovers. On the completion of recrystallization, the material essentially attains its original soft and ductile condition (see Fig. 28–6).

Grain Growth. The recrystallized structure has a certain average grain size, depending on the number of nuclei. The more severe the cold working, the greater the number of such nuclei. Thus, the grain size for the completely recrystallized material can range from rather fine to fairly coarse.

If the fine grain structure is further annealed, the grains begin to grow, as illustrated in Figure 28–5. It can be shown that this grain growth process is simply a process of minimizing the boundary energy. In effect, the large grains consume the smaller grains. The process of grain growth does not progress indefinitely to the ultimate formation of a single crystal. Rather, an ultimate coarse grain structure is produced, and then, for all practical purposes, the grain growth process is finished.

Excessive annealing can lead to larger grains. This phenomenon occurs only in wrought materials. When a large grain structure is present in a casting, it is primarily the result of excessive casting and mold temperatures.

A large grain structure is generally detrimental to the strength properties of a metal. As previously noted, the grain boundary is a barrier to the movement of dislocations. With small or fine grains, the concentrations of inhibited dislocations per grain are greater. Consequently, with small grains, a greater increase in strength, hardness, and proportional limit occurs during cold work than with large grains. However, under such a condition, a lower ductility results for the smaller grain size.

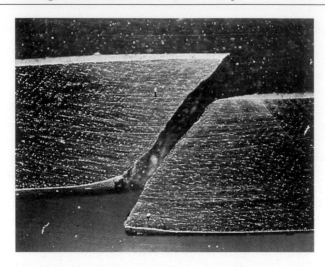

Figure 28–7. A cast rod showing a shear fracture through one large grain that occupied the entire cross-sectional area of the rod. Although ductility was high, fracture occurred because of a high stress concentration. ×24.

On the other hand, with a sufficiently large grain size, particularly in a dental appliance of small cross-sectional thickness, the space lattice of one large grain may be oriented in such a manner to produce high ductility and a low proportional limit.

A low proportional limit, large grain size, and high stress concentration at the grain boundary can lead to catastrophic fracture, as shown in Figure 28–7 for a cast 9.5 mm-diameter gold alloy rod. One of the grains occupied the entire cross section of the rod. From a standpoint of the stress distribution uniformity during cold work, the small grain size is preferred because grain orientation is more equally distributed.

Cast Structure Versus Wrought Structure. Generally, all metals and alloys are produced from castings. Castings can be machined, forged, drawn, extruded, or worked in some manner to provide the required article or appliance. It then becomes a wrought metal in contrast with a cast metal.

The influence of grain size on the physical properties of the metal is equally important in both cases. However, the grain size of the cast metal is normally established at the time of solidification. Apparently, the cast structure is so close to equilibrium conditions that heat treatments are virtually ineffective in changing the grain size.

Most dental appliances are cast, not wrought. Consequently, the factors that affect the grain size of the casting are important. However, if the dentist bends a cast clasp or burnishes a cast crown margin sufficiently during adjustment, the structure may be cold worked sufficiently to be converted to a wrought metal structure.

In the dental applications in which wrought materials are used, such as orthodontic bands and wires, pedodontic appliances, and partial denture clasp arms, the strength values depend on the wrought structure. An extended anneal into the recrystallization stage could seriously reduce the fracture resistance. Prolonged heating of stainless steel to high temperatures can also markedly reduce its corrosion resistance.

Such considerations become important during the soldering operations discussed later and during similar procedures in which a high temperature is employed. Also, before heating any instrument such as a rubber dam clamp (retainer), the dentist should consider the possibility that it might be ruined by grain growth or by other metallographic changes.

CARBON STEELS

As has been pointed out, stainless steels are the major alloy system used in orthodontics. However, the metallurgy and terminology of these alloys are intimately connected to those of the simpler binary iron-carbon alloy system and to carbon steel alloys. Therefore, this discussion begins with a brief outline of the metallurgy of the iron-carbon system.

Steels are iron-based alloys that usually contain less than 1.2% carbon. The different classes of steels are based on three possible lattice arrangements of iron. Pure iron at room temperature has a body-centered cubic (BCC) structure and is referred to as *ferrite*. This phase is stable in temperatures as high as 912° C. The spaces between atoms in the BCC structure (interstices) are small and oblate; hence, carbon has a very low solubility in ferrite (maximum of 0.02 wt%).

At temperatures between 912° C and 1394° C, the stable form of iron is a face-centered cubic (FCC) structure called *austenite*. The interstices in the FCC lattice are larger than those in the BCC structure. However, the size of the carbon atom limits the maximum carbon solubility to 2.1 wt%.

When austenite is cooled slowly from high temperatures, the excess carbon that is not soluble in ferrite forms iron carbide (Fe_3C). This hard, brittle phase adds strength to the relatively soft and ductile ferritic and austenitic forms of iron. However, this transformation requires diffusion and a defined period of time. If the austenite is cooled rapidly (quenched), it will undergo a spontaneous, diffusionless transformation to a body-centered tetragonal (BCT) structure called *martensite*. This lattice is highly distorted and strained, resulting in an extremely hard, strong, brittle alloy.

The formation of martensite is an important strengthening mechanism for carbon steels. The cutting edges of carbon steel instruments are ordinarily martensitic, because the extreme hardness allows for grinding a sharp edge that is retained in use. Martensite decomposes to form ferrite and carbide. This process can be accelerated by appropriate heat treatment to reduce the hardness, but this is counterbalanced by an increase in toughness. Such a heat treatment process is called *tempering*.

STAINLESS STEELS

Chromium-containing Steels. When 12% to 30% chromium is added to steel, the alloy is commonly called *stainless steel*. Elements other than iron, carbon, and chromium may also be present, resulting in a wide variation in composition and properties of the stainless steels. For example, room temperature yield strengths may range from 211 MPa to more than 1760 MPa.

These steels resist tarnish and corrosion primarily because of the passivating effect of the chromium. For passivation to occur, a thin, transparent, but tough and impervious oxide layer of Cr_2O_3 forms on the surface of the alloy when it is subjected to an oxidizing atmosphere such as room air. This protective oxide layer prevents further tarnish and corrosion. If the oxide layer is ruptured by mechanical or chemical means, a temporary loss of protection against corrosion will occur. However, the passivating oxide layer eventually forms again in an oxidizing environment.

There are essentially three types of stainless steels, evolving from the possible

TABLE 28–2. Composition (Percentages) of Three Types of Stainless Steel*

Type (Space Lattice)	Chromium	Nickel	Carbon
Ferritic (BCC)	11.5–27	0	0.20 max
Austenitic (FCC)	16.0–26	7–22	0.25 max
Martensitic (BCT)	11.5–17	0–2.5	0.15–1.20

*Silicon, phosphorus, sulfur, manganese, tantalum, and niobium may also be present in small amounts. The balance is iron.

BCC, body-centered cubic; FCC, face-centered cubic; BCT, body-centered tetragonal.

lattice arrangements of iron previously described. This classification, with approximate compositions, is given in Table 28–2.

Ferritic Stainless Steels. These alloys are often designated as American Iron and Steel Institute (AISI) Series 400 stainless steels. This series number is shared with the martensitic alloys. The ferritic alloys provide good corrosion resistance at a low cost, provided that high strength is not required. Because temperature change induces no phase change in the solid state, the alloy is not hardenable by heat treatment. Also, ferritic stainless steel is not readily work hardenable. This series of alloys finds little application in dentistry.

Martensitic Stainless Steels. As noted, martensitic stainless steel alloys share the AISI 400 designation with the ferritic alloys. They can be heat treated in the same manner as plain carbon steels, with similar results. Because of their high strength and hardness, martensitic stainless steels are used for surgical and cutting instruments.

The yield strength of a high-carbon martensitic stainless steel may range from 492 MPa in the annealed condition to 1898 MPa in the hardened (quenched and tempered) state. The corresponding hardness ranges from a Brinell hardness value of 230 to 600.

Corrosion resistance of the martensitic stainless steel is less than that of the other types and is reduced further following a hardening heat treatment. As usual, when the strength and hardness increase, ductility decreases. It may decrease to as low as 2% elongation for a high carbon martensitic stainless steel.

Austenitic Stainless Steels. The austenitic stainless steel alloys are the most corrosion resistant of the stainless steels. AISI 302 is the basic type, containing 18% chromium, 8% nickel, and 0.15% carbon. Type 304 stainless steel has a similar composition, but the chief difference is its reduced carbon content (0.08%). Both 302 and 304 stainless steel may be designated as *18-8 stainless steel*; they are the types most commonly used by the orthodontist in the form of bands and wires. Type 316L (0.03% maximum carbon) is the type ordinarily employed for implants.

Generally, austenitic stainless steel is preferable to ferritic stainless steel because of the following characteristics:

- Greater ductility and ability to undergo more cold work without fracturing
- Substantial strengthening during cold working (some transformation to a body-centered lattice)
- Greater ease of welding
- Ability to fairly readily overcome sensitization

- Less critical grain growth
- Comparative ease in forming

CORROSION RESISTANCE

Sensitization of 18-8 Stainless Steel. The 18-8 stainless steel may lose its resistance to corrosion if it is heated between 400° C and 900° C, the exact temperature depending on its carbon content. Such temperatures are definitely within the range used by the orthodontist in brazing, soldering and welding; therefore, this effect merits further discussion. The difference between brazing and soldering is the temperature at which the procedure is performed. According to the 1992 *Metals Handbook* published by the American Society for Metals, brazing is performed using a filler metal with a liquidus temperature above 450° C and below the solidus temperature of the base materials. Soldering is performed with a filler metal having a liquidus temperature that is 450° C or less. For simplicity, we refer to all such operations subsequently as soldering procedures.

The reason for a decrease in corrosion resistance is the precipitation of chromium carbide at the grain boundaries at the high temperatures. The small, rapidly diffusing carbon atoms migrate to the grain boundaries from all parts of the crystal to combine with the large, slowly diffusing chromium atoms at the periphery of the grain, where the energy is highest. The formation of Cr_3C is most rapid at 650° C. Below this temperature the diffusion rate is less, whereas above it a decomposition of Cr_3C occurs. When the chromium combines with the carbon in this manner, its passivating qualities are lost, and, as a consequence, the corrosion resistance of the steel is reduced. Because that portion of the grain adjacent to the grain boundary is generally depleted to produce chromium carbide, intergranular corrosion occurs, and a partial disintegration of the metal may result with a general weakening of the structure.

There are several methods by which this condition can be minimized. One method would be to reduce the carbon content of the steel to an extent that such carbide precipitation cannot occur. However, this remedy is not economically feasible.

If the stainless steel is severely cold worked, the carbides precipitate along the slip planes. As a result, the areas deficient in chromium are less localized and the carbides are more uniformly distributed so that the resistance to corrosion is greater than when they precipitate only along the grain boundaries. Such a method is presumably used in the processing of orthodontic stainless steel wires.

Stabilization of Stainless Steel. The method employed most successfully is the introduction of some element that precipitates as a carbide in preference to chromium. Titanium is often used for this purpose. If titanium is introduced in an amount approximately six times the carbon content, the precipitation of chromium carbide can be inhibited for a short period at the temperatures ordinarily encountered in soldering procedures. Stainless steels that have been treated in this manner are said to be stabilized. Few, if any, of the stainless steels used in orthodontics are so stabilized.

General Causes of Corrosion. As previously noted, the function of the chromium is to prevent corrosion by oxidation. With respect to the prevention of electrolytic corrosion, the situation is somewhat analogous to that of dental amalgam discussed in Chapter 17.

Any surface inhomogeneity is a potential source of tarnish or corrosion. Severe strain hardening may produce localized electric couples in the presence of an electrolyte such as saliva. Any surface roughness or unevenness may allow corrosion cells to form. A stainless steel orthodontic appliance should be polished not only for the comfort of the patient but also so that it remains cleaner and less susceptible to tarnish or corrosion during use.

A common cause of the corrosion of stainless steel is the incorporation of bits of carbon steel or similar metal in its surface. For example, if the stainless steel wire is manipulated carelessly with carbon steel pliers, it is conceivable that some of the steel from the pliers may become embedded in the stainless steel. Or if the stainless steel appliance is abraded or cut with a carbon steel bur or similar steel tool, some of the steel from the tool may also become embedded in the stainless steel. Such a situation results in an electric couple that may cause considerable corrosion.

Brazed or soldered joints in orthodontic appliances also lead to a galvanic couple. In addition, austenitic stainless steels are susceptible to attack by solutions containing chlorine. Chlorine-containing cleansers should not be used to clean removable appliances fabricated from stainless steel.

Mechanical Properties of Stainless Steels. The general range of the mechanical properties of 18-8 stainless steel is presented in Table 28–3. In orthodontic wires, strength and hardness may increase with a decrease in the diameter because of the amount of cold working induced in forming the wire. Tensile strengths of 2100 MPa, yield strengths of 1400 MPa, and Knoop hardness values of 600 may be expected. Cold working during the fabrication of stainless steel orthodontic wires contributes a substantial proportion to the strength values shown in Table 28–3.

The property of being readily strain hardened is a characteristic of austenitic stainless steel. Part of this increase in hardness is caused by strain hardening, but a considerable amount is the result of phase change from a face-centered to a body-centered lattice. This phase change can be readily demonstrated, because the body-centered lattices (ferrite and martensite) are ferromagnetic at room temperature, whereas austenite is nonmagnetic. It is unfortunate that after strain hardening, a stainless steel wire can become fully annealed in a few seconds at a temperature of 700° C to 800° C. After such an annealing procedure, it has lost much of the range of elasticity or working range that is necessary to produce a satisfactory orthodontic appliance. Because the annealing temperatures involved are in the soldering and welding temperature ranges normally employed, an unavoidable softening of the wire during normal heating operations is a decided disadvantage.

TABLE 28–3. Mechanical Properties of Orthodontic Wires

Alloy	Modulus of Elasticity (10^3 MPa [GPa])	0.2% Offset Yield Strength (MPa)	Ultimate Tensile Strength (MPa)	Number of 90-Degree Cold Bends Without Fracture*
Stainless steel	179	1579	2117	5
Cobalt-chromium nickel	184	1413	1682	8
Nickel-titanium	41.4	427	1489	2
β Titanium	71.7	931	1276	4

*American Dental Association Specification No. 32 for orthodontic wires.
GPa = gigapascal = 10^3 MPa.

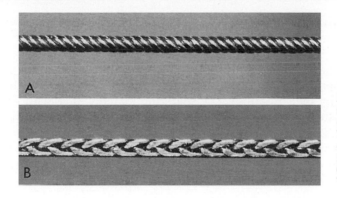

Figure 28–8. Multistranded stainless steel wires for orthodontic applications. *A,* Twisted form with overall diameter of 0.44 mm. *B,* Braided form with overall dimensions of 0.44 × 0.63 mm. (Courtesy of J. Y. Morton and J. Goldberg.)

This disadvantage can be minimized by using low-fusing solders and by confining the time for soldering and welding procedures to a minimum. Any softening that occurs under such conditions of heating can be remedied considerably by the strain hardening incurred in subsequent operations, such as may occur during contouring and polishing.

Braided and Twisted Wires. Very-small-diameter stainless steel wires can be braided or twisted together by the manufacturer to form larger wires for clinical orthodontics. The separate strands may be as small as 0.178 mm, but the final intertwined wires may be either round or rectangular in shape, and their cross-sectional dimension is between 0.406 mm and 0.635 mm. Figure 28–8 shows a magnified cross section of two such wires.

Braided or twisted wires are able to sustain large elastic deflections in bending. Because of their low "apparent" elastic modulus in bending, these types of wire apply low forces for a given deflection when compared with solid stainless steel wire.

Solders (brazing materials) for Stainless Steel. It is important that the stainless steel wire not be heated to too high a temperature so as to minimize carbide precipitation and to prevent an excessive softening of the wire so that its usefulness is lost. The requirement of a low-temperature soldering (brazing) technique generally rules out of consideration any of the gold soldering (brazing) materials normally employed with gold alloy wires because their melting points are generally too high. Instead, silver solders are used. As stated previously, the term *soldering* is the preferred general term (rather than *brazing*) for such joining processes because of its common usage in dentistry.

Silver solders are essentially alloys of silver, copper, and zinc to which elements such as tin and indium may be added to lower fusion temperatures and improve solderability. Although such solders definitely corrode in use because they are anodic to the stainless steel, in orthodontic appliances such a condition is not too objectionable. The appliance is a temporary structure, not usually worn in the mouth for more than 6 to 30 months, and frequent inspections by the orthodontist are necessary.

The soldering temperatures for orthodontic silver solders are in the range of 620° C to 665° C. The solidus-liquidus ranges of the soldering materials should be small. This is an important characteristic of the soldering materials for free-hand soldering as normally practiced by the orthodontist. In free-hand soldering, the joint metal should harden promptly when the work is removed from the flame. Otherwise, the operator may unavoidably move the work before the soldering material has completely solidified, and the joint will be weakened.

Soldering Fluxes. In addition to the usual reducing and cleaning agents, a flux used for soldering stainless steel also contains fluoride to dissolve the passivating film formed by the chromium. The soldering material (solder) does not wet the metal when such a film is present. Potassium fluoride is one of the most active chemicals in this respect.

The flux is similar to that recommended for gold soldering, with the exception of the addition of potassium fluoride. The boric acid is used in a greater ratio to the borax than in the flux for gold soldering because it lowers the fusion temperature.

Technical Considerations for Soldering. The free-hand soldering operation with stainless steel is not greatly different from that of gold soldering described in Chapter 27.

A needlelike, nonluminous, gas-air flame may be used. The thinner the diameter of the flame, the less the metal surrounding the joint is annealed. The work should be held about 3 mm beyond the tip of the blue cone, in the reducing zone of the flame. The soldering should be observed in a shadow, against a black background, so that the temperature can be judged by the color of the work. The color should never exceed a dull red.

If possible, before soldering, the parts should be tack-welded together to hold them in alignment during the soldering procedure. Then flux should be applied, and the heavier gauge part should be heated first. Flux must cover all of the areas to be soldered before heat is applied. As soon as the flux fuses, soldering alloy should be added and heating continued until the metal flows around the joint. After the metal has flowed, the work should be immediately removed from the heat and quenched in water. Based on the metallurgy of the austenitic stainless steels, it should be evident that the objective during soldering is to use as little heat as possible, as briefly as possible.

In addition to the conventional gas-air torch method, a number of other techniques can be used to supply the heat for soldering, including a hydrogen-oxygen torch, electric resistance heating, and indirect heating using a brass wire intermediary. Gas-air and hydrogen-oxygen torch heating have been shown to produce comparable joints in terms of strength.

A photomicrograph of a cross section of stainless steel wire–silver solder junction is shown in Figure 28–9. Although intimate contact between the metals is seen, present evidence indicates that no measurable amount of atomic diffusion occurs at the interface and that the bond is strictly mechanical. The tensile strength of a good silver solder joint can exceed that of the bulk silver soldering alloy. Interfacial constraint between the thin layer of solder alloy and the harder wire could conceivably account for the higher strength of the joint.

Welding. Although soldering of orthodontic wires is not uncommon, flat structures such as bands and brackets are usually joined by welding. The electric spot welding apparatus produces a large electric current that is forced to flow through a limited area (spot) on the overlapped materials that are to be welded. The resistance of the material to the flow of current produces intense localized heating and fusion of the overlapped metals. No solder is employed. Ideally, the melting is confined to the junction area and can be observed metallographically in cross section as a nugget of resolidified cast structure. The grain structure of

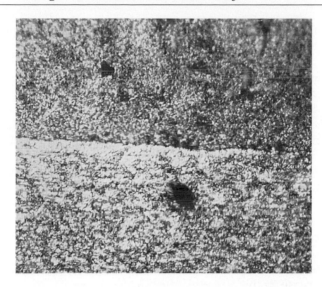

Figure 28–9. Photomicrograph of a soldered joint between a stainless steel orthodontic wire and a silver solder. ×800.

the surrounding alloy should not be affected. The strength of the welded joint is decreased with increasing recrystallization of the wrought structure. The strength becomes greater by an increase in the weld area. However, the weld joint area becomes susceptible to corrosion, primarily because of chromium carbide precipitation and consequent loss of passivation.

COBALT-CHROMIUM-NICKEL ALLOYS

Cobalt-chromium-nickel alloys drawn into wire can be used successfully in orthodontic appliances. These alloys were originally developed for use as watch springs (Elgiloy), but their properties are also excellent for orthodontic purposes.

The wires are furnished to the orthodontist in different gauges and cross-sectional shapes, with differing physical properties as well. Their resistance to corrosion and tarnish in the mouth is excellent. Furthermore, they can be subjected to the same welding and soldering procedures as described for the stainless steel orthodontic wires.

Composition. A representative composition (by mass) for such an alloy is cobalt (40%), chromium (20%), nickel (15%), molybdenum (7%), manganese (2%), carbon (0.16%), beryllium (0.04%), and iron (15.8%).

Heat Treatment. A cobalt-chromium-nickel alloy may be softened by heat soaking at 1100° C to 1200° C, followed by a rapid quench. The age-hardening temperature range is 260° C to 650° C. For the alloy Elgiloy, the alloy should be held at 482° C for 5 hours, according to the manufacturer.

Ordinarily, the wires are heat-treated before being supplied to the user and may be ordered in several degrees of hardness (soft, ductile, semispring temper, and spring temper). In addition, the orthodontist can heat-treat the wires by placing them in an oven or by passing an electric current through them with certain types of spot welders. A typical cycle would be 482° C for 7 to 12 minutes. This heat treatment would increase the yield strength and decrease the ductility.

Wires made from this alloy should not be annealed. The resulting softening effect cannot be reversed by subsequent heat treatment. Moreover, if only a portion of a wire is annealed, severe embrittlement of adjacent sections may occur.

Physical Properties. Tarnish and corrosion resistance are excellent. Hardness, yield strength, and tensile strength are approximately the same as those of 18-8 stainless steel. Typical mechanical properties of orthodontic wires are shown in Table 28–3. Ductility in the softened condition is greater than that of the 18-8 stainless steel alloys and less than the alloys in the hardened condition.

Recovery Heat Treatment. An increase in the measured elastic properties of a wire can be affected by heating it to comparatively low temperatures (370° C to 480° C) after it has been cold worked. This *stress-relief heat treatment* removes residual stresses during recovery without pronounced alteration in mechanical properties. Such a treatment also stabilizes the shape of the appliance.

For an 18-8 stainless steel wire, the apparent effect is a slight increase in the modulus of elasticity, a somewhat greater increase in the yield strength, and a considerable increase in the modulus of resilience.

If the wire is bent into tight loops of 180 degrees, or a spiral of small radius, the measured increase in elastic strength may be as great as 50%. A phase change during the heat treatment in the temperature range of 370° C to 480° C cannot account for this strength increase. A release of residual stress is the explanation generally given.

When a force is applied to a wire in bending, tension, or torsion, the total stresses that are present are the sum of the residual stresses and those induced by the load. Thus, when a wire has been bent sharply or coiled, the residual stresses are much higher and more concentrated than in a straight piece of wire. Therefore, less additional stress from the external force is required to produce plastic deformation than is required in a straight wire. Also, the measured increase in the yield strength after a stress-relief heat treatment is greater for the formed appliance.

Cobalt-chromium-nickel wires are more responsive than the 18-8 stainless wires to the low-temperature heat treatment. A reduction in ductility accompanies the increase in yield strength. A phase change as well as stress relief is probably responsible. As noted earlier, caution must be used to avoid excessive embrittlement.

Although the optimum temperature range for the stress-relief heat treatment is most often reported as 370° C to 480° C, there appears to be no reason to exceed the low temperature limit of 370° C when the wire is a nonstabilized grade of austenitic stainless steel. Eleven minutes at approximately 370° C results in a maximum proportional limit for a severely cold-worked appliance. This temperature is also below the lower limit (425° C) of the sensitization temperature range.

A stress-relief heat treatment not only improves the working elastic properties of a wire appliance but also can reduce failure caused by corrosion, which may occur in areas of high localized stress.

NICKEL-TITANIUM ALLOYS

The alloys previously discussed in this chapter generally have similar mechanical properties. Although processing, stress relieving, and heat-treating allow for small product differences, those wrought base metals have elastic moduli in the range of 152 to 200 GPa, whereas yield strengths range between 1170 and 2070

MPa. The wires with lower strength usually have superior formability. Nitinol, a nickel-titanium alloy, represents the first product with significantly different properties than those of other base metal orthodontic alloys used for wires.

Mechanical Properties. The modulus of elasticity of Nitinol wire is 41.4 GPa, the yield strength is 427 MPa, and the ultimate tensile strength is 1489 MPa. These properties result in very low orthodontic forces when compared with similarly constructed and activated stainless steel appliances (see Table 28–3). The low stiffness in combination with moderately high strength account for the large elastic deflections, or working range. The alloy has limited formability as judged by the small number of 90-degree bends that can be made before fracture occurs

Composition, Shape Memory, and Superelasticity. The nickel-titanium alloys used in dentistry contain approximately 54% nickel, 44% titanium, and generally 2% or less cobalt. This composition results in a 1:1 atomic ratio of the two major components. As with other systems, this alloy can exist in various crystallo-graphic forms. At high temperatures, a BCC lattice, referred to as the *austenitic phase,* is stable, whereas appropriate cooling can induce a transformation to a close-packed hexagonal martensitic phase. This transformation can also be induced by the application of stress. There is a volumetric change associated with the transition, and an orientation relation is developed between the phases. These characteristics of the austenite to martensite phase transition result in two unique features of potential clinical relevance: *shape memory* and *superelasticity (pseudoelasticity).*

The *memory* effect is achieved by first establishing a shape at temperatures near 482° C. If the appliance, such as an orthodontic archwire, is then cooled and formed into a second shape and heated through a lower transition temperature, the wire will return to its original shape. The cobalt content is used to control the lower transition temperature, which can be near mouth temperature (37° C).

Inducing the austenite to martensite transition by stress can produce *superelasticity,* a phenomenon that is employed with some nickel-titanium orthodontic wires and some endodontic files. As shown in Figure 28–10, application of a bending stress (through a bending moment) to such an alloy initially results in the standard proportional stress-strain behavior (line ab). However, at a stress sufficient to induce the phase transformation, there is a significant increase in strain (bc), referred to as *superelasticity,* or *pseudoelasticity.* This additional strain is caused by the volume change that results from the change in crystal structure. At the completion of the phase transformation at point c (Fig. 28–10), the behavior reverts to conventional elastic and plastic strain with increasing stress (cd). Unloading results in the reverse transition and recovery. This characteristic is desirable in some orthodontic situations because it results in low forces and a large working range or springback. For an endodontic file, the markedly increased strain, bc, for a small increase in bending stress would facilitate its adaptation along a sharply curving root canal, thereby minimizing the risk for perforation of the root by the file.

Thus, nickel-titanium alloys that can be produced with either the austenitic or the martensitic structure may have varying degrees of cold work and variations in transition temperatures. A number of products, reflecting these variations, are available. Generally, nickel-titanium wires have relatively low modulus values

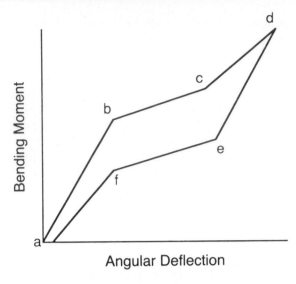

Figure 28–10. Schematic bending moment versus angular deflection curve, showing region of superelasticity, bc. Such behavior imparts a large working range to an orthodontic archwire. (Courtesy of J. Goldberg.)

and large working ranges. The wires are difficult to form and have to be joined by mechanical crimps, because the alloy cannot be soldered or welded.

β-TITANIUM ALLOYS

Crystallographic Forms. Like stainless steel and Nitinol, pure titanium has different crystallographic forms at high and low temperatures. At temperatures lower than 885° C, the hexagonal close-packed (HCP), or α-crystal, lattice is stable, whereas at higher temperatures, the metal rearranges into a BCC, or β-crystal, lattice. The HCP lattice has room-temperature modulus and yield strength values of 110 GPa and 379 MPa, respectively.

Titanium 6%–aluminum 4% alloy, a representative commercial product based on the HCP lattice, can have a yield strength as high as 965 MPa. These properties in a wrought wire, however, do not result in improved springback characteristics when compared with austenitic stainless steel, so that α titanium has not been used in orthodontic applications.

Through the addition of alloying elements such as molybdenum, the β form of titanium can be stabilized down to room temperature. An alloy with the composition of titanium-11% molybdenum-6% zirconium-4% tin is produced in wrought wire form for orthodontic applications.

Mechanical Properties of β-Titanium Wire. Wrought β-titanium orthodontic wire has an elastic modulus of 71.7 GPa and a yield strength between 860 and 1170 MPa. These properties produce several clinically desirable characteristics. The low elastic modulus yields large deflections for low forces. The high ratio of yield strength to elastic modulus produces orthodontic appliances that can sustain large elastic activations when compared with stainless steel devices of the same geometry.

β Titanium can be highly cold worked. The wrought wire can be bent into various orthodontic configurations and has formability comparable to that of austenitic stainless steel.

The mechanical properties of many titanium alloys can be altered by heat treatments that use the transformation from the α to the β lattice structure.

However, heat treatment of the current orthodontic β-titanium wire is not recommended.

Welding. Clinically satisfactory joints can be made by electrical resistance welding of β titanium. Such joints need not be reinforced with solder. A weld made with insufficient heat fails at the interface between the wires, whereas overheating may cause a failure adjacent to the weld joint. Figure 28–11 is a cross section of a welded β-titanium joint, showing minimum distortion of the original cold-worked structure.

Corrosion Resistance. Both forms of titanium have excellent corrosion resistance and environmental stability. These features have stimulated the use of titanium alloys in chemical processing, as well as biologic applications, including heart valves, hip implants, and orthodontic appliances.

GOLD ALLOYS

Wire is the principal form in which wrought gold dental alloy is used. Gold alloy wires are occasionally employed in the construction of removable partial denture clasps. They are also used in fabricating orthodontic appliances and as retention pins for restorations.

When wrought wire is used as a direct retainer in a removable partial denture, it may be attached to the restoration by soldering, by casting the framework to the wire, or by embedding a portion of the wire in the resin denture base. Such wires are ductile and easily adjusted and have superior resistance to fracture as compared with cast clasps. However, the wrought wire clasps require extra laboratory steps and therefore are more expensive. As the current generation of partial denture alloys are more ductile, the need for wrought wire clasps has decreased significantly.

Composition. Many gold wires resemble the Type IV gold casting alloys in composition, but typically they contain less gold. The composition limits of some dental gold alloy wires are given in Table 28–4. As the gold content decreases to 30% or less, the platinum and palladium content increases, and the composition is similar to that of the "white gold" alloys.

Two types of gold wire are recognized in American Dental Association (ADA)

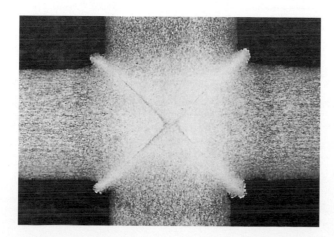

Figure 28–11. Photomicrograph of a weld joint between two 0.43 × 0.63-mm β-titanium orthodontic wires showing minimum distortion of the original cold-worked microstructure. (Courtesy of T. C. Lahnski and J. Goldberg.)

TABLE 28–4. Composition Limits of Some High-Strength Wires Used in Dentistry

Wire Type	Gold	Platinum	Palladium	Silver	Copper	Nickel	Zinc
ADA Type I	54–63	7–18	0–8	9–12	10–15	0–2	0–0.6*
ADA Type II	60–67	0–7	0–10	8–21	10–20	0–6	0–1.7*
P-G-P	25–30	40–50	25–30		16–17		†
P-S-C		0–1	42–44	38–41		0	†

*Dentists Desk Reference: Materials, Instruments and Equipment, 1st ed, Metals and Alloys: Precious Metal Wrought Wire. Chicago, American Dental Association, 1981.
†Lyman T: Metals Handbook, 8th ed, Vol 1, Properties and Selection of Metals. Metal Park, OH, American Society for Metals, 1964.
P-G-P, palladium-gold-platinum; P-S-C, palladium-silver-copper.

Specification No. 7. Type I wire according to the ADA classification of 1984 are *high noble* or *noble* metal alloys. According to ADA Specification No. 7, they must contain at least 75% gold and platinum group metals. Similarly, Type II wires are high noble or noble metal alloys that must contain at least 65% of the same noble metals.

The palladium-gold-platinum (P-G-P) wires, because of their high fusion temperature, and therefore high recrystallization temperatures, are especially useful as wires to be cast against and obviously meet the composition requirements for an ADA Type I wire. Some of them also satisfy the mechanical requirements (Table 28–5) for a Type I wire, even though they are not age hardenable (the mechanical properties listed are for the wire in the quenched condition).

The palladium-silver-copper (P-S-C) alloy wires are neither Type I nor Type II gold wires, but their mechanical properties would meet the requirements for an ADA Type I or II wire. The corrosion resistance of palladium-silver or even silver-palladium dental alloys, both in cast and wrought forms, is generally satisfactory.

General Effects of the Constituents. The contributions of the individual metals are essentially the same as those for the casting gold alloys. The increased palladium and platinum content ensures that the wire does not melt or recrystal-

TABLE 28–5. Physical Properties of Some Wires Used in Dentistry

Type	Yield Strength Oven-Cooled (min)		Tensile Strength Oven-Cooled (min)		Elongation		Fusion Temperature (min)	
					Quenched (min)	Oven-Cooled (min)		
	(MPa)	*(1000 psi)*	*(MPa)*	*(1000 psi)*	%	%	° C	° F
ADA Type I	862	125	931	135	15	4	955	1750
ADA Type II	690	100	862	125	15	2	871	1600

Type	Proportional Limit		Tensile Strength		Elongation		Fusion Temperature	
					Quenched (min)	Oven-Cooled (min)		
	(MPa)	*(1000 psi)*	*(MPa)*	*(1000 psi)*	%	%	° C	° F
P-G-P	552–1034	80–150□	862–1241	125–180□	14–15		1500–1530	2730–2790
P-S-C	690–793	100–115△	965–1070	140–155△	16–24	8–15	1050–1080	1910–1970

□ = Quenched—Alloy does not age harden. △ = Hardened.
References: 1) Dentists Desk Reference: Materials, Instruments and Equipment, 1st ed. Metals and Alloys: Precious Metal Wrought Wire. Chicago, American Dental Association, 1981. 2) Lyman T: Metals Handbook, 8th ed, Vol 1. Properties and Selection of Metals. Metal Park, OH, American Society for Metals, 1964.
ADA, American Dental Association; P-G-P, palladium-gold-platinum; P-S-C, palladium-silver-copper.

lize during soldering procedures. Also, these two elements ensure a fine grain structure.

Copper contributes to the ability of the alloy to age harden. When copper is present, silver may be added to balance the color.

Nickel is sometimes included in small amounts as a strengthener of the alloy, although it tends to reduce the ductility. The presence of a large quantity of nickel tends to decrease the tarnish resistance and change its response to age hardening. In the amounts represented in Table 28–4, any deleterious effects are not likely to be present.

Zinc is added as a scavenger agent to obtain oxide-free ingots from which the wires are drawn.

Fusion Temperature. The minimum fusion temperature of an alloy is usually taken as the temperature halfway between the liquidus and solidus temperature. Fusion temperatures of wrought wires must be known to ensure that the wires do not melt or lose their wrought structure during normal soldering procedures. According to ADA Specification No. 7 for a Type I wire, this temperature is 955° C or higher; for the Type II wire, the minimum fusion temperature must be 871° C.

Mechanical Properties of Noble Alloy Wires. A wire of a given composition is generally superior in mechanical properties to a casting of the same composition. The casting contains unavoidable porosity, which has a weakening effect. When the cast ingot is drawn into a wire, the small pores and surface projections may be collapsed, and welding may occur so that such defects disappear. Any defects of this type that are not eliminated will weaken the wire. Some of the mechanical properties of the alloys whose compositions are shown in Table 28–4 are indicated in Table 28–5.

The relationship between the Brinell hardness number and the proportional limit or tensile strength of gold alloy wires is the same as described for the casting gold alloys. Also, there appears to be a relationship between the proportional limit and the strength of these alloys when they are tested under tension. As a rule, the value for the proportional limit is approximately two thirds that of the tensile strength.

The modulus of elasticity of wrought gold wires is in the range of 97 to 117 GPa, which is slightly higher than that for the gold casting alloys. It increases by approximately 5% after a hardening heat treatment.

Heat Treatment of Gold Alloy Wires. Both types of gold alloy wires that contain copper are heat treatable in the same manner as described for the casting gold alloys. The considerations for solution heat treatment and age hardening are also the same.

Microstructure. The microstructural appearance of cold-worked or wrought alloys is fibrous with extremely elongated crystals. It results from the deformation of the grains during the drawing operation to form the wire. Such a structure generally exhibits enhanced mechanical properties as compared with a corresponding cast structure. Specifically, the wrought material possesses increased tensile strength and hardness.

There is a tendency for wrought alloys to recrystallize during heating operations. The extent of recrystallization is related directly to the duration of heating, the temperature employed, and the cold work or strain energy imparted to the alloy when the wire was drawn. Recrystallization is inversely related to the fusion temperature of the wire when heating temperature and time are constant. Because there is a concomitant decrease in the mechanical properties of the alloy as recrystallization increases, sufficient platinum and palladium should be present to increase the fusion temperature of the wrought gold alloy wire. Therefore, of those wires listed, the P-G-P wires are the most resistant to recrystallization.

This is especially important when casting an alloy against the wire. The wire may be held at the mold burnout temperature for an extended period, and the temperature of the molten casting alloy is greater than that of a gold solder, especially if the casting alloy is one to which porcelain is to be fused.

SELECTED READING

Andreasen GF, and Morrow RE: Laboratory and clinical analyses of Nitinol wire. Am J Orthod 73:143, 1978.
Description of the laboratory properties and clinical uses of the first commercially available nickel-titanium orthodontic wire.

Asgharnia MK, and Brantley WA: Comparison of bending and tension tests for orthodontic wires. Am J Orthod 89:228, 1986.
A complete set of bending and tensile data for various sizes of the four common orthodontic archwire alloys.

Burstone CJ: Application of bioengineering to clinical orthodontics. In: Graber TM, and Swain BF (eds): Orthodontics: Current Principles and Techniques. St. Louis, CV Mosby, 1985, pp 193.
Presents the application of mechanics to clinical orthodontics and the relationship among alloy properties, wire geometry, and appliance force systems.

Burstone CJ, and Goldberg AJ: Beta titanium: A new orthodontic alloy. Am J Orthod 77:121, 1980.
Brief review of the various alloys used in orthodontics and clinical applications for β-titanium wires.

Burstone CJ, and Goldberg AJ: Maximum forces and deflections from orthodontic appliances. Am J Orthod 84:95, 1983.
Actual maximum properties of various orthodontic wire sizes and alloys, related to theoretically predicted values, assuming complete elastic behavior.

Kusy RP, and Greenberg AR: Effects of composition and cross section on the elastic properties of orthodontic archwires. Angle Orthop 51:325, 1981.
A comprehensive derivation of the effects of wire shape, wire size, and alloy type on the strength, stiffness, and range properties in the elastic region.

Miura R, Masakuni M, Ohura Y, et al: The superelastic property of the Japanese Ni-Ti alloy wire for use in orthodontics. Am J Ortho Dent Orthoped 90:1, 1986.
Describes the metallurgy, mechanical properties, and clinical applications of nickel-titanium orthodontic wires that possess superelastic characteristics.

Parr JG, and Hanson A: An Introduction to Stainless Steel. Metals Park, OH, American Society for Metals, 1971.
An easy-to-read review of the applications, metallurgy, mechanical properties, and corrosion principles of stainless steel.

Perkins J (ed): Shape Memory Effects in Alloys. New York, Plenum Press, 1975.
Thirty-two monographs from the first symposium on the subject, providing detailed discussions of metallurgical transitions, properties, and possible applications for shape memory and superelastic alloys.

Pickering FB (ed): The Metallurgical Evolution of Stainless Steels. Metals Park, OH, American Society for Metals; and London, The Metals Society, 1979.
A series of 22 original articles highlighting important developments in stainless steel. The introductory chapter is an extensively referenced review of stainless steel metallurgy.

Sarkar NK, Redmond W, Schwaninger B, et al: The chloride corrosion behavior of four orthodontic wires. J Oral Rehabil 10:121, 1983.
Characterization of the in vitro potentiodynamic cyclical polarization of stainless steel, nickel-chromium-cobalt, β-titanium, and nickel-titanium orthodontic wires.

Eisenstadt MM: Introduction to Mechanical Properties of Materials. New York, Macmillan, 1971.
Chapter 8, pp 217–266: Review of elastic deformation and strain hardening effects.
Chapter 9, pp 286–294: Influence of strain rate dependence, temperature, and annealing on strength and plastic deformation.

Van Vlack LH: Elements of Materials Science and Engineering, 5th ed. Reading, MA, Addison-Wesley, 1985, pp 514–517.
Principles of ductile-brittle behavior, temperature, and strain rate dependence.

29 *Dental Implants*

- **Evolution of Dental Implants**
- **Implant Types**
- **Materials**

EVOLUTION OF DENTAL IMPLANTS

Practicing dentists spend much of their time replacing partially missing tooth structure. However, researchers have long searched for improved methods of anchoring prosthetic materials within the jaw to reconstruct an entire tooth either as a single restoration or as a support for a removable partial denture or for a fixed partial denture. The desire to provide a substitute for a single tooth or an entire arch began in ancient civilizations, where gold and ivory were common materials for such purposes. In more modern times, a host of biomaterials have been employed to replace the roots of natural teeth, with varying degrees of success. Metals such as platinum, lead, silver, steel, cobalt alloys, and titanium have been used, in addition to porcelain, carbon, sapphire, alumina, calcium phosphates, and dental acrylic resin.

Through the years, it has become obvious that this complex field of *dental implantology* would require the optimization of several important variables to enhance the chances of success. These include proper material selection and design; an understanding and evaluation of the biologic interaction at the interface between the implant and tissue; an evaluation of the quality of the existing bone; a careful and controlled surgical technique; and a joint approach between the various specialties to optimize patient selection, implant spacing, load distribution, prosthodontic geometry, and follow-up care.

This knowledge has evolved at the expense of many failed implants, in part because clinical treatment often preceded controlled experimental studies in animals and humans. The safety and efficacy aspects of preliminary studies ensure that only truly biocompatible materials are employed in human clinical trials and that the widespread use of such implants does not proceed until efficacy has been established. Vitreous carbon is a good example of a material that showed great promise as a dental implant after trials in baboons but failed in controlled human studies. It is unfortunate that many of these implants had already been placed clinically by the time research results had been presented to the dental community.

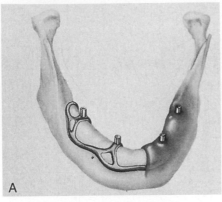
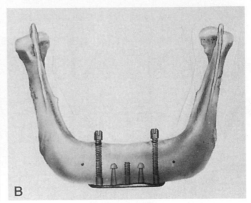
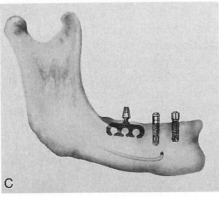

Figure 29–1. Three types of dental implants: *A*, subperiosteal; *B*, transosteal; and *C*, endosseous. (*A* to *C* from Taylor TD: Dental Implants: Are They for Me? Chicago, Quintessence, 1990.)

IMPLANT TYPES

The three main types of dental implants are illustrated in Figure 29–1. These include the subperiosteal implant, a framework that rests on the bony ridge but does not penetrate it; the transosteal implant, which penetrates completely through the mandible; and the endosseous implant, which is partially submerged and anchored within the bone.

The subperiosteal implant has had the longest history of clinical trials, but its long-term success rate is suspect (54% survival rate over 15 years). There has been considerable success reported for the transosteal mandibular staple—survival rates of 90% over an 8- to 16-year period—but its use is limited to the mandible. The endosseous implant appears to offer the best solution in terms of fewer clinical limitations and greater success. Reports suggest a high success rate over a 15-year period for a specific type of cylindrical-shaped screw implant, when careful attention is paid to the surgical technique and follow-up. The encouraging results for this implant have paved the way for the introduction of a variety of endosseous implants of varying design and composition. These implants have been shaped as blades, spirals, screws, hollow cylinders, cones, or cylinders with porous surfaces.

The threaded cylindrical implants are placed into the prepared bony plate and are almost immediately anchored in the cortical bone. However, to produce an effective stabilization requires the growth of new bone completely surrounding the entire submerged implant, a phenomenon requiring a period of several months, during which the implant must remain immobile and unstressed. Once bone has grown into intimate contact with the implant, the device readily transmits forces to the bone, distributing them over a large area in the absence of virtually any movement at the interface. This provides stability for the prosthesis supported by the implant. Implants with porous or irregular surfaces are usually cylindrical in shape. The openings, pores or irregularities (such as sintered beads) are added to allow bone ingrowth. Although this bone ingrowth within the intentional porosities on the implant surface seems to be a logical concept, the results for certain smooth-surfaced screw-shaped implants suggest that the added mechanical retention is not required for long-term success.

Other advances have included the production of endosseous implants with polymeric inserts to act as *shock absorbers* instead of the usual *all rigid* design. This insert is designed to serve as a pseudoperiodontal ligament. However, clinical evidence seems to suggest a significant occurrence of fatigue failure of the plastic inserts, which must then be removed and replaced. These designs, as well as other options, are now being manufactured with metallic substructures that have been coated with ceramics, such as hydroxyapatite, or a titanium-plasma spray, to enhance their interaction with the biologic environment. The ability of living bone to grow into direct contact and potentially bond with the implant before function has been proved at both the light and electron microscopic levels. This interaction between the bone and the implant has been called *osseointegration,* which connotes a stable, biocompatible interface void of "fibrous connective tissue." There has been much debate over the nature of this "bony" interface, in that some researchers believe that it is a dense, fibrous tissue and not a true calcified structure. However, regardless of its actual biology, it appears to provide a successful support mechanism for the material and is an absolute requirement for a successful implant. Its attainment is predicated on several factors, including the choice of a material with a stable surface structure, such as an oxide; a surgical procedure that ensures a predictable biologic response; and proper design and follow-up for the prosthetic attachments to ensure long-term function. The materials used for these implants, as well as for other nonendosseous implants, are described in the following sections.

MATERIALS

Metals. Most commonly, metals and alloys are used for dental implants. Initially, surgical grade stainless steel and a cobalt-chromium alloy were used because of their acceptable physical properties and relatively good corrosion resistance and biocompatibility. However, it is currently more common to use implants made of pure titanium or titanium alloys, because of the excellent biocompatibility of titanium.

Stainless Steel. Surgical austenitic steel is an iron-carbon (0.05%) alloy with approximately 18% chromium to impart corrosion resistance and 8% nickel to stabilize the austenitic structure. Because nickel is present, its use in patients allergic to nickel is contraindicated. The alloy is most frequently used in a wrought and heat-treated condition. It has high strength and ductility; thus, it is resistant to brittle fracture.

Surface passivation is required to maximize corrosion-biocorrosion resistance. Of all alloys, this one is the most subject to crevice and pitting corrosion. Therefore, care must be taken to use and retain the passivated (oxide) surface. Because of the galvanic potential that enhances corrosion, some situations create a problem. For example, if a bridge of a noble or base metal alloy touches the abutment heads of a stainless steel implant, an electrical circuit is created through the tissues. If the bridge and implant are not in contact, no couple exists and each device functions independently.

Cobalt-Chromium-Molybdenum Alloy. These alloys are most often used in an as-cast or cast and annealed condition. This permits the fabrication of custom designs, such as subperiosteal frames. Their composition is approximately 63% cobalt, 30% chromium, and 5% molybdenum and they contain small concentrations of carbon, manganese, and nickel. The molybdenum serves to stabilize the structure, and carbon acts as a hardener. All of these elements are critical, as are their concentrations and the need for proper fabrication techniques. These alloys possess outstanding resistance to corrosion and they have a high modulus. However, they are the least ductile of all the alloy systems, and bending must be avoided. Because many of these devices are fabricated by dental laboratories, all aspects of quality control must be followed for casting and finishing. When proper quality control is ensured, this alloy group exhibits excellent biocompatibility.

Because of the requirements of low cost and long-term clinical success, both stainless steel and cobalt-chromium alloys have been used extensively in many areas of surgery and dentistry. However, the greater corrosion resistance and tissue compatibility of titanium have made it a particularly effective metal for dental implants.

Titanium and Titanium-Aluminum-Vanadium Alloy. Commercially pure titanium (cpTi) has become one of the materials of choice because of its predictable interaction with the biologic environment. Titanium is a highly reactive metal—it oxidizes (passivates) on contact with air or normal tissue fluids. This reactivity is favorable for implant devices because it minimizes biocorrosion. An oxide layer 10 Å thick forms on the cut surface of pure titanium within a millisecond. Thus, any scratch or nick in the oxide coating is essentially self-healing. Typically, titanium is further passivated by placement in a bath of nitric acid to form a thick, durable oxide coating.

Pure titanium also contains oxygen (0.5% maximum) and minor amounts of impurities such as nitrogen, carbon, and hydrogen. In its most common alloyed form, it contains 90 wt% titanium, 6 wt% aluminum, and 4 wt% vanadium. Titanium has a density of approximately 4.5 g/cm^3, making it about 40% lighter than steel. The metal possesses a high strength:weight ratio. Titanium has a modulus of elasticity approximately one half that of stainless steel or cobalt-chromium alloys. However, this is still 5 to 10 times higher than that of bone, as shown by the differences in the slopes in Figure 29–2. Nonetheless, design of the implant is important to distribute stress transfer properly. The mechanical properties of the alloy exceed those of the cpTi.

Although titanium is a biologically compatible metal with high corrosion resistance, the titanium oxide surface does release titanium ions at a low rate into electrolytes such as those in blood and saliva. Elevated levels of titanium, as well as other elements present in stainless steel and cobalt-chromium alloys, have been determined in tissues immediately surrounding implants and in major organs. Although there are still questions that remain to be answered, the long-term clinical applications of these alloys in orthopedic and dental implants suggest that these levels have not been associated with significant sequelae.

Despite the desirable properties of titanium, through the years it has become obvious that the surface characteristics of the material are the main determinants of the biologic response to the implant. Therefore, in addition to composition, the

Elastic Modulus Comparison

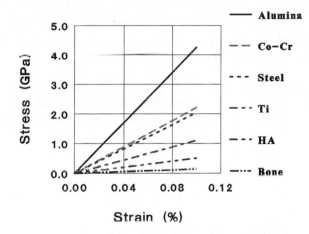

Figure 29–2. Stress strain curves for various materials used in dental implant devices, as compared with that of bone. The slopes represent the elastic moduli.

mode of fabrication and preparation of the implant surface must be controlled. It has been proposed that the high dielectric properties of titanium oxide, which exceed those of most metal oxides, may in part be responsible for the positive biologic response to these implants because they make the surface more reactive to biomolecules via enhanced electrostatic forces. Therefore, any contamination or adulteration of this surface before placement will surely have a negative effect on the success of the implant. In recent years, efforts to characterize and modify the implant surface to enhance clinical success have been made. These efforts have led to a variety of new implants.

Metal with Surface Coatings. The design of some of the new implants makes use of a titanium substructure that has either been plasma-sprayed or coated with a thin layer of a calcium phosphate ceramic. The rationale for coating the implant with tricalcium phosphate or hydroxyapatite, both rich in calcium and phosphorus, is to produce a bioactive surface that promotes bone growth and induces a direct bond between the implant and the hard tissue. The term *bioactive* is applied to inorganic materials that develop an adherent, bonded interface with bone. Such materials, like other ceramics, tend to have a moderately high elastic modulus but low ductility and tensile strength, making them relatively unsuitable for use as a structural component unless placed under purely compressive stresses. Because this is not feasible in the dental environment, the biologic benefits of such materials are usually achieved when the materials have been applied via a flame or plasma-spraying technique as a thin, uniform coating to a metal substructure, such as titanium. These coatings have clearly enhanced the bond strength of the implant to bone, and they have accelerated the rate at which attachment occurs.

The long-term success of these implants is dictated by the durability of the ceramic-metal bond during function, as well as the characteristics and uniformity of the coating. These data are not yet available. However, cpTi with a plasma-sprayed coating of titanium has been evaluated in clinical trials for 5 years, and it has shown good results. The rationale behind a plasma-sprayed surface is to provide a roughened, though biologically acceptable, surface for bone ingrowth to ensure anchorage in the jaw. Some brands of these implants employ a screw shape, whereas others are nonthreaded cylinders. In any case, sufficient time must pass between the time of placement and the loading of the implant through a prosthetic appliance to ensure adequate bone growth and immobilization. Early movement of the implant before it becomes solidly anchored to the bone is considered to be one of the main reasons for failure of the implant, because it disrupts the interfacial attachment.

Ceramics. Although they are brittle and susceptible to flexural fracture, ceramics are logical materials to employ for dental implants because of their outstanding biocompatibility and inert behavior. At least two types of ceramic materials have been developed. One type is designated as bioactive. As noted earlier, hydroxyapatite is a bioactive material; Bioglass is another. The second type is the nonreactive family of ceramics, which include alumina and sapphire. They do not have the necessary composition to actively participate in the process of bone deposition.

The bioactive materials are ceramics or glasses that are rich in calcium and phosphate. Hydroxyapatite is a mineral with the formula, $Ca_{10}(PO_4)_6(OH)_2$, that is similar to that of bone and teeth. It has mainly been used as an implant material for augmenting alveolar ridges or filling bony defects. For these uses, it is produced in a block or granular form that is packed or fitted into the bony site, providing a scaffold for new bone growth. One of the major problems with the use of the material in a granular form has been the difficulty in keeping it localized at the site of implantation. Materials have been developed in which collagen has been used as a matrix to hold the particles together in the defect, thus providing a more stable environment for new bone formation. The material can be synthesized in either a dense or porous form, the latter containing porosity of 100 to 300 μm in size, which is adequate for bone ingrowth.

However, the inadequate strength and ductility of this ceramic when bending or tensile forces are developed has limited its use to very-low-stress applications. As mentioned previously, the use of hydroxyapatite as a coating for titanium substructures addresses the mechanical deficiencies of the material while realizing the benefits of its bioactivity.

Another bioactive material is Bioglass, a dense ceramic material made from CaO, Na_2O, P_2O_5, and SiO_2. The mechanism by which these bioactive materials bond to bone has been described as follows and is depicted in Figure 29–3. Local pH changes near the Bioglass surface cause sodium, calcium, and phosphate ions to be dissolved from it. At the same time, hydrogen ions from the local tissue fluids replace the lost sodium in the Bioglass. At the surface, a silica-rich gel forms because of the selective dissolution of elements that are lost from the surface including an abundance of silica. This silicon depletion is followed by the migration of calcium and phosphate ions to the silica gel surface from within both the Bioglass and the tissue fluids, to form a calcium-phosphorus layer. Once a sufficient concentration of phosphorus is present at the surface, osteoblasts begin to proliferate, thereby producing collagen fibrils that become incorporated into the calcium-phosphorus gel and are anchored by the calcium-phosphorus crystals. This strong bonding layer has been shown to be 100 to 200 μm thick, roughly 100 times the thickness of comparable layers formed on hydroxyapatite. The bond has been shown to be so strong that when tested to failure, fracture occurs within the bone or Bioglass material, leaving the interface intact. Thus, the brittle nature of the Bioglass becomes the limiting factor in its use as a stress-bearing dental implant material. If the mechanical properties of this material can be improved, it will be considered as a valuable addition to the dental implant armamentarium.

One type of nonreactive ceramic implant that has shown evidence of success

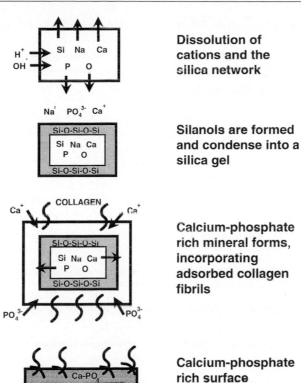

Dissolution of cations and the silica network

Silanols are formed and condense into a silica gel

Calcium-phosphate rich mineral forms, incorporating adsorbed collagen fibrils

Calcium-phosphate rich surface crystallizes into a hydroxy, carbonate, fluorapatite layer, locking in the collagen fibrils

Figure 29–3. Bonding mechanism for bioactive ceramic. *Top,* The outer region of ceramic dissolves; *Top-Middle,* silica-rich gel is formed; *Bottom-Middle,* collagen fibrils develop and become incorporated in calcium-phosphorus gel; and *Bottom,* calcium-phosphorus surface crystallizes and locks in collagen fibrils.

in clinical studies is made from aluminum oxide (Al_2O_3), either as a polycrystalline form or as a single crystal (sapphire). Although this ceramic is well tolerated by bone, it is not bioactive, because it does not promote the formation of bone as do the calcium phosphate ceramics and bioactive glasses. However, it does possess high strength, stiffness (see Fig. 29–2), and hardness. These implants are designed with either a screw or blade shape and appear to work optimally when they are used as abutments for prostheses in partially edentulous mouths.

Polymers and Composites. The application of polymers and composites continues to expand. Polymers have been fabricated in porous and solid forms for tissue attachment and replacement augmentation, and as coatings for force transfer to soft and hard tissues. Some are extremely tough. Thus, they have been used principally for internal force distribution connectors for osseointegrated implants when the connector is intended to better replicate normal tooth functions.

Other Implant Materials. A variety of other materials have been used for dental implants, some of which are still employed today. Early implants were made of gold, palladium, tantalum, platinum, and alloys of these metals. More recently, zirconium and tungsten have been evaluated. Carbon compounds were used for root replacement in the 1970s. They are also marketed as coatings for metallic and ceramic devices.

The trend for conservative treatment of oral diseases continues to accelerate. Thus, it can be anticipated that dental implants will become a frequent first-option treatment and increased research activity on implant materials will grow.

SELECTED READING

Albrektsson T, Zarb G, Worthington P, and Eriksson AR: The long-term efficacy of currently used dental implants: A review and proposed criteria of success. Int J Oral Maxillofac Implantol 1:11–25, 1986.
This article provides a well-written, comprehensive review of most of the currently used dental implants. These materials are described in terms of their composition, background, indications, complications, and clinical results to date.

Hench JW, and Hench LL: Tissue response to surface-active material. In: McKinney RV, and Lemons JE (eds): The Dental Implant. Littleton, MA, PSG Publishing, 1985, pp 181–196.
This review of bioactive glass provides a description of the formulation and properties of these series of glasses and discusses the mechanism by which bonding to bone is realized with these materials.

Kasemo B: Biocompatibility of titanium implants: Surface science aspects. J Prosthet Dent 49:832–837, 1983.
The methods used to prepare and characterize implant surfaces on a molecular level are discussed. Emphasis is placed on the manner in which this surface influences the formation of the interface between the bone and the implant.

Kay JF: Bioactive surface coatings: Cause for encouragement and caution. J Oral Implantol 14:43–54, 1988.
This article reviews the composition and mode of fabrication of calcium-phosphate–coated metal implants, with emphasis on both the positive and negative aspects of these new composite structures.

Lemons JE, and Phillips RW: Biomaterials for dental implants. In: Misch CE (ed): Contemporary Implant Dentistry: Diagnosis and Treatment. St. Louis, CV Mosby, 1990, pp 259–278.

Parr GR, Gardner LK, and Toth RW: Titanium: The mystery metal of implant dentistry—dental materials aspects. J Prosthet Dent 54:410–414, 1985.
This report provides a succinct but inclusive review of the properties and characteristics of titanium used in dental implants.

Schnitman PA, and Shulman LB: Vitreous carbon implants. Dent Clin North Am 24:441–463, 1980.
A review of the properties, manufacture, placement, and evaluation of vitreous carbon implants. It also details reports on the successes of this material in baboon trials and its ultimate failure in human studies.

Skalak R: Biomechanical considerations in osseointegrated prostheses. J Prosthet Dent 49:843–848, 1983.
The biomechanics involved in anchoring a dental implant into bone are discussed, with emphasis on the stress patterns generated by prosthetic appliances supported by several implants.

Williams DF (ed): Biocompatibility of Clinical Implant Materials, Vol 1. Boca Raton, FL, CRC Press, 1981.
This book (262 pages) outlines the composition, the mechanical and physical properties, and the biocompatibility of the materials used as dental and medical implants.

30 *Finishing and Polishing Materials*

- Benefits of Finishing Restorative Materials
- Finishing, Cutting, Grinding, and Polishing Processes
- Abrasive and Erosive Wear
- Abrasive Instrument Design
- Types of Abrasives
- Dentifrices

BENEFITS OF FINISHING RESTORATIVE MATERIALS

Dental restorations are finished before placement in the oral cavity to provide three benefits of dental care: oral health, function, and aesthetics. A well-contoured and polished restoration promotes oral health by resisting the accumulation of food debris and pathogenic bacteria. This is accomplished through a reduction in total surface area and reduced roughness of the restoration surface. Smoother surfaces are easier to maintain in a hygienic state when preventive oral home care is practiced because dental floss and the toothbrush can gain more complete access to all surfaces and marginal areas. With some dental materials, tarnish and corrosion activity can be significantly reduced if the entire restoration is highly polished. Oral function is enhanced with a well-polished restoration because food glides more freely over occlusal and embrasure surfaces during mastication. More important, smooth restoration contacts minimize wear rates on opposing and adjacent teeth. This is particularly true for restorative materials such as ceramics that contain phases that are harder than tooth enamel and dentin. Rough material surfaces lead to the development of high-contact stresses that can cause the loss of functional and stabilizing contacts between teeth. Finally, aesthetic demands may require the dentist to handle highly visible surfaces of restorations differently than those that are not accessible. Although a high mirrorlike polish is preferred for the previously mentioned reasons, this type of surface may not be aesthetically compatible with adjacent teeth in highly visible areas such as the labial surfaces of the maxillary anterior teeth. Fortunately, these surfaces are not subject to high-contact stresses, and they are easily accessible for cleaning. Subtle anatomic features and textures may be added to these areas without affecting oral health or function.

FINISHING, CUTTING, GRINDING, AND POLISHING PROCESSES

The processes of finishing, cutting, grinding, and polishing have not been differentiated well in dentistry. Perhaps, the confusion lies in the manner in which some of the terms are used. For example, the finishing process transforms a material object from a rough form to a more refined form. A finish can mean the final surface achieved or applied to a material. Examples include a rough finish (as shown in Fig. 30–1), a satin finish, and a glossy finish. It is helpful to consider *finishing* as a general process and *finish* as the final surface character obtained on an object. If the general nature of finishing is accepted, then cutting, grinding, and polishing can be considered as a series of steps completed within the process of finishing any given material. The term *polish* would remain an operative term, whereas *finish* would be the preferred term used to describe the type and character of a final surface. Not all finishes are achieved by polishing. In some instances, the finish of a material is a coating that has been placed. Electroplated deposits, pit and fissure sealants covering etched *white-spot* areas on tooth enamel, and thermally processed ceramic overglazes are examples of finishes produced by coatings. Polished ceramic surfaces can be thermally processed to produce a naturally glazed surface where no overglaze material is used. This type of glaze, called an *autoglaze* or *self-glaze,* is an example of a finish that is not achieved by polishing or coating.

The finishing process usually removes material such that (1) surface blemishes and imperfections are removed; (2) the material is shaped to an ideal form; and (3) the outermost surface of the material is developed to a desired state. Cutting, grinding, and polishing occur through similar processes. Particles of a substrate material (workpiece) are removed by the action of a harder material that comes into frictional contact with the substrate. This contact must generate sufficient

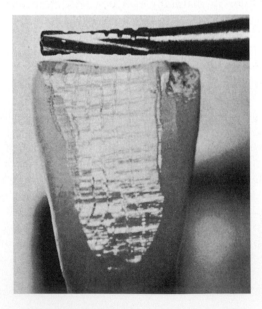

Figure 30–1. Tooth cut by a carbide bur. Note the regular pattern of tooth structure removal that corresponds to the regular arrangement of blades on the bur.

tensile and shear stresses to break atomic bonds and release a particle from the substrate. With rotary instrumentation, the blades of a carbide bur or the abrasive points on a bonded abrasive stone transfer the force to the substrate. Remember that these tensile and shear stresses are induced within both the substrate *and* the rotary instrument. This is an important point because the instrument will fail to cut, grind, or polish if the stress that develops in any part of the instrument exceeds its strength compared with the stress developed in the substrate (work-piece) relative to its strength. Blade edges will become dull and abrasive particles will fracture or tear away from their binder. Such degradation of finishing instruments is discussed further in the section on hardness.

There are subtle differences among cutting, grinding, and polishing processes. A *cutting operation* usually refers to the use of a bladed instrument or the use of any instrument in a bladelike fashion. Substrates may be divided into large separate pieces or they may sustain deep notches and grooves by a cutting operation. High-speed tungsten carbide burs have numerous regularly arranged blades that remove small shavings of the substrate as the bur rotates. Figure 30–1 illustrates the unidirectional cutting pattern of the regularly arranged blades on a carbide bur. Whereas 30-fluted finishing burs have been used on a surface, the regular pattern of the cutting blades is only discernible if the surface is magnified for inspection. A separating wheel is an example of an instrument that can be used in a blade-like fashion. A separating wheel does not contain individual blades, but its shape allows it to be used in a rotating blade-like fashion to slice through casting sprues and die stone materials. A *grinding operation* removes small particles of a substrate through the action of bonded or coated abrasive instruments. Grinding instruments contain many randomly arranged abrasive particles. Each particle may contain several sharp points that run along the substrate surface and remove particles of material. For example, a diamond-coated rotary instrument may contain thousands of sharp diamond particles that pass over a tooth during each revolution of the instrument. Because these particles are randomly arranged, innumerable unidirectional scratches are produced on the material surface, as illustrated in Figure 30–2A, which shows a

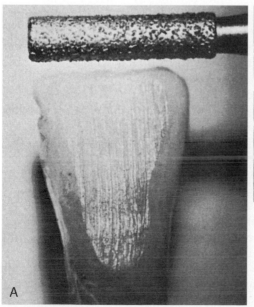

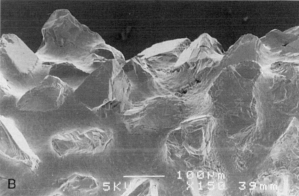

Figure 30–2. Tooth ground by a diamond bur. *A,* Note the multiple scratches formed by the random arrangement of abrasive particles on the diamond bur. *B,* Photomicrograph of the bonded diamond particles on a coarse diamond bur. ×150.

tooth surface ground by a diamond bur. Cutting and grinding are both considered to be predominantly *unidirectional* in their course of action. This means that a cut or ground surface would exhibit cuts and scratches oriented in one predominant direction.

A *polishing operation*, the most refined of the finishing processes, produces the finest of particles; it acts on an extremely thin region of the substrate surface. Polishing produces scratches so fine that they are not visible unless greatly magnified. Examples of polishing instruments are rubber abrasive points, fine-particle disks and strips, and fine-particle polishing pastes. Polishing pastes are applied with soft felt points, muslin wheels, prophy cups, or buffing wheels. *Buffing* refers to the process that is controlled by the use of abrasives carried via bristle brushes, treated leather, and cloth materials. The ideally polished surface would be atomically smooth with no surface imperfections. This condition is virtually impossible to achieve because most restorative materials are brittle and easily acquire surface flaws during cutting and grinding procedures. Polishing is considered to be *multidirectional* in its course of action. This means that the final surface scratches are oriented in many directions. Shown in Figure 30–3 are examples of ground and polished surfaces. Note that the differences in surface appearance are subtle because of the transitional nature of the grinding and polishing processes. If there were larger differences in the size of particles removed, the surface change would be more easily detected.

Aerosol Hazards of the Finishing Process. Aerosols, the dispersions of solid and liquid particles in air, are generated whenever finishing operations are performed. Dental aerosols may contain tooth structure, dental materials, and micro-organisms. They have been identified as potential sources of infectious and chronic diseases of the eyes and lungs and present a hazard to dental personnel and their patients. *Silicosis*, also called *grinder's disease,* is a major aerosol hazard in dentistry because a number of silica-based materials are used in the processing and finishing of dental restorations. Silicosis is a fibrotic pulmonary disease that severely debilitates the lungs and doubles the risk of lung cancer. The risk of silicosis is substantial because 95% of generated aerosol particles are smaller than 5 µm in diameter and can readily reach the pulmonary alveoli during normal respiration. Additionally, 75% of aerosol particles are potentially contaminated with infectious micro-organisms. Finally, aerosols can remain airborne for more than 24 hours before settling and are therefore capable of cross-contaminating other areas of the treatment facility. A concise and informative source of information on aerosol hazards has been written by Cooley (1984). The conclusion from the previous discussion is that aerosol sources, in both the dental operatory and laboratory environments, must be controlled whenever finishing procedures are performed.

Aerosols that are produced during finishing procedures may be controlled in three ways. First, they may be controlled at the source through the use of adequate infection control procedures, water spray, and high-volume suction. Second, personal protection, such as safety glasses and disposable face masks, can protect the eyes and respiratory tract from aerosols. Masks should be chosen to provide the best filtration along with ease of breathing for the wearer. Third, the entire facility should have an adequate ventilation system that efficiently removes any residual particulates from the air. Many systems are also capable of controlling chemical contaminants such as mercury vapor from amalgam scrap and monomer vapor from acrylic resin.

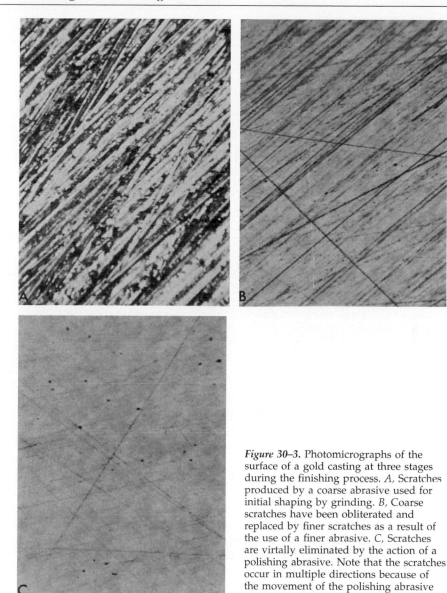

Figure 30–3. Photomicrographs of the surface of a gold casting at three stages during the finishing process. *A,* Scratches produced by a coarse abrasive used for initial shaping by grinding. *B,* Coarse scratches have been obliterated and replaced by finer scratches as a result of the use of a finer abrasive. *C,* Scratches are virtally eliminated by the action of a polishing abrasive. Note that the scratches occur in multiple directions because of the movement of the polishing abrasive in more than one general direction.

ABRASIVE AND EROSIVE WEAR

Abrasive Wear. Wear is a material removal process that can occur whenever surfaces slide against each other. The process of finishing a restoration involves abrasive wear through the use of hard particles. In dentistry, the outermost particles or surface material of an abrading instrument is referred to as the *abrasive*. The material being finished is called the *substrate*. In the case of a diamond bur abrading a tooth surface, such as that illustrated in Figure 30–4, the diamond particles bonded to the bur represent the abrasive and the tooth is the substrate. Also notice that the bur in the high-speed handpiece rotates in a *clockwise* direction as observed from the head of the handpiece. It is important to observe the rotational direction of a rotary abrasive instrument to control its action on the substrate surface. When a handpiece and bur are translated in a

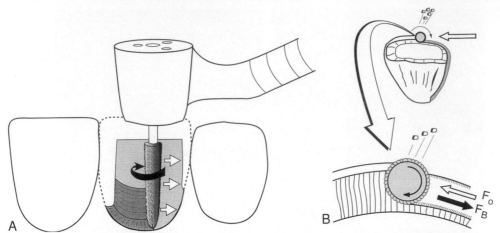

Figure 30–4. Illustration of the mechanics of high-speed rotary instrumentation. *A,* The *black arrow* indicates that the high-speed diamond bur rotates in a clockwise direction when viewed from the head of the handpiece. The *open white arrows* indicate the direction that the instrument should be drawn to counteract the rotational force of the bur and to achieve optimal control of the abrasive action of the bur. *B,* Incisal view of the forces generated during high-speed rotary tooth preparation. As the bur rotates in a clockwise direction, it generates a rotational tangential force at the tooth surface, F_B (represented by the *large black arrow*). The operator of the instrument must generate an opposing force, F_O (*open white arrows*), that exceeds the rotational force of the bur, F_B, and carries the instrument against the tooth surface where the surface will be abraded.

direction opposite to the rotational direction of the bur at the surface being abraded, a smoother grinding action is achieved. However, when the handpiece and bur are translated in the same direction as the rotational direction of the bur at the surface, the bur tends to "run away" from the substrate, thereby producing a more uncontrolled grinding action and a rougher surface.

Abrasive wear is further divided into the processes of two-body and three-body wear. *Two-body wear* occurs when abrasive particles are firmly bonded to the surface of the abrasive instrument and no other abrasive particles are used. A diamond bur abrading a tooth represents an example of two-body wear. *Three-body wear* occurs when abrasive particles are free to translate and rotate between two surfaces. Dental prophylaxis, which involves the use of a rotating rubber cup and an abrasive paste on a tooth or material surface, is an example of three-body wear. These two processes are not mutually exclusive. Diamond particles may debond from a diamond bur and cause three-body wear. Likewise, some abrasive particles in the abrasive paste can become trapped in the surface of a rubber cup and cause two-body wear. Lubricants are often used to minimize the risk for these unintentional shifts from two-body to three-body wear and vice versa.

Erosive Wear. Erosive wear is caused by hard particles impacting a substrate surface, carried either by a stream of air or a stream of liquid. Figure 30–5 illustrates schematically two-body abrasion, three-body abrasion, and hard-particle erosion. Most dental laboratories have air-driven grit-blasting units that employ *hard-particle erosion* to remove surface material. A distinction must be made between this type of erosion and *chemical erosion,* which involves chemicals such as acids and alkalis instead of hard particles to remove substrate material. *Acid etching* is a familiar term that is used more commonly than chemical erosion. Chemical erosion is not used as a method of finishing dental materials. It is used primarily to prepare surfaces to enhance bonding or coating.

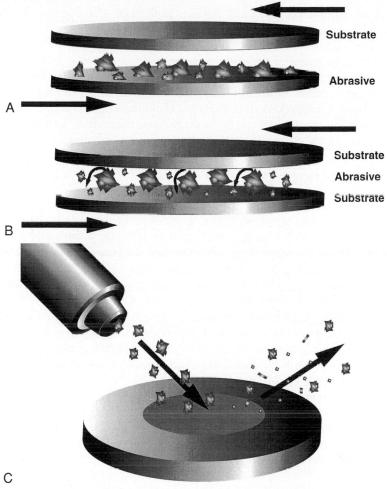

Figure 30–5. Illustrations of two-body abrasion, three-body abrasion, and hard-particle erosion. *A*, Two-body abrasion occurs when abrasive particles are tightly bonded to the abrasive instrument that is removing material from the substrate surface. *B*, Three-body abrasion occurs when abrasive particles are free to translate and rotate between two surfaces. *C*, Hard-particle erosion is produced when abrasive particles are propelled against a substrate by air pressure. (Illustrations courtesy of Joel Anusavice.)

Hardness of Abrasives. As stated previously, the inherent strength of cutting blades or abrasive particles on a dental instrument must be great enough to remove particles of substrate material without becoming dull or fracturing too rapidly. The strength of an abrasive is often measured by the *hardness* of its particles or surface material. Hardness is a surface measurement of the resistance of one material to plastic deformation by another material. The first ranking of hardness was published by Friedrich Mohs, a German mineralogist, in 1820. He ranked 10 minerals by their relative scratch resistance to one another. The least scratch-resistant mineral (talc) received a score of 1 and the most scratch-resistant mineral (diamond) received a score of 10. Mohs' scale was later expanded in the 1930s to accommodate several new abrasive materials that received scores in the 9 to 10 range. Knoop and Vickers hardness tests are based on indentation methods that quantify the hardness of materials. The tip of a Knoop diamond indenter has an elongated pyramid shape, whereas the Vickers diamond indenter has an equilateral pyramid design. Both tests involve the application of the indenter to a test surface under a known load (usually 100 N). The depth of surface penetration is reported as hardness in units of force per unit area. Although a number of other factors affect a material's abrasivity, the farther apart a substrate and an abrasive are in hardness, the more efficient is the abrasion process. Based on a comparison of hardness values for several dental materials in Table 30–1, it is expected that silicon carbide and diamond abrasives will abrade dental porcelain more readily than does garnet, even though the abrasive particles for all three materials have very sharp edge characteristics.

ABRASIVE INSTRUMENT DESIGN

Abrasive Grits. Abrasive grits are derived from materials that have been crushed and passed through a series of mesh screens to obtain different particle-size ranges. Table 30–2 lists grit and particle sizes for commonly used dental abrasives. Dental abrasive grits are classified as coarse, medium coarse, medium, fine, and superfine according to particle size ranges. Experience generally indicates which grades of an abrasive give the best results in finishing a given material. Keep in mind that the rate of material removal is not the only important factor. The surface finish obtained with each abrasive is just as important. If too hard an abrasive is used, or the grain size is too coarse for use on a given material, deep scratches result in the substrate that cannot be removed easily in subsequent finishing operations. Additionally, if an abrasive does not have the proper particle shape, or it does not break down in a manner that creates or exposes new sharp-edged particles, it will tend to *gouge* the substrate.

Bonded Abrasives. Bonded abrasives consist of abrasive particles that are incorporated through a binder to form grinding tools such as points, wheels, separating disks, and a wide variety of other abrasive shapes. Particles are

TABLE 30–1. Hardness Values for Dental Materials and Abrasives

Material	Mohs Hardness	Knoop Hardness (kg/mm^2)	Vickers Hardness (kg/mm^2)
Calcite	3	—	—
Denture resins	—	20	—
Microfill composite	—	30	—
Hybrid composite	—	55	—
Dentin	—	70	—
Dental amalgam	—	—	120 (silver-mercury phase)
			15 (tin-mercury phase)
Type III gold	3	—	135
Type IV gold	4	—	250
Enamel	5	340	—
Glass-ceramics	—	360	—
Pumice	6–7	460	—
Porcelain	6–7	560	430
Sand	7	—	—
Cuttle	7	800	—
Quartz	7	820	—
Garnet	8–9	1350	—
Emery	7–9	2000	—
Corundum	9	2000	—
Aluminum oxide	9	2100	—
Silicon carbide	9–10	2500	—
Diamond	10	7000–10,000	—

TABLE 30–2. Abrasive Particle Sizes*

Grit/Mesh (USA)	Aluminum Oxide, Silicon Carbide, and Garnet (μm)	Coated-disk Grade†	Diamond (μm)	Diamond Bur Grade and Diamond Polishing Paste
120	142	Coarse	142	Supercoarse-coarse
150	122		122	Coarse-regular
180	70–86		86	
240	54–63		60	Fine
320	29–32	Medium	52	
400	20–23		40	Fine-superfine-coarse finishing
600	12–17	Fine	14	Superfine-medium finishing
800	9–12		8	Ultrafine-fine finishing
1200	2–5	Superfine	6	Milling pastes
1500	1 2		4	Polishing pastes (2–5 μm)
2000	1		2	

*Average particle sizes. Grades vary among manufacturers.
†Popular brand of aluminum oxide–coated disks. Silicon carbide and garnet may vary among manufacturers.

bonded by four general methods: (1) *sintering*; (2) *vitreous bonding* (glass or ceramic); (3) *resinoid bonding* (usually phenolic resin); and (4) *rubber bonding* (usually silicone rubber). Sintered abrasives are the strongest type because the abrasive particles are fused together. Vitreous-bonded abrasives are mixed with a glassy or ceramic matrix material, cold-pressed to the instrument shape, and fired to fuse the binder. Resin-bonded abrasives are cold-pressed or hot-pressed and then are heated to cure the resin. Hot pressing yields an abrasive binder with extremely low porosity. Rubber-bonded abrasives are made in a manner similar to that for resin-bonded abrasives.

The type of bonding method employed for the abrasive greatly affects the grinding behavior of the tool on the substrate. Bonded abrasives that tend to disintegrate rapidly against a substrate are too weak and result in increased abrasive costs because of the reduced instrument life. Those that tend to degrade too slowly clog with grinding debris and result in the loss of abrasive efficiency, increased heat generation, and increased finishing time. An ideal binder holds the abrasive particles in the tool sufficiently long enough to cut, grind, or polish the substrate, yet release the particle either before its cutting efficiency is lost or before heat build-up causes thermal damage to the substrate. Binders are specifically formulated for substrate specific applications. Several examples of bonded abrasives are illustrated in Figure 30–6.

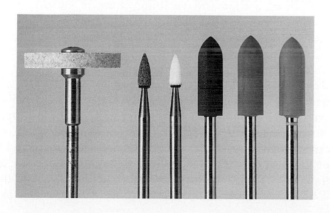

Figure 30–6. Typical bonded abrasive instruments that are used in the dental laboratory include vitreous-bonded abrasive wheels and points (left three instruments) and rubber-bonded abrasive bullets (right three instruments).

A bonded abrasive instrument should always be trued and dressed before its use. *Truing* is a procedure through which the abrasive instrument is run against a harder abrasive block until the abrasive instrument rotates in the handpiece without eccentricity or runout when placed on the substrate. The *dressing procedure*, like truing, is used to shape the instrument but accomplishes two different purposes. First, the dressing procedure reduces the instrument to its correct working size and shape. Second, it is used to remove clogged debris from the abrasive instrument to restore grinding efficiency during the finishing operation. The clogging of the abrasive instrument with debris is called *abrasive blinding*. Abrasive blinding occurs when the debris generated from grinding or polishing occludes the small spaces between the abrasive particles on the tool and reduces the depth that particles can penetrate into the substrate. As a result, abrasive efficiency is lost and greater heat is generated. A blinded abrasive appears to have a coating of the substrate material on its surface. Frequent dressing of the abrasive instrument during the finishing operation on a truing instrument, such as that illustrated in Figure 30–7, maintains the efficiency of the abrasive in removing the substrate material.

Binders for diamond abrasives are manufactured specifically to resist abrasive particle loss rather than to degrade at a certain point and release particles. One reason for this is that diamond is the hardest material known, so that diamond abrasive particles do not lose their cutting efficiency against substrates. There is no need for new abrasive particles to be exposed during the grinding process. Another reason is that diamond grits are expensive and must be used in limited quantities for instrument manufacture. Special bonding processes have been designed to allow for extended instrument life by keeping the abrasive particles firmly bound to the instrument shank yet with maximal particle exposure. Diamond particles are bonded to metal wheels and bur blanks with special heat-resistant resins such as polyimides. The supercoarse through fine grades are then plated with a refractory metal film such as nickel. The nickel plating provides improved particle retention and acts as a heat sink during grinding. Titanium nitride coatings are used as an additional layer on some of the recent diamond abrasive instruments to further extend their longevity. *Finishing diamonds* used for resin-based composites contain diamond particles 40 μm or less in diameter, and many are not nickel plated. Therefore, they are highly susceptible to abuse and should always be used with light force and copious water spray to preserve the very-fine diamond coatings.

Diamond instruments are preshaped and trued and are not treated like the other bonded abrasives. *Diamond cleaning stones* are used on the supercoarse through fine grades to remove debris build-up and to maintain grinding efficiency. An example of a diamond cleaning stone is shown in Figure 30–8. Cleaning stones should not be used on finishing diamonds because their bonded particles are quickly removed. Manufacturers provide special operating and cleaning instructions for these instruments.

Coated Abrasive Disks and Strips. Coated abrasives are fabricated by securing abrasive particles to a flexible backing material (heavyweight paper or Mylar) with a suitable adhesive material. These abrasives typically are supplied as disks and finishing strips. Disks are available in different diameters and with thin and very thin backing thicknesses. A further designation is made with regard to whether or not the disk or strip is moisture resistant. It is advantageous to use abrasive disks or strips with moisture-resistant backings because their stiffness is not reduced by water degradation. Furthermore, moisture acts as a lubricant

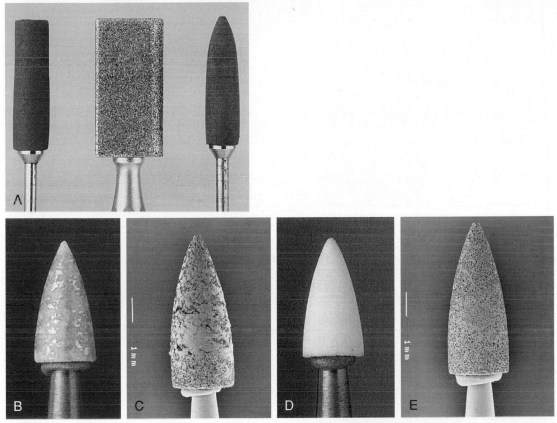

Figure 30–7. A dressing tool is used to true, shape, and clean bonded abrasive instruments before and during the finishing procedure. *A,* A rubber-bonded abrasive cylinder *(left)* shows irregular external contours that cause it to run eccentrically. The cylinder is first trued against a diamond-coated abrasive dressing tool *(center)* to make it rotate around the central axis of the instrument. Once trued, the abrasive is further dressed to a desired working shape *(right). B,* Instruments that are blinded with debris lose cutting efficiency and generate more heat during operation. Note the coating of debris on the abrasive surface. *C,* A scanning electron micrograph of the same instrument reveals the significant amount of debris that is clogging the instrument surface. *D,* Frequent dressing of the abrasive on the dressing tool shown in *A* removes accumulated debris and restores cutting efficiency. *E,* A scanning electron micrograph of the blinded abrasive after dressing reveals that the debris has been removed and the abrasive surface has been restored.

to improve cutting efficiency. Examples of coated abrasives are shown in Figure 30–9.

TYPES OF ABRASIVES

Many types of abrasive materials are available, but only those that are commonly used in dentistry are discussed in this section. *Natural abrasives* include Arkansas stone, chalk, corundum, diamond, emery, garnet, pumice, quartz, sand, tripoli, and zirconium silicate. Cuttle and kieselguhr are derived from the remnants of living organisms. *Manufactured abrasives* are synthesized materials that are generally preferred because of their more predictable physical properties. Silicon carbide, aluminum oxide, synthetic diamond, rouge, and tin oxide are examples of manufactured abrasives.

Arkansas Stone. Arkansas stone is a semitranslucent, light gray, siliceous sedimentary rock mined in Arkansas. It contains microcrystalline quartz and is dense, hard, and uniformly textured. Small pieces of this mineral are attached

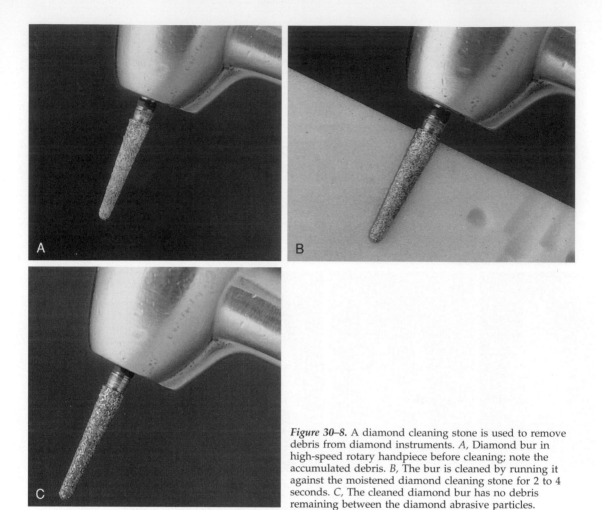

Figure 30–8. A diamond cleaning stone is used to remove debris from diamond instruments. *A,* Diamond bur in high-speed rotary handpiece before cleaning; note the accumulated debris. *B,* The bur is cleaned by running it against the moistened diamond cleaning stone for 2 to 4 seconds. *C,* The cleaned diamond bur has no debris remaining between the diamond abrasive particles.

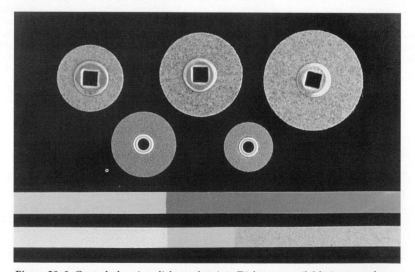

Figure 30–9. Coated abrasive disks and strips. Disks are available in several sizes and with both paper and moisture-resistant backings. Paper-backed disks are represented by the upper row of disks and moisture-resistant Mylar-backed disks are shown in the lower row. Mylar-backed abrasive strips may be coated with two different grades of abrasive. The coatings are separated in the center of the strip by an uncoated area that allows the strip to be passed between teeth.

to metal shanks and trued to various shapes for fine grinding of tooth enamel and metal alloys.

Chalk. One of the mineral forms of calcite is called *chalk*. Chalk is a white abrasive composed of calcium carbonate. It is used as a mild abrasive paste to polish tooth enamel, gold foil, amalgam, and plastic materials.

Corundum. This mineral form of aluminum oxide is usually white. Its physical properties are inferior to those of manufactured α-aluminum oxide, which has largely replaced corundum in dental applications. Corundum is used primarily for grinding metal alloys and is available as a bonded abrasive in several shapes. It is most commonly used in an instrument known as a *white stone*.

Diamond. Diamond is a transparent, colorless mineral composed of carbon. It is the hardest substance known. Diamond is called a *superabrasive* because of its ability to abrade any other known substance. Diamond abrasives are supplied in several forms, including bonded abrasive rotary instruments, flexible metal-backed abrasive strips, and diamond polishing pastes. They are used on ceramic and resin-based composite materials.

Emery. This abrasive is a grayish-black corundum that is prepared in a fine-grain form. Emery is used predominantly in the form of coated abrasive disks and is available in a variety of grit sizes. It may be used for finishing metal alloys or plastic materials.

Garnet. The term *garnet* includes a number of different minerals that possess similar physical properties and crystalline forms. These minerals are the silicates of aluminum, cobalt, iron, magnesium, and manganese. The garnet abrasive used in dentistry is usually dark red. Garnet is extremely hard and, when fractured during the grinding operation, forms sharp, chisel-shaped plates, making garnet a highly effective abrasive. Garnet is available on coated disks and arbor bands. It is used in grinding metal alloys and plastic materials.

Pumice. Volcanic activity produces this light-gray, highly siliceous material. It is used mainly in grit form but can be found in some rubber-bonded abrasives. Both forms are used on plastic materials. Flour of pumice is an extremely fine-grained volcanic rock derivative from Italy and is used in polishing tooth enamel, gold foil, dental amalgam, and acrylic resins.

Quartz. The most commonly used form of quartz is very hard, colorless, and transparent. It is the most abundant and widespread of minerals. Quartz crystalline particles are pulverized to form sharp, angular particles that are useful in making coated abrasive disks. Quartz abrasives are used mostly to finish metal alloys and may be used to grind dental enamel.

Sand. Sand is a mixture of small mineral particles predominantly composed of silica. The particles represent a mixture of colors, making sand abrasives distinct in appearance. Sand particles have a rounded to angular shape. They are applied under air pressure to remove refractory investment materials from base metal alloy castings. They are also coated onto paper disks for grinding of metal alloys and plastic materials.

Tripoli. This abrasive is derived from a lightweight, friable siliceous sedimentary rock. It can be white, gray, pink, red, or yellow. The gray and red types are most frequently used in dentistry. The rock is ground into very fine particles and is formed with soft binders into bars of polishing compound. It is used for polishing metal alloys and some plastic materials.

Zirconium Silicate. Zircon or zirconium silicate is supplied as an off-white mineral. This material is ground to various particle sizes and is used to make coated abrasive disks and strips. It is frequently used as a component of dental prophylaxis pastes.

Cuttle. *Cuttlefish, cuttle bone,* or *cuttle* are the common names for this abrasive. It is a white calcareous powder made from the pulverized internal shell of a Mediterranean marine mollusk of the genus *Sepia.* It is available as a coated abrasive and is useful for delicate abrasion operations such as polishing of metal margins and dental amalgam restorations.

Kieselguhr. This material is composed of the siliceous remains of minute aquatic plants known as *diatoms.* The coarser form is called *diatomaceous earth,* which is used as a filler in many dental materials, such as the hydrocolloid impression materials. It is an excellent mild abrasive. The risk of respiratory silicosis caused by chronic exposure to airborne particles of this material is significant, and appropriate precautions should always be taken.

Silicon Carbide. This extremely hard abrasive was the first of the *synthetic abrasives* to be made. Both green and blue-black types are produced and have equivalent physical properties. The green form is often preferred because substrates are more visible against the green color. Silicon carbide is extremely hard and brittle. Particles are sharp and break to form new sharp particles. This results in highly efficient cutting of a wide variety of materials, including metal alloys, ceramics, and plastic materials. Silicon carbide is available as an abrasive in coated disks and vitreous-bonded and rubber-bonded instruments.

Aluminum Oxide. Fused aluminum oxide was the second synthetic abrasive to be developed after silicon carbide. Synthetic aluminum oxide (alumina) is made as a white powder. It can be much harder than corundum (natural alumina) because of its purity. Alumina can be processed with different properties by slight alteration of the reactants in the manufacturing process. Several grain sizes are available and alumina has largely replaced emery for several abrasive uses. Aluminum oxide is widely used in dentistry. It is used to make bonded abrasives, coated abrasives, and air-propelled grit abrasives. White stones are made of sintered aluminum oxide and are popular for adjusting dental enamel and for finishing both metal alloys and ceramic materials.

Pink and ruby variations of aluminum oxide abrasives are made by adding chromium compounds to the original melt. These variations are sold in a vitreous-bonded form as noncontaminating mounted stones for the preparation of metal-ceramic alloys to receive porcelain. Any remnants of these abrasives should not interfere with porcelain bonding to the metal alloy. A review by Yamamoto (1985) suggests that carbide burs are the most effective instrument for finishing this type of alloy because they do not contaminate the metal surface with entrapped abrasive particles.

Synthetic Diamond Abrasives. Manufactured diamond is used almost exclusively as an abrasive and is produced at five times the level of natural diamond abrasive. This abrasive is used in the manufacture of diamond saws, wheels, and burs. Blocks with embedded diamond particles are used to true other types of bonded abrasives. Diamond polishing pastes are also produced from particles smaller than 5 μm in diameter and are useful in polishing ceramic materials. Synthetic diamond abrasives are used primarily on tooth structure, ceramic materials, and resin-based composite materials.

Rouge. Iron oxide is the fine, red abrasive component of rouge. It is blended, like tripoli, with various soft binders into a cake form. It is used to polish high noble metal alloys.

Tin Oxide. This extremely fine abrasive is used extensively as a polishing agent for polishing teeth and metallic restorations in the mouth. It is mixed with water, alcohol, or glycerin to form a mildly abrasive paste.

DENTIFRICES

Dentifrices are made in three forms: toothpastes, gels, and powders. They provide three important functions. Their abrasive and detergent actions provide efficient removal of debris, plaque, and stained pellicle compared with a toothbrush alone. They polish teeth to provide increased light reflectance and superior aesthetic appearance. The high polish, as an added benefit, enables teeth to resist the accumulation of micro-organisms and stains better than rougher surfaces. Finally, dentifrices act as vehicles for the delivery of therapeutic agents that provide known benefits. Examples of therapeutic agents are fluorides, tartar control agents, and desensitizing agents. Fluorides improve caries resistance and may, under a proper oral hygiene regimen, enhance the remineralization of incipient noncavitated enamel lesions. Tartar control agents such as potassium and sodium pyrophosphates can reduce the rate at which new calculus deposits form supragingivally. Desensitizing agents with proven clinical efficacy are strontium chloride and potassium nitrate. The therapeutic benefits of other additives such as peroxides and bicarbonates are under investigation.

Composition. Typical dentifrice components are listed in Table 30–3. The abrasive concentrations in paste and gel dentifrices are 50% to 75% lower than those of powder dentifrices. Therefore, powders should be used more sparingly and with greater caution by patients (especially where cementum and dentin are exposed) to avoid excessive dentinal abrasion and pulpal sensitivity.

Abrasivity. The ideal dentifrice would provide the greatest possible cleaning action on tooth surfaces with the lowest possible abrasion rates. Dentifrices do not need to be highly abrasive to clean teeth effectively. This is fortunate because exposed root surface cementum and dentin are abraded at rates of 35 and 25 times, respectively, that of enamel. Standardized laboratory tests have been developed to measure the cleaning ability and the abrasivity of a dentifrice. Only the abrasivity test is discussed in this section. Currently, the preferred means of evaluating dentifrice abrasivity is to employ irradiated dentin specimens and brush them for several minutes with both test and reference dentifrices. An abrasivity ratio is then calculated by comparing the amounts of radioactive phosphorus (^{32}P) released by each dentifrice, and this value is

TABLE 30–3. Typical Dentifrice Components*

| Component | Composition (%) | | Materials | Purpose |
	Pastes and Gels	Powders		
Abrasive	20–55	90–98	Calcium carbonate Dibasic calcium phosphate dihydrate Hydrated alumina Hydrated silica Sodium bicarbonate Mixtures of listed abrasives	Removal of plaque/stain, polish tooth surface
Detergent	1–2	1–6	Sodium lauryl sulfate	Aids debris removal
Colorants	1–2	1–2	Food colorants	Appearance
Flavoring	1–2	1–2	Oils of spearmint, peppermint, wintergreen, or cinnamon	Flavor
Humectant	20–35	0	Sorbitol, glycerine	Maintains moisture content
Water	15–25	0	Deionized water	Suspension agent
Binder	3	0	Carrageenan	Thickener, prevents liquid-solid separation
Fluoride	0–1	0	Sodium monofluorophosphate, sodium fluoride, stannous fluoride	Dental caries prevention
Tartar control agents	0–1	0	Disodium pyrophosphate, tetrasodium pyrophosphate, tetrapotassium pyrophosphate	Inhibits formation of calculus above the gingival margin
Desensitization agents	0–5	0	Potassium nitrate, strontium chloride	Promotes occlusion of dentinal tubules

*Percentages (data) are given in w/w and are adapted from both manufacturers' product information and Stookey G, Burkhard TA, and Schemehorn BR: In vitro removal of stain with dentifrices. J Dent Res 61:1236, 1982.

multiplied by 1000. A dentifrice must obtain an abrasivity score of 200 to 250 or less to meet the safe abrasivity standards established by the American Dental Association (ADA) and the International Organization for Standardization (ISO). This means that a test dentifrice must abrade dentin at 20% to 25% of the rate of the reference standard to be considered safe for normal usage. A problem with this laboratory test is that it does not account for all variables that would affect abrasivity under *in vivo* conditions. Some of the factors affecting dentifrice abrasivity are listed in Table 30–4.

Another problem is that not all dentifrices respond in a similar manner under this test. For example, dentifrices that contain sodium bicarbonate yield poor test results because the particles completely dissolve approximately 1 minute into the 8-minute test. This illustrates that it is very difficult, if not impossible, to use a laboratory test to predict the actual abrasivity of various dentifrices *in vivo*. Patients should experience similar relative amounts of wear from the various dentifrices as those found in the laboratory tests. It is safe to say that the great majority of modern dentifrices are not exceedingly abrasive. In fact,

TABLE 30-4. Factors Affecting Dentifrice Abrasivity

Extraoral Factors
Abrasive particle type, size, and quantity in dentifrice
Amount of dentifrice used
Toothbrush type
Toothbrushing method and force applied during brushing
Toothbrushing frequency and duration
Patient's coordination ability

Intraoral Factors
Saliva consistency and quantity (normal variations)
Xerostomia induced by drugs, salivary gland pathology, and radiation therapy
Presence, quantity, and quality of existing dental deposits (pellicle, plaque, calculus)
Exposure of dental root surfaces
Presence of restorative materials, dental prostheses, and orthodontic appliances

one published document has rated four dozen dentifrices with regard to cleaning ability and abrasiveness. The products are ranked as high, moderate, or low in abrasiveness. It is highly probable that most of the evaluated products meet the ADA and ISO standards. Thus, these rankings should be considered as a guide to products that do not exceed a maximum acceptable (safe) abrasivity value.

ADA Acceptance Program. A discussion of dentifrices would not be complete without mention of the American Dental Association (ADA) acceptance program for these materials. The ADA designates a dentifrice as "Accepted" only if the dentifrice meets specific requirements. First, the abrasivity of the dentifrice must not exceed the maximum acceptable abrasivity value of 250 (also a limit for the ISO standard). Second, the manufacturer must produce scientific data, usually from clinical trials, that verifies any claims the manufacturer wishes to make on the product package or in commercial advertisements. The manufacturer's advertisements are also periodically reviewed by the appropriate ADA Council.

In advertising the product, a manufacturer may not claim or imply that the dentifrice confers benefits that have not been specifically proven. Many manufacturers produce excellent dentifrice products but do not seek ADA acceptance simply because they do not want such restrictions placed on their advertisements. For products that receive the ADA seal, a unique and individual statement for each product is written on the container that states exactly what the dentifrice does and does not do.

Toothbrushes. Toothbrush bristle stiffness alone has been shown to have no effect on abrasion of hard dental tissues. However, when a dentifrice is used, there is evidence that more flexible toothbrush bristles bend more readily and bring more abrasive particles into contact with tooth structure, albeit with relatively light forces. This interaction should produce more effective abrasion and cleaning action on areas that the bristles can reach.

SELECTED READING

Cooley RL: Aerosol hazards: In: Goldman HS, Hartman KS, and Messite J (eds): Occupational Hazards in Dentistry. Chicago, Yearbook Medical, 1984, pp 21–33.
Sources of dental aerosols, their hazards, and preventive measures are presented.
Hefferren JJ: Laboratory method for assessment of dentifrice abrasivity. J Dent Res 55:563, 1976.
This reference describes the dentifrice abrasivity test.
Hutchings IM: Tribology: Friction and Wear of Engineering Materials. Boca Raton, FL, CRC Press, 1992.

This publication thoroughly discusses the scientific basis of friction, wear, and lubrication in a readable format.

Kroschwitz JI, and Howe-Grant M (eds): Kirk-Othmer Encyclopedia of Chemical Technology, 4th ed, Vol 1. New York, John Wiley and Sons, 1991, pp 17–37.
This encyclopedia presents a thorough review of specific abrasives, their physical properties, and their methods of manufacture.

Mackert JR: Side effects of dental ceramics. Adv Dent Res 6:90–93, 1992.
Presents information on silicosis and the potential hazards of porcelain dust generation during grinding procedures.

Powers JM, and Bayne SC: Friction and wear of dental materials: In: Henry SD (ed): Friction Lubrication and Wear Technology, ASM Handbook, Vol 18, pp 665–681. Materials Park, American Society of Metals International, 1992.
This article presents a review of friction and wear as they relate to human dental tissues and restorative materials. It is a compilation of information from more than 200 sources.

Ratterman E, and Cassidy R: Abrasives: In: Lampman SR, Woods M, and Zorc TP (eds): Engineered Materials Handbook, Vol 4, Ceramics and Glasses. Materials Park, ASM International, 1991, pp 329–335.
Presents a system for selecting abrasives for glasses and ceramics based on a comparison of physical properties. Mechanical property tables are presented for several materials.

Stookey GK, Burkhard TA, and Schemehorn BR: *In vitro* removal of stain with dentifrices. J Dent Res 61:1236, 1982.
The method used to measure the cleaning effectiveness of a dentifrice is presented.

Toothpastes. Consumer Reports, September 1992, pp 602–606.
This reporting agency sent 48 toothpastes to independent laboratories for an analysis of abrasivity and cleaning effectiveness. All toothpastes were subsequently ranked for these criteria. The American Dental Association no longer provides a ranking according to laboratory tests. Thus, this report may serve as a screening guide in light of the fact that the tests were done in vitro *instead of in a clinical environment.*

Yamamoto M: Metal-Ceramics. Chicago, Quintessence, 1985, pp 124–130.
Discusses the preparation of metal-ceramic alloys for porcelain application, using several excellent photographs.

Index

Note: Page numbers in *italics* refer to illustrations; page numbers followed by t refer to tables.